BRAUNWALD'S
HEART DISEASE

Review and Assessment
(To Accompany Braunwald's Heart Disease, 5th Edition)

Michael E. Mendelsohn, M.D., F.A.C.C.

Director, Molecular Cardiology Research Center
Director, Preventive Cardiology
Associate Professor of Medicine and Physiology
New England Medical Center
Boston, Massachusetts

W.B. SAUNDERS COMPANY

A Division of Harcourt Brace & Company

PHILADELPHIA / LONDON / TORONTO / MONTREAL / SYDNEY / TOKYO

W.B. SAUNDERS COMPANY
A Division of Harcourt Brace & Company

The Curtis Center
Independence Square West
Philadelphia, Pennsylvania 19106

NOTICE

Medicine is an ever-changing field. Standard safety precautions must be followed, but as new research and clinical experience broaden our knowledge, changes in treatment and drug therapy become necessary or appropriate. Readers are advised to check the product information currently provided by the manufacturer of each drug to be administered to verify the recommended dose, the method and duration of administration, and contraindications. It is the responsibility of the treating physician relying on experience and knowledge of the patient to determine dosages and the best treatment for the patient. Neither the Publisher nor the editor or authors assume any responsibility for any injury and/or damage to persons or property.

THE PUBLISHER

PREFACE

The Third Edition of *Heart Disease: Review and Assessment* consists of 706 multiple-choice questions designed to provide a comprehensive review of the broad field of cardiology. It is a companion study guide to the fifth edition of Braunwald's *Heart Disease: A Textbook of Cardiovascular Medicine*. *Heart Disease: Review and Assessment* is designed to aid in the education of cardiology fellows and cardiologists, as well as residents in internal medicine, internists, and other physicians who wish to attain a high level of expertise in cardiology and the ability to solve clinical problems in cardiology. It should be especially helpful to cardiology fellows and others preparing for Subspecialty Examination in Cardiovascular Disease of the American Board of Internal Medicine.

The basic question types are in the format of the aforementioned examination. Each question is followed by an answer, sometimes quite detailed, and is referenced to specific pages, tables, and figures in Braunwald's *Heart Disease, 5th Edition*, and frequently to other pertinent references as well. By allowing two and a half minutes to answer each question, the time constraints of the board examination may be simulated. This new edition of *Heart Disease: Review and Assessment* again was prepared in response to a number of requests. We hope that it will be useful. The author and the publisher, W.B. Saunders, invite comments and suggestions from the reader.

For this Third Edition, I am especially indebted and grateful to four talented cardiologists from my institution: Ayman Al-Khadra, M.D., Jeffrey Kuvin, M.D., Nasser Mahdi, M.D., and Howard Surks, M.D. Each of these physicians applied their excellent clinical skills and knowledge of cardiovascular disease to the design of the many new questions contained in this Third Edition.

Mrs. Patricia Nayak rendered invaluable assistance in the preparation of the manuscript for the Third Edition. Dr. Bradford C. Berk was a co-author of the first edition of this book. A number of the excellent questions that he prepared for the original book remain in this edition, and we are indebted to him for this contribution. The Members of the Cardiology Division of the New England Medical Center also gave generously of their time and provided new primary materials for this Edition, and we are grateful for their help. Finally, Dr. Eugene Braunwald, my co-author for the first two editions of *Heart Disease: Review and Assessment*, has contributed greatly to every facet of all three editions of this book. I am especially grateful to him for his help with this project and for the generous support and mentoring he has provided me throughout my career.

MICHAEL E. MENDELSOHN, M.D.

CONTENTS

ABBREVIATIONS

A_2 = second aortic sound
AF = atrial fibrillation
APC = atrial premature contraction
ASD = atrial septal defect
AV = atrioventricular
BP = blood pressure
CHF = congestive heart failure
CT = computed tomography
CVP = central venous pressure
CXR = chest x-ray
EKG = electrocardiogram
ETT = exercise tolerance testing
HCM = hypertrophic cardiomyopathy
HR = heart rate
JVP = jugular venous pressure
LA = left atrium
LAHB = left anterior hemiblock
LBBB = left bundle branch block

LPHB = left posterior hemiblock
LV = left ventricle
LVH = left ventricular hypertrophy
LVOT = left ventricular outflow tract
MI = myocardial infarction
MRI = magnetic resonance imaging
P_2 = second pulmonic sound
PTCA = Percutaneous Transluminal Coronary Angioplasty
PVC = premature ventricular contractions
RA = right atrium
RBBB = right bundle branch block
RV = right ventricle
S_1 = first heart sound
S_2 = second heart sound
S_3 = third heart sound
S_4 = fourth heart sound
VSD = ventricular septal defect

Part I
Examination of the Patient

CHAPTERS 1 THROUGH 11

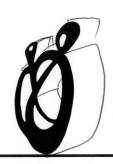

DIRECTIONS: Each question below contains five suggested responses. Select the ONE BEST response to each question.

1. Each of the following statements concerning the history in congenital heart disease is true EXCEPT:

   A. Murmurs due to aortic or pulmonic stenosis are often apparent within the first 48 hours of life
   B. A large left-to-right shunt may lead to frequent episodes of pneumonia in early infancy
   C. Rubella in the first 2 months of pregnancy is associated with several cardiac malformations, including patent ductus arteriosus and supravalvular aortic stenosis
   D. A history of squatting is most frequently associated with valvular pulmonic or aortic stenosis
   E. A maternal viral illness in the third trimester may lead to neonatal myocarditis

2. True statements about continuous murmurs include all of the following EXCEPT:

   A. A continuous murmur must occupy the entirety of the diastolic portion of the cardiac cycle
   B. A holosystolic murmur followed by a holodiastolic murmur is not a continuous murmur
   C. The murmur of patent ductus arteriosus usually peaks just around the second heart sound
   D. Arteriovenous fistulas often generate continuous murmurs
   E. The ''mammary souffle'' heard during late pregnancy may be a continuous murmur

3. Each of the following are true statements about physical maneuvers that may aid in auscultatory diagnosis EXCEPT:

   A. Hyperextension of the shoulders is a useful positional maneuver

   B. The left lateral decubitus position may be helpful in identifying the right ventricular impulse
   C. The click and murmur of mitral valve prolapse occur earlier in systole during the strain phase of the Valsalva maneuver
   D. The Muller maneuver occasionally increases the murmurs of tricuspid valve regurgitation or stenosis
   E. Isometric exercise by sustained handgrip may delay the click of mitral valve prolapse

4. All of the following statements about pulsus paradoxus are true EXCEPT:

   A. A reduction in the systolic arterial pressure of up to 8 mm Hg during inspiration is within normal limits and reflects a small reduction in LV stroke volume and a transmission of negative intrathoracic pressure to the aorta
   B. Pulsus paradoxus is observed frequently in cardiac tamponade
   C. Pulsus paradoxus is observed in patients with pulmonary disease associated with wide swings in intrathoracic pressure
   D. In the presence of aortic regurgitation, pulsus paradoxus is less likely to develop, despite the presence of tamponade
   E. Pulsus paradoxus may occur in hypertrophic cardiomyopathy (HCM)

5. True statements about left anterior fascicular block (LAFB) on the ECG include all of the following EXCEPT:

   A. The duration of the QRS complex is less than 0.12 sec
   B. The QRS axis varies from −20 degrees to −60 degrees

C. LAFB may be mistaken for an anteroseptal MI
D. A prominent S wave is seen in leads V_5 and V_6
E. LAFB is often an indication of underlying organic heart disease

---

6. True statements about the blood pressure response during exercise testing include all of the following EXCEPT:

   A. Normal subjects will display a progressive increase in systolic blood pressure to a peak level between 160 and 220 mm Hg
   B. Black subjects tend to have higher systolic blood pressure responses than white subjects
   C. An elevation of diastolic blood pressure >20 mm Hg is a relatively sensitive indicator for underlying myocardial or coronary disease
   D. Hypertrophic cardiomyopathy may lead to a fall in systolic blood pressure during exercise
   E. Postexercise hypotension is less suggestive of severe underlying coronary artery disease than is exertional hypotension

---

7. True statements about technetium 99m (^{99m}Tc) sestamibi and myocardial imaging include all of the following EXCEPT:

   A. ^{99m}Tc-sestamibi images are of better quality than those obtained with thallium-201 (^{201}Tl)
   B. ^{99m}Tc-sestamibi may be especially useful in the evaluation of successful reperfusion following thrombolysis
   C. ^{99m}Tc-sestamibi is superior to ^{201}Tl for myocardial perfusion imaging
   D. ^{201}Tl is superior to ^{99m}Tc-sestamibi for the simultaneous evaluation of left ventricular (LV) function and perfusion
   E. ^{201}Tl allows for assessment of myocardial viability at rest and following redistribution, while ^{99m}Tc-sestamibi does not

---

8. True statements about exercise testing in an asymptomatic population include all of the following EXCEPT:

   A. Middle-aged asymptomatic men demonstrate a prevalence of abnormal exercise ECGs ranging from 5 to 12 per cent
   B. The most common sequela during the 5 years following a positive exercise test is the development of angina
   C. A positive exercise test is highly correlated with the occurrence of subsequent nonfatal myocardial infarctions

D. The presence of cardiac risk factors makes a positive exercise test in an asymptomatic subject a better predictor of subsequent cardiac events
E. Approximately half of asymptomatic subjects with both an abnormal exercise ECG and an abnormal thallium scan will sustain a cardiac event in the subsequent 4 years

---

9. True statements regarding bundle branch block and exercise testing include *all* of the following EXCEPT:

   A. Patients with left bundle branch block (LBBB) demonstrating ST-segment depression ≥0.3 mV (3 mm) are more likely to have underlying ischemia
   B. Patients with exercise-induced LBBB who demonstrate ST-segment depression after resolution of the conduction defect during recovery are more likely to have underlying ischemia
   C. LBBB develops in approximately 0.4 per cent of patients during exercise testing
   D. Exercise-induced ST-segment depression in right precordial leads in the setting of RBBB is nondiagnostic
   E. Exercise-induced RBBB is seen in approximately 0.1 per cent of exercise tests

---

10. Each of the following statements about the measurement of cardiac output is true EXCEPT:

    A. The Fick principle states that the total uptake or release of a substance by an organ is the product of blood flow to the organ and the arteriovenous difference of the substance measured
    B. A disadvantage of the Fick method is the difficulty of obtaining steady-state conditions for measurement of oxygen consumption
    C. Angiographic measurement of LV end-diastolic and end-systolic volumes permits calculation of stroke volume, which may be used with heart rate to calculate cardiac output
    D. In patients with low cardiac output, the thermodilution method provides a more accurate measurement of cardiac output than the Fick O_2 method
    E. Provided that no intracardiac shunt is present, measurement of pulmonary blood flow and the difference between systemic and pulmonary arterial O_2 content allows calculation of the systemic blood flow

11. Each of the statements below concerning the ECG and location of myocardial infarction are true EXCEPT:

   A. Q waves may be absent in transmural infarction
   B. Q waves do not appear in nontransmural infarction
   C. An anterolateral infarct is defined as Q waves present in leads I and aV$_1$ and V$_3$ through V$_6$
   D. Lead V$_4$R is especially useful in establishing the diagnosis of right ventricular infarction
   E. Infarction of the posterior left ventricular wall may be difficult to detect by ECG

12. Using Doppler ultrasound methods, the following values are obtained for a patient with a restrictive VSD and MR: systolic mitral flow velocity = 5.8 m/sec, systolic flow velocity at the site of the VSD = 5.1 m/sec. The patient's blood pressure is 144/78. The estimated RV systolic pressure is (choose the single best answer):

   A. 35
   B. 40
   C. 45
   D. 50
   E. 55

13. True statements about left bundle branch block (LBBB) include all of the following EXCEPT:

   A. LBBB is a predictor of cardiovascular mortality
   B. The QRS duration in complete LBBB is between 0.12 and 0.18 second
   C. The small septal Q wave due to septal depolarization is absent in LBBB
   D. A T-wave vector concordant with the QRS vector in LBBB may suggest a primary myocardial abnormality such as ischemia
   E. The septal Q wave is preserved in incomplete LBBB

14. Each of the following statements concerning cyanosis is true EXCEPT:

   A. The bluish discoloration of cyanosis results from either an increased amount of reduced hemoglobin or the presence of abnormal hemoglobin pigments
   B. Central cyanosis is characterized by decreased arterial oxygen saturation
   C. Patients with marked polycythemia become cyanotic at higher levels of arterial oxygen saturation than patients with normal hematocrit
   D. Peripheral cyanosis most commonly results from impaired pulmonary function
   E. Localization of peripheral cyanosis to a single extremity may suggest arterial or venous obstruction

15. Echocardiographic predictors of successful mitral balloon valvuloplasty include all of the following EXCEPT:

   A. Presence of valve mobility
   B. Normal left atrial size
   C. Lack of calcification
   D. Minimal valve thickening
   E. Subvalvular disease

16. True statements about the effects of calcium on the ECG include all of the following EXCEPT:

   A. Hypocalcemia may cause ST-segment prolongation
   B. Hypocalcemia does not affect the T wave
   C. Hypercalcemia may lead to a shorter Q-T interval
   D. Hypercalcemia may cause a prominent "J" wave
   E. Calcium affects primarily phase 4 of the action potential

17. All of the following statements about the ECG depicted *below* are correct EXCEPT:

   A. The basic rhythm is atrial fibrillation
   B. The abnormal beat is an example of the Ashman phenomenon
   C. The Ashman phenomenon is based on the fact that the refractory period is directly related to the length of the preceding R-R interval
   D. RBBB morphology is more commonly associated with this type of aberrancy
   E. Because the bundle of His has the longest refractory period, it is the likely anatomic location of the conduction delay

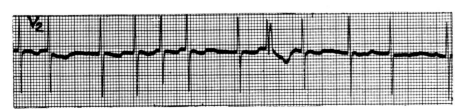

From Marriott, H.J.L.: Rhythm Quizlets: Self Assessment. Philadelphia, Lea & Febiger, 1987, p. 14.

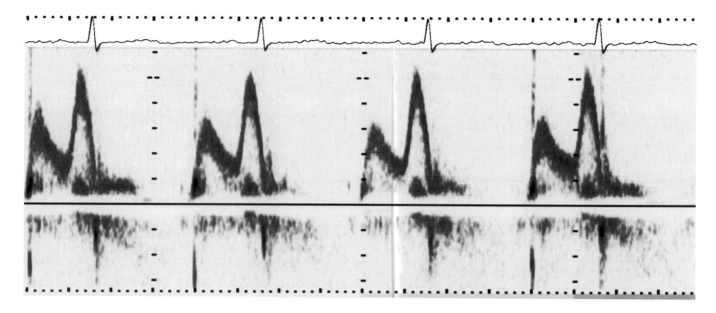

18. True statements about early and late systolic murmurs include all of the following EXCEPT:

    A. Acute mitral regurgitation is characterized by an early systolic murmur
    B. An early systolic murmur characterizes mitral valve prolapse
    C. With normal right ventricular systolic pressures, tricuspid regurgitation is heard as an early systolic murmur
    D. The Valsalva maneuver is helpful in characterizing the murmur of mitral valve prolapse
    E. Elevated pulmonary vascular resistance in the setting of a nonrestrictive ventricular septal defect leads to an early systolic murmur

19. True statements about the jugular venous tracing include all of the following EXCEPT:

    A. The height of the H wave reflects the stiffness of the right atrium
    B. Kussmaul's sign is characterized by a rise in venous pressure with inspiration
    C. The a wave is prominent in LVH
    D. Cannon a waves are found in atrioventricular dissociation
    E. Abdominal-jugular reflux is characterized by transient elevation of the jugular venous pulse while abdominal pressure is maintained

20. Each of the following statements about cardiac catheterization is true EXCEPT:

    A. Patients with ball-cage prosthetic aortic valves can safely undergo retrograde left ventricular catheterization

    B. Transseptal left-heart catheterization should not be attempted in patients with suspected severe mitral valve obstruction
    C. Catheterization of outpatients has been demonstrated to be a safe and cost-effective alternative in appropriately selected patients
    D. A percutaneous brachial arterial approach may be used in adults provided that the catheters used are of small size
    E. Porcine heterograft valves in the aortic position can safely be crossed in the course of performing a retrograde left ventricular catheterization

21. Causes for this type of mitral inflow Doppler pattern shown *above* include all of the following EXCEPT:

    A. LVH
    B. Normal aging
    C. Severe heart failure
    D. Myocardial ischemia
    E. Pulmonary hypertension

22. All of the following statements regarding the use of exercise testing in the postmyocardial infarction patient are true EXCEPT:

    A. Patients who complete 80 per cent of the age-predicted maximum exercise protocol without ECG or blood pressure abnormalities have a 1-year mortality of 2 per cent or less
    B. Approximately 30 per cent of postinfarction patients have exercise test abnormalities
    C. Exertional hypotension is the most specific marker for severe underlying coronary artery disease in postinfarction patients

D. Asymptomatic ST-segment depression in patients completing a low-level exercise test following MI is of uncertain prognostic significance

E. Exercise testing at 6 or more months after an acute infarction is more useful in risk stratification than testing at 6 weeks after MI

23. All of the following information can be deduced from the accompanying Doppler tracing EXCEPT:

A. The severity of mitral stenosis
B. The severity of mitral regurgitation
C. The suitability of the mitral valve for percutaneous mitral valvuloplasty
D. An assessment of left ventricular systolic performance
E. The transmitral pressure gradient

24. A patient with a long history of pulmonary emboli undergoes noninvasive assessment of cardiac status by Doppler echocardiography. Assuming the following values:

RA pressure = 4 mm Hg
Peak Doppler flow signal across the tricuspid valve = 4 m/sec

The patient's right ventricular systolic pressure is:

A. 64 mm Hg
B. 68 mm Hg

C. 50 mm Hg
D. 20 mm Hg
E. Insufficient information to determine the value

25. All of the following are true of the physiology of exercise in healthy people EXCEPT:

A. Both stroke volume and increased heart rate contribute to augmentation of cardiac output throughout the exercise period
B. Diastolic blood pressure does not change significantly during exercise
C. Anaerobic threshold is reached at approximately 50 per cent of maximal workload
D. An exercise capacity of 9 METs is equivalent to heavy physical labor or strenuous exercise
E. The pulmonary vasculature can accommodate a sixfold increase in cardiac output without a significant increase in pulmonary artery pressure

26. All of the following diseases may be accompanied by a mid-diastolic murmur EXCEPT:

A. Tricuspid stenosis
B. Mitral regurgitation
C. Complete heart block

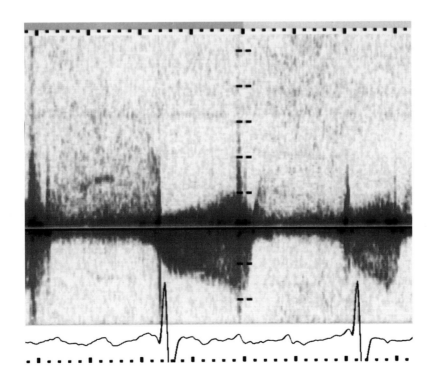

D. Pulmonic regurgitation associated with pulmonary hypertension
E. Tricuspid regurgitation

---

27. All of the following are true regarding the echocardiographic assessment of mitral regurgitation EXCEPT:

A. Color flow Doppler echocardiography provides an accurate quantitative assessment of MR
B. Pulse Doppler can provide an indirect assessment of MR
C. Regurgitant color flow Doppler jets directed towards the atrial wall underestimate the severity of MR
D. Echocardiography may be used to assess the hemodynamic consequences of MR
E. Determining the etiology of MR is one of the most important applications of echocardiography

---

28. Findings easily shown on *both* two-dimensional and M-mode echocardiography in mitral stenosis include all of the following EXCEPT:

A. Doming of the mitral valve leaflets
B. Inadequate separation of the anterior and posterior leaflets of the valve during diastole
C. Increased thickness of the valve leaflets
D. The presence of fibrosis and calcifications as revealed by an increase in the number of echoes
E. An increase in left atrial size due to left atrial hypertension

---

29. True statements regarding ST-segment changes during exercise protocols include all of the following EXCEPT:

A. J-point (junctional) depression is a normal finding during exercise
B. The ischemic response recorded during an exercise test occurs only during the recovery phase in 30 to 40 per cent of patients
C. ≥1 mm of J-point depression with a flat ST-segment depression, persisting ≥0.10 mV for 60 to 80 msec after the J-point in three consecutive beats is considered to be an abnormal ST-segment response
D. In patients with early repolarization on the resting electrocardiogram, abnormal

ST-segment depression should be measured from the PQ junction
E. Exercise-induced ST-segment depression does not localize the coronary artery involved

---

30. The electrocardiogram depicted on page 7 is consistent with

A. reversal of the limb leads
B. left posterior hemiblock
C. right ventricular hypertrophy
D. counterclockwise rotation and left anterior hemiblock
E. none of the above

---

31. True statements about exercise protocols include all of the following EXCEPT:

A. The heart rate and blood pressure responses to a given workload of arm ergometric exercise usually are less than those for leg exercise
B. One limitation of bicycle protocols is early fatigue in subjects unconditioned to or unfamiliar with bicycle exercise
C. The modified Bruce protocol is useful in older individuals
D. The standard Bruce protocol is characterized by a relatively large increase in oxygen consumption between stages
E. Heart rate−adjusted indices of ST-segment depression are more reliably estimated by decreasing the length of the Bruce protocol stages

---

32. Each of the following statements about early diastolic murmurs is false EXCEPT:

A. The murmur of aortic regurgitation most commonly radiates to the right sternal edge
B. The early diastolic murmur of acute, severe aortic regurgitation is usually relatively short
C. The early diastolic murmur of aortic regurgitation is usually quite loud
D. The Graham Steell murmur is often heard in pulmonary stenosis
E. The murmur of chronic severe aortic regurgitation rarely decreases in intensity during diastole

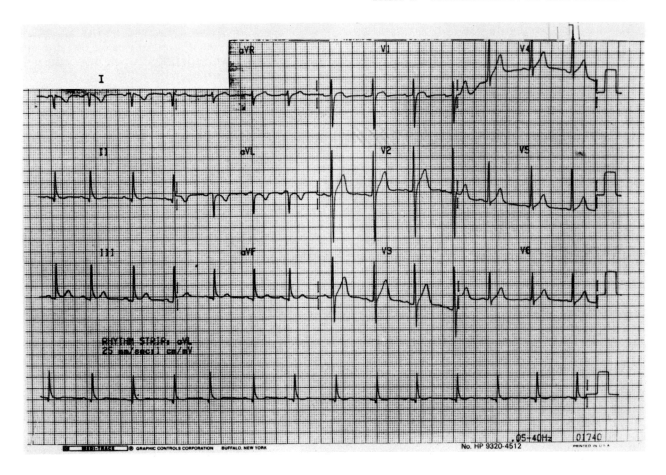

33. Each of the following is a true statement about the ECG in chronic obstructive lung disease EXCEPT:

A. Right-axis deviation of the P wave may occur

B. An increase in Ta-segment wave amplitude may lead to pseudo–ST-segment depression

C. Left-axis deviation is seen in the majority of cases

D. If biventricular hypertrophy is present, left ventricular forces often predominate

E. When pulmonary hypertension and right ventricular hypertrophy (RVH) occur, prominent R waves may appear in right precordial leads

34. All of the following statements concerning myocardial perfusion imaging and acute MI are true EXCEPT:

A. After an acute MI, the size of a myocardial perfusion defect may decrease over time

B. Thallium-201 imaging is an impractical method of assessing efficacy of thrombolytic therapy

C. Myocardial perfusion defects during unstable angina reverse with resolution of chest pain

D. Patients with ECG abnormalities and chest pain have larger myocardial perfusion defects than patients with chest pain who do not have ECG abnormalities

E. The size of the myocardial perfusion defect after an MI correlates directly with prognosis and survival

35. Which of the following statements concerning ST-segment elevation during exercise is *false*?

A. Exercise-induced ST-segment elevation in a lead with an abnormal Q wave is correlated with poor left ventricular function

B. Exercise-induced ST-segment elevation in patients undergoing annual testing following myocardial infarction is correlated with poor left ventricular function

C. ST-segment elevation in leads with abnormal Q waves is a marker of ongoing myocardial ischemia

D. ST-segment elevation in a non–Q wave lead in a patient without prior myocardial infarction is correlated with coronary vasospasm or a high-grade coronary stenosis

E. The ECG site of ST-segment elevation during exercise is relatively specific for the coronary artery involved

36. All of the following are true of prognosis as determined by myocardial perfusion imaging EXCEPT:

    A. Patients with normal perfusion in the presence of angiographically documented coronary artery disease have low rates of cardiac events
    B. The prognostic predictive value of myocardial perfusion is independent of imaging technique or isotope used
    C. The sensitivity of a high-risk pattern of myocardial perfusion is approximately 70 per cent
    D. The combination of clinical and cardiac catheterization data provides more prognostic information than the combination of clinical and myocardial perfusion data
    E. Both the number and extent of myocardial perfusion defects and the magnitude of defect reversibility are predictors of future cardiac events

37. All of the following statements concerning radiographic contrast agents are true EXCEPT:

    A. Ionic contrast-induced nephrotoxicity occurs in about 1 to 2 per cent of patients receiving ionic contrast media
    B. Nonionic, low osmolar contrast agents cause fewer acute adverse hemodynamic and arrhythmic side effects than ionic agents
    C. There is no advantage of low osmolar contrast over ionic contrast in the prevention of nephrotoxicity in patients with normal renal function
    D. Saline hydration is less effective than furosemide and mannitol for prevention of contrast-induced nephrotoxicity in patients with baseline renal insufficiency
    E. Diabetes mellitus is an indication for using low osmolar contrast agents

38. All of the following statements about cardiac myosin structure are true EXCEPT:

    A. Each myosin filament contains two heavy chains and four light chains
    B. Mutation of the β-MHC gene may be responsible for a type of hypertrophic cardiomyopathy
    C. β-MHC has lower ATPase activity and is less commonly found in humans than α-MHC
    D. MLC-1 may inhibit the contractile process by interactions with actin
    E. Phosphorylation of MLC-2 may accelerate contraction by increasing the affinity of myosin for actin

39. All of the following statements concerning the accompanying Doppler study are true EXCEPT:

    A. Diastolic mitral flow is characteristically abnormal in this disease

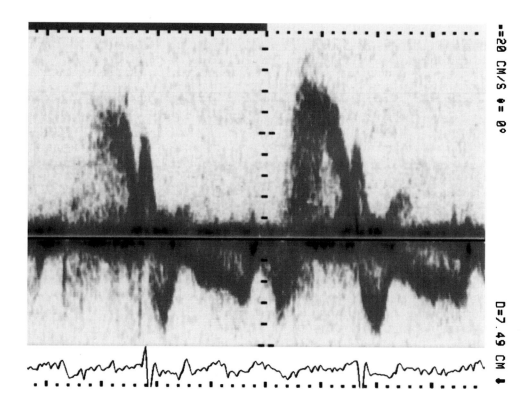

B. This Doppler echocardiogram could be from a 22-year-old patient with a family history of sudden death

C. This Doppler echocardiogram could be from a 73-year-old patient with longstanding hypertension

D. Systolic anterior motion of the mitral valve is specific for this disorder

E. M-mode echocardiography might demonstrate midsystolic closure of the aortic valve in this patient

---

DIRECTIONS: Each question below contains suggested answers. For EACH of the alternatives, you are to respond either TRUE (T) or FALSE (F). In a given item, ALL, SOME, OR NONE OF THE ALTERNATIVES MAY BE CORRECT.

40. Which of the following statements about the echocardiographic evaluation of mitral valve prolapse are true?

    A. The direction of the mitral leaflet tips in systole distinguishes between mitral valve prolapse and flail mitral leaflet

    B. Posterior buckling of the mitral valve by more than 3 mm is a specific sign of mitral valve prolapse

    C. Two-dimensional evaluation of mitral valve prolapse is more likely to provide a false-positive in the apical four-chamber view than in the parasternal long axis view

    D. M-mode echocardiography reliably distinguishes mitral valve prolapse from a normal variant, especially when holosystolic buckling is noted

    E. Mitral leaflet thickening and redundancy help to confirm the diagnosis of mitral valve prolapse

41. For each of the following statements about radionuclide angiocardiography, indicate true (T) or false (F).

    A. First-pass radionuclide angiocardiography studies are favored over equilibrium radionuclide angiocardiography for evaluation of right ventricular performance

    B. Radionuclide angiocardiography is a useful technique for assessing prognosis after acute MI

    C. Serial radionuclide angiocardiographic studies are indicated for patients receiving doxorubicin chemotherapy

    D. Ambulatory radionuclide angiocardiograXphy may play a major role in the detection of silent ischemia

    E. Diastolic ventricular function may be assessed by either first-pass or equilibrium radionuclide angiocardiography

42. Which of the following statements concerning the echocardiographic evaluation of aortic valve disease are *true*?

    A. The peak instantaneous pressure gradient provides a good estimation of the peak-to-peak gradient found at cardiac catheterization

    B. An aortic flow velocity of 2.5 m/sec indicates mild AS

    C. A gradual decline in the velocity of the AR jet is consistent with mild AR

    D. Premature closure of the mitral valve in AR is a marker of high left ventricular diastolic pressure

    E. The mean aortic gradient is invariably higher when measured by Doppler echocardiography than when measured by cardiac catheterization

43. With reference to intracardiac shunts, which of the following statements are true?

    A. In normal subjects, O_2 content in different portions of the right atrium may vary by as much as 2 volumes per cent (20 ml O_2/liter), reflecting that streaming of blood received from the superior vena cava, the inferior vena cava, and the coronary sinus occurs in the right atrium

    B. Atrial septal defect, anomalous pulmonary venous drainage, and ruptured sinus of Valsalva may all lead to significant step-up in O_2 saturation values between the venae cavae and the right atrium

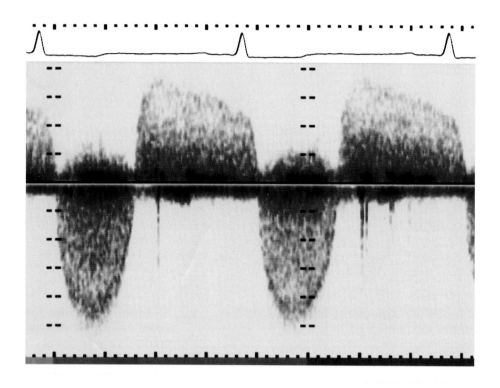

C. Because of the normal variability in O_2 saturation, shunts with pulmonary-to-systemic flow ratios (Qp/Qs) ≤ 1.3 at the level of the pulmonary artery or right ventricle may escape detection by oximetry run analyses

D. When a shunt is unidirectional (e.g., left-to-right only), its magnitude is calculated as the difference between the pulmonary and systemic blood flows as determined using the appropriate variations of the Fick equation

E. In patients with a pure right-to-left shunt, such as in tetralogy of Fallot, the calculated left-to-right shunt will be a negative value

---

44. Which of the following findings of an exercise test are associated with multivessel (or left main) coronary artery disease?

    A. Early onset of ST-segment depression
    B. Persistence of ST-segment changes late into the recovery phase
    C. ST-segment elevation in lead aV_r
    D. Multifocal premature ventricular contractions
    E. Failure to increase systolic blood pressure by at least 10 mm Hg

---

45. Which of the following statements about the accompanying Doppler flow tracing are true?

    A. The probability of critical aortic stenosis in this patient is high
    B. The estimated aortic valve gradient is 60 mm Hg
    C. The aortic insufficiency is not severe
    D. Based on the Doppler findings, one would expect to find premature closure of the mitral valve on M-mode echocardiographic examination of this patient
    E. One would expect the 2-D echocardiogram of this patient to reveal left ventricular hypertrophy

---

46. Which of the following imaging techniques are capable of correctly identifying acutely necrotic myocardial tissue?

    A. ^{99m}Tc-pyrophosphate scintigraphy
    B. echocardiography
    C. monoclonal antimyosin-specific antibody scintigraphy
    D. coronary angiography
    E. positron emission tomography (PET)

---

47. Which of the following statements about heart murmurs are TRUE?

    A. There are three basic types of murmur: systolic, diastolic, and continuous

B. Systolic murmurs may be further characterized as early, midsystolic, late systolic, or holosystolic

C. Holosystolic murmurs end in most instances with the pulmonic component of the second heart sound

D. Systolic murmurs are characterized as crescendo, decrescendo, diamond-shaped, plateau, or variable

E. A continuous murmur begins in systole and decreases in intensity with the second heart sound, only to increase again throughout the entirety of diastole

---

48. Correct statements on the utility of echocardiography in evaluation of myocardial ischemia and myocardial infarction include which of the following?

A. During systole, the left ventricle normally increases in thickness

B. At 1 year following a transmural myocardial infarction, ventricular wall thickness remains normal in diastole, but systolic thickening is abolished, indicative of infarction

C. The presence of a ventricular aneurysm is suggested echocardiographically by identification of a thrombus in the left ventricular inferior wall surrounded by a pericardial sac

D. LV mural thrombi occur most commonly with anterior myocardial infarctions

E. M-mode echocardiography is a sensitive way to detect a ventricular septal defect during acute MI

---

49. Which of the following statements regarding pericardial rubs are true?

A. The pericardial friction rub usually has three components

B. Deep inspiration may augment the pericardial rub during auscultation

C. Atrial fibrillation leads to loss of the presystolic component in pericardial rubs

D. Pericardial rubs are heard frequently following open heart surgery

E. Hamman's sign is a classic finding in patients with pericardial rub

---

50. Which of the following are true statements about coronary artery anatomy?

A. The left coronary artery is dominant in 10 to 23 per cent of humans

B. The interventricular septum is the most densely vascularized area of the heart

C. Over 90 per cent of patients have between one and three diagonal vessels branching off the left anterior descending artery

D. A ramus medianus branch arising between the left anterior descending coronary (LAD) and circumflex arteries is present in approximately 10 per cent of patients

E. The position of the coronary sinus identifies the position of the circumflex artery, which runs in or near the atrioventricular groove

---

51. Which of the following are true examples of *noncoronary* causes of ST-segment depression during exercise testing?

A. left ventricular hypertrophy

B. preexcitation syndrome

C. mitral valve prolapse

D. cardiomyopathy

E. digitalis therapy

---

52. Which of the following statements concerning the echocardiographic findings in hypertrophic cardiomyopathy (HCM) are true? (One or more choices may be true.)

A. The presence of systolic anterior motion of the mitral valve is a sensitive and specific finding in HCM

B. Early systolic closure of the aortic valve, while indicative of significant outflow obstruction, is not a specific sign of HCM

C. Asymmetric septal hypertrophy (ASH) is defined echocardiographically as a ratio of septal to posterior wall thickness of 1.3:1.0

D. The absence of ASH excludes the diagnosis of HCM

E. The Doppler mitral inflow pattern is typically normal in HCM

---

53. With reference to the electrocardiographic diagnosis of myocardial infarction, which of the following are true?

A. Less than 75 per cent of patients have a diagnostic ECG initially

B. Serial ECGs will increase the diagnostic sensitivity to greater than 80 per cent

C. About 30 per cent of patients with old Q-wave myocardial infarction will eventually "lose" their Q wave

D. Patients with inferior myocardial infarctions from right coronary artery lesions and reciprocal ST depressions in leads V_1 to V_4 usually have associated circumflex artery disease

E. Right ventricular infarction can be diagnosed with high sensitivity (>75 per cent) by ST-segment elevation in V_4R

54. True statements about abnormal splitting of the second heart sound include

    A. Persistent splitting is not commonly heard in ostium secundum atrial septal defect
    B. Persistent splitting may be due to early timing of the aortic component or a delay in the pulmonic component of the second heart sound
    C. Paradoxical splitting of the second heart sound may be due to a left ventricular pacemaker
    D. An increase in the intensity of the aortic component is common in hypertension
    E. In aortic root dilatation, the pulmonic sound may be more prominent

55. With reference to the jugular venous pulse (JVP), true statements include which of the following?

    A. Two principal observations made from examination of the neck veins include the level of venous pressure and the type of venous wave pattern
    B. Tricuspid regurgitation and right ventricular failure respond to the abdomino-jugular reflex test with a sustained rise in jugular venous pressure
    C. The *v* wave results from right atrial pressure rise in response to blood flow into the right atrium during ventricular systole when the tricuspid valve is shut
    D. Cannon (giant) *a* waves are observed when the right atrium contracts against a closed tricuspid valve, as in atrioventricular dissociation
    E. Kussmaul's sign is a paradoxical fall in the height of the jugular venous pulse during inspiration that occurs frequently in patients with chronic constrictive pericarditis

56. With reference to complications of cardiac catheterization, which of the following statements are true?

    A. The likelihood of death occurring from cardiac catheterization is less than 0.5 per cent
    B. The likelihood of acute MI occurring from cardiac catheterization is less than 0.5 per cent
    C. The incidence of death from cardiac catheterization is greater in patients under 1 year of age
    D. Mortality from catheterization of patients with significant left main coronary artery disease is less than 0.5 per cent

    E. The presence of valvular disease is associated with a higher risk of death at cardiac catheterization

57. True statements about the second heart sound include:

    A. Whereas the pulmonic component is heard primarily at the second left intercostal space, the aortic component of the second heart sound can be heard at the sternal edge, as well as at the base and apex
    B. Splitting of the second heart sound is primarily due to a delay in the aortic component
    C. Earlier onset of the aortic component may contribute to inspiratory splitting
    D. The aortic and pulmonic components are heard at different frequencies
    E. Splitting of the second heart sound is best heard at the second left intercostal space

58. Correct statements regarding the clinical interpretation of exercise stress tests include which of the following?

    A. A finding of 0.1 mV of ST-segment depression *after* exercise is more specific than 0.1 mV ST-segment depression *during* exercise
    B. A patient with a 50 per cent stenosis in the right coronary artery will probably develop ischemic ECG changes in leads II, III, and aV_f at a peak-pressure product of $\leq 15,000$ mm Hg $\times$ beats/min
    C. In most exercise protocols the systolic blood pressure rises about 8 to 10 mm Hg per stage
    D. Maximal predicted exercise heart rate is approximately 220 minus the patient's age
    E. In normal exercise there may be ≥ 0.1 mV J-point depression

59. Which of the following statements comparing first-pass and equilibrium angiocardiography are true?

    A. Both techniques yield accurate measurements of global left ventricular ejection fraction
    B. Regional wall motion abnormalities are assessed with equal accuracy
    C. Physiological or pharmacological interventions are better assessed by the equilibrium technique
    D. The number of studies is more limited by first-pass technique
    E. Interventions that result in rapid changes in heart rate are assessed better by equilibrium technique

60. True statements about digitalis-induced arrhythmias include all of the following EXCEPT:

    A. Atrial tachycardia with block is usually due to digitalis toxicity
    B. Nonparoxysmal junctional tachycardia may be a sign of digitalis excess
    C. Ventricular bigeminy with varying morphology and regular coupling may be a sign of digitalis toxicity
    D. AV dissociation in a patient taking digitalis is a strong indication of digitalis toxicity
    E. Ventricular premature contractions are not highly specific for toxicity in the patient on digitalis therapy

61. Abnormalities that may enter into the differential diagnosis of chest pain or discomfort include:

    A. pulmonary hypertension
    B. Mallory-Weiss syndrome
    C. scalenus anticus syndrome
    D. congenital absence of the pericardium

62. Which of the following statements regarding exercise testing in symptomatic patients are true (T) and which are false (F)?

    A. Patients with known chronic ischemic heart disease should undergo exercise testing before angiography unless specific contraindications exist
    B. In the presence of chronic stable angina pectoris, an excellent exercise tolerance is not as precise a predictor of prognosis as the anatomical extent of coronary artery disease
    C. Symptomatic patients who are unable to exercise past Bruce stage I and who exhibit 1 mm or more of ST-segment depression have an annual mortality of 5 per cent or more based on the CASS study
    D. In the presence of documented coronary artery disease, exercise-induced ischemic ST-segment changes predict increased risk even in patients who do not experience chest pain (i.e., with silent ischemia)
    E. In the CASS study, patients stratified by coronary anatomy and left ventricular function had similar survival rates regardless of whether their ischemia was silent or symptomatic

63. Which of the following statements regarding cardiac arrhythmias during exercise testing are true (T) and which are false (F)?

    A. In patients who have undergone ambulatory monitoring and electrophysiological studies, exercise testing does not add any incremental diagnostic information
    B. Patients demonstrating Q-T$_c$ interval prolongation with exercise in the setting of known ventricular arrhythmias are likely to demonstrate a better response to type IA antiarrhythmic drugs
    C. Sustained supraventricular tachycardias occur in approximately 10 per cent of normal subjects during an exercise test
    D. Patients with atrial fibrillation almost always have an increased exercise capacity once ventricular rate control is achieved
    E. Up to 50 per cent of patients with sick sinus syndrome will have a normal exercise heart rate response

64. True statements concerning ejection sounds include:

    A. Ejection sounds or aortic origin are most prominent in association with a deformed aortic valve, such as a bicuspid valve, or in congenital or rheumatic aortic stenosis (AS)
    B. While aortic ejection sounds due to a di.lated aortic root may be less prominent than those associated with valvular disease, they have a similar timing early in systole
    C. A decrease in intensity of the pulmonic ejection sound with inspiration is heard in pulmonic valve stenosis
    D. It can be shown by echophonocardiography that high-frequency ejection sounds start before the aortic or pulmonic valve is completely open

65. Which of the following are true statements about the electrocardiogram in acute pulmonary embolism?

    A. The ECG in acute pulmonary embolism is entirely normal in the majority of cases
    B. The $S_1Q_3T_3$ pattern is seen in approximately half of patients who sustain an acute pulmonary embolism
    C. Atrial arrhythmias are rare in acute pulmonary embolism
    D. Nonspecific ST- and T-wave changes are common in acute pulmonary embolism
    E. The pathophysiology that leads to ECG changes in acute pulmonary embolism is primarily acute pulmonary hypertension

66. Which of the following are true statements (T) about right ventricular hypertrophy (RVH) and which are false (F)?

    A. Unlike left ventricular hypertrophy, the sensitivity of the ECG pattern for RVH is relatively high

B. Based on the QRS pattern in lead V_1, RVH can be separated into four distinct types
C. The QRS morphology in lead V_1 may allow some estimate of the right ventricular pressure relative to that in the left ventricle
D. ST-segment depression in right precordial leads with accompanying T-wave inversion is consistent with moderate or severe RVH
E. Isolated right-axis deviation is a less sensitive indicator of RVH

67. The cardiac catheterization tracing illustrated *below* could be associated with the following features:

A. A large systolic pressure gradient between left ventricle and aorta
B. A bifid aortic pulse contour
C. Increased ventricular stiffness resulting in an elevated left ventricular end-diastolic pressure
D. A slow and delayed rise in the aortic pressure as compared with that of the left ventricle

68. Which of the following statements about holosystolic murmurs are true (T) and which are false (F)?

A. Holosystolic murmurs may be generated by a communication between the ventricles
B. The radiation of the murmur of mitral regurgitation is independent of the direction of the intraatrial jet of regurgitant blood
C. Carvallo's sign is a selective inspiratory increase in the loudness of the murmur of tricuspid regurgitation
D. Carvallo's sign is present primarily during right ventricular failure

E. Patent ductus arteriosus may generate a holosystolic murmur

69. Which of the following are true statements regarding systolic arterial murmurs?

A. Systolic arterial murmurs are heard at nonprecordial sites
B. Systolic arterial murmurs are usually crescendo-decrescendo in configuration
C. The "supraclavicular systolic murmur" is heard in many normal older adults
D. Duroziez's sign in aortic regurgitation results from the same underlying vascular pathology that generates common systolic arterial murmurs in older adults
E. Aortic coarctation may lead to a systolic arterial murmur

70. Rotation of the heart within the chest cavity results in the following changes in the ECG:

A. A "horizontal" heart leads to a QRS complex in aV_1 that resembles leads V_5 and V_6
B. "Clockwise rotation" causes the "rS" portions of the QRS complex to be present in leads V_2 to V_5
C. A "vertical" heart leads to a QRS complex in lead aV_f that resembles leads V_5 and V_6
D. "Counterclockwise rotation" can mimic right ventricular hypertrophy

71. True statements about the ECG in ischemic heart disease include which of the following?

A. Ischemia and infarction cannot be diagnosed in the presence of a left bundle branch block (LBBB)

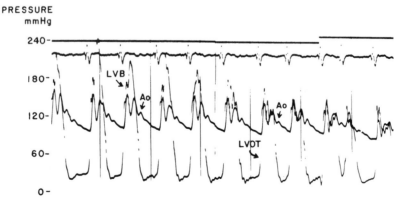

From Levinson, G.E.: Aortic stenosis. *In* Dalen, J.E., and Alpert, J.S. (eds.): Valvular Heart Disease. 2nd ed. Boston, Little, Brown & Company, 1987, p. 257.

B. The appearance of a negative U wave during an exercise test is highly specific for left anterior descending coronary artery disease
C. Loss of Q waves following an anterior MI is correlated with smaller areas of infarction
D. The sensitivity of the Q wave is lowest for inferior MI
E. Right bundle branch block (RBBB) obscures an ECG infarction pattern in approximately 30 per cent of subjects

72. Which of the following statements concerning the cardiac catheterization laboratory evaluation of valve orifice areas are true?

A. Valve area in cm^2 is calculated as: Flow (in ml/sec) $\div$ K $\times$ (mean pressure gradient in mm Hg)$^{1/2}$ where K is an empirical constant for the valve in question
B. The presence of valvular regurgitation will result in a falsely low calculated valve area because actual flow across the valve is greater than the flow calculated from the systemic cardiac output
C. Calculation of mitral valve area often relies on substitution of a confirmed pulmonary capillary wedge pressure for left atrial pressure
D. Valve area calculation is more strongly influenced by errors in the pressure gradient measurement than by errors in cardiac output measurement

73. The myocardial scintigrams in A are from a normal patient. The scintigrams in B demonstrate the following features:

A. a perfusion defect that is partly reversible
B. an inferior perfusion defect
C. an irreversible perfusion defect
D. an increase in lung uptake of the radioisotope on the initial image

74. Which of the statements below concerning the ECG in myocardial infarction (MI) are true (T) and which are false (F)?

A. In patients presenting early with an MI, the initial ECG is nondiagnostic in the majority of patients
B. The time of onset of Q waves varies between several hours and 1 or 2 days
C. The classic pattern of ECG evolution in MI begins with T-wave changes
D. Infarction of an electrocardiographically silent area of the heart is one of several

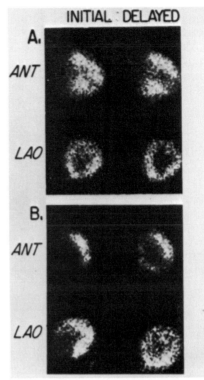

From Okada, R.D., Boucher, C.A., Strauss, H.W., and Pohost, G.M.: Exercise radionuclide imaging approaches to coronary artery disease. Am. J. Cardiol. *46*:1188, 1980.

explanations for a normal ECG in patients with evolving MI
E. ST-segment depression in leads V_1 to V_4 in the presence of an inferior infarction is usually an indication of ischemia in the distribution of the left anterior descending artery

75. Which of the following statements regarding the effect of the potassium concentration on the ECG are true (T) and which are false (F)?

A. The earliest ECG sign of hyperkalemia is a slight reduction in P-wave amplitude
B. There is a good correlation between plasma potassium level and the surface ECG in patients
C. Hyperkalemia may mimic right bundle branch block or left bundle branch block
D. Hypokalemia is marked by a prominent U wave but a normal Q-T interval

76. Computed tomography of the pericardium can delineate or differentiate the following features:

A. loculated pericardial effusions and hemopericardium from transudative fluid

B. congenital absence of the pericardium
C. constrictive pericarditis with thickened pericardium from restrictive cardiomyopathy
D. mucoid-secreting pericardial cysts from solid tumors

77. Which of the following are potential causes of noninfarction Q waves?

A. Cardiac amyloidosis
B. Hypertrophic cardiomyopathy
C. Chronic obstructive pulmonary disease
D. Spontaneous pneumothorax
E. Wolff-Parkinson-White syndrome

DIRECTIONS: The group of questions below consists of lettered headings followed by a set of numbered items. For each numbered item select the ONE lettered heading with which it is MOST closely associated. Each lettered heading may be used ONCE, MORE THAN ONCE, OR NOT AT ALL.

For each of the chest roentgenograms shown on page 17 (A–D), match the most appropriate cardiac diagnosis:

78. mitral stenosis

79. aortic regurgitation

80. atrial septal defect

81. pericardial effusion

Match the following cardiac muscle proteins with their properties:

A. A calcium storage protein in the sarcoplasmic reticulum
B. Negatively inhibits the activity of the calcium-pumping ATPase of the sarcoplasmic reticulum
C. Its presence in myofibrils helps to explain the stress-strain elastic relation of striated muscle
D. A regulatory protein of the troponin complex
E. A complex structure that includes the calcium release channel

82. Titin

83. Ryanodine

84. Calsequestrin

85. Phospholamban

86. Calrectulin

For each statement or definition, match the appropriate sign on physical examination:

A. Hill's sign
B. de Musset's sign
C. Duroziez's sign
D. Quincke's sign
E. Traube's sign

87. "Pistol shot" sounds heard over the femoral artery when a stethoscope is placed on it

88. Systolic blood pressure in the popliteal artery exceeds that in the brachial artery by more than 20 mm Hg

89. Bobbing of the head in synchrony with each heartbeat

90. A systolic murmur heard upon gradual compression of the proximal femoral artery, with a diastolic murmur heard upon compression of the artery distally

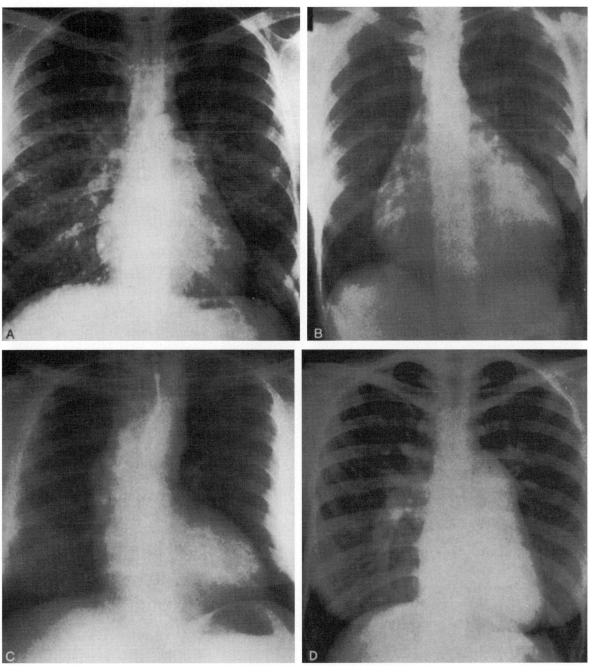

A, From Daves, M.L.: Cardiac Roentgenology. Chicago, Year Book Medical Publishers, 1981, p. 397.
B, From Daves, M.L.: Cardiac Roentgenology. Chicago, Year Book Medical Publishers, 1981, p. 470.
C, From Daves, M.L.: Cardiac Roentgenology. Chicago, Year Book Medical Publishers, 1981, p. 413.
D, From Daves, M.L.: Cardiac Roentgenology. Chicago, Year Book Medical Publishers, 1981, p. 271.

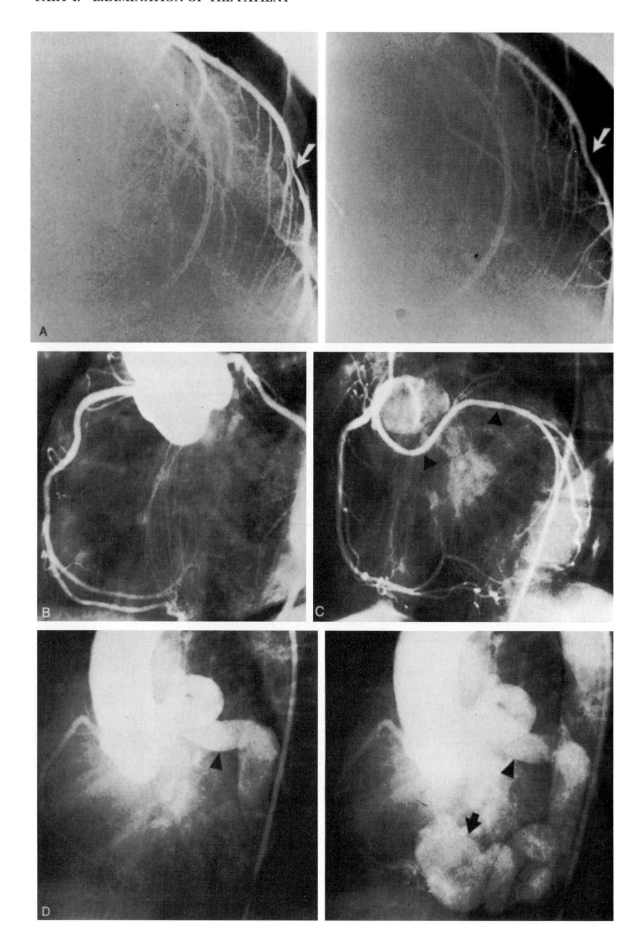

For each arteriogram or set of arteriograms on these 2 pages (A–E), match the appropriate descriptive phrase.

91. RAO projection; LAD artery, demonstrating myocardial bridging with narrowing in systole and near-normal caliber in diastole

92. LAO projection; right coronary arteriogram demonstrating anomalous origin of the left circumflex artery from the proximal RCA

93. LAO projection; collateral vessels arising from the distal right coronary artery and supplying an occluded LAD artery

94. RAO projection; catheter-induced coronary spasm and restoration of normal caliber with introduction of nitroglycerin

95. LAO projection; showing early filling of a markedly dilated left circumflex artery and subsequent coronary sinus opacification due to a congenital fistula

For each statement below, match the clinical trial of pharmacologic therapy for systolic dysfunction that yielded the information in the statement.

A. CONSENSUS-1
B. TRACE
C. V-HeFT-II
D. SOLVD
E. SAVE

96. Showed a benefit of enalapril versus the combination of hydralazine and isosorbide dinitrate for patients with mild to moderate heart failure

97. Found a reduction in mortality and rate of progression to severe heart failure in patients with recent MI and reduced ejection fraction who were treated with captopril

98. Found a significant reduction in mortality among patients with *severe* heart failure treated with enalapril

99. A reduction in mortality was found in patients with *mild to moderate* heart failure and ejection fractions <35 per cent who were treated with enalapril

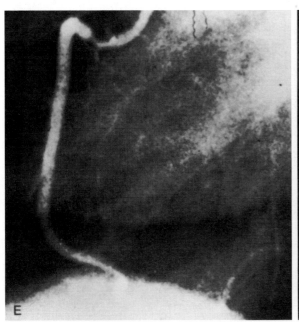 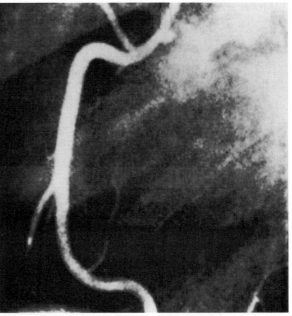

A, From Levin, D.C.: Pitfalls in coronary arteriography. *In* Abrams, H.L. (ed.): Coronary Arteriography: A Practical Approach. Boston, Little, Brown & Company, 1983, p. 251.

B, From Paulin, S.: Coronary angiography: A technical anatomic and clinical study. Acta Radiol. Suppl. 233:142, 1964.

C, From Levin, D.C.: Anomalies and anatomic variations of the coronary arteries. *In* Abrams, H.L. (ed.): Coronary Arteriography: A Practical Approach. Boston, Little, Brown & Company, 1983, p. 290.

D, From Levin, D.C., Fellows, K.E., and Abrams, H.L.: Hemodynamically significant primary anomalies of the coronary arteries. Angiographic aspects. Circulation *58*:25, 1978. Reprinted by permission of the American Heart Association, Inc.

E, From Abrams, H.L.: Angiography in coronary disease. *In* Abrams, H.L. (ed.): Coronary Arteriography: A Practical Approach. Boston, Little, Brown & Company, 1983, p. 225.

For each electrocardiogram, match the appropriate interpretation.

100. left posterior hemiblock

101. Wolff-Parkinson-White syndrome

102. right bundle branch block and left anterior hemiblock

103. right ventricular hypertrophy

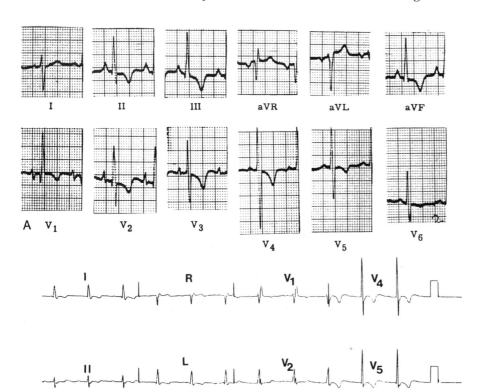

A, From Goldman, M.J.: Principles of Clinical Electrocardiography. 11th ed. Los Altos, CA, Lange Medical Publications, 1982, p. 363.

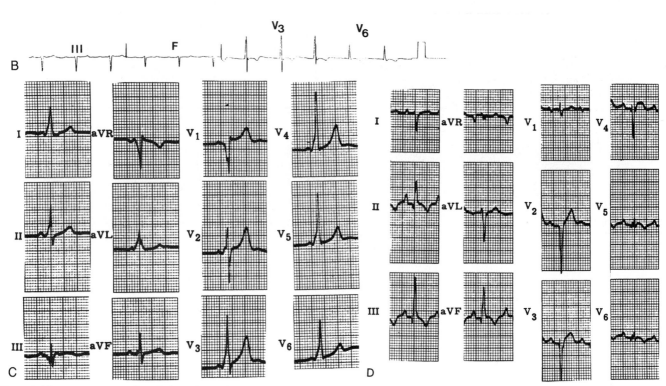

From Goldman, M.J.: Principles of Clinical Electrocardiography. 11th ed. Los Altos, CA, Lange Medical Publications, 1982, p. 277.

From Goldman, M.J.: Principles of Clinical Electrocardiography. 11th ed. Los Altos, CA, Lange Medical Publications, 1982, p. 131.

ELECTROCARDIOGRAMS

DIRECTIONS: Each of the 12-lead ECGs *below* is introduced by a brief descriptive phrase. For each electrocardiogram, perform a systematic reading. Begin by noting any atrial, AV junctional, or ventricular rhythms present and point out whether any AV conduction abnormalities or atrial-ventricular interactions exist. Determine whether criteria are met for abnormal voltage, ventricular hypertrophy, or intraventricular conduction disturbances. Continue by noting abnormal ST- and/or T-wave changes as well as any Q-wave MI that may be apparent. Conclude by citing any suggested clinical abnormality compatible with each tracing.

104. An elderly man was seen in a nursing home with a complaint of occasional dizziness

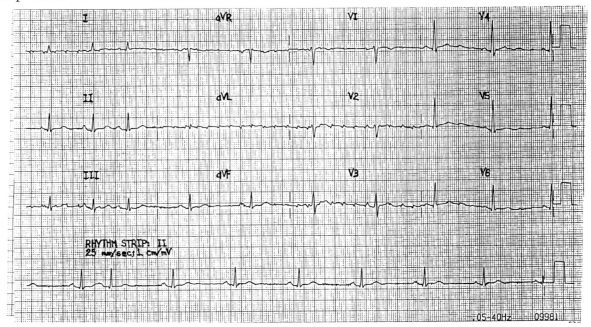

105. A 71-year-old man with symptoms of dizziness and shortness of breath in the emergency department

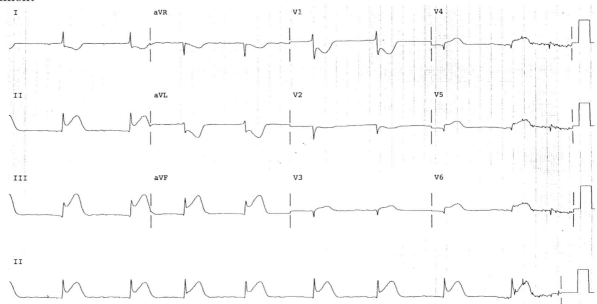

106. A 54-year-old woman with weight loss

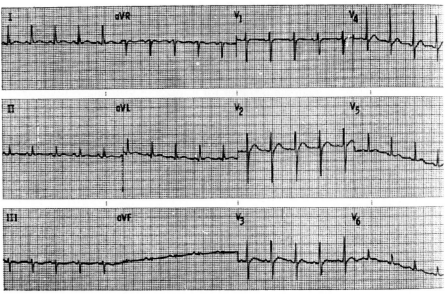

From Chung, E.K.: Electrocardiography: Practical Applications with Vectorial Principles. 3rd ed. Boston, Appleton-Century-Crofts, 1985, p. 532.

107. An exercise tolerance test tracing from a 46-
     year-old man

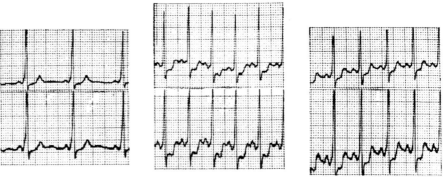

Left, Preexercise; *center,* during exercise; *right,* postexercise. From Chung, E.K. Electrocardiography: Practical Applications with Vectorial Principles. 3rd ed. Boston, Appleton-Century-Crofts, 1985, p. 456.

108. A 23-year-old woman with a history of a heart
murmur seen in cardiology clinic

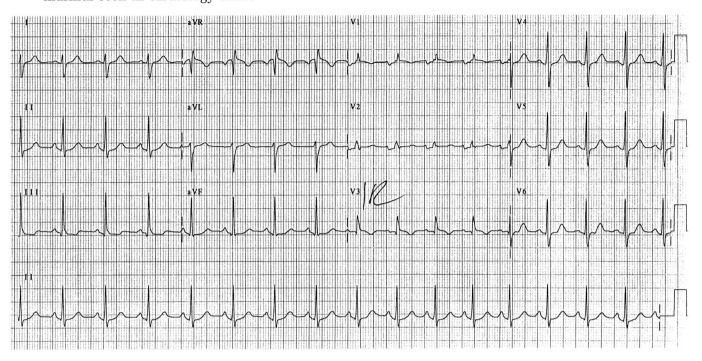

109. A 29-year-old man with a history of a heart
transplant seen in clinic

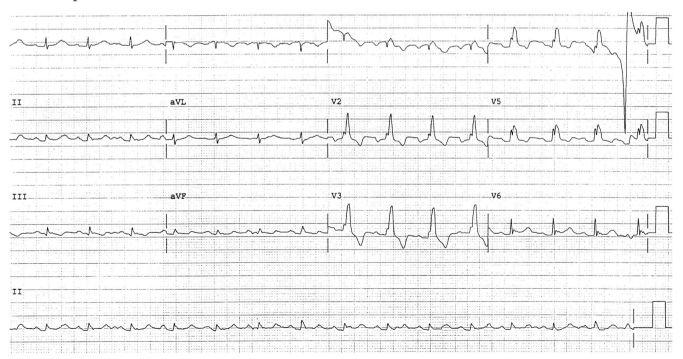

110. An 18-year-old woman in the emergency room
     with chest pain

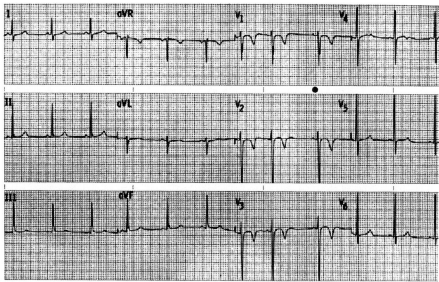

From Chung, E.K.: Electrocardiography: Practical Applications with Vectorial Principles. 3rd ed. Boston, Appleton-Century-Crofts, 1985, p. 692.

111. A 20-year-old man with a heart murmur

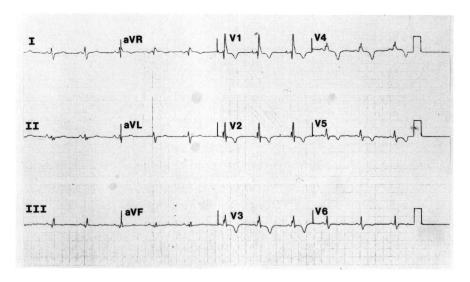

112. A 35-year-old woman with shortness of breath
      seen in cardiology clinic

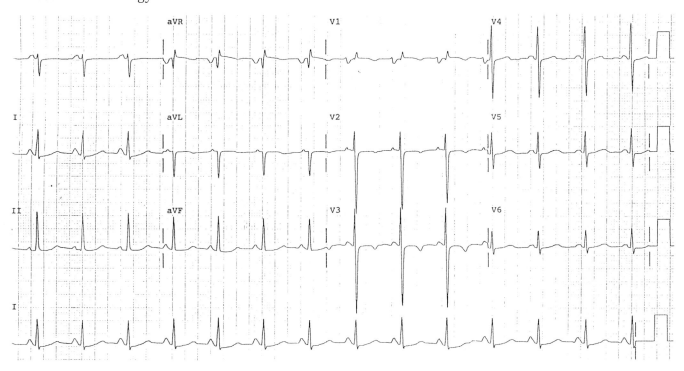

113. An 86-year-old woman with an extensive his-
      tory of cigarette smoking presents to the emer-
      gency department with shortness of breath

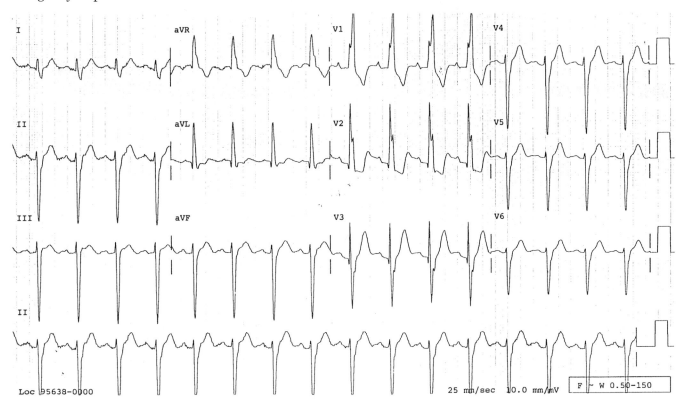

114. An 18-year-old woman with a history of
     syncope

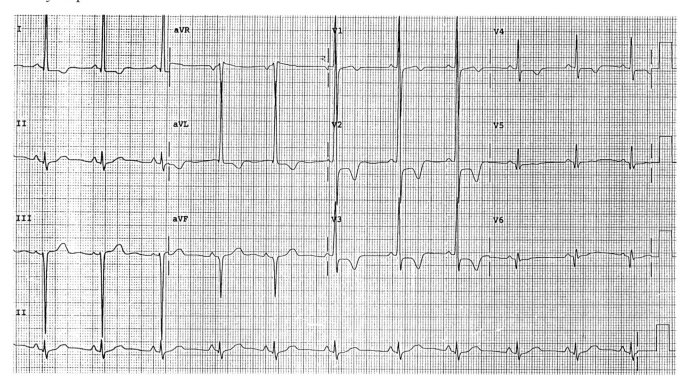

115. An 18-year-old woman with dyspnea and
     cyanosis

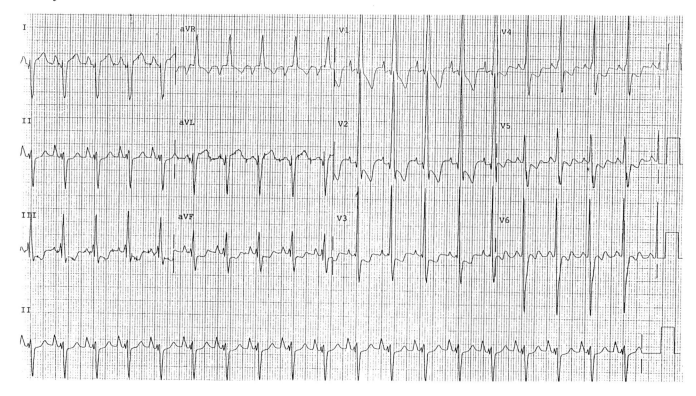

116. An 85-year-old woman during her routine
    clinic appointment

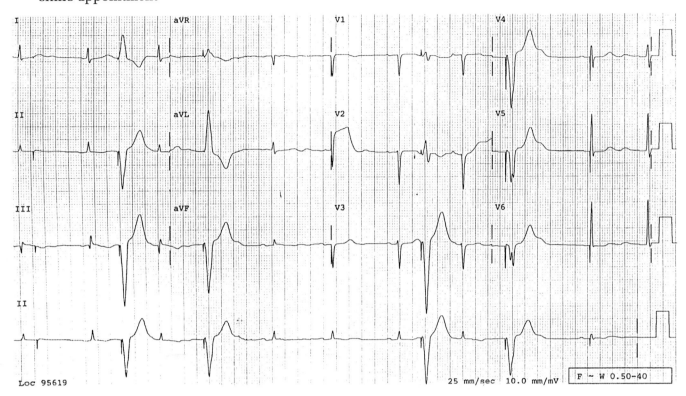

117. A 15-year-old boy with episodes of palpita-
    tions

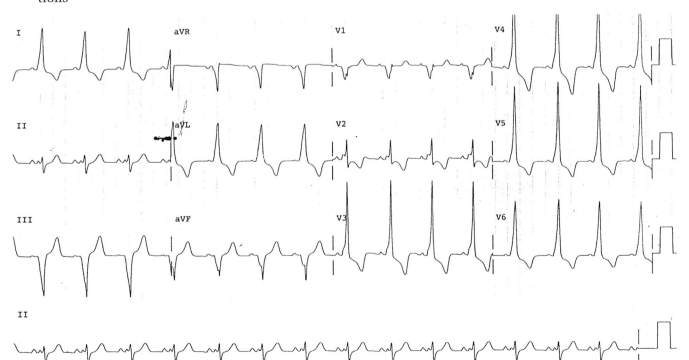

118. A 44-year-old asymptomatic woman having a
     routine evaluation

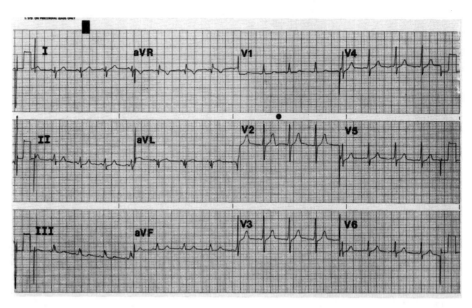

119. A 63-year-old man with symptoms of palpi-
     tations and chest pressure

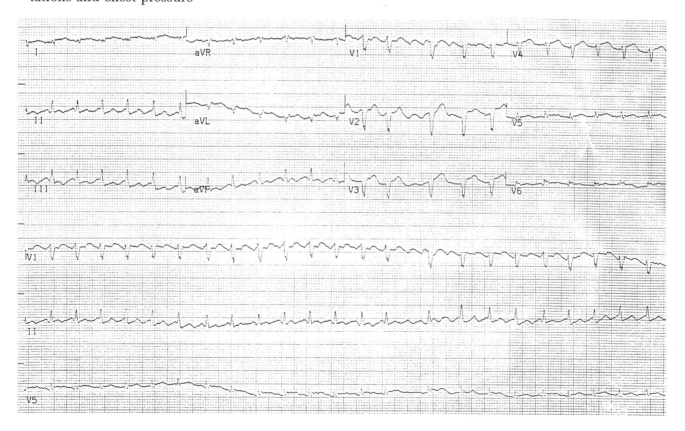

120. A 58-year-old man with a history of a prior
MI presents to the emergency department
with symptoms of palpitations

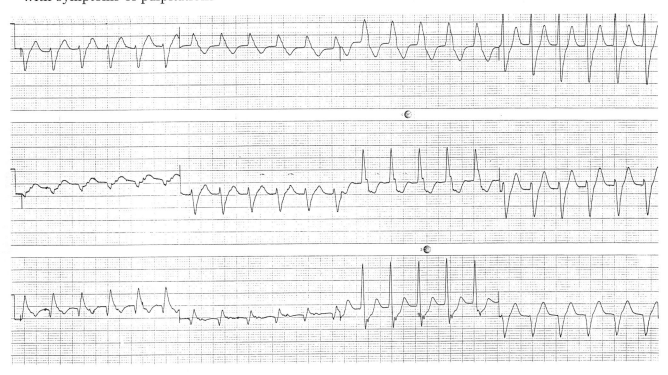

121. A 21-year-old woman with symptoms of palpitations and presyncope

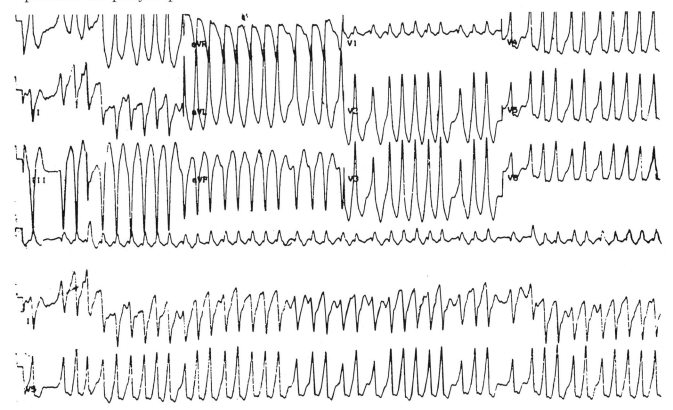

122. A 72-year-old man seen in cardiology clinic
with chronic dyspnea on exertion

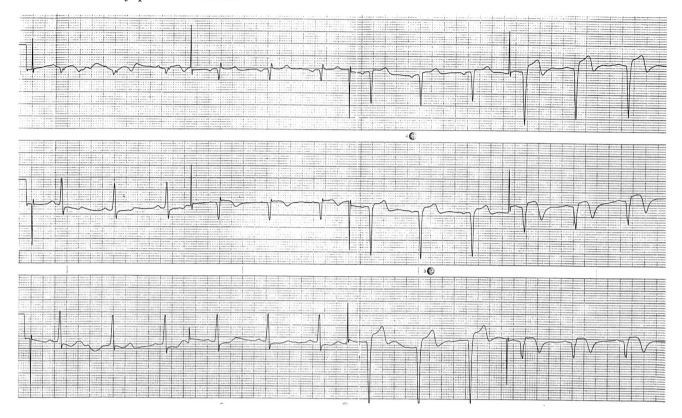

123. A young man in the cardiology clinic

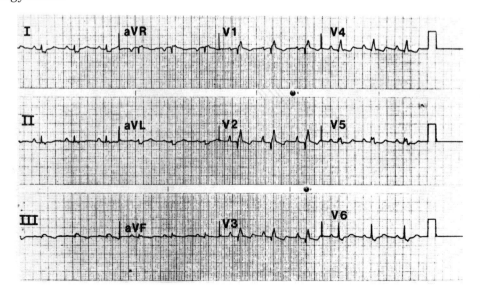

124. A 56-year-old man in the CCU

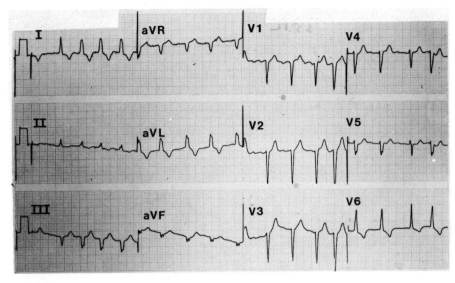

125. A 42-year-old man in the emergency room
with palpitations

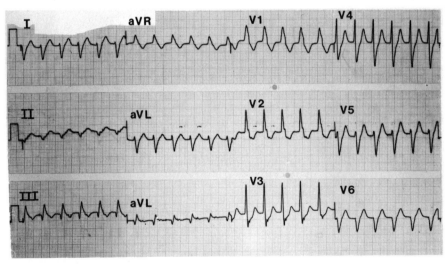

126. A 72-year-old man in the CCU

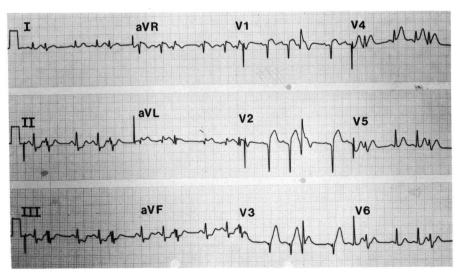

127. An asymptomatic 52-year-old man

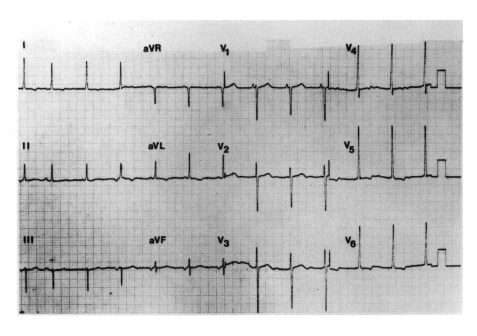

128. A 75-year-old man with symptoms of exertional dizziness

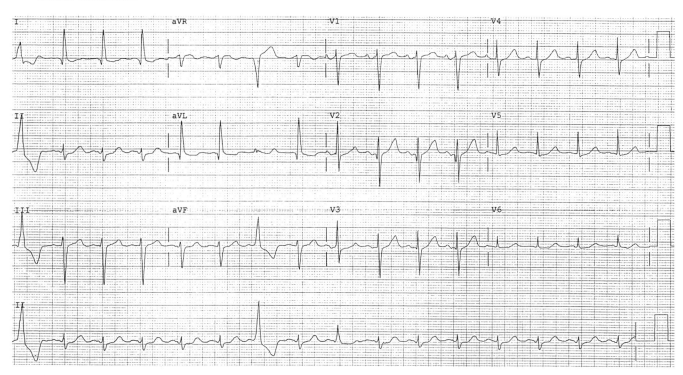

129. A 43-year-old woman presents to the emergency department with symptoms of palpitations

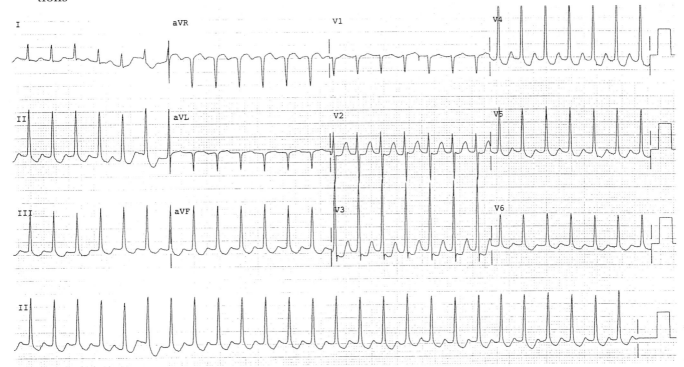

Part I
Examination of the Patient

CHAPTERS 1 THROUGH 11

ANSWERS

1-D   *(Braunwald, p. 11)*

In infants or children with cardiac murmurs, knowing the age at which a murmur was first appreciated may be helpful diagnostically. Murmurs of aortic or pulmonic stenosis are usually audible within the first 2 days of life, whereas the murmur of a ventricular septal defect (VSD) usually appears a few days or weeks later. Frequent episodes of pneumonia early in infancy should suggest the presence of a sizable left-to-right shunt. Excessive diaphoresis may occur in LV failure in this age group, most often due to the presence of a VSD. Squatting, which appears to improve O_2 saturation by increasing systemic vascular resistance, is most frequently noted in tetralogy of Fallot or tricuspid atresia, especially after exertion.[1]

Maternal illness may lead to cardiac disease in the developing fetus. Rubella in the first trimester is associated with patent ductus arteriosus, atrial and ventricular septal defect, tetralogy of Fallot, and supravalvular aortic stenosis, whereas a maternal viral illness in the last trimester may be responsible for neonatal myocarditis.

REFERENCE

1. Guntheroth, W.G., et al.: Physiologic studies of paroxysmal hyperpnea in cyanotic congenital heart disease. Circulation *31*:70, 1965.

2-A   *(Braunwald, pp. 43–45;*
Figs. 2–45 through 2–47)

Continuous murmurs begin in systole and continue without interruption through the second heart sound. However, they need not extend completely through diastole. In contrast, a holosystolic murmur that is followed by a holodiastolic murmur but does not encompass the second heart sound represents two distinct murmurs, not a continuous murmur. The classic example of a continuous murmur is that generated by a patent ductus arteriosus. The murmur peaks with the second heart sound and may be absent in late diastole.[1] Connections between the arterial and venous systems may be congenital or acquired. Such connections may lead to continuous murmurs that vary a great deal in their configuration and location. Coronary arterial fistulas into the pulmonary trunk, right atrium, or right ventricle may generate a continuous murmur. Rupture of a congenital aortic sinus aneurysm into the right heart also results in such a murmur, but there is no peak around the second heart sound in this instance; rather, the murmur of a ruptured congenital aortic sinus aneurysm tends to be louder in either systole or diastole and may even give a to-and-fro impression.

The "mammary souffle" that is heard in pregnancy and the early postpartum period is an arterial murmur that is usually louder in systole and heard best over one of the breasts. This murmur may, on occasion, be continuous and may be augmented with light pressure on the stethoscope, which brings out the continuous features. Continuous murmurs are also found in tetralogy of Fallot with pulmonary atresia and in other instances of congenital cyanotic heart disease in which large systemic to pulmonary arterial collaterals are present. Continuous venous murmurs (see Braunwald, Figs. 2–45 through 2–47, pp. 44–45) are best represented by the cervical venous hum, which is found in most normal healthy children and is also frequently heard in young adults, especially during pregnancy. The cervical venous sound is continuous, and typically louder in diastole, although the mechanism of this auscultatory finding remains obscure.

REFERENCE

1. Perloff, J.K.: The Clinical Recognition of Congenital Heart Disease. Philadelphia, W.B. Saunders Co., 1987.

Each answer in this Review and Assessment for *Heart Disease* contains page references to the 5th edition of the textbook.

3-B *(Braunwald, pp. 47–49)*

Specific physical maneuvers may be of great help in the differential diagnosis of cardiac auscultatory findings at the bedside. The left lateral decubitus position may be quite helpful in identifying the *left* ventricular impulse and may allow soft systolic and diastolic sounds to be heard more easily. Hyperextension of the shoulders often decreases the intensity of supraclavicular systolic murmurs that arise in a benign manner from the brachiocephalic arteries, presumably due to anatomical positional changes.

The classic Valsalva maneuver consists of four distinct phases. Phase I, the transient increase in systemic blood pressure, cannot be identified at the bedside easily. Phase II is accompanied by a small decrease in blood pressure and pulse pressure, with a concomitant reflex tachycardia. Phase III begins with the cessation of the straining maneuver and is associated with an abrupt transient decrease in blood pressure. This phase is also generally not perceived at the bedside but is followed promptly by phase IV, which is easily identified and characterized by the obvious reflex bradycardia and mild increase in systemic arterial pressure that precedes a return to the rest state. During the decreased stroke volume that occurs in phase II, the murmurs of pulmonic or aortic stenosis, and mitral or tricuspid regurgitation become softer. The murmur of hypertropic cardiomyopathy will become louder and the click and systolic murmur of mitral valve prolapse will occur earlier in systole.

Muller's maneuver is the forcible inspiration of air against a nose, mouth, and glottis that are firmly closed. Although the maneuver is generally not of great help in bedside diagnosis, it may occasionally augment tricuspid valve murmurs.[1] Isometric exercise through sustained handgrip is a useful bedside maneuver. It leads to an increase in systemic blood pressure and afterload, resulting in an increase in left ventricular systolic and diastolic pressure as well as heart rate. Murmurs of aortic and mitral regurgitation may be augmented, the click of mitral valve prolapse may be moved later into systole, and the late systolic murmur of this condition may be increased in intensity and shortened in duration by the handgrip maneuver. In addition, the murmur of hypertrophic cardiomyopathy may be decreased by handgrip. As a general principle, any newly encountered systolic murmur should be examined by at least two positions, and with the aid of several physical maneuvers.

REFERENCE

1. Rothman, A., and Goldberger, A.L.: Aids to cardiac auscultation. Ann. Intern. Med. *99*:346, 1983.

4-E *(Braunwald, p. 23)*

Pulsus paradoxus is an exaggeration of the normal tendency for arterial pulse strength to fall with inspiration, resulting from a reduced LV stroke volume and the transmission of negative intrathoracic pressure to the aorta. A fall of more than 8 to 10 mm Hg with inspiration is considered abnormal and can be observed in a variety of conditions. Pulsus paradoxus is characteristic of patients with cardiac tamponade, is seen in approximately half of patients with chronic constrictive pericarditis, and is noted as well in patients with wide intrapleural pressure swings (e.g., bronchial asthma and emphysema), pulmonary embolism, pregnancy, extreme obesity, and hypovolemic shock. Notably, aortic regurgitation tends to prevent the development of pulsus paradoxus even in the presence of tamponade. In HCM an inspiratory *rise* in arterial pressure may occur, leading to *reversed* pulsus paradoxus.[1] Interestingly, pulsus paradoxus may also be present occasionally in patients with right ventricular infarction, perhaps due to a combination of right ventricular dysfunction and the restricting effects of the pericardium, in a manner analogous to that occurring in constrictive pericardial disease.

REFERENCE

1. Massumi, R.A., et al.: Reversed pulsus paradoxus. N. Engl. J. Med. *289*:1272, 1973.

5-B *(Braunwald, pp. 121–122)*

Left anterior fascicular block leads to a distinct pattern of ventricular activation that is easily recognized on the surface electrocardiogram. Because of the block in the anterior division of the left fascicle, initial septal activation begins inferiorly and is then followed subsequently by an anterior vector of depolarization, right-sided activation, activation of the inferior and apical areas, and finally, activation of the anterolateral and posterobasal left ventricular wall. Lead I therefore records a large dominant R wave that may be preceded by a small initial Q wave (qR pattern). The Q wave represents initial septal activation and is inscribed when the inferiorly directed initial vector is directed slightly toward the right. The QRS axis in left anterior fascicular block is, by definition, between −45 degrees and −90 degrees, with a QRS duration which is less than 0.12 sec.[1] The QRS forces are displaced superiorly, resulting in small r waves in the anterior precordial leads.[2] The small anterior r waves may appear as delayed transition or poor r wave progression, and may be mistaken for an anteroseptal MI. Prominent S waves may be seen in the lateral precordial leads consistent with the orientation of the net left ventricular vector in a superior direction. While left anterior fascicular block is usually an acquired abnormality due to underlying organic heart disease, the underlying disorder is often subclinical.

REFERENCES

1. Willems, J.L., Robles de Medina, E., Bernard, R., et al.: WHO task force on criteria for intraventricular conduction dis-

turbances and preexcitation. J. Am. Coll. Cardiol. *5*:1261, 1985.
2. Chou, Te-Chuan, and Knilans, T.K.: Electrocardiography in Clinical Practice, Adult and Pediatric. 4th ed. Philadelphia, W.B. Saunders Co., 1996, p. 104.

6-C   *(Braunwald, pp. 153, 163–164)*

In normal subjects, diastolic blood pressure does not change significantly during exercise. A large change in diastolic blood pressure is distinctly uncommon and has not been shown to correlate specifically with underlying coronary artery disease. The normal systolic blood pressure response during exercise is a progressive increase to a peak value between 160 and 220 mm Hg. The higher end of this range is more commonly observed in older patients; in general, black patients tend to have a higher systolic blood pressure response to exercise than do white patients.[1] A failure to increase systolic blood pressure to at least 120 mm Hg, or a decrease in systolic blood pressure below resting values, is considered distinctly abnormal. It may occur due to inadequate elevations of cardiac output because of left ventricular dysfunction or a marked reduction in systemic vascular resistance.[2] Exertional hypotension occurs in between 3 and 9 per cent of patients and is suggestive of underlying multivessel or left main coronary disease. Several other causes of a decrease in systolic blood pressure or a failure to increase systolic blood pressure with exercise have been noted. These include cardiomyopathy, vasovagal episodes, ventricular outflow obstruction, antihypertensive agents, hypovolemia, cardiac arrhythmias, or prolonged and vigorous exercise.[3] Subjects who demonstrate a fall in blood pressure in the *post*exercise period are less likely to have severe underlying coronary artery disease: about 3 per cent of normal subjects <55 years old have such a response.[4]

REFERENCES

1. Ekelund, L.G., Suchindran, C.M., Karon, J.M., et al: Black-white differences in exercise blood pressure. Circulation *31*:1568, 1990.
2. Fisman, E.Z., Pines, A., Ben-Ari, E., et al.: Left ventricular exercise echocardiographic abnormalities in apparently healthy men with exertional hypotension. Am. J. Cardiol. *63*:81, 1989.
3. Froelicher, V.F.: Exercise and the Heart. Clinical Concepts. 2nd ed. Chicago, Year Book Medical Publishers, Inc., 1987.
4. Fleg, J.L., and Lakatta, E.G.: Prevalence and significance of postexercise hypotension in apparently healthy subjects. Am. J. Cardiol. *57*:1380, 1986.

7-D   *(Braunwald, pp. 274, 286–287, 290 and 294–295; Table 9–1)*

[99m]Tc-sestamibi is a member of the isonitrile family, which has a similar initial distribution to that of ^{201}Tl, entering the myocardium in a manner proportional to blood flow. However, myocardial distribution of ^{99m}Tc-sestamibi remains relatively fixed following myocardial uptake, without significant redistribution, and thus the distribution of myocardial blood flow is "frozen" at the time of injection for a number of hours. This property confers unique clinical applications to the agent. For example, ^{201}Tl is not a practical radiopharmaceutical for imaging myocardial perfusion in the setting of thrombolytic therapy because of the relatively rapid redistribution of this agent that occurs following injection. However, ^{99m}Tc-sestamibi can be injected before the initiation of thrombolytic therapy, and subsequent imaging to assess myocardial perfusion may be performed several hours later. Thus, this agent may be used to demonstrate perfusion of myocardium after successful thrombolysis.[1,2] Because of the relatively high photon flux that is obtained with ^{99m}Tc-sestamibi, images with this agent are consistently better than those obtained with [201]Tl. Interpretation of these images is consistently easier and they are more reproducible. In addition, because of its unique uptake and redistribution kinetics, ^{99m}Tc-sestamibi may be used for the simultaneous assessment of left ventricular function and perfusion, which is not possible with [201]Tl. Because the timing of imaging after injection is not crucial, ^{99m}Tc-sestamibi is particularly suited for use in acutely ill patients and also lends flexibility to the scheduling of patients who are clinically stable. [201]Tl remains the agent of choice for dynamic assessment of myocardial viability, allowing imaging of the myocardium at rest and following redistribution with exercise in a manner that is not possible with ^{99m}Tc-sestamibi.

REFERENCES

1. Wackers, F.J.T., Gibbons, R.J., Verani, M.S., et al: Serial quantitative planar technetium-99m-isonitrile imaging in acute myocardial infarction. Efficacy for noninvasive assessment of thrombolytic therapy. J. Am. Coll. Cardiol. *14*: 861, 1989.
2. Gibbons, R.J., Verani, M.S., Behrenback, T., et al.: Possibility of tomographic 99m-Tc-hexakis-2-methoxy-2-methylpropyl-isonitrile imaging for the assessment of myocardial area at risk and the effect of treatment in acute and myocardial infarction. Circulation *80*:1277, 1989.

8-C   *(Braunwald, pp.164–165)*

As stated, an abnormal exercise ECG is found in between 5 and 12 per cent of middle-aged asymptomatic men.[1] While the risk of developing a cardiac event over the next 5 years is ninefold greater in these subjects, only one quarter of these men will suffer a cardiac event, and in many cases, this proves to be the development of chronic stable angina. In the Lipid Research Clinics (LRC) prevention trial, 3 per cent of the 3806 middle-aged asymptomatic men who had an elevated total cholesterol level had a strongly positive test, and this group demonstrated a 2 per cent per year event rate over the subsequent 4 years.[2] However, there was no association between a positive exercise test and nonfatal myocardial infarction in this study. In the Seattle Heart Watch Study (SHW), no increase in cardiac events was noted in asymptomatic men who had an abnormal ST-segment response unless concomitant cardiovascular risk factors were present.[3] In another study of an asymptomatic population, Fleg and colleagues noted that the combination of thallium scintigraphy and an abnormal exercise ECG predicted a cardiac event in approximately half of the subjects over the subsequent 4 years.[4] While the lead set studied and the criteria for an abnormal ECG response differs among the studies noted here, a general relationship between the number of underlying risk factors, the degree of abnormality on the exercise ECG, and subsequent cardiac events is demonstrable in all.

REFERENCES

1. Rautaharju, P.M., Prineas, R.J., Eifler, W.J., et al.: Prognostic value of exercise electrocardiogram in men at high risk of future coronary heart disease. Multiple Risk Factor Intervention Trial experience. J. Am. Coll. Cardiol. 8:1, 1986.
2. Ekelund, L.G., Suchindran, C.M., McMahon, R.P., et al.: Coronary heart disease morbidity and mortality in hypercholesterolemic men predicted from an exercise test. The Lipid Research Clinics Coronary Primary Prevention Trial. J. Am. Coll. Cardiol. 14:556, 1989.
3. Bruce, R.A., and Fisher, L.D.: Exercise-enhanced assessment of risk factors for coronary heart disease in healthy men. J. Electrocardiol. (Suppl. October):62, 1987.
4. Fleg, J.L., Gerstenblith, G., Zonderman, A.B., et al.: Prevalence and prognostic significance of exercise-induced silent myocardial ischemia detected by thallium scintigraphy and electrocardiography in asymptomatic volunteers. Circulation 81:428, 1990.

9-A *(Braunwald, pp. 168–169; Fig. 5–17)*

Most patients with LBBB demonstrate exercise-induced ST-segment depression, and in patients with RBBB such depression in right precordial leads is also common. These changes are *not* useful as diagnostic or prognostic markers. Approximately 0.1 per cent of subjects will develop exercise-induced RBBB, 0.3 per cent will develop transient left fascicular block, and 0.4 per cent will develop full LBBB.[1] However, in patients with ischemic ST-segment depression before LBBB appears or after it resolves in recovery, the ST-segment changes are of similar significance in any exercise test (see Braunwald, Fig. 5–18, p. 169). Exercise-induced ST-segment depression in lateral precordial leads in a patient with RBBB is predictive of coronary artery disease, but similar changes in right precordial leads may result from the RBBB and therefore are not diagnostic.

REFERENCE

1. Williams, M.A., Esterbrooks, D.J., Nair, C.K., et al.: Clinical significance of exercise-induced left bundle branch block. Am. J. Cardiol. 61:346, 1988.

10-D *(Braunwald, pp. 191–192; Fig. 6–11)*

The two methods routinely used to measure cardiac output at cardiac catheterization are the Fick O_2 method and the indicator dilution technique.[1] The Fick principle, as applied to measurement of systemic blood flow, states that the total uptake of O_2 (O_2 consumption) divided by the difference in O_2 content between arterial and mixed venous blood gives a measure of pulmonary blood flow which, in the absence of intracardiac shunting, is equal to systemic blood flow. This is expressed mathematically as:

Cardiac index (ml/min/m^2)

$$= \frac{O_2 \text{ consumption (ml/min/m}^2)}{\text{arterio-mixed venous } O_2 \text{ difference}}$$

The normal range for cardiac index is 2.6 to 4.2 L/min/m^2. (The cardiac output is divided by body surface area to correct for differences in O_2 consumption rates caused by variations in body size.) Of the available measures of cardiac output, the Fick method is most accurate in patients with a low cardiac output and corresponding wide arteriovenous O_2 difference. A difficulty of the Fick method is the necessity of obtaining O_2 consumption measurements under steady-state conditions. Because the method assumes a mean flow over a given period of time, changes in flow during the O_2 consumption recording period will reduce the accuracy of the measurement.

Angiographic cardiac output can be calculated as described in statement C; the calculation is limited by the accuracy with which the systolic and diastolic volumes can be extrapolated from the angiographic data.

REFERENCE

1. Winniford, M.D., Lambert, C.R.: Blood measurement. In Pepine, C.J., Hill, J.A., Lambert, C.R. (eds): Diagnostic and Therapeutic Cardiac Catheterization. 2nd ed. Baltimore, Williams & Wilkins, 1994, pp. 321–334.

11-B *(Braunwald, p. 132; Fig. 4–35)*

Correlation of autopsy findings with ECG evidence of myocardial infarction (MI) suggests that transmural MI may occur in the absence of Q waves and, conversely, nontransmural lesions may generate a Q wave on the electrocardiogram.[1] In fact, the presence of a Q wave in nontransmural MI may be quite common. Conventionally, the location of an infarct by ECG criteria is based upon typical ECG patterns or distributions of T waves. An anterior MI is described when Q waves are present in leads V_3 and V_4; a septal MI when a Q wave appears in leads V_1 and V_2; an anteroseptal MI when Q waves exist from V_1 through V_4; lateral when Q waves are present in leads I, aV_1, and V_6; anterolateral when present in these leads and V_3 through V_5 as well; and an extensive anterior MI is considered present when Q waves are found in leads I, aV_1, and across the precordium. In addition, a high lateral MI is described by Q waves in leads I and aV_1 alone; an inferior MI by Q waves in leads II, III, and aV_f; and an anteroinferior or apical infarct when present in leads II, III, and aV_f and in one or more of leads V_1 through V_4 (see Braunwald, Fig. 4–35, p. 131).

In the presence of an inferior MI, a posterior infarction is recognized by prominent R waves in leads V_1 and/or V_2. Infarction of the right ventricle may be suspected in patients with evolving inferior MI and abnormalities of right-sided precordial leads, especially V_4R. ST-segment elevation ≥ 1 mm in this lead has a high sensitivity and specificity for right ventricular infarction.[2] The appearance of RBBB may be noted in patients with ischemia of the right ventricle in the presence of ST-segment elevation. In contrast, it is quite difficult to make a diagnosis of infarction of the posterior portion of the left ventricular wall because this region is explored poorly by the surface electrocardiogram.

REFERENCES

1. Andre-Fouet, X., Pillot, M., Leizorovicz, A., et al.: "Non-Q-wave," alias "nontransmural" myocardial infarction. A specific entity. Am. Heart. J. *117*:892, 1989.
2. Andersen, H.R., Falk, E., and Nielsen, D.: Right ventricular infarction. J. Electrocardiol. *22*:181, 1989.

12-B   *(Braunwald, pp. 68–70; Figs. 3–39 through 3–41*

One of the most clinically important applications of Doppler technology is the estimation of pressure gradients across stenotic orifices or septal defects in the cardiovascular system. The Bernoulli equation relates the pressure difference across a narrowed area to the convective acceleration, flow acceleration, and viscous friction (see Braunwald, Fig. 3–40, p. 69). By modifying the Bernoulli equation, a more clinically useful simplified formula is derived. The simplified Bernoulli equation states that the pressure difference across a flow-limiting orifice = $4V^2$, where V is the peak velocity distal to the obstruction.

In Question 12, we are given the information that the patient's systolic blood pressure is 144, which, in the absence of left ventricular outflow obstruction, is also the left ventricular systolic pressure. If the VSD flow is 5.1 m/sec, then using the modified Bernoulli equation, we calculate the pressure gradient across the VSD to be 104 mm Hg. The RV systolic pressure is then 144–104, or 40 mm Hg.

If the patient's blood pressure was not given, it would still be possible to estimate the LV systolic pressure using the MR velocity. If the MR velocity is 5.8 m/sec, then we know, using the modified Bernoulli equation, that the pressure difference across the mitral valve in systole is 135 mm Hg. An estimate of the left atrial pressure is then made using 2-D and Doppler parameters, and this value is added to the transmitral systolic gradient to derive an estimate of LV systolic pressure. Thus, if the estimated left atrial pressure is 10 mm Hg, then the estimated LV systolic pressure will be 145 mm Hg.

The same method may be used to estimate RV systolic pressures when TR velocity is known.

REFERENCE

Feigenbaum, H.: Echocardiography. 5th ed. Malvern, PA, Lea & Febiger, 1994, pp. 195–198.

13-E   *(Braunwald, pp. 119–121; Fig. 4–17)*

When the left bundle branch is interrupted, transseptal activation from left to right no longer occurs through the bundle branch itself and is instead transmyocardial, resulting in loss of the septal Q wave. In addition, ventricular activation proceeds from right to left, and the lateral wall and basal portions of the left ventricle are the last ventricular tissue to be activated. LBBB has been shown to be strongly associated with an increase in cardiovascular mortality.[1] Complete LBBB leads to a QRS complex between 0.12 and 0.18 sec in duration, a frontal axis that is either normal or leftward, and ST-segment and T-wave vectors opposite in direction to the QRS vector. In addition, the prolonged QRS often has a distinct pattern, which may include an upright notched or slurred R wave due to the slow right-to-left myocardial activation, a pattern seen most prominently in leads I and V_6. If the T-wave vector becomes concordant with that of the QRS complex, it suggests an underlying myocardial abnormality such as ischemia, although this is not a very specific sign. Incomplete LBBB also demonstrates a loss of the septal Q wave; nevertheless, the left bundle itself ultimately provides some portion of the septal and left ventricular wall activation, and the net duration of the QRS complex is therefore between 0.10 and 0.12 sec. In incomplete LBBB, large voltages of the QRS complexes are often present.

REFERENCE

1. Freedman, R.A., Alderman, E.L., Sheffield, L.T., et al.: Bundle branch block in patients with chronic coronary artery disease: Angiographic correlates and prognostic significance. J. Am. Coll. Cardiol. *10*:673, 1987.

14-D   *(Braunwald, pp. 7–8)*

Cyanosis is a bluish discoloration of the skin and mucous membranes which results from either an increased amount of reduced hemoglobin or from abnormal hemoglobin perfusing these areas. Two forms of cyanosis are recognized: (1) peripheral cyanosis, which most commonly is due to cutaneous vasoconstriction (e.g., cold air or water exposure or low cardiac output), and (2) central cyanosis, characterized by a decreased arterial oxygen saturation (in Caucasians, arterial saturation is usually ≤ 85 per cent), caused by right-to-left shunting or abnormal pulmonary function. It is the *absolute* quantity of reduced hemoglobin in the blood that produces the characteristic blue discoloration. Therefore, patients with polycythemia become cyanotic at higher levels of arterial oxygen saturation, and those with severe anemia may resist cyanosis despite marked arterial desaturation.[1] Localized peripheral cyanosis involving one extremity may be due to arterial or venous occlusion.

REFERENCE

1. Lisler, G., and Talner, N.S.: Oxygen transport in congenital heart disease. In Engle, M.A. (ed.): Pediatric Cardiovascular Disease. Philadelphia, F. A. Davis, 1981.

15-B *(Braunwald, pp. 71, 1016–1017, 1385)*

Balloon valvuloplasty has become an excellent treatment option for patients with severe mitral stenosis. However, not all patients are suitable candidates for this procedure. Echocardiography is used in evaluating both the severity of mitral stenosis and the suitability for balloon mitral valvuloplasty.

There are four major criteria correlated with successful valvuloplasty that are therefore used to judge the suitability of the mitral valve for balloon valvuloplasty. Mobility of the mitral valve is one criteria that can be evaluated by both M-mode and 2-D echo. Mobility can be determined by measuring the movement of the belly of the anterior mitral valve leaflet.[2] Another criterion that can be evaluated by both M-mode and 2-D echo is the degree of mitral valve calcification. The two final predictors of successful mitral valvuloplasty include minimal valvular thickening and involvement of the sub-valvular apparatus.

Although determination of left atrial size is one important correlate of mitral stenosis severity, it is not helpful in estimating the suitability of the valve for balloon valvuloplasty. It is, however, important to evaluate the left atrium for the presence of thrombus before proceeding to balloon valvuloplasty, which may dislodge any thrombi present. Many clinicians routinely employ transesophageal echocardiography to determine whether there is left atrial thrombus before balloon mitral valvuloplasty. Transesophageal echocardiography is more sensitive than transthoracic echocardiography for detecting small left atrial thrombi as well as thrombus within the left atrial appendage.[3]

REFERENCES

1. Feigenbaum, H.: Echocardiography. 5th ed. Malvern, PA, Lea & Febiger, 1994, pp. 249–251.
2. Reid, C.L., Chandraratna, A.N., Kawanishi, D.T., et al.: Influence of mitral valve morphology on double-balloon, catheter balloon valvuloplasty in patients with mitral stenosis. Circulation 80:515, 1989.
3. Thomas, R.R., Monaghan, M.J., Smyth, D.W., et al.: Comparative value of transthoracic and transesophageal echocardiography before balloon dilatation of the mitral valve. Br. Heart J. 68:493, 1992.

16-E *(Braunwald, p. 142; Fig. 4–52)*

The effect of an increase or a decrease in circulating calcium ions on the duration of phase II of the transmembrane action potential leads to alterations in the ST segment and the Q-T interval. Elevations of circulating calcium lead to shortening of phase II and therefore of the Q-T interval itself. A prominent J wave similar to that seen in hypothermia has also been observed in this setting.[1] Conversely, hypocalcemia leads to prolongation of phase II, with a lengthening of the Q-T interval due to a prolonged ST segment. The interval between the Q wave and the apex of the T wave can be used as the most accurate correlate of this change, and the Q-Tc interval itself rarely exceeds 140 per cent of normal due to hypocalcemia. In patients with chronic renal disease, a combination of hypocalcemia with hyperkalemia may occur and may lead to both ST-segment prolongation and tenting of the T wave (see Braunwald, Fig. 4–52, p. 142). Administration of magnesium may also lead to shortening of the Q-T interval, but electrocardiographic changes due to magnesium are not usually identified because calcium plays the dominant role.

REFERENCE

1. Sridharan, M.R., and Horan, L.G.: Electrocardiographic T wave of hypercalcemia. Am. J. Cardiol. 54:672, 1984.

17-E *(Braunwald, p. 125; Fig. 4–24)*

The Ashman phenomenon is aberrancy caused by changes in the preceding cycle length. Since the duration of the refractory period is a function of the immediate preceding cycle length, the longer the preceding cycle the longer the ensuing refractory period and the more likely that the next impulse will be conducted with delay.[1] Normally the refractory periods of the conduction system components are right bundle branch > left bundle branch = AV node >> His bundle. Therefore, it would be unusual for the bundle of His to be the site of conduction delay.

REFERENCE

1. Gouaaux, J.L., and Ashman, R.: Auricular fibrillation with aberration simulating ventricular paroxysmal tachycardia. Am. Heart J. 34: 366, 1947.

18-B *(Braunwald, pp. 38–40; Fig. 2–33)*

Mitral regurgitation, tricuspid regurgitation, and ventricular septal defects may, with the appropriate pathophysiology, lead to an early systolic murmur. In acute severe mitral regurgitation, the murmur is early in systole in many instances, although it may also be a holosystolic decrescendo murmur[1] (see Braunwald, Fig. 2–33, p. 39). So-called low-pressure tricuspid regurgitation, in which abnormal right ventricular systolic pressure is present, leads to an early systolic murmur as well.[2] This may be seen in the tricuspid regurgitation that accompanies tricuspid endocarditis in intravenous drug abusers. In ventricular septal defect, an early systolic murmur may be generated either by a very small defect, in which the shunt is confined to early systole, or may result when a nonrestrictive ventricular septal defect exists with pulmonary vascular resistance elevations that lead to a decrease in late systolic shunting.[3] Late systolic murmurs are most frequently caused by mitral valve prolapse; the murmur may be preceded by one or more systolic clicks. Decreases in left ventricular volume, such as with prompt standing after squatting or by Valsalva, may cause the late systolic murmur to become longer, although they may also lead to a decrease in intensity. Occasionally, a musical, high-frequency sound ("whoop"), which is thought to arise from the high-frequency vibrations of the mitral leaflets and chordae,[4] accompanies mitral valve prolapse.

REFERENCES

1. Sutton, G.C., and Craige, E.: Clinical signs of acute severe mitral regurgitation. Am. J. Cardiol. 20:141, 1967.
2. Rios, J.C., Massumi, R.A., Breesman, W.T., and Sarin, R.K.: Ausculatory features of acute tricuspid regurgitation. Am. J. Cardiol. 23:4, 1969.
3. Perloff, J.K.: The Clinical Recognition of Congenital Heart Disease. Philadelphia, W.B. Saunders Co., 1987.
4. Osler, W.: On a remarkable heart murmur: Heard at a distance from the chest wall. Med. Times Gax. Lond. 2:432, 1908.

19-E   (Braunwald, pp. 19–20; Fig. 2–5)

The pressure waveforms in the jugular venous tracing reflect events in the cardiac cycle. Important hemodynamic information can be obtained from analyzing these waveforms. The a wave in the jugular venous tracing reflects right atrial systole. The x descent occurs as the right atrial pressure declines following atrial systole. Following the x descent, the v wave represents increasing right atrial pressure from atrial filling during ventricular systole. The y descent then occurs as the tricuspid valve opens and the right atrial pressure declines. Following the y descent and before the ensuing a wave is a period of relatively slow filling or diastasis termed the H wave. The H wave height reflects the stiffness of the right atrium (see Braunwald, Fig. 2–5, p. 18).

During inspiration, the height of the jugular venous pulse normally falls. In conditions such as chronic constrictive pericarditis there may be a paradoxical rise in jugular venous pressure with inspiration. This phenomenon is known as Kussmaul's sign.

Prominence in the a wave may occur in a number of disease states, including tricuspid stenosis, pulmonary hypertension, and right ventricular hypertrophy. In addition, tall a waves may occur in LVH as a result of impedance to right ventricular filling by a thickened ventricular septum. In atrioventricular dissociation, large Cannon a waves are noted in the jugular venous pulse for those beats when the right atrium contracts against a closed tricuspid valve.

Abdominal-jugular reflux is elicited by applying firm pressure in the periumbilical region for 10 to 30 sec. In pathological states, such as heart failure or tricuspid regurgitation, there is a sustained rise in the jugular venous pulse by more than 3 cm H_2O.

20-B   (Braunwald, pp. 185–186)

Most cardiac catheterizations at present are performed using either direct exposure of the artery and vein (e.g., brachial vessels) or by the percutaneous approach (brachial or femoral vessels, including transseptal catheterizations). In selected patients, outpatient catheterization is now being used because it is practical, cost-effective, and safe. In this setting the brachial approach is most often used because the patient may ambulate easily shortly after the procedure. The brachial approach may be used either with direct exposure of the appropriate vessels or percutaneously, utilizing the Seldinger technique and No. 5 French catheters.[1] In patients in whom the aortic valve should not be crossed by a retrograde approach from the aorta, including those with a tilting-disc prosthetic aortic valve,[2] transseptal catheterization may be utilized. This approach may also be used when a severely stenotic aortic valve cannot be crossed, as well as in patients with suspected mitral valve stenosis in whom a confirmed wedge pressure cannot be obtained. Transseptal left heart catheterization is not necessary with bioprostheses or ball-and-cage prosthetic valves in the aortic position, which can be crossed safely in retrograde fashion.

REFERENCES

1. Fergusson, D.J.G., and Karnada, R.O.: Percutaneous entry of the brachial artery for left heart catheterization using an arterial sheath: Further experience. Cathet. Cardiovasc. Diagn. 12:209, 1986.
2. Karsh, D.L., et al.: Retrograde left ventricular catheterization in patients with an aortic valve prosthesis. Am. J. Cardiol. 41:893, 1978.

21-C   (Braunwald, p. 67; Figs. 3–33 and 3–38)

Diastolic Doppler mitral flow patterns are measured with the transducer located at the tips of the mitral leaflets. The mitral diastolic flow profile is composed of two flow velocity peaks; the early or E wave and the A wave. In the normal profile, the E wave is taller than the A wave in a 60:40 relationship. The E wave represents early ventricular filling, whereas the A wave occurs as a result of atrial systole.

In a number of disease states and in normal aging, the E:A relationship may be reversed, with a taller A wave than E wave. This usually occurs in conjunction with prolongation of the isovolumic relaxation time and the deceleration time. This pattern is usually associated with abnormal ventricular relation and occurs in conditions such as left ventricular hypertrophy, myocardial ischemia, cardiomyopathy, and normal aging. In addition to abnormal relaxation, low left atrial pressures may cause the pattern of E:A reversal. In conditions such as pulmonary hypertension or hypovolemia, low left atrial pressure may result in reduced early filling of the left ventricle.

When the left ventricular diastolic pressure is very high, the pattern of mitral flow is the reverse of the abnormal relaxation pattern, with a tall E wave and shorter A wave. This may occur in congestive heart failure, severe mitral regurgitation, or in restrictive filling patterns such as in constrictive or restrictive cardiomyopathy.

REFERENCE

Feigenbaum, H.: Echocardiography. 5th ed. Malvern, PA, Lea & Febiger, 1994, p. 152.

22-C   (Braunwald, pp. 165–167)

A submaximal exercise protocol performed by patients with a recent myocardial infarction is helpful for a variety of reasons. Predischarge testing gives a clear baseline regarding hemodynamic response, functional capacity, the presence or absence of ventricular arrhythmia, and the possibility of residual ischemia. Patients who complete 80 per cent of the age-predicted exercise test maximum without any ECG or blood pressure abnormalities have a low 1-year mortality in the range of 1 to 2 per cent. [1] About one third of postinfarction patients demonstrate an exercise-induced ischemia ST-segment depression, and another 15 per cent of patients have exertional hypotension. However, in the weeks just after an infarction, a drop in blood pressure with exercise is not as specific prognostically as the same finding in patients with chronic ischemic heart disease. In fact, patients retested 6 weeks after the infarction may demonstrate resolution of this hypotensive response. A repeat exercise test 6 weeks following infarction is useful in clearing patients for a return to work in strenuous occupations, as well as for estimating cardiovascular reserve at greater exercise levels. However, the prognostic value of a 6-week postdischarge exercise test is small when clinical variables and a low-level in-hospital test are taken into account. [2] Risk stratification is better accomplished by a full exercise test performed 6 or more months following the acute infarction. [3]

Left ventricular function is an important prognostic determinant of mortality following acute MI in at least one study. Patients with an ejection fraction of <35 per cent by gated radionuclide scans in the month following an acute MI who also demonstrate a diminished exercise capacity have a threefold greater risk of dying than similar patients with a preserved exercise capacity. [4]

REFERENCES

1. Froelicher, V.F., Perdue, S., Pewen, W., and Risch, M.: Application of meta-analysis using an electronic spread sheet to exercise testing in patients after myocardial infarction. Am. J. Med. 83:1045, 1987.
2. Senaratne, M.P., Hsu, L., Rossall, R.E., and Kappagoda, T.: Exercise testing after myocardial infarction: Relative values of the low level predischarge and the postdischarge exercise test. J. Am. Coll. Cardiol. 12:1416, 1988.
3. Stone, P.H., Turi, Z.G., Muller, J.E., et al.: Prognostic significance of the treadmill exercise test performance 6 months after myocardial infarction. J. Am. Coll. Cardiol. 8:1007, 1986.
4. Pilote, L., Silberberg, J., Lisbona, R., and Sniderman, A.: Prognosis in patients with low left ventricular ejection fraction after myocardial infarction. Circulation 80:1636, 1989.

23-C   (Braunwald, pp. 71–73; Fig. 3–14)

In this patient with mitral valve disease, the severity of mitral stenosis can be assessed by calculating the transmitral gradient, and the mitral valve area. The transmitral gradient can be determined by using the modified Bernoulli equation (pressure gradient = $4V^2$). [1] The mitral valve area can be calculated by measuring the time required for the peak diastolic mitral velocity to reach one half of its initial level. This technique, known as the pressure half-time, correlates reasonably well with the mitral valve area in most cases, but may be less accurate in certain situations, such as after percutaneous balloon mitral valvuloplasty. [2,3] The suitability of the mitral valve for percutaneous balloon valvuloplasty may be assessed by 2-D echocardiographic methods, but *not* by Doppler echocardiography. 2-D echocardiographic predictors of successful balloon mitral valvuloplasty include adequate valve mobility, minimal valve thickening and calcification, and lack of involvement of the subvalvular apparatus. [4,5]

The severity of mitral regurgitation is best determined using Doppler color flow mapping. Pulsed Doppler may be used to visualize the density of the regurgitant jet. In this case, the faint jet implies mild mitral regurgitation. All Doppler techniques to quantitate mitral regurgitation have only a limited correlation with the severity of regurgitation. [6] Additional methods include measurement of stroke volume to calculate regurgitant volume and regurgitant fraction and assessment of the hemodynamic consequences of mitral regurgitation, such as left atrial enlargement and reversal of systolic venous flow in the pulmonary veins. The mitral regurgitant jet as visualized by Doppler echocardiography may be used to determine dP/dt, and thus assess left ventricular contractility. [7]

REFERENCES

1. Nishimura, R.A., Rihal, C.S., Tajik, A.J., et al.: Accurate measurement of the transmitral gradient in patient with mitral stenosis: A simultaneous catheterization and Doppler echocardiography study. J. Am. Coll. Cardiol. 24:152, 1994.

2. Loyd, D., Ask, P., and Wranne, B.: Pressure half-time does not always predict mitral valve area correctly. J. Am. Soc. Echocardiogr. *1*:313, 1988.
3. Thomas, J.D., Wilkins, G.T., Choong, C.Y.P., et al.: Inaccuracy of mitral pressure half-time immediately after percutaneous mitral valvotomy. Circulation *78*:980, 1988.
4. Reid, C.L., McKay, C.R., Chandraratna, P.A.N., et al.: Mechanisms of increase in mitral valve area and influence of anatomic features in double-balloon, catheter balloon valvuloplasty in adults with rheumatic mitral stenosis: A Doppler and two-dimensional echocardiographic study. Circulation *76*:628, 1987.
5. Reid, C.L., Otto, C.M., Davis, K.B., et al.: Influence of mitral valve morphology on mitral balloon commissurotomy: Immediate and six-month results from the NHLBI balloon valvuloplasty registry. Am. Heart J. *124*:657, 1992.
6.. McCully, R.B., Enriquez-Sarano, M., Tajik, A.J., et al.: Overestimation of severity of ischemic/function mitral regurgitation by color Doppler jet area. Am. J. Cardiol. *74*:790, 1994.
7. Chen, C., Rodriguez, L., Lethord, J.P., et al.: Continuous wave Doppler echocardiography for non-invasive assessment of left ventricular dP/dt and relaxation time constant from mitral regurgitant spectra in patients. J. Am. Coll. Cardiol. *23*:970, 1994.

24-B   (Braunwald, pp. 68–70)

Calculation of the pressure gradient across a cardiac value is determined by the following equation. Δ Pressure $= 4 \times$ (velocity)^2. In this instance, the pressure gradient is 64 mm Hg (4×4^2). With a right atrial pressure of 4 mm Hg and a pressure gradient of 64 mm Hg, the right ventricular pressure equals 68 mm Hg ($64 + 4 = 68$ mm Hg). Pressure gradients across other cardiac valves can be calculated in a similar manner.

25-A   (Braunwald, pp. 153–155)

During the early phase of exercise, cardiac output is increased by augmenting heart rate and stroke volume. Increases in stroke volume occur via the Frank-Starling mechanism. In the later phase of exercise, stroke volume augmentation becomes maximal and further increases in cardiac output primarily via increases in heart rate. During exercise, elevation in systolic blood pressure, mean arterial pressure, and pulse pressure occur. Diastolic blood pressure remains essentially unchanged, though it may vary by approximately 10 mm Hg. The pulmonary vascular bed can accommodate up to six times the baseline cardiac output without a significant increase in pulmonary artery pressure, pulmonary capillary wedge pressure, or right atrial pressure in healthy subjects.

Anaerobic threshold is the theoretical point during exercise when tissues begin to utilize anaerobic metabolism as an additional energy source.[1,2] Not all tissues in the body reach this point at the same time. When anaerobic metabolism begins, lactic acid builds up in the tissues. The excess lactic acid is buffered by bicarbonate with subsequent increases in ventilation to facilitate CO_2 excretion. The anaerobic threshold is reached at 50 to 60 per cent of maximal aerobic capacity.

The term *MET*, or metabolic equivalent, is used to denote a resting oxygen consumption in a 70-kg, 40-year-old male of 3.5 ml/min/kg. METs can be used to standardize workload for exercise testing. Mild activity, such as casual walking, is considered approximately 3 to 5 METs. Heavy manual labor, or strenuous exercise, will generate as much as 9 to 10 METs.

REFERENCES

1. Weber, K.T., Janicki, J.S., McElroy, P.A., and Reddy, H.K.: Concepts and applications of cardiopulmonary exercise testing. Chest *93*:843, 1988.
2. Cohen-Solal, A., Aupetit, J.F., Gueret, P., et al.: Can anaerobic threshold be used as an end-point for therapeutic trials in heart failure? Lessons from a multicentre randomized placebo-controlled trial. The V French Study Group. Eur. Heart J. *15*:236, 1994.

26-D   (Braunwald, pp. 41–43; Fig. 2–42)

Most mid-diastolic murmurs arise from flow across the mitral or tricuspid valves during the rapid filling phase of diastole. In rheumatic mitral stenosis, the mid-diastolic murmur characteristically occurs following the opening snap and is generated by the gradient between the left atrial pressure and the diastolic left ventricular pressure. Similarly, a mid-diastolic murmur may exist in tricuspid stenosis. The murmur in tricuspid stenosis differs from that in mitral stenosis in two ways. First, an increase in the tricuspid murmur intensity is noted with inspiration, and second, the tricuspid stenosis murmur is usually confined to the lower left sternal border rather than to the apex. Mid-diastolic murmurs may also occur across atrioventricular valves that are not stenotic when the volume and flow velocities present are abnormally increased. This type of mid-diastolic murmur is heard in severe tricuspid or mitral regurgitation, often preceded by a third heart sound. When atrial contraction occurs simultaneously with the rapid diastolic filling phase of the cardiac cycle in complete heart block, a short mid-diastolic flow murmur may result. The murmurs are thought to arise directly from antegrade flow across an antrioventricular valve that is closing rapidly during ventricular filling.[1] This is a mechanism analogous to that thought to be responsible for the Austin-Flint murmur (see Braunwald, Fig. 3–31, p. 64).

A mid-diastolic murmur may also be found in pulmonary regurgitation *in the presence of normal or low pulmonary arterial pressures*. Under these circumstances, the regurgitation accelerates slightly as right ventricular pressure dips below the diastolic pressure present in the pulmonary trunk, leading to a mid-diastolic occurrence of the sound (see Braunwald, Fig. 3–32, p. 64). Pulmonary regurgitation associated with pulmonary hypertension (Graham Steell murmur) is heard as an *early* diastolic murmur because a pressure gradient between the pulmonary artery and the right ventricle is established early in diastole. However, in pulmonic regurgitation in the absence of pulmonary hypertension, the pulmonary artery pressure is low and regurgitant flow is minimal until the right ventricular diastolic pressure falls below the pulmonary artery diastolic pressure and flow can accelerate across the incompetent pulmonic valve causing a mid-diastolic murmur (see Braunwald, Fig. 2–42B, p. 43).

27-A *(Braunwald, pp. 72–73; Figs. 3–49 and 3–50)*

Two-dimensional echocardiography is an extremely useful procedure for the detection of mitral regurgitation, the assessment of the severity of mitral regurgitation, and the evaluation of mitral valve morphology. Doppler echocardiography is the technique that is most useful in detecting MR. In assessing the severity of MR, both Doppler and 2-D echocardiography are useful. Mitral valve morphology is accurately determined using 2-D and M-mode techniques.

Color flow Doppler readily identifies the mitral regurgitant jet within the left atrium (LA). The direction and size of the jet are easily determined. Although rough estimates of the degree of mitral regurgitation can be made by color flow Doppler, there are many pitfalls to this method. Alterations in instrument settings and variability between machines can affect the nature of the detected regurgitant jet. Because the jet is not symmetrical in all planes, numerous views are necessary. The jet also will vary with hemodynamic factors such as afterload (in fact, varying loading conditions may be employed to help assess the severity of the MR). Whereas the full profile of centrally directed MR jets may be appreciated, asymmetrical or LA wall-directed jets are more difficult to evaluate due to distortion of the jet by the atrial wall. Because of these multiple limitations of color Doppler MR assessment, accurate quantitative measurements are difficult to make with this method.

Pulse Doppler also can provide information about the hemodynamic effects of MR. For example, examination of the mitral inflow to the left ventricle may reveal a prominent E wave and small A wave in MR. In cases of severe MR, the pulmonary venous flow pattern actually may show reversal of the systolic venous flow and an increase in early diastolic flow.

Two dimensional echocardiography is very useful in evaluating the secondary effects of chronic mitral regurgitation. Left atrial enlargement, exaggerated septal motion, and left ventricular enlargement are all found in chronic severe MR. Careful evaluation of left ventricular size and function are important in the timing of mitral valve repair or replacement.

Two-dimensional echocardiography also may be helpful in determining the etiology of MR. Rheumatic mitral valve disease usually presents with thickening and fibrosis of the mitral leaflets and some degree of mitral stenosis. Myxomatous degeneration is appreciated as thickening and redundancy of the mitral leaflets. Mitral valve prolapse and flail mitral leaflet are also often detectable by 2-D echocardiography.

REFERENCE

Feigenbaum, H.: Echocardiography. 5th ed. Malvern, PA, Lea & Febiger, 1994, pp. 251–262.

28-A *(Braunwald, p. 71; Fig. 3–46)*

The echocardiographic hallmarks of mitral stenosis are the same for M-mode and 2-D echocardiography and consist of decreased valve motion, increased thickness of the valve leaflets, inadequate separation of the anterior and posterior leaflets of the valve during diastole, and increase in left atrial size. However, doming of the mitral leaflets, which is indicative of restricted motion, is a characteristic sign of stenosis seen only on 2-D echocardiography. The presence of doming is particularly helpful because it may distinguish a valve that is truly stenotic from one that opens poorly because of low flow.

29-B *(Braunwald, p. 157; Figs. 5–4 through 5–6, 5–8 and 5–10)*

Several different types of ST-segment displacement may be observed during exercise protocols. In normal subjects, the PR segment becomes progressively more downsloping in the inferior leads, and junctional depression (J-joint depression) is a normal finding (see Braunwald, Fig. 5–4, p. 157). In patients developing myocardial ischemia, the ST segment usually becomes more flattened or downsloping as the severity of ischemia worsens. ST-segment displacement may occur only during exercise, during both exercise and recovery, or only during recovery. The last situation is observed as the ischemic response in approximately 10 per cent of patients.[1]

The isoelectric point, by convention, is taken to be the PQ junction for a given beat on the electrocardiogram. By definition, the development of ≥ 0.10 mV (1 mm) of J-point depression measured from the PQ junction with a relatively flat (or downsloping) ST-segment slope, depressed ≥ 0.10 mV for 60 to 80 msec after the J point, in three consecutive beats, with a stable baseline, is considered to be an abnormal exercise response. If the ST segment is depressed at rest, an additional 0.10 mV of depression in the manner just defined is required to meet abnormal criteria.

Patients with normal early repolarization should be evaluated with respect to the ST segment by measuring from the PQ junction. It is important to emphasize that exercise tests demonstrating ST-segment depression neither localize the site of myocardial ischemia nor provide any clue as to which coronary artery is involved.[2] In contrast, exercise-induced ST-segment elevation is relatively specific for the specific artery involved (see Braunwald, Fig. 5–10, p. 160).

REFERENCES

1. Lachterman, B., Lehmann, K.G., Abrahamson, D., and Froelicher, V.F.: "Recovery only" ST-segment depression and the predictive accuracy of the exercise test. Ann. Intern. Med. *112*:11, 1990.
2. Mark, D.B., Hlatky, M.A., Lee, K.L., et al.: Localizing coronary artery obstructions with the exercise treadmill test. Ann. Intern. Med. *106*:53, 1987.

30-A *(Braunwald, pp. 112–113; Fig. 4–7)*

Limb lead reversal is a relatively common cause of a bizarre QRS axis. It is useful to remember Einthoven's law, which allows one to derive the relationship that a complex in lead 2 is equal to the sum of the corresponding complexes in leads 1 and 3 (2 = 1 + 3). Thus, if the P wave is upright in all three leads, the lead with the tallest P is lead 2. The most common technical error is reversal of the arm leads (as shown). This is readily detected as inversion of all complexes in lead I. Thus, "I" is the mirror image of I, and aV_r and aV_l are reversed.

31-A *(Braunwald, pp. 155–156; Fig. 5–2)*

Exercise protocols may be either dynamic or static. In general, dynamic protocols are most useful clinically to assess cardiovascular reserve and function. The protocol should be chosen with the patient in mind, with a goal of achieving 6 to 10 minutes of continuous and progressive exercise, during which the myocardial oxygen demand is sequentially elevated to the patient's maximal level. The protocol should also include a recovery, or "cool-down," period.[1] Arm ergometry protocols in general result in heart rate and blood pressure responses at a given workload that are somewhat *greater* than those for leg exercise. They are most useful for patients who cannot perform either treadmill or bicycle protocols. Bicycle protocols may be quite useful in appropriately selected subjects, although persons unfamiliar with this form of exercise will not have the appropriate muscle development required for optimal performance of the test, and early fatigue may lead to limitations in interpretation. Bicycle ergometry leads to a lower maximal oxygen consumption and anaerobic threshold than treadmill protocols, although maximal heart rates are similar. In addition, less motion artifact for precordial measurement is present with bicycle ergometry than with treadmill protocols.

The standard Bruce protocol treadmill test is the most widely used and studied of the exercise protocols. In older patients, or those with a decreased exercise capability, modification of the initial two stages of the Bruce protocols may be useful. The first two 3-minute segments may be completed at a speed of 1.7 mph with first no incline and then

with a 5 per cent grade. Thus, stage III of the *modified* Bruce protocol is equivalent to stage I of the *standard* Bruce protocol. One limitation of the Bruce protocols is the relatively large increase in oxygen consumption occurring between stages. This may in part be avoided by using the so-called *Cornwell* protocol, which is a modification of the Bruce regimen, with smaller increments based on 2-minute stages, allowing a better estimate of heart rate–adjusted indices of ST-segment depression.[1]

REFERENCE

1. Okin, P.M., and Kligfield, P.: Effect of exercise protocol and lead selection on the accuracy of heart rate–adjusted indices of ST-segment depression for detection of three-vessel coronary artery disease. J. Electrocardiol. *22*:187, 1989.

32-B *(Braunwald, pp. 40–41; Fig. 2–37)*

Aortic regurgitation is the most common cause of an early diastolic murmur originating from the left side of the heart. The murmur is initiated when the aortic component of the second heart sound occurs, and tends to be decrescendo due to a progressive decline in the volume and rate of regurgitation during the course of diastole. This is the norm in chronic severe aortic regurgitation. Selective radiation of the murmur of aortic regurgitation to the right sternal border is consistent with the aortic root being dilated, as occurs in the Marfan syndrome. When acute severe aortic regurgitation occurs, the murmur is somewhat different from that just described: a short diastolic murmur results because of the early equilibration of aortic diastolic pressure and the existing diastolic pressure in the low-compliance left ventricle. The murmur may be quite soft and less high-pitched than the murmur of chronic aortic regurgitation (see Braunwald, Fig. 2–37, p. 41). Graham Steell first described the murmur of pulmonary regurgitation resulting from elevated pulmonary artery pressure in 1888. The murmur commences with the pulmonic component of the second heart sound, which may be prominent, and may be associated with any form of pulmonary hypertension, including that accompanying rheumatic mitral valvular disease.

33-C *(Braunwald, pp. 118–119; Fig. 4–AE1, p. 146)*

In chronic lung disease, a variety of ECG changes may occur. Right-axis deviation, increased size, and peaking of the P wave may all appear in the limb leads, and a biphasic P wave may be more obvious in lead V_1. When the P-wave axis becomes rightward (> +90 degrees), chronic obstructive lung disease is suggested. The underlying cause of this finding is overinflation of the lungs and not the increased pulmonary artery pressures that may accompany the disorder. For this reason, right-axis deviation of the P wave is not observed in interstitial fibrosis.[1] Because the magnitude of the Ta segment is directly proportional to the area of the P wave, while its orientation is opposite to that of the P wave, the early portion of the ST segment may appear depressed due to the Ta segment in the presence of chronic obstructive lung disease and cor pulmonale with right atrial enlargement. This may lead to a "pseudo−ST-segment depression" pattern. In chronic obstructive lung disease, the amplitude of the R wave is often reduced in leads V_5 and V_6, while prominent R waves may appear in the right precordial leads. The latter changes are thought to be due to the unopposed activation of the right ventricular free wall and crista terminalis. In biventricular hypertrophy, however, left ventricular forces usually dominate the electrocardiographic pattern and may obscure ECG criteria for RVH.

REFERENCE

1. Ikeda, K., Kubota, I., Takahashi, K., and Yasui, S.: P-wave changes in obstructive and restrictive lung diseases. J. Electrocardiol. *18*:233, 1985.

34-C *(Braunwald, pp. 285–287)*

Myocardial perfusion imaging is a useful technique for assessing the adequacy of reperfusion after thrombolytic therapy. Serial studies of myocardial perfusion both before and after thrombolytic therapy demonstrate a reduction in size of the resting defect after successful thrombolysis.[1,2] The size of the resting myocardial perfusion defect may continue to decrease over the ensuing days in some patients. Myocardial perfusion imaging prior to administration of a thrombolytic agent is impractical with ^{201}Tl. Because of the redistribution properties of ^{201}Tl, the patient would have to be imaged prior to thrombolytic therapy, resulting in an unacceptable delay. However, ^{99m}Tc-sestamibi can be administered prior to thrombolysis with imaging performed at a time when therapy will not be interrupted.

Myocardial perfusion imaging is a strong predictor of morbidity and mortality following MI. Patients with large perfusion defects have poorer prognosis and long-term survival than patients with small defects.[3] Additional indicators of a poor prognosis include visualization of the right ventricle and lung uptake at rest. In some patients, the size of the myocardial perfusion defect after acute MI appears to decrease over time. This may be related to spontaneous thrombolysis, which occurs in approximately 20 per cent of patients.

Myocardial perfusion imaging in patients with unstable angina reveals defects that are reversible. Myocardial perfusion defects are demonstrable during the episode of chest pain and for a variable period of time after resolution of chest pain. Patients who have ECG abnormalities during chest pain have larger perfusion defects than patients who have chest pain without ECG abnormalities.[4]

REFERENCES

1. Gibbons, R.J., Verani, M.S., Behrenbeck, T., et al.: Feasibility of tomographic ^{99m}Tc-hexakis-2-methoxy-2-methylpropyl-isonitrile imaging for the assessment of myocardial area at risk and the effect of treatment in acute myocardial infarction. Circulation *80*:177, 1989.
2. Wackers, F.J. Th., Gibbons, R.J., Verani, M.S., et al.: Serial quantitative planar technetium-99m-isonitrile imaging in acute myocardial infarction: Efficacy for noninvasive assessment of thrombolytic therapy. J. Am. Coll. Cardiol. *14*: 861, 1989.
3. Silverman, K.J., Becker, L.C., Bulkley, B.H., et al.: Value of early thallium-201 scintigraphy for predicting mortality in patients with acute myocardial infarction. Circulation *61*: 996, 1980.
4. Bilodeau, L., Theroux, P., Gregoire, J., et al.: Technetium-99m sestamibi tomography in patients with spontaneous chest pain: Correlations with clinical, electrocardiographic and angiographic findings. J. Am. Coll. Cardiol. *18*:1684, 1991.

35-C *(Braunwald, p. 163; Fig. 5–10)*

Data from the Coronary Artery Surgery Study (CASS) supports earlier indications that ST-segment elevation in the setting of exercise in a lead containing an abnormal Q wave is a marker for both decreased left ventricular function and an adverse prognosis.[1] A finding of ST-segment elevation may be seen in patients following myocardial infarction, provided that the testing is given within the first 2 weeks after the index event. The occurrence of exercise-induced ST-segment elevation in the post-MI setting decreases in frequency by 6 weeks, however.[2] The occurrence of exercise-induced ST-segment elevation in leads with a Q wave is not a marker of more extensive coronary artery disease or active myocardial ischemia. If ST-segment elevation occurs during exercise in a lead that does not contain a Q wave in a patient without a previous MI, the finding is correlated with underlying vasoplasm or a high-grade stenosis and may be considered a marker of ischemia (see Braunwald, Fig. 5−10, p. 160). The latter situation occurs in approximately 1 per cent of patients with obstructive coronary artery disease. The ECG site of exercise-induced ST-segment elevation is well correlated with the underlying coronary artery involved (in contrast to ST-segment depression), and thallium scintigraphy or coronary angiography will often demonstrate a defect in the predicted territory.

REFERENCES

1. Bruce, R.A., Fisher, L.D., Pettinger, M., et al.: ST-segment elevation with exercise: A marker for poor ventricular function and poor prognosis. Coronary Artery Surgery Study (CASS) confirmation of Seattle Heart Watch Results. Circulation*77*:897, 1988.
2. Haines, D.E., Beller, G.A., Watson, D.D., et al.: Exercise-induced ST segment elevation 2 weeks after uncomplicated myocardial infarction: Contributing factors and prognostic significance. J. Am. Coll. Cardiol. *9*:996, 1987.

36-D *(Braunwald, pp. 291–292)*

Myocardial perfusion imaging is an important source of prognostic information in coronary artery disease. Stress myocardial perfusion imaging has been shown to be the most powerful available indicator of subsequent cardiac events.[1] The combination of clinical and myocardial perfusion data is more predictive than the combination of clinical and cardiac catheterization data in recent analyses.[2-4]

Stress perfusion defects in multiple locations corresponding to multiple vascular territories are suggestive of left main or three-vessel coronary artery disease. Other indicators of high-risk coronary artery disease include large defects, transient pulmonary uptake of tracer, and LV cavity dilatation after exercise. A high-risk pattern has a specificity of approximately 95 per cent, whereas the sensitivity is only approximately 70 per cent. The severity of a myocardial perfusion defect can be assessed both in terms of its size and the extent of its reversibility. A severe defect is one that has little or no uptake with stress imaging, whereas a mild defect may have only a slight reduction in counts with stress. The severity of defects as well as their number and size are important indicators of prognosis. The predictive value of myocardial perfusion imaging is independent of the imaging technique (planar or SPECT) and the imaging agent used (^{201}Tl or ^{99m}Tc-sestamibi).[5,6]

Just as the presence of stress-induced myocardial perfusion defects can predict a poor prognosis, the absence of such defects reflects a good prognosis. This principle is maintained even in the presence of angiographically documented coronary artery disease. Such patients who do not have perfusion abnormalities have a low risk of subsequent cardiac events, despite their angiographic abnormalities.[7-9]

REFERENCES

1. Bodenheimer, M.M., Wackers, F.J.Th., Schwartz, R.G., et al.: Prognostic significance of a fixed thallium defect one to six months after onset of acute myocardial infarction or unstable angina. Am. J. Cardiol. *74*:1196, 1994.
2. Pollock, S.G., Abbott, R.D., Boucher, C.A., et al.: Independent and incremental prognostic value of tests performed in hierarchical order to evaluate patients with suspected coronary artery disease. Circulation *85*:237, 1992.
3. Melin, J.A., Robert, A., Luwaert, R., et al.: Additional prognostic value of exercise testing and thallium-201 scintigraphy in catheterized patients without previous myocardial infarction. Int. J. Cardiol. *27*:235, 1990.
4. Iskandrian, A.S., Chae, S.C., Heo, J., et al.: Independent and incremental prognostic value of exercise single-photon emission computed tomographic (SPECT) thallium imaging in coronary artery disease. J. Am. Coll. Cardiol. *22*: 665, 1993.
5. Miller, D.D., Stratmann, H.G., Shaw, L., et al.: Dipyridamole technetium-99m-sestamibi myocardial tomography as an independent predictor of cardiac event-free survival after acute ischemic events. J. Nucl. Cardiol. *1*:172, 1994.
6. Stratmann, H.G., Williams, G.A., Wittry, M.D., et al.: Exercise technetium-99m sestamibi tomography for cardiac risk stratification of patients with stable chest pain. Circulation *89*:615, 1994.
7. Brown, K.A., Altland, E., and Rowen, M.: Prognostic value of normal Tc-99m sestamibi cardiac imaging. J. Nucl. Med. *35*:554, 1994.
8. Raiker, K., Sinusas, A.J., Zaret, B.L., et al.: One year prognosis of patients with normal Tc-99m-sestamibi stress imaging. J. Nucl. Cardiol. *1*:449, 1994.
9. Berman, D.S., Kiat, H., Cohen, J., et al.: Prognosis of 1044 patients with normal exercise Tc-99m sestamibi myocardial perfusion SPECT. J. Am. Coll. Cardiol. *1A*:63A, 1994.

37-D *(Braunwald, pp. 245–246)*

Radiographic contrast agents used during cardiac catheterization have been a source of hemodynamic, arrhythmic, and renal side effects. It is believed that most of the side effects that occur with ionic contrast agents are related to their osmolality, sodium content, and calcium binding properties. Toxicity due to use of ionic contrast agents occurs in 1.4 to 2.3 per cent of patients who receive them. Newer nonionic, low osmolar contrast agents are associated with fewer side effects. There has been controversy over when to use nonionic, low osmolar contrast agents, since they are considerably more expensive than the traditional ionic contrast agents. Some frequently used criteria for selecting nonionic low osmolar contrast agents include diabetes mellitus, unstable ischemic syndromes, congestive heart failure, history of contrast allergy, severe valvular heart disease, internal mammary artery injection, hypotension, and bradycardia (see Braunwald, Table 6–3, p. 180). Although low osmolar, nonionic contrast agents may cause less renal toxicity in those patients at highest risk (those with preexisting renal insufficiency), there is no evidence that they have any advantage over traditional contrast agents in patients with normal renal function. In patients with renal insufficiency, preventing decreases in renal perfusion during cardiac catheterization may diminish the incidence of acute renal failure. In patients with baseline renal insufficiency, saline hydration was superior to both furosemide and mannitol in preventing acute worsening in renal function.[1]

REFERENCE

1. Solomon, R., Werner, C., Mann, D., et al.: Effects of saline, mannitol and furosemide on acute decreases in renal function induced by radiocontrast agents. N. Engl. J. Med. *331*:1416, 1994.

38-C *(Braunwald, p. 363; Fig. 12–6)*

The structure of cardiac myosin is such that two myosin heavy chains (MHC) and four myosin light chains (MLC) combine to form one unit. Myosin heavy chains contain the head and neck structures involved in crossbridge formation with actin. Each myosin filament contains two MHCs intertwined. Each MHC is associated with two MLCs, so that one filament contains two myosin head containing heavy chains and four MCLs.

MHC molecules exist in two isoforms, α-MHC and β-MHC. Despite having the same molecular weight, their ATPase activity is different. β-MHC, the predominant form in humans, has less ATPase activity than the alpha isoform. It is thought that mutations in the β-MHC isoform may be responsible for some types of congenital hypertrophic cardiomyopathy.[1]

MLC molecules serve a regulatory function in the interaction between actin and myosin. The essential MLC, or MLC-1, has recently been found to have an inhibitory role in actin and myosin binding.[2] MCL-2 contains a phosphorylation site that promotes crossbridge formation by enhancing actin and myosin binding.

REFERENCES

1. Watkins, H., McKenna, W.J., Thierfelder, L., et al.: Mutations in the genes for cardiac troponin-T and alpha-tropomyosin in hypertrophic cardiomyopathy. N. Engl. J. Med. *332*:1058–1064, 1995.
2. Morano, I., Ritter, O., Bonz, A., et al.: Myosin light chain-actin interation regulates cardiac contractility. Circ. Res. *76*:720–725, 1995.

39-D (Braunwald, pp. 91–92)

This Doppler echocardiogram demonstrates findings characteristic for hypertrophic cardiomyopathy. The Doppler recording of the left ventricular outflow tract shows a late peaking systolic flow of increased velocity that is abruptly terminated as obstruction occurs.[1] Abnormalities in mitral flow are common due to left ventricular hypertrophy and reduced left ventricular compliance. Diastolic mitral flow often reveals an abnormal relaxation pattern with reversal of the normal relationship of predominant E wave and smaller A wave.[2]

Hypertrophic cardiomyopathy frequently presents in young adults who may present with syncope, angina, dyspnea, or sudden death. This disorder has autosomal dominant transmission with variable penetrance. A similar clinical syndrome may occur in elderly patients with long histories of hypertension. Hypertensive hypertrophic cardiomyopathy of the elderly is a sporadic disease that usually results from symmetrical left ventricular hypertrophy.[3,4]

Systolic anterior motion of the mitral valve (SAM) is an echocardiographic finding that may be associated with hypertrophic cardiomyopathy. The degree of SAM appears to be related to the severity of left ventricular outflow obstruction.[5] SAM may be found in clinical situations unrelated to hypertrophy, such as anemia, hypovolemia, and hyperdynamic states.[6] Midsystolic closure of the aortic valve may be detected by M-mode echocardiography in patients with hypertrophic cardiomyopathy. Although not specific for hypertrophic cardiomyopathy, it is usually correlated with significant obstruction.

REFERENCES

1. Panza, J.A., Petrone, R.K., Fananapazir, L., et al.: Utility of continuous wave Doppler echocardiography in the non-invasive assessment of left ventricular outflow tract pressure gradient in patients with hypertrophic cardiomyopathy. J. Am. Coll. Cardiol. *19*:91, 1992.
2. Spirito, P., and Maron, B.J.: Relation between extent of left ventricular hypertrophy and diastolic filling abnormalities in hypertrophic cardiomyopathy. J. Am. Coll. Cardiol. *15*: 808, 1990.
3. Topol, E.J., Traill, T.A., and Fortuin, N.J.: Hypertensive hypertrophic cardiomyopathy of the elderly. N. Engl. J. Med. *312*:277, 1985.
4. Pearson, A.C., Gudipati, C.V., and Labovitz, A.J.: Systolic and diastolic flow abnormalities in elderly patients with hypertensive hypertrophic cardiomyopathy. J. Am. Coll. Cardiol. *12*:989, 1988.
5. Pollick, C., Rakowski, H., and Wigle, E.D.: Muscular subaortic stenosis: The quantitative relationship between systolic anterior motion and the pressure gradient. Circulation *69*:43, 1984.
6. Mintz, G.S., Kotler, M.N., Segal, B.L., et al.: Systolic anterior motion of the mitral valve in the absence of asymmetric septal hypertrophy. Circulation *57*:256, 1978.

40 A-T, B-F, C-T, D-F, E-T (Braunwald, pp. 73–74; Figs. 3–51 and 3–52)

M-mode and 2-D echocardiography are particularly useful in diagnosing mitral valve prolapse. In both mitral valve prolapse and flail mitral valve there can be an anatomical abnormality in the mitral valve or submitral apparatus with accompanying mitral regurgitation. In mitral valve prolapse, the leaflet tips point toward the left ventricle during systole, whereas in flail mitral valve the leaflet tip of the flail leaflet points towards the left atrium. The classic M-mode finding in mitral valve prolapse is posterior displacement of the mitral valve late in systole, also known as the hammock sign. However, some degree of posterior bowing can be seen in normal variants. Using the criteria of 3 mm of posterior displacement is sensitive for the diagnosis of mitral valve prolapse, but is less specific, since such displacement occurs in up to 18 per cent of healthy young females.[2] Therefore, most clinicians are reluctant to make the diagnosis on this criterion alone. Under certain loading conditions, late systolic mitral valve prolapse may become holosystolic. Holosystolic prolapse may be difficult to differentiate from a normal variant.

Mitral valve prolapse can be detected on a 2-D echocardiographic study by noting that the mitral leaflet moves to the atrial side of the mitral annular plane during systole. In the parasternal long-axis view, the plane of the mitral annulus is at an angle and is therefore more difficult to determine. In the apical four-chamber view, the mitral annular plane is horizontal and is easier to determine. However, the mitral annulus in the four-chamber view is saddle-shaped rather than planar and therefore a false-positive mitral valve prolapse diagnosis occurs more commonly in this view than in the parasternal long axis view. Other 2-D characteristics of the myxomatous mitral valve, such as thickening and redundancy of the mitral leaflets, may help make the diagnosis of prolapse when they are present.

REFERENCES

1. Feigenbaum, H.: Echocardiography. 5th ed. Malvern, PA, Lea & Febiger, 1994, pp. 262–269.
2. Markiewicz, W., Stoner, J., London, E., et al.: Mitral valve prolapse in one hundred presumably healthy young females. Circulation 53:464, 1976.

41 A-T, B-T, C-T, D-T, E-T *(Braunwald, pp. 297 and 300–301; Figs. 9–32 through 9–34)*

Radionuclide angiocardiography (RNA) uses ^{99m}Tc to assess cardiac performance. RNA utilizes either a first-pass (FPRNA) or equilibrium (ERNA) method with ECG gating to provide information about right and left ventricular systolic and diastolic function, regional ventricular function, and cardiac volumes. FPRNA involves visualization of only the first transit of radiopharmaceutical agent through the circulation, whereas ERNA reveals analysis of ventricular function after the radiopharmaceutical has reached equilibrium in the circulation. Each technique has its relative advantages. Because ERNA allows visualization of cardiac performance over a more prolonged period of time, it is less susceptible to the effect of transient arrhythmias on ventricular function. ERNA also facilitates the evaluation of multiple views and serial studies. Because of radiopharmaceutical activity in overlying structures, right ventricular function may be difficult to assess by ERNA. For this reason, FPRNA is preferable for evaluation of RV function. FPRNA is also the method of choice for shunt studies. Diastolic function may be assessed by either FPRNA or ERNA. Indices measured by RNA in the evaluation of diastolic function include peak filling rate, time-to-peak filling rate, and filling fraction.[1,2]

Important prognostic information is obtained from RNA in several clinical situations. Most notably, in patients who have suffered an acute MI, the left ventricular ejection fraction is an extremely important prognostic indicator. In addition to overall prognosis, LV ejection fraction can predict which patients with three-vessel coronary artery disease will enjoy increased survival after coronary bypass surgery. An unrelated condition where RNA may provide considerable prognostic information is in patients with cancer who are treated with the chemotherapeutic agent doxorubicin. Doxorubicin has been associated with cardiotoxicity that may be severe, irreversible, and lethal. There are now guidelines for management of doxorubicin therapy based on the results of serial RNA (see Braunwald, Table 9–5, p. 303)[3].

Recent developments have resulted in an instrument known as the VEST which can provide several hours of ambulatory RNA monitoring following blood pool labeling.[4] RNA and ECG data are stored on tape. Analysis of these data yields trends in ventricular function during the recording period. Since myocardial ischemia results in transient ventricular dysfunction, this technique may yield important information regarding silent ischemia.

REFERENCES

1. Bonow, R.O., Bacharach, S.L., Green, M.V., et al.: Impaired left ventricular diastolic filling in patients with coronary artery disease: Assessment with radionuclide angiography. Circulation 64:315, 1981.
2. Bashore, T.M., Leithe, M.E., and Shaffer, P.: Diastolic function. In Gerson, M.C. (ed): Cardiac Nuclear Medicine. New York, McGraw-Hill Book Co., 1991, p. 195.
3. Schwartz, R.G., McKenzie, W.B., Alexander, J., et al.: Congestive heart failure and left ventricular dysfunction complicating doxorubicin therapy: Seven-year experience using serial radionuclide myocardiography. Am. J. Med. 82: 1109, 1987.
4. Tamaki, N., Yasuda, T., Moore, R., et al.: Continuous monitoring of left ventricular function by an ambulatory radionuclide detector in patients with coronary artery disease. J. Am. Coll. Cardiol. 12:669, 1988.

42 A-F, B-F, C-T, D-T, E-F *(Braunwald, pp. 74–76; Figs. 3–54, 3–56, 3–58 and 3–59)*

The peak instantaneous gradient measured by Doppler echocardiography and the peak-to-peak gradient measured in the cardiac catheterization laboratory are both used as estimates of the pressure gradient between the left ventricle and the aorta in aortic stenosis. The peak-to-peak gradient is measured by taking the difference between the maximum left ventricular pressure and the maximum aortic pressure for a given cardiac cycle. These two values do not occur at the same point in time due to the delay in aortic pressure generation from aortic valve stenosis. The peak instantaneous gradient measured by Doppler echocardiography reflects the maximum gradient at one instant of time, and is therefore a real-time pressure difference measurement. The peak instantaneous gradient invariably is greater than the peak-to-peak pressure gradient (see Braunwald, Fig. 3–56, p. 75). The mean gradient is determined by measuring the integral of either the difference in the left ventricular and aortic pressure tracings by cardiac catheterization or the aortic flow profile by Doppler echocardiography. This value is similar when measured by either technique.

The pressure gradient across a stenotic aortic valve can be determined by Doppler echocardiography using the modified Bernoulli equation (pressure difference across a stenotic orifice = $4V^2$). Using the modified Bernoulli equation, an aortic velocity of 2.5 m/sec is equivalent to a pressure gradient of 25 mm Hg. It must be emphasized, however, that the pressure gradient alone does not estimate the severity of aortic stenosis. A small pressure gradient in the setting of low cardiac output may still reflect severe aortic stenosis. To provide a better estimate of aortic stenosis severity, the aortic valve area should be calculated by the Gorlin formula.

When estimating the severity of aortic regurgitation (AR) by echocardiography, the most accurate approach combines color flow Doppler, continuous wave Doppler (CW), and M-mode methods. Color flow Doppler is used to estimate the width of the aortic regurgitant jet compared to the width of the aortic orifice in systole. When measuring the aortic regurgitant flow by CW Doppler, the rate of decline in velocity of the regurgitant blood provides an estimation of the severity of AR. In severe AR, the left ventricular diastolic pressure quickly rises, decreasing the pressure gradient between the left ventricle and the aorta. The rate of decline is rapid and the slope of the regurgitant flow decline by CW Doppler measurement is steep. In mild AR, the opposite is true and the slope of the regurgitant flow decline by CW Doppler is less steep (see Braunwald, Fig. 3–59, p. 76). In severe, usually acute AR, the M-mode recording may show premature closure of the mitral valve. In particularly severe AR, there may even be premature opening of the aortic valve. Both of these M-mode findings indicate elevated left ventricular diastolic pressure.

REFERENCE

Feigenbaum, H.: Echocardiography. 5th ed. Malvern, PA, Lea & Febiger, 1994, pp. 273–291.

43 A-T, B-T, C-T, D-T, E-T   *(Braunwald, pp. 196–197)*

Detection and localization of intracardiac shunts is usually possible at catheterization by the traditional oximetry run, in which samples are drawn at numerous sites in the right side of the heart and adjacent vessels. The technique involves measurement of O_2 saturations in order to identify a significant step-up between consecutive chambers. Using averaged samples, an O_2 saturation step-up of ≥ 7 per cent is necessary to diagnose a left-to-right shunt at the atrial level, while ≥ 5 per cent suffices at the level of the right ventricular or pulmonary artery levels. Because of normal variability in O_2 saturation, shunts with QP/QS ≤ 1.3 at the pulmonary artery or right ventricular levels and those with QP/QS < 1.5 at the atrial level are not detected. The data obtained in the course of an oximetry run may be used to quantify shunt size. Pulmonary and systemic blood flows can be calculated using the standard Fick equation appropriately written for the system in question. For unidirectional shunts, the magnitude is given by QP/QS; from this it can be deduced that a negative value will occur with pure right-to-left shunts, as often is seen in tetralogy of Fallot. More sensitive techniques, including hydrogen-sensitive electrode placement used with inhaled hydrogen gas or indocyanine green dye curve methods, may be used to detect small shunts.

44 A-T, B-T, C-F, D-F, E-T   *(Braunwald, p. 162; Table 5–4)*

The exercise electrocardiogram is more likely to be abnormal in patients with severe coronary artery disease. There are several abnormalities of the exercise ECG that are suggestive of multivessel coronary artery disease and/or an adverse prognosis. These include the early onset of ischemic ST-segment depression, such as that occurring during the first stage of a standard Bruce protocol. In addition, ST-segment depression of ≥ 2 mm (0.20 mV), which involves five or more leads and/or persists five or more minutes into recovery is suggestive of more severe underlying coronary atherosclerosis. Exercise-induced ST-segment elevation is also consistent with multivessel coronary artery disease, except in lead aV$_r$, which may demonstrate ST-segment elevation in a variety of circumstances, including cases of less severe coronary disease. A failure to increase systolic blood pressure by 10 mm Hg, or a sustained decrease in systolic blood pressure of 10 mm Hg or more, is suggestive of multivessel (or left main) coronary artery disease and an adverse prognosis. Multifocal premature ventricular contractions occurring during exercise in and of themselves are not correlated with extensive disease, but reproducible sustained or symptomatic ventricular tachycardia is highly suggestive of multivessel coronary disease.

45 A-T, B-F, C-T, D-F, E-T   *(Braunwald, pp. 74–76; Fig. 3–55)*

The Doppler tracing is from a patient with combined aortic stenosis and aortic insufficiency. The Doppler aortic outflow tracing shows a characteristic delayed onset of peak velocity, consistent with significant aortic stenosis. The pressure gradient across the aortic valve can be calculated by using the modified Bernoulli equation (pressure difference $= 4V^2$). Using a peak aortic velocity of 4.8 estimates the maximum instantaneous aortic gradient to be 92. In general, when the aortic flow velocity is more than 4 m/sec, the probability of critical aortic stenosis is high. Similarly, a normal or slightly elevated aortic flow velocity is usually associated with mild aortic stenosis. For aortic flow velocities that are intermediate, additional hemodynamic data are often needed.[1]

The diastolic flow on this tracing represents aortic insufficiency. Severe aortic insufficiency is associated with a rapidly declining flow velocity, and mild aortic insufficiency with a gradually declining velocity (see Braunwald, Fig. 3–59, p. 76). Therefore, the aortic insufficiency in this patient is likely mild. Mild aortic insufficiency is not associated with premature closure of the mitral value. Premature closure of the mitral valve may be found on M-mode examination of patients with severe, acute aortic insufficiency due to elevated diastolic left ventricular pressure.[2]

Additional findings on the echocardiogram that may help assess the severity of aortic value disease include left ventricular size, shape, and thickness. In this patient with severe aortic stenosis and mild aortic insufficiency, one might expect to find left ventricular hypertrophy on 2-D echocardiography.

REFERENCES

1. Yeager, M., Yock, P.G., and Popp, R.L.: Comparison of Doppler-derived pressure gradient to that determined at cardiac catheterization in adults with aortic valve stenosis: Implications of management. Am. J. Cardiol. 57:644, 1986.
2. Botvinick, E.H., Schiller, N.B., Wickramasekaran, R., et al.: Echocardiographic demonstration of early mitral valve closure in severe aortic insufficiency. Its clinical implications. Circulation 51:836, 1975.

46 A-T, B-F, C-T, D-F, E-T   (Braunwald, pp. 296–297 and 305–306)

The use of infarct-avid scintigraphy may be a useful method to identify acutely necrotic myocardial tissue in the appropriate patient. Current methods have not found widespread clinical applicability because of the somewhat poor spatial resolution they afford. This limits the clinician's ability to assess the size of a given myocardial infarction. The only imaging methods currently available for the identification of acutely infarcted myocardial tissue are ^{99m}Tc pyrophosphate scintigraphy and labeled monoclonal antimyosin specific–antibody scintigraphy.[1] The appearance of regional wall motion abnormalities on echocardiography may, in some patients, permit estimate of infarct size, provided a baseline study is available. However, this technique is somewhat indirect and is complicated by the known variation of contractile patterns in normal subjects[2] as well as the load-dependence of regional wall motion patterns.[3] Two further techniques, metabolic imaging with PET and MRI spectroscopy, show great promise for identifying acutely necrotic myocardial tissue. In the former technique, the combination of preserved or increased glucose uptake in a region of decreased perfusion suggests the presence of viable myocardial tissue, while a decrease in perfusion and glucose uptake appears to identify irreversibly damaged cardiac tissue[4]; the necrosis may be of short or long duration.

REFERENCES

1. Khaw, B.A., Gold, H.K., Yasuda, T., et al.: Scintigraphic quantification of myocardial necrosis in patients after intravenous injections of myosin-specific antibody. Circulation 74:501, 1986.
2. Pandian, N.G., Skorton, D.J., Collins, S.M., et al.: Heterogeneity of left ventricular segmental wall thickening and excursion in two-dimensional echocardiograms of normal humans. Am. J. Cardiol. 51:1667, 1983.
3. Weiss, R.M., Shonka, M., Kinzey, J.E., and Marcus, M.L.: Effects of loading alterations on the pattern of heterogeneity of regional left ventricular function (abstr) FASEBJ 2:1494A, 1988.
4. Tillisch, J., Brunken, R., Marshall, R., et al.: Reversibility to cardiac wall motion abnormalities predicted by positron tomography. N. Engl. J. Med. 314:884, 1986.

47 A-T, B-T, C-F, D-T, E-F   (Braunwald, pp. 35–36)

Cardiac murmurs are characterized by their intensity, shape, pitch, and timing in the cardiac cycle, as well as by duration, direction of radiation, and the overall "quality" of the sound. Murmur frequencies, or pitch, may vary from high to low. Systolic murmurs usually have a distinct shape that is best characterized as crescendo, decrescendo, diamond-shaped (crescendo-decrescendo), even (plateau), or uneven (variable). The chief classification of a cardiac murmur, however, is made from the timing of the sound during the cardiac cycle. There are three categories of murmurs: systolic, diastolic, and continuous. Continuous murmurs begin in systole and continue without interruption throughout the second heart sound. A systolic murmur begins at or following the first heart sound and ends at the component of the second heart sound corresponding to the ventricle of origin of the murmur. Thus, in murmurs originating in the left side of the heart, the sound is heard to end before the aortic component of the second heart sound, while murmurs originating on the right side of the heart continue through the aortic component and end before or at the pulmonic component of the second heart sound. Holosystolic murmurs begin with the first heart sound, continue in a plateau-like fashion throughout systole, and end with the second heart sound on the side of origin of the murmur. A loud murmur may radiate from a site of maximal intensity to a number of locations across the precordium and into the neck, and the radiation may sometimes provide diagnostic information. The duration of a murmur may vary from short to long and often provides more useful diagnostic information than the intensity of the murmur.

48 A-T, B-F, C-F, D-T, E-F   (Braunwald, pp. 85–86; Fig. 3–87)

The ventricular wall normally thickens during systole. During ischemia the ability of the myocardium to thicken during systole is impaired. Myocardial infarction is manifested by a decrease in diastolic wall thickness and an increase in the echo intensity consistent with the presence of scar. Echocardiography is only moderately sensitive in the detection of ventricular aneurysms, which are localized areas of dilated ventricular wall. A pseudoaneurysm (Statement C) is a serious complication representing rupture of the free wall; in this condition the blood actually escapes from the myocardium and is trapped within the pericardial sac. This occurs most commonly in inferior wall infarctions. Indications for surgery are urgent with pseudoaneurysm; the diagnosis is crucial.

Mural thrombi are a common complication of MI and are especially common following anterior MI. When these thrombi are elongated they have a higher incidence of embolizing; more typically they are flat and line the ventricular wall. In general, reendothelialization of mural thrombi occurs within 2 weeks after acute MI. Although perforation of the ventricular septum is commonly observed in 2-D echocardiography, the best technique for making the diagnosis is Doppler echocardiography. Sampling on the RV side of the interventricular septum, one can record a high-velocity systolic flow in a positive direction—that is, moving from the LV to the RV through the ruptured septum.

49 A-T, B-F, C-T, D-T, E-F *(Braunwald, p. 45)*

As described by McGuire and colleagues, the classic pericardial friction rub has three distinct phases in sinus rhythm, including midsystolic, mid-diastolic, and presystolic.[1] The scratching quality of the sounds is generated by the abnormal apposition and rubbing of the visceral and parietal pericardial surfaces against each other during the contractile cycle of the heart. With a patient in the supine position, pressure with the diaphragm of the stethoscope during a complete expiration serves to accentuate the rub. This technique may be used to even greater advantage with the patient sitting up and leaning forward or resting on elbows and knees. The systolic phase of a pericardial friction rub is heard most commonly, with the presystolic phase the next most common. This presystolic component is often lost if atrial fibrillation intervenes. Following cardiac surgery, a pericardial rub is frequently heard. The rub must be distinguished from the "crunch" that may be heard due to the presence of air in the mediastinum (Hamman's sign).

REFERENCE

1. McGuire, J., Kotte, J.H., and Helm, R.A.: Acute pericarditis. Circulation *9*:425, 1954.

50 A-T, B-T, C-T, D-F, E-T *(Braunwald, pp. 250–253; Figs. 8–10 and 8–11)*

A knowledge of the anatomy of the human coronary circulation is important in the diagnosis and management of ischemic syndromes. The left main coronary artery gives rise to the left anterior descending artery (LAD) and the left circumflex artery and, in approximately 37 per cent of patients, a branch lying between these two vessels called the ramus medianus branch.[1] The major components of the LAD are the septal and diagonal branches. The septal branches supply the interventricular septum, the most densely vascularized area of the heart, and the first septal serves as the most important potential collateral channel. Over 90 per cent of patients have one to three diagonal branches that arise from the LAD; the absence of identifiable diagonal branches on angiography should suggest the possibility of one or more diagonal occlusions. The circumflex artery runs in or near the atrioventricular groove and supplies the lateral free wall of the left ventricle via obtuse marginal branches. While the majority of patients have a right dominant system, in 10 to 23 per cent of humans the posterior diaphragmatic myocardium is supplied via branches of the left coronary system.

REFERENCE

1. Levin, P.C., Harrington, D.P., Bettman, M.A., et al.: Anatomic variations of the coronary arteries supplying the anterolateral aspect of the left ventricle. Invest. Radiol. *17*:458, 1982.

51 A-T, B-T, C-T, D-T, E-T *(Braunwald, pp. 161–162; Table 5–3)*

The sensitivity of exercise stress testing for single-vessel coronary artery disease ranges from 25 to 71 per cent. The test is most sensitive for left anterior coronary artery disease. Approximately 75 to 80 per cent of all of the diagnostic information that may be obtained from exercise-induced ST-segment depression is found in leads V_4 through V_6. In a large series analyzing patients who had both exercise stress testing and coronary angiography, the mean sensitivity of ST-segment depression was 68 per cent, and the mean specificity was 77 per cent.[1] The test was 86 per cent sensitive and 53 per cent specific for left main or three-vessel coronary artery disease.

A number of noncoronary causes of ST-segment depression can give a false-positive test and thus decrease specificity. Most notable among these are left ventricular hypertrophy and digitalis therapy. Other noncoronary causes of ST-segment depression include mitral valve prolapse, hyperventilation, severe aortic stenosis, hypertension, cardiomyopathy, and preexcitation syndromes. In addition, sudden excessive exercise, supraventricular tachycardias, volume overload due to aortic or mitral regurgitation, interventricular conduction disturbances, and anemia or hypokalemia all may lead to noncoronary ST-segment depression.

REFERENCE

1. Gianrossi, R., Dotrano, R., Mulvihill, D., et al.: Exercise-induced ST depression in the diagnosis of coronary artery disease. A meta analysis. Circulation *80*:87, 1989.

52 A-F, B-T, C-T, D-F, E-F *(Braunwald, pp. 91–92; Figs. 3–99 and 3–100)*

In HCM, the mitral valve apparatus moves toward the interventricular septum during systole, producing what is termed systolic anterior motion of the mitral valve. This can be identified by 2-D echocardiography or by characteristic findings on M-mode echocardiograms. SAM may play an integral role in the development of outflow obstruction in HCM. However, some patients may demonstrate SAM without evidence of hypertrophic cardiomyopathy. Given the fact that SAM may occur in the absence of ASH, it may be that SAM is a nonspecific reaction to ventricular hypertrophy or distortion of the LV cavity.[2–4] Midsystolic closure of the aortic valve can be detected by M-mode echocardiography in patients with HCM. This finding is suggestive of significant outflow obstruction. It is not, however, specific for

HCM and may be found in patients with discrete subaortic stenosis. A proposed mechanism for this finding is that late in systole, when obstruction worsens, eddy currents form in the ascending aorta that precipitate closure of the aortic valve leaflets.[5]

Although ASH has become almost synonymous with HCM, it is well recognized that HCM can occur without ASH. Dynamic ventricular outflow obstruction can be found in patients who have concentric hypertrophy, isolated proximal septal hypertrophy, apical hypertrophy, and posterior wall hypertrophy.

The Doppler mitral inflow pattern in HCM can be quite variable, but usually reflects the abnormal diastolic function of the hypertrophied ventricle. Quite often, an abnormal relaxation pattern, with a diminished E wave and prominent A wave, can be seen. Variability may occur in the presence of severe mitral regurgitation, or a restrictive pattern of ventricular hypertrophy, both of which would result in an accentuated E wave.

REFERENCES

1. Feigenbaum, H.: Echocardiography. 5th ed. Malvern, PA, Lea & Febiger, 1994, pp. 511–526.
2. Buckley, B.H., and Fortuin, J.J.: Systolic anterior motion of the mitral valve without asymmetric septal hypertrophy. Chest 69:694, 1976.
3. Maron, B.J., Epstein, S.E., Bonow, R.O., et al.: Obstructive hypertrophic cardiomyopathy associated with minimal left ventricular hypertrophy. Am. J. Cardiol. 53:377, 1984.
4. Wei, J.Y., Weiss, J.L., and Bulkley, B.H.: Nonspecificity of the echocardiographic diagnosis of idiopathic hypertrophic subaortic stenosis: A clinicopathologic study (abstr.) Circulation 58(Suppl. II):237, 1978.
5. Yock, P.G., Hatle, L., and Popp, R.L.: Patterns and timing of Doppler-detected intracavitary and aortic flow in hypertrophic cardiomyopathy. J. Am. Coll. Cardiol. 8:1047–1058, 1986.

53 A-T, B-T, C-T, D-F, E-T *(Braunwald, pp. 128–130)*

Various studies have shown that ECGs in the emergency room are diagnostic in 50 to 70 per cent of patients with myocardial infarction and that serial ECGs increase the sensitivity significantly to >80 per cent.[1] Within 6 to 12 months about 30 per cent of patients with Q-wave infarcts will lose Q waves. Patients with inferior infarcts and anterior ST-segment depressions have been shown to have a worse prognosis than those with inferior MI without such ST-segment depressions. The mechanism of this finding is controversial. Some authors have suggested that this is due to an increased probability of associated left anterior descending artery disease in this situation.[2,3] Others suggest the worsening prognosis results from more extensive ischemia in the primary distribution.[4] ST-segment elevation ≥1 mm in V_4R has a sensitivity and specificity for right ventricular infarction of approximately 90 per cent.[5]

REFERENCES

1. Cooperating investigation from the MILIS study group: Electrocardiographic, enzymatic and scintigraphic criteria of acute myocardial infarction as determined from study of 726 patients (MILIS study). Am. J. Cardiol. 55:1463, 1985.
2. Tzivoni, D., Chenzbraun, A., Keren, A., et al.: Reciprocal electrocardiographic changes in acute myocardial infarction. Am. J. Cardiol. 56:23, 1986.
3. Pierard, L.A., Sprynger, M., Gilis, F., and Carlier, J.: Significance of precordial ST segment depression in inferior acute myocardial infarction as determined by echocardiography. Am. J. Cardiol. 57:82, 1986.
4. Ruddy, T.D., Yasuda, T., Gold, H.K., et al.: Anterior ST segment depression in acute inferior myocardial infarction as a marker of greater inferior, apical, and posterolateral damage. Am. Heart J. 112:1210, 1986.
5. Lopez-Sendon, J., Coma-Canella, I., Alcasena, S., et al.: Electrocardiographic findings in acute right ventricular infarction. Sensitivity and specificity of electrocardiographic alterations in right precordial leads V_4R, V_3R_1V, V_2 and V_3. J. Am. Coll. Cardiol. 6:1273, 1985.

54 A-F, B-T, C-F, D-T, E-F *(Braunwald, pp. 32–33)*

Splitting of the second heart sound may provide important diagnostic information in pathological situations. Persistent splitting of the second heart sound implies that both the aortic and pulmonic components may be heard during inspiration as well as expiration. Fixed splitting of the second heart sound means that the two components are not only persistent but that they remain unchanged in their wide separation throughout the respiratory cycle. In contrast, paradoxical splitting is the term used to describe separation of the aortic and pulmonic components of the second heart sound during expiration, with their simultaneous occurrence during inspiration. Persistent splitting may be due to either a delay in the pulmonic component as occurs in complete right bundle branch block or to early timing of the aortic sound, as may sometimes occur when left ventricular emptying is quite rapid in mitral regurgitation.[1] Fixed splitting is considered to be the hallmark of uncomplicated ostium secundum atrial septal defect and is due to changes in the capacitance of the pulmonary bed. An increase in pulmonary vascular capacitance leads to a delay in the pulmonic component (wide splitting), and because of the large increase in capacitance, little or no additional increase in pulmonary capacitance is achieved in inspiration. Therefore, no further inspiratory delay in the pulmonic component of the second sound is possible.

When the pulmonic component precedes the aortic component, the term "paradoxical splitting" of the second heart sound is used. This may occur in situations during which delayed activation of the left ventricle occurs, such as left bundle branch block, or with a right ventricular pacemaker.[2] Upon inspiration, the delay that occurs in the pulmonic component leads to fusion of the aortic and pulmonic components into a single sound. Situations that increase the force with which the aortic valve closes, such as systemic hypertension, may lead to an increase in the intensity of the aortic component of the second heart sound. In addition, pathological changes leading to a location of the aorta closer to the anterior chest wall, such as aortic root dilatation and transposition of the great arteries, may also increase the intensity of the aortic component of the second heart sound. A loud pulmonic component is similarly heard in patients with any of the various causes of pulmonary hypertension.[3]

REFERENCES

1. Perloff, J.K., and Harvey, W.P.: Auscultatory and phonocardiographic manifestations of pure mitral regurgitation. Prog. Cardiovasc. 5:172, 1962.
2. Hultgren, H.N., Craige, E., Nakamura, T., and Bilisoly, J.: Left bundle branch block and mechanical events of the cardiac cycle. Am. J. Cardiol. 52:755, 1985.
3. Perloff, J.K.: Auscultatory and phonocardiographic manifestations of pulmonary hypertension. Prog. Cardiovasc. Dis. 9:303, 1967.

55 A-T, B-T, C-T, D-T, E-F   *(Braunwald, pp. 18–20)*

The JVP is best examined on the right side of the neck, with the patient lying in the 45-degree position. The JVP, which reflects the distention of the internal jugular vein, provides a measure of right-sided cardiac dynamics, including the level of venous pressure and the pattern of the venous waves, which may give important information about the underlying cardiac pathology.[1] Whereas the *a* wave results from venous distention in response to atrial systole, the *v* wave is created by venous return to the right atrium when the tricuspid valve is closed (i.e., during ventricular systole). Giant (cannon) *a* waves are seen when atrial systole occurs against a closed tricuspid valve in the presence of atrioventricular dysynchrony. During inspiration, the height of the JVP normally declines while the amplitude of the pulsations increases.

In Kussmaul's sign, inspiration leads to a paradoxical *rise* in the height of the JVP with inspiration; it is seen frequently in chronic constrictive pericarditis and may also occur in congestive heart failure and tricuspid stenosis. A positive abdominojugular reflux augments already elevated right-sided pressures (as might be seen in RV failure or tricuspid regurgitation) and leads to a sustained elevation in the jugular venous column. Interestingly, an elevated JVP and Kussmaul's sign have been shown to be sensitive indicators for the bedside diagnosis of RV infarction.[2]

REFERENCES

1. Swartz, M.H.: Jugular venous pressure pulse: Its value in cardiac diagnosis. Primary Cardiol. 8:197, 1982.
2. Dell'italia, L.J., Sterling, M.R., and O'Rourke, R.A.: Physical examination for exclusion of hemodynamically important right ventricular infarction. Ann. Intern. Med. 99:608, 1983.

56 A-T, B-T, C-T, D-F, E-T   *(Braunwald, pp. 179–180; Table 6–2)*

The Registry for the Society for Cardiac Angiography has reported the incidence of various complications in 53,581 patients undergoing cardiac catheterization over a 14-month period beginning October, 1979.[1] The overall death rate was 0.14 per cent, the rate of acute MI was 0.07 per cent, and the greatest incidence of death occurred in patients under 1 year of age (1.75 per cent). Coronary angiography led to a mortality of 0.86 per cent in patients with significant left main coronary artery disease, in contrast to zero in patients with normal coronary arteries. The mortality rate was also increased in patients over 60 (0.25 per cent). Other patient characteristics that have been associated with an increased mortality from catheterization include elevated functional class and valvular heart disease (especially if coexisting with CAD, left ventricular dysfunction, or severe noncardiac disease). Of note, patients with an LV ejection fraction < 30 per cent have a risk of death more than ten times those with a normal ejection fraction. Strict attention to technique, use of low volumes of radiographic contrast medium, and careful therapeutic intervention when arrhythmias or abnormal hemodynamics occur all may help minimize morbidity and mortality from the procedure.

REFERENCE

1. Kennedy, J.W.: Complications associated with cardiac catheterization and angiography. Cathet. Cardiovasc. Diagn. 8: 5, 1982.

57 A-T, B-F, C-T, D-F, E-T   *(Braunwald, p. 32)*

Analysis of the second heart sound, which is composed of the "aortic" component and the "pulmonic" component (contributed by closure of the aortic pulmonic valves, respectively) may provide a great deal of diagnostic information. Splitting of the second heart sound primarily results from a delay in the pulmonic component owing to an inspiratory increase in the capacitance of the pulmonary vascular bed.[1] A smaller contribution to splitting during inspiration is made by the slight decrease in left ventricular volume during inspiration, which allows left ventricular emptying to reach completion at a slightly earlier time. The amplitude of the aortic component of the second heart sound is usually greater because of the higher systemic arterial closing pressure. The frequency compositions of the two components of the second heart sound are quite similar. Therefore, splitting of the second heart sound is best heard in the second left intercostal space, where the pulmonic component may be best appreciated. Whereas the softer pulmonic component is usually confined to the second left intercostal space, the louder aortic component may be appreciated at the sternal border, base and apex.

REFERENCE

1. Shaver, J.A., Nadolny, R.A., O'Toole, J.D., et al.: Sound-pressure correlates of the second heart sound. Circulation 49:316, 1974.

58 A-T, B-F, C-T, D-T, E-T   *(Braunwald, pp. 153 and 157)*

The conventional criterion for ECG diagnosis of ischemia (0.1 mV ST-segment depression) was standardized postexercise and does not necessarily apply to tracings recorded during exercise. However, some authors have proposed that during exercise greater degrees of ST-segment depression ($\geq$0.2 mV), perhaps proportional to heart rate, are more specific for ischemia.[1] During normal exercise there is frequently J-point depression, but this is associated with an upsloping ST segment. Because of the large coronary vasodilator reserve which normally exists, patients with a 50 per cent stenosis are unlikely to develop characteristic symptoms or ECG changes. The normal peak-pressure product (HR $\times$ systolic BP) is 20,000 to 35,000 mm Hg $\times$ beats/min. Heart rate is linearly related to cardiac output and hence to exercise capacity. As maximal aerobic capacity is approached, heart rate approaches a plateau just as oxygen consumption does. Maximal heart rate decreases linearly with age over 20.[2]

REFERENCES

1. Hlatky, M.A., Pryor, D.B., Harrell, F.E., Jr., et al.: Factors affecting sensitivity and specificity of exercise electrocardiography. Am. J. Med. 77:64, 1984.
2. Gould, F.L., Nordstrom, L.A., Nelson, R.R., et al.: The rate-pressure product as an index of myocardial oxygen consumption during exercise in patients with angina pectoris. Circulation 57:549, 1978.

59 A-T, B-F, C-T, D-T, E-F   *(Braunwald, pp. 297, and 299–301)*

Both first-pass and equilibrium angiography provide reliable measures of global function. However, equilibrium techniques, which yield high counts by virtue of "gating" strategies, provide greater spatial resolution and accuracy for regional wall motion abnormalities. Thus, alterations in systolic function in response to inotropes or vasodilators maintained over several minutes can be assessed using an equilibrium study. On the other hand, rapid changes in left ventricular function are better assessed by first-pass techniques, which require only five or six cardiac cycles, in contrast to at least 2 minutes for gated studies. Furthermore, because a radiopharmaceutical must be administered each time for a first-pass study, background counts and radiation dosage limits preclude serial studies.

60 A-F, B-T, C-T, D-T, E-T   *(Braunwald, pp. 482, 484)*

Although almost any arrhythmia may be caused by digitalis toxicity, some are seen more frequently in therapy with this drug, and/or may be a more specific sign of toxicity. Atrial tachycardia with block may be caused by excess digitalis but is equally likely to occur in the setting of underlying heart disease without digitalis toxicity. The rhythm must be distinguished from atrial flutter, and because the amplitude of the atrial depolarization may be low, this rhythm is sometimes quite difficult to recognize. A nonparoxysmal junction tachycardia may be highly specific for digitalis excess,[1] although the less common causes of this rhythm must be excluded, including acute myocardial infarction, open heart surgery, general anesthesia, and myocarditis. The term "nonparoxysmal" refers to the gradual appearance and disappearance of the rhythm. The majority of patients with this arrhythmia demonstrate AV dissociation due to the acceleration of the AV junctional pacemaker.

AV dissociation appearing in the course of digitalis therapy must be considered a sign of digitalis intoxication until proven otherwise. The most common manifestation of excess digitalis is the appearance of ventricular premature contractions (VPCs). However, because these are morphologically identical to VPCs of other causes, they are not highly specific for digitalis toxicity. When ventricular bigeminy occurs, the presence of VPCs with varying morphology is suggestive of digitalis excess. Some ventricular tachycardias are also more suggestive of digitalis toxicity. These include ventricular tachycardia with exit block and a bidirectional ventricular tachycardia. AV conduction delay and an accelerated junctional escape both may be due to an excess of digitalis as well.

REFERENCE

1. Pick, A., and Dominiquez, P.: Nonparoxysmal AV nodal tachycardia. Circulation 16:1022, 1957.

61 A-T, B-T, C-T, D-T   *(Braunwald, p. 7; Fig. 1–2; Table 1–2)*

Chest pain or discomfort may arise from a variety of cardiac and noncardiac structures, either intrathoracic or subdiaphragmatic in location. The history is the single most important mode of examination providing data for the differential diagnosis of chest pain.[1] The chest discomfort of pulmonary hypertension may be caused by dilatation of the pulmonary arteries, acute pulmonary embolism, or right ventricular ischemia and may be identical to that of typical angina.[2] A lower esophageal tear due to protracted vomiting (the Mallory-Weiss syndrome) may elicit a chest pain syndrome that is difficult to distinguish from acute MI without a careful history. The thoracic outlet, or scalenus anticus syndrome, is an uncommon cause of chest or arm discomfort due to compression of the neurovascular bundle by a cervical rib or the anterior scalenus muscle. Paresthesias may occur along the ulnar distribution of the forearm in this syndrome and may be confused with angina despite the non-exertional nature of the pain. Congenital absence of the pericardium is a rare anomaly that may produce fleeting chest pain precipitated by lying on the left side and relieved by changing position. While difficult, the diagnosis may be made by standard chest roentgenography.[3]

REFERENCES

1. Walsh, R.A., and O'Rourke, R.A.: Clues to the evaluation of chest pain in the patient's history. Pract. Cardiol. 4:41, 1978.
2. Viar, W.M., and Harrison, T.R.: Chest pain in association with pulmonary hypertension; its similarity to the pain of coronary disease. Circulation 5:1, 1952.
3. Glover, L.B., Barcia, A., and Reeves, T.J.: Congenital absence of the pericardium. Am. J. Roentgenol. 82:125, 1959.

62 A-T, B-F, C-T, D-T, E-T   (Braunwald, p. 165)

Patients with chronic ischemic heart disease are excellent candidates for functional assessment before coronary angiography, which should be completed in subjects who do not have a contraindication for the test. The presence of excellent exercise tolerance is highly predictive of an excellent prognosis. The predictive value of this functional assessment was well supported in the CASS study,[1] in which a high-risk patient subset unable to complete Bruce stage I and demonstrating ST-segment depression had an annual mortality of 5 per cent or more per year. Conversely, in the same study, patients who exercised into Bruce stage III with a normal exercise ECG had an annual mortality of <1 per cent over the subsequent 4 years, regardless of the underlying coronary anatomy. Silent myocardial ischemia in patients with documented coronary artery disease predicts an increased risk of subsequent cardiac events. In the CASS databank, 7-year survival was similar in patients stratified by anatomy and ventricular function, regardless of the presence of silent or symptomatic exercise-induced ECG changes. In the Duke data bank, the presence of symptoms tended to predict more severe coronary artery disease and a worse 5-year survival.[3] Differences in these series include a prior history of angina in all patients in the Duke series as compared to 65 per cent of the CASS series and a higher prevalence of prior myocardial infarction in the CASS study.

REFERENCES

1. Weiner, D.A., Ryan, T.J., McCabe, C.H., et al.: Prognostic importance of a clinical profile and exercise test in medically treated patients with coronary artery disease. J. Am. Coll. Cardiol. 3:772, 1984.
2. Weiner, D.A., Ryan, T.J., McCabe, C.H., et al.: Significance of silent myocardial ischemia during exercise testing in patients with coronary artery disease. Am. J. Cardiol. 59:725, 1987.
3. Mark, D.B., Hlatky, M.A., Califf, R.M., et al.: Painless exercise ST deviation on the treadmill: Long-term prognosis. J. Am. Coll. Cardiol. 14:885, 1989.

63 A-F, B-F, C-F, D-F, E-T   (Braunwald, pp. 167–168)

A number of cardiac arrhythmias and conduction disturbances are noted during exercise testing. Approximately 20 per cent of patients with known heart disease and 50 to 75 per cent of those who have had sudden cardiac death will have repetitive ventricular beats induced by exercise protocols. Exercise-induced ventricular arrhythmias are found more frequently during recovery, in part because catecholamine responses to exercise continue to increase several minutes after exercise when vagal tone is high.[1] Exercise testing adds valuable information in the assessment of patients with ventricular rhythm disturbances, even if ambulatory monitoring and electrophysiological studies have been performed.[2] The test may be used to evaluate patients for drug toxicity and for the general ability of the chosen agent to control the rhythm disturbance, as well as to detect supraventricular arrhythmias. While supraventricular premature beats may be induced by exercise in up to 10 per cent of normal subjects, and up to 40 per cent of patients with known heart disease, a sustained supraventricular tachycardia occurs in only 1 or 2 per cent of patients. No apparent correlation exists between the presence of such arrhythmias and underlying ischemic heart disease. In patients with atrial fibrillation, the underlying cardiac disease often determines exercise capacity and therefore better ventricular rate control does not necessarily lead to a significant increase in exercise capacity. In patients with sick sinus syndrome, a lower heart rate during exercise is often noted in comparison to normal subjects. However, 40 to 50 per cent of such patients will have a normal heart rate response to exercise. In patients with identified atrioventricular block, exercise testing may allow some determination of the need for AV sequential pacing. Exercise can occasionally bring out a more advanced AV block in such subjects as well.

REFERENCES

1. Sokoloff, N.M., Spielman, S.R., Greenspan, A.M., et al.: Plasma norepinephrine in exercise-induced ventricular tachycardia. J. Am. Coll. Cardiol. 8:11, 1986.
2. Podrid, P.J., Venditti, F.J., Levine, P.A., and Klein, M.D.: The role of exercise testing in evaluation of arrhythmias. Am. J. Cardiol. 62:24H, 1988.

64 A-T, B-T, C-T, D-F   (Braunwald, pp. 30–31)

Ejection sounds are high-frequency "clicks" that occur in early systole. They may be either aortic or pulmonic in origin, require a mobile valve for their generation, and begin at the exact time of maximal opening of the semilunar valve in question.[1] If the valve is abnormal, as is frequently the case, the ejection sound is "valvular," and it is generally accepted that halting of the "doming" valve generates the sound. If the valve associated with the ejection sound is normal, it is called a "vascular" ejection sound; the origin of the sound is not clearly defined. In either case, the ejection sound starts at the moment of full opening of the aortic (0.12 to 0.14 sec after the Q wave on the ECG) or pulmonic (0.09 to 0.11 sec after the Q wave) valve. In valvular pulmonic stenosis, the ejection sound is loudest during expiration. With inspiration, increased venous return augments atrial systole and results in partial opening of the pulmonic wave before ventricular systole commences. In contrast, with expiration, the pulmonic valve opens quickly from a fully closed position, generating a louder ejection sound from the sudden halt to the valve's opening movement.[1]

REFERENCE

1. Mills, P.G., Brodie, B., McLaurin, L.P., et al.: Echocardiographic and hemodynamic relationships of ejection sounds. Circulation 56:430, 1977.

65 A-F, B-F, C-F, D-T, E-T *(Braunwald, p. 118; Fig. 4–13)*

While ECG abnormalities may be seen in the majority of episodes of pulmonary embolism, the most common abnormalities are nonspecific, such as T-wave changes and ST-segment elevation or depression. The ECG proves to be normal in between 6 and 23 per cent of patients, depending upon the severity of the embolism.[1] Acute pulmonary hypertension may lead to both right ventricular and right atrial dilatation, as well as hypoxia and even myocardial ischemia, and it is these pathophysiological abnormalities that lead to the electrocardiographic manifestations of the disorder. The classic $S_1Q_3T_3$ pattern that describes changes in the three limb leads is seen in only 25 per cent of patients. Acute atrial pressure and volume changes may lead to atrial dilatation; this along with myocardial ischemia is believed to be responsible for the common occurrence of atrial arrhythmias in pulmonary embolism. It is important to obtain serial ECG tracings for comparative purposes from patients with suspected pulmonary embolism; this allows for more sensitive evaluation of the ECG abnormalities that may arise during such an event.

REFERENCE

1. National Comparative Study: The urokinase-pulmonary embolism trial. Circulation 47(Suppl. II):1, 1973.

66 A-F, B-F, C-T, D-T, E-T *(Braunwald, pp. 117–118; Fig. 4–12)*

Much like left ventricular hypertrophy, the ECG pattern of RVH is relatively specific, but also relatively insensitive, despite the criteria used.[1] The QRS pattern in lead V_1 may be helpful in both diagnosing RVH and in suggesting the underlying pathophysiology. Three principal patterns for the QRS pattern in lead V_1 are described. These include the type "A" variant, or a dominant "R" wave (qR, rR, rsR'); the RS variant (Rs, Rsr'); and the rS or rsr' complex. When right ventricular pressure is equal to or greater than left ventricular pressure, the type A or dominant R wave variant is commonly seen. More specifically, when systolic pressure in the right ventricle exceeds that in the left ventricle, a qR pattern is more common, as in severe pulmonary stenosis or pulmonary hypertension. Relative equivalence between right and left ventricular systolic pressures, as in tetralogy of Fallot or the Eisenmenger complex, may lead to an R or rR pattern in V_1. When right ventricular systolic pressure remains less than that in the left ventricle, but RVH intervenes, an incomplete right bundle branch block (rsR') pattern may appear, as in atrial septal defect.

ST-segment depression and T-wave inversion in lead V_1 and occasionally V_2 may accompany RVH and are consistent with moderate to severe elevations in right ventricular pressure. Right-axis deviation alone is sometimes used to suggest the presence of RVH but is a less sensitive criterion. Similarly, an R/S ratio greater than 1 in lead V_1 alone may be seen in situations besides RVH, including posterior infarction and occasionally as a normal variant. The combination of right-axis deviation, prominent R wave in V_1, and an R/S ratio ≥ 1 in V_1 is highly specific for underlying RVH.

REFERENCE

1. Surawicz, B.: Electrocardiographic diagnosis of chamber enlargement. J. Am. Coll. Cardiol. 8:714, 1986.

67 A-T, B-T, C-T, D-F *(Braunwald, p. 195)*

Pressure tracing recordings at cardiac catheterization remain the "gold standard" for diagnosis of hypertrophic obstructive cardiomyopathy (HCM). In the tracing provided, a large gradient between the body of the left ventricle (LVB) and the root of the aorta (Ao) is seen on the left of the tracing. As the catheter is withdrawn into the LV outflow tract (LVOT), the gradient is no longer present and the diagnosis is confirmed, while that of *valvular* aortic stenosis is excluded. The bifid aortic pulse contour with a characteristic notch on the upstroke and a rapid initial upstroke of the LVB tracing is also demonstrated. This is in marked contrast to the slow and delayed rise in the aortic pressure pulse in valvular aortic stenosis.

In HCM, left ventricular diastolic dysfunction is often present; this may lead to a prominent *a* wave and an elevation of left ventricular end-diastolic pressure. Interestingly, recent studies of LV diastolic function in this condition have identified abnormalities in both LV distensibility and relaxation leading to impaired diastolic filling.[1] Although controversial, many investigators believe that the outflow tract gradient in HCM results from true mechanical impedance to ejection by anterior movement of the mitral valve across the outflow tract and subsequent contact of the valve with the ventricular septum in early systole.[2]

REFERENCES

1. Maron, B.J., et al.: Hypertrophic cardiomyopathy. N. Engl. J. Med. *316*:780, 1987.
2. Moro, E., tenCate, F.J., Leonard, J.J., et al.: Genesis of systolic anterior motion of the mitral valve in hypertrophic cardiomyopathy: An anatomical or dynamic event? Eur. Heart J. *8*:1312, 1987.

68 A-T, B-F, C-T, D-F, E-T *(Braunwald, p. 38; Figs. 2–31 and 2–32)*

Holosystolic murmurs begin with the first heart sound and continue throughout systole up to the component of the second sound generated from the side of origin of the murmur. The flow of blood from a chamber or vessel whose pressure or resistance is higher than the pressure or resistance of the recipient chamber throughout systole generates a holosystolic murmur. Murmurs caused by mitral and tricuspid regurgitation are classic examples of such murmurs. A holosystolic murmur may also be generated from a restrictive ventricular septal defect and from a communication between the great arteries, such as an aortopulmonary window or patent ductus arteriosus, provided that the elevated pulmonary vascular resistance eliminates any diastolic flow (murmur). In other words, when the pulmonary vascular resistance is high enough to prevent the diastolic portion of a continuous murmur, a murmur that sounds holosystolic is present.[1]

In murmurs of mitral regurgitation, the direction of radiation of the intraatrial jet may determine the location of the murmur for auscultation.[2] If the intraatrial jet is forward and medial against the atrial septum, the murmur may radiate to the left sternal edge and even into the neck. In contrast, when the intraatrial jet is directed posterolaterally into the left atrial cavity, the murmur may radiate to the axilla, left scapula, and occasionally even to the vertebral column of the spine (see Braunwald, Fig. 2–32, p. 39). When right ventricular systolic pressures are elevated, the murmur of tricuspid regurgitation becomes holosystolic. In such instances, an increase in the loudness of the murmur with inspiration is an important finding and is known as Carvallo's sign.[3] This occurs because the inspiratory increase in right ventricular volume results in an increase in right ventricular stroke volume and in the velocity of regurgitant tricuspid flow. Carvallo's sign is lost during right ventricular failure, in which the inspiratory increase in stroke volume and regurgitant flow velocity is comprised. In an uncomplicated ventricular septal defect, the left ventricular systolic pressure and systemic resistance exceed right ventricular systolic pressure and pulmonary resistance throughout the duration of systole. In such situations, a holosystolic murmur is also generated.

REFERENCES

1. Perloff, J.K.: The Clinical Recognition of Congenital Heart Disease. Philadelphia, W.B. Saunders Co., 1987.
2. Perloff, J.K., and Harvey, W.P.: Auscultatory and phonocardiographic manifestations of pure mitral regurgitation. Prog. Cardiovasc. Dis. *5*:172, 1962.
3. Rivero-Carvallo, J.M.: Sitno para el diagnostico de las insuficiencies tricuspidas. Arch. Inst. Cardiol. Mexico *16*:531, 1946.

69 A-T, B-T, C-F, D-F, E-T *(Braunwald, pp. 40–41; Fig. 2–35)*

Systolic arterial murmurs are heard at nonprecordial sites due to increases in flow in a normal artery or because of turbulent flow in a diseased artery. The supraclavicular systolic murmur (see Braunwald, Fig. 2–35, p. 40) is a murmur that is often heard in normal children and adolescents and is believed to originate in the brachiocephalic arteries.[1] These murmurs may be made to decrease or vanish when the shoulders are hyperextended by bringing the elbows back until the shoulder girdle muscles are taut. In older adults, the common cause of a systolic arterior murmur is turbulence due to narrowing of the carotid, subclavian, and/or iliofemoral arteries by atherosclerosis. When aortic regurgitation exists, compression of the femoral artery generates a systolic murmur that may continue into diastole if further compression is applied. In this case, the systolic and diastolic sounds originate from the compression itself, which is an extrinsic cause of flow irregularity analogous to but distinct from that caused by the intraluminal changes of atherosclerosis. Finally, in coarctation of the aorta, a systolic arterial murmur may be present and heard most prominently between the scapulae at a site corresponding to the site of the coarctation itself.

REFERENCE

1. Nelson, W.P., and Hall, R.J.: The innocent supraclavicular arterial bruit—utility of shoulder maneuvers in its recognition. N. Engl. J. Med. *278*:778, 1968.

70 A-T, B-T, C-T, D-T *(Braunwald, pp. 112–113)*

The heart may be considered to maintain two axes—an anteroposterior axis, which defines whether the apex of the heart faces the left arm (horizontal) or the left foot (vertical), and a longitudinal, apex-to-base axis, which defines whether the left ventricle is anterior or posterior. The direction of rotation for the latter axis is described by viewing the heart from a position below the diaphragm. Clockwise rotation results in a more posterior position of the left ventricle and the right ventricular QRS complex (rS) is displaced to the left precordial leads. Counterclockwise rotation results in a more anterior shift of the left ventricle, and the left ventricular QRS (qR) pattern is observed in the right precordial leads.

71 A-F, B-T, C-T, D-F, E-F   *(Braunwald,*
pp. 132–133)

Although LBBB may obscure ischemia and infarction, a number of criteria are specific and predictive for myocardial infarction. These include a
Q wave in at least two leads aV_1, I, V_5, V_6; R-wave
regression from leads V_1 through V_4; notching of
the S wave in at least two leads V_3 through V_6; primary ST-T changes in two or more adjacent leads.[1]
In addition, studies of patients during angioplasty
reveal that coronary occlusion in the presence of
LBBB results in ST-segment elevation over the ischemic area. A recent analysis of patients enrolled
in the GUSTO-1 trial who had LBBB and anterior
MI revealed three ECG criteria for acute MI that had
independent diagnostic value. These included ST-
segment elevation of 1 mm or more that was concordant with the QRS complex; ST-segment depression of 1 mm or more in lead V_1, V_2, or V_3; and
ST-segment elevation of 5 mm or more that was
discordant with the QRS complex.[2]

An abnormal U wave is often a marker of underlying ischemic heart disease. For example, negative
or biphasic U waves are present in up to 30
per cent of patients with chronic stable angina. The
appearance of a negative U wave during exercise-
induced ischemia is highly specific for disease of
the left anterior descending coronary artery.[3] In addition, the appearance of a negative U wave may
be one of the earliest findings of evolving myocardial infarction. In one large study that correlated
myocardial infarction patterns on ECG with findings on autopsy, the sensitivity and specificity of
the Q wave on the electrocardiogram were 61 and
89 per cent, respectively.[4] The presence of any anterior or inferior Q wave proved to be falsely positive in 46 per cent of subjects. However, when diagnostic criteria for the Q wave were stricter and
included a duration >0.03 sec, or Q waves in more
than one "electrocardiographic zone," only 4 per
cent were false-positive. The sensitivity for diagnosis of infarction by Q-wave criterion was lowest
in the lateral basal portion of the left ventricle, an
area explored by leads I and aV_1.

In general, RBBB does not alter the diagnosis of
myocardial infarction, since the initial activation of
the ventricle is normal. In rare instances, the onset
of RBBB has allowed unmasking of a previously
undetected infarction in anteroseptal territories.[5]

REFERENCES

1. Hands, M.E., Cook, E.F., Stone, P.H., et al.: Electrocardiographic diagnosis of myocardial infarction in the presence
   of complete left bundle branch block. Am. Heart J. *116*:
   23, 1988.
2. Sgarbossa, E.B., Pinski, S.L., et al.: Electrocardiographic diagnosis of evolving acute myocardial infarction in the
   presence of left bundle-branch block. N. Engl. J. Med. *33*:
   481–487, 1996.
3. Gerson, M.C., Phillips, J.F., Morris, S.N., and McHenry, P.L.:
   Exercise-induced U wave inversion as a marker of stenosis
   of the left anterior descending coronary artery. Circulation
   60:1014, 1979.
4. Horan, L.G., Flowers, N.C., and Johnson, J.C.: Significance
   of the diagnostic Q wave of myocardial infarction. Circulation *43*:428, 1971.
5. Rosenbaum, M.B., Girotti, L.A., Lazzari, J.O., et al.: Abnormal Q waves in right sided chest leads provoked by onset
   of right bundle branch block in patients with anteroseptal
   infarction. Br. Heart J. *47*:227, 1982.

72 A-T, B-T, C-T, D-F   *(Braunwald, pp. 193–195;*
Figs. 6–12 and 6–13)

The pioneering work of Gorlin and Gorlin[1] has
provided equations using measured pressure gradient and flow across the stenotic valve that allow
for calculation of valve orifice area by the following
formula:

$$\text{Valve area} = F/K \times (P)^{1/2}$$

where F is flow in ml/sec, P is the mean pressure
gradient in mm Hg across the orifice, and K is an
empirical constant for the valve in question.

There are assumptions and potential pitfalls in
determination of valve area by catheterization techniques.[2] Since flow in the Gorlin equation is as-
sumed to be systemic (forward) cardiac output, the
presence of valvular regurgitation results in a
falsely low value for transvalvular flow in the Gorlin equation. The valve area calculated is falsely
low. Thus, in measuring the valve area of a stenotic
orifice, the calculated valve area represents the
lower limit of the true valve area, since any coexisting regurgitation would provide for a larger flow
than the calculated cardiac output used as F in the
equation above.

In calculations of mitral valve area, a confirmed
pulmonary capillary wedge pressure may be sub-
stituted for left atrial pressure. This confirmation
requires that (1) the measured mean wedge pressure is lower than the mean pulmonary artery pressure, and (2) the blood drawn from a wedged catheter has an O_2 saturation ≥ 95 per cent (or at least
equal in saturation to arterial blood).

Accurate and simultaneous determinations of
cardiac output and mean pressure gradient are essential in the determination of a stenotic orifice
area. Both the cardiac output and mean pressure
gradient measurements are subject to error. Since
the square root of the mean pressure gradient is
used in the Gorlin formula, the valve area calculation is more strongly influenced by errors in the
cardiac output determination than in the mean gradient measurement.

REFERENCES

1. Gorlin, R., and Gorlin, G.: Hydraulic formula for calculation
   of area of stenotic mitral valve, other valves, and central
   circulatory shunts. Am. Heart J. *41*:1, 1951.
2. Kolansky, D.M., Hirshfeld, J.W.: Valve function: Stenosis
   and regurgitation. In Pepine, C.J., Hill, J.A., and Lambert,
   C.R. (eds.): Diagnostic and Therapeutic Catheterization.
   2nd ed. Baltimore, Williams & Wilkins, 1994, pp. 443–
   467.

73 A-T, B-T, C-T, D-F *(Braunwald, pp. 281–282)*

In the normal scintigram (*A*) there is homogeneous distribution of tracer in the apical and apical-inferior segments, in which activity can normally be slightly lower. In the abnormal scintigram (*B*), inferior and apical defects are seen on the initial anterior (ANT) view and septal and apical-inferior defects on the initial left anterior oblique (LAO) view. There is complete redistribution into the septal and apical-inferior segments (transient defect), partial redistribution into the inferior segment, and no redistribution into the apical defect (persistent defect). When an increase in lung activity is observed, it correlates both with increased pulmonary capillary wedge pressure and multivessel disease.

The images can be evaluated as follows: (1) a reversible or transient defect corresponds to transient ischemia; (2) an irreversible defect, interpreted as scar, corresponds to prior infarct (segments involving the apex can normally have reduced activity because of myocardial thinning and must be interpreted with caution); and (3) normal anatomical variations such as apical thinning and decreased perfusion at the base as occurs with the aortic and mitral valves.

74 A-F, B-T, C-T, D-T, E-F *(Braunwald, pp. 129–130)*

One of the most important uses of the 12-lead ECG is in establishing the diagnosis of a myocardial infarction (MI) and following its evolution. Classic or "diagnostic" changes of MI are seen in 60 per cent of patients upon presentation, while nondiagnostic changes will be seen in approximately 25 per cent and a normal ECG is present in the remaining 15 per cent. Several explanations for a normal initial ECG are possible, including a delay in the evolution of the characteristic pattern, a small infarct or one that is obscured electrocardiographically, or transient normalization of the ECG as evolution of the MI proceeds. However, serial ECGs make the diagnostic specificity of the test quite high, and form a cornerstone of diagnosis of MI.

The classic evolution of MI on ECG begins with T-wave abnormalities and is followed by ST-segment changes (elevation in areas of injury), and only subsequently by the appearance of Q waves. Q waves may occur within the first hours of an infarction or may not evolve for 1 or 2 days. ST-segment depression may be a reflection of subendocardial ischemia or may be due to "reciprocal" changes secondary to infarction at a different site.[1,2] Current evidence suggests that the ST-segment depression in anterior precordial leads in the presence of an inferior or posterolateral MI is the result of changes that are proportional to the severity of ischemia in the primary distribution rather than ischemia in the anterior myocardium.[3] Recent review of the data from the GUSTO trials has yielded further prognostic information regarding precordial ST-segment depression in the setting of inferior MI. Patients with precordial ST-segment depression had larger MIs, more complications, and higher mortality than those who did not.[4,5] In addition, the early mortality increased by 36 per cent for every 0.5 mV of precordial ST-segment depression in this study.[4]

REFERENCES

1. Becker, R.C., and Alpert, J.S.: Electrocardiographic ST segment depression in coronary artery disease. Am. Heart J. *115*:862, 1988.
2. Kracoff, O.S., Adelman, A.G., Marquis, J.F., et al.: Twelve lead electrocardiogram recording during percutaneous transluminal coronary angioplasty. J. Electrocardiol. *23*:191, 1990.
3. Sato, H., Kodama, K., Masuyama, T., et al.: Right coronary artery occlusion: Its role in the mechanism of precordial ST segment depression. J. Am. Coll. Cardiol. *14*:297, 1989.
4. Peterson, E.D., Hathaway, K., Zabel, M., et al.: Prognostic significance of precordial ST segment depression during inferior myocardial infarction in the thrombolytic era: Results in 16,521 patients. J. Am. Coll. Cardiol. *28*:305, 1996.
5. Birnbaum, Y., Herz, I., Sclarovsky, S., et al.: Prognostic significance of precordial ST segment depression on admission electrocardiogram in patients with inferior wall myocardial infarction. J. Am. Coll. Cardiol. *28*:313, 1996.

75 A-F, B-F, C-T, D-T *(Braunwald, pp. 141–142; Fig. 4–51)*

A series of characteristic changes in the electrocardiogram are noted in hyperkalemia, although the correlation between plasma potassium levels in each of these changes is not strictly reliable. The earliest ECG abnormality in hyperkalemia is peaking of the T wave in a symmetrical and "tented" manner (see Braunwald, Fig. 4–51, p. 141). Peaked T waves are usually best seen in inferior and right precordial leads. The *shape* of the T wave is probably more characteristic of hyperkalemia than is the absolute *height* of the complex. As the potassium continues to increase, a series of changes may occur, including a decrease in the amplitude of the R wave, appearance of a prominent S wave, depression of the ST segment, and a series of changes in the P wave and P-R interval. These latter changes include a decrease in the height of the P wave, prolongation of P-wave duration, and lengthening of the P-R interval. In addition, hyperkalemia may directly depress intraventricular conduction and, combined with the changes just described, lead to patterns of right bundle branch block, left bundle branch block, left anterior or posterior fascicular block, or any combination of these.

By contrast, hypokalemia is characterized by a gradual depression of the ST segment, a decrease in the height of the T wave, and the appearance of a prominent U wave. The Q-T interval itself, however, does not change significantly (see Fig. 4–51). Prominent U waves may also be observed in ventricular hypertrophy and are not of pathophysiological significance.

76 A-T, B-T, C-T, D-F *(Braunwald, pp. 339–342; Figs. 10–40 and 10–41)*

Computed tomography (CT) provides distinct visualization of the pericardium based on the presence of the pericardial line, which is probably due to epicardial fat and is less than 4 mm in width. Thus, the presence or absence of pericardium, its thickness and density, and fluid collections outside the pericardium can readily be discerned. CT is particularly useful for differentiating benign from malignant tumors on the basis of density, but mucoid-secreting pericardial cysts have the same density as solid tumors and usually cannot be distinguished. CT can aid in the diagnosis of constrictive pericarditis by documentation of increased pericardial thickness (>4 mm) and coexisting effusions and calcification.[1]

REFERENCE

1. Hackney, D., Mattrey, R., Peck, W.W., et al.: Experimental pericardial inflammation evaluated by computed tomography. Radiology *151*:145, 1984.

77 A-T, B-T, C-T, D-T, E-T *(Braunwald, pp. 135–136; Figs. 4–42 and 4–43)*

A number of disease processes may lead to Q waves on the ECG that are independent of myocardial infarction. The most common cause of so-called noninfarction Q waves is intrinsic myocardial disease as is seen in the myocarditides, infiltrative diseases such as cardiac amyloidosis, neuromuscular disorders such as progressive muscular dystrophy, and the various cardiomyopathies, especially hypertrophic cardiomyopathy[1] (Fig. 4–43). The ECG abnormality in hypertrophic cardiomyopathy is believed to be due to abnormal depolarizations caused by the underlying abnormality in the myocardial structure and/or the increase in septal mass present in the disorder. Chronic pulmonary disease is responsible for a downward displacement of both the diaphragm and the heart, with clockwise rotation, leading to the appearance of a QS complex in anterior leads, which may simulate anterior infarction. The onset of acute cor pulmonale in pulmonary embolism may also lead to abnormal Q waves. A spontaneous pneumothorax may stimulate anterior infarction as well, in part by decreasing or entirely ablating the R wave normally seen in precordial leads. In the Wolff-Parkinson-White syndrome, a negative complex in right precordial leads (type B pattern) may simulate anteroseptal infarction. Other potential causes of noninfarction Q waves include left bundle branch block, severe metabolic disturbances, such as in shock or pancreatitis, and left ventricular hypertrophy.

REFERENCE

1. Pelliccia, F., Cianfrocca, C., Cristofani, R., et al.: Electrocardiographic findings in patients with hypertrophic cardiomyopathy. J. Am. Coll. Cardiol. *23*:213, 1990.

78-A, 79-C, 80-D, 81-B *(Braunwald, pp. 225–227, 232–233 and 235)*

The chest roentgenogram in patients with abnormalities of the mitral valve commonly displays evidence of dilatation of the left atrium, whether the lesion in question is mitral stenosis or mitral regurgitation. The characteristic chest film in mitral stenosis displays a heart that is often normal in size, except for the enlargement of the left atrium, which is more prominent in patients with atrial fibrillation. Extensive calcification of the mitral valve may also be visible on chest films and must be distinguished from calcification of the mitral valve annulus. Severe mitral stenosis commonly occurs with pulmonary hypertension, which may be associated with right ventricular dilatation that is often reflected on the chest roentgenogram. In many patients with progressive mitral stenosis, a sequence of alterations in the pulmonary vascular pattern up to and including frank interstitial edema is seen.

More unusual findings on the chest roentgenogram that are relatively specific for mitral stenosis include calcification of the left atrium, pulmonary hemosiderosis from chronic intraalveolar hemorrhages, and pulmonary ossification, probably also from intraalveolar hemorrhage.

A number of findings may be present on the chest roentgenogram in patients with aortic regurgitation. Enlargement of the left ventrical causing elongation and dilatation of the chest film may be present. This results in displacement of the cardiac apex downward, to the left, and posteriorly. In addition, the ascending aorta may be dilated, and fluoroscopic examination in such cases may reveal an increase in the amplitude of the aortic pulsations. In contrast, aortic stenosis tends to be more difficult to recognize on plain chest films. Abnormalities in the shape of the heart, while sometimes present, tend to be subtle. Significant left ventricular dilatation occurs only with myocardial failure in end-stage aortic stenosis. While calcification of the aortic valve is common in aortic stenosis, it may not be appreciated on routine chest films. Similarly, such routine views may obscure the poststenotic dilatation of the ascending aorta that occurs in this disease.

The ostium secundum type of atrial septal defect is a congenital cardiac lesion commonly seen in adults. This lesion may be difficult to diagnose from chest roentgenograms in younger patients, but as time passes the characteristic findings of the ASD appear. These include dilatation of the main pulmonary artery, enlargement of the right ventricle, and a generalized increase in the pulmonary vascularity. Right atrial enlargement may be present as well. It is usually not possible to distinguish between an ostium primum ASD and an ostium secundum ASD on the plain chest film. Although the chest film in patients with a secundum ASD may be similar to that of the patient with mitral stenosis, in the latter condition there is usually left atrial enlargement and redistribution of pulmonary blood flow with dilatation of upper lobe vessels and constriction of the vessels at the lung bases. In contrast, when significant left-to-right shunting is present in an ASD, all the pulmonary vessels—including those at the bases—are dilated.

The presence of pericardial fluid leads to a characteristic set of changes in the chest roentgenogram. With increasing volumes of pericardial fluid, enlargement of the cardiac silhouette with smoothing out and loss of the normal cardiac contours occurs, leading to a smoothly distended flask-shaped cardiac shadow. While such a pattern may be seen with the generalized dilatation that occurs in heart failure, the appearance of the pulmonary hila distinguishes between these two conditions. In pericardial effusion, the pericardial sac tends to cover the shadows of the hilar vessels as it is further distended. In contrast, the failing heart is usually associated with abnormally prominent hilar vessels in the setting of pulmonary vascular congestion. In some instances displacement of the epicardial fat line may be visible, a sign that is pathognomonic of pericardial effusion.

82-C, 83-E, 84-A, 85-B, 86-A *(Braunwald, pp. 361, 367–369; Figs. 12–1 and 12–3)*

Titin, also called connectin, is a third myofibrillar protein in addition to actin and myosin. The largest protein yet described, it performs two known functions in the sarcomere. It acts to anchor myosin to the Z line and, as it stretches, it helps to explain the stress-strain elastic characteristics of striated muscle. It has both an inextensible segment that binds to myosin, and an elastic segment that stretches as the sarcomere extends (see Braunwald, Fig. 12–4, p. 364).

The ryanodine receptor is a complex structure that functions as the calcium release channel in the sarcoplasmic reticulum. Part of the ryanodine receptor, known as the foot structure, extends from the sarcoplasmic reticulum and is in contact with the adjacent T tubule. When an action potential occurs, the voltage-gated calcium channels in the sarcolemma open and calcium enters the cardiac myocyte. The cytosolic calcium causes a conformational change in the foot structure of the ryanodine receptor, which results in opening of the calcium release channel and extrusion of calcium ion into the myocyte cytosol (see Braunwald, Fig. 12–10, p. 367).

The sarcoplasmic reticulum is the structure in cardiac myocytes that stores calcium ions for release into the cytosol during a cardiac action potential. Calcium ion is stored in the highly charged protein, calsequestrin. Calsequestrin is found primarily in the areas of the sarcoplasmic reticulum close to the T tubules. Another calcium storage protein, calrectulin, is similar in structure and, likely, in function to calsequestrin.

Following an action potential, calcium ions are removed from the cytosol into the sarcoplasmic reticulum by a calcium pump known as the calcium-pumping ATPase of the SR, or SERCA. This pump moves two molecules of calcium for each molecule of ATP hydrolyzed. Found in a 1:1 relationship with SERCA is a regulatory protein known as phospholamban. Phospholamban has an inhibitory affect on SERCA. The inhibition of SERCA by phospholamban can be diminished by its phosphorylation by a number of protein kinases (see Braunwald, Fig. 12–12, p. 368).

87-E, 88-A, 89-B, 90-C *(Braunwald, pp. 22, 1049–1050)*

Chronic, severe AR may lead to a variety of characteristic physical signs, most of which have eponyms. In each instance these physical findings arise as a direct consequence of the widened pulse pressure that characterizes AR. The most predictive such sign is *Duroziez's sign*,[1] demonstrated by placing a stethoscope over the femoral artery in the groin and applying first proximal and then distal pressure to hear, respectively, a systolic murmur and then a diastolic one. Placing a stethoscope over the femoral artery may also reveal the "pistol shot" sounds described by *Traube*. The exaggerated pulse pressure of AR may lead to transmission of a visible bobbing pulsation to the entire head with each heartbeat, known as *de Musset's sign*. *Hill's sign*, a systolic pressure in the legs that is >20 mm Hg of that in the arms, usually indicates the presence of AR. *Quincke's pulse* or *sign*, which was not described above, is the alternating blanching and flushing of the skin as observed, for instance, in the nail beds, in response to wide swings in arterial pulse pressure.[2] While it is most commonly seen in patients with AR, it is rarely observed in normal subjects with vasodilation as well.

REFERENCES

1. Rowe, G.G., et al.: The mechanism of the production of Duroziez's murmur. N. Engl. J. Med. *272*:1207, 1965.
2. Sapira, J.D.: Quincke, de Musset, Duroziez, and Hill: Some aortic regurgitations. South Med. J. *74*:459, 1981.

91-A, 92-C, 93-B, 94-E, 95-D *(Braunwald, pp. 258–265; Figs. 8–29, 8–31)*

Coronary arteriography remains the benchmark by which the coronary anatomy and circulation may be assessed. Coronary artery spasm may be due to organic disease or may be induced by the mechanical stimulation of the coronary artery by the catheter tip. In 1 to 3 per cent of patients who do not receive vasodilators (e.g., nitroglycerin) prior to arteriography, spasm may be seen.[1] While the major coronary arteries usually pass along the epicardial surface of the heart, occasional short segments pass down into the myocardium, leading to myocardial bridging, as demonstrated in example

A above. Edwards et al. identified such bridging in 5.4 per cent of human hearts at autopsy.[2] Angiographic identification of a myocardial bridge usually occurs in the LAD artery.

Intercoronary collaterals in the interventricular septum are normally <1 mm in diameter, are characterized by moderate tortuosity, and tend to serve as connections between numerous septal branches of the LAD and smaller posterior septal branches that arise from the posterior descending artery. Recruitment and development of such collaterals due to occlusion of the LAD artery are demonstrated in *B* above.

The most prevalent hemodynamically significant congenital coronary artery anomaly is the coronary arteriovenous fistula. When the fistula drains into any of several areas—the coronary sinus, SVC, pulmonary artery, or a right-sided cardiac chamber—a left-to-right shunt is created. Seen in infancy and childhood, approximately half of such patients develop symptoms of CHF, but the majority come to catheterization at some point due to the presence of a loud continuous murmur.[3]

The most common *anomalous* aortic origin of a coronary artery is anomalous origin of the circumflex artery from the right sinus of Valsalva. The artery passes around the posterior aspect of the aortic root toward the left atrioventricular groove and resumes a normal circumflex course. This anomaly accounts for between one-half and two-thirds of all anomalous coronary artery origins from the aorta.

REFERENCES

1. Bertrand, M.E., LaBlanche, J.M., Tilmant, P.Y., et al.: Frequency of provoked coronary arterial spasm in 1089 consecutive patients undergoing coronary arteriography. Circulation *65*:1299, 1982.
2. Edwards, J., et al.: Arteriosclerosis in intramural and extramural portions of coronary arteries in the human heart. Circulation *13*:235, 1956.
3. Levin, D.C., Fellows, K.E., and Abrams, H.L.: Hemodynamically significant primary anomalies of the coronary arteries. Angiographic aspects. Circulation *58*:25, 1978.

96-C, 97-E, 98-A, 99-D *(Braunwald, pp. 495–496, 498)*

After an earlier trial demonstrated that both enalapril and the combination of hydralazine and isosorbide nitrate could reduce mortality in patients with mild to moderate heart failure, the second Veterans Administration Cooperative Vasodilator Heart Failure Trial (V-HeFT-II) was designed to compare these treatment regimes.[1] There was a small incremental benefit found in the cohort of patients assigned to enalapril rather than hydralazine plus isosorbide dinitrate.

In the Survival and Ventricular Enlargement (SAVE) trial, patients who had an MI and ejection fraction of 40 per cent or less were randomized to captopril versus placebo.[2] Patients enrolled in this study had no symptoms of heart failure. After 4 years of follow-up, there was a 20 per cent reduc-

tion in mortality and a 36 per cent reduction in progression to severe heart failure in the captopril-treated group.

CONSENSUS-1, the COoperative Northern Scandinavian ENalapril SUrvival Study, studied patients with severe heart failure.[3] Patients taking diuretics, digoxin, and vasodilators were randomized to receive either enalapril or placebo. The patients in the enalapril group had a 40 per cent reduction in mortality at 6 months.

The treatment arm of the Studies On Left Ventricular Dysfunction (SOLVD) trial was designed to evaluate the effect of enalapril on mortality in patients with mild to moderate symptoms of heart failure and ejection fractions <35 per cent.[4] Patients in the enalapril-treatment group had a 16 per cent reduction in overall mortality compared to patients taking placebo.

REFERENCES

1. Cohn, J.N., Johnson, G., Ziesche, S., et al.: A comparison of enalapril with hydralazine-isosorbide dinitrate in the treatment of chronic congestive heart failure. N. Engl. J. Med. *325*:303, 1991.
2. Pfeffer, M.A., Braunwald, E., Moye, L.A., et al.: Effect of captopril on mortality and morbidity in patients with left ventricular dysfunction after myocardial infarction. N. Engl. J. Med. *327*:669, 1992.
3. CONSENSUS Trial Study Group: Effects of enalapril on mortality in severe congestive heart failure. Results of the Cooperative North Scandinavian Enalapril Survival Group (CONSENSUS). N. Engl. J. Med. *316*:1429, 1987.
4. SOLVD Investigators: Effect of enalapril on survival in patients with reduced left ventricular ejection fractions and congestive heart failure. N. Engl. J. Med. *325*:293, 1991.

100-D, 101-C, 102-B, 103-A *(Braunwald, pp. 117–118, 122–123 and 126–127)*

In contrast to left ventricular (LV) hypertrophy, right ventricular (RV) hypertrophy is not simply an exaggeration of normal; rather, the RV mass must become so large as to overcome the LV forces. Thus, the specificity of the ECG pattern of RV hypertrophy is high but the sensitivity is low, varying from 25 to 40 per cent. In RV hypertrophy there is right axis deviation ($\geq$110 degrees), a vertical position with rS pattern in leads I, II, and III and rS pattern in V_5 and V_6, and counterclockwise rotation (R/S ratio in $V_1 \geq 1$, R/S V_5: R/S $V_1 \leq 0.4$, qR in V_1, R in V_5 or $V_6 \leq 5$ mm). Based on the QRS pattern in lead V_1, RVH can be generally separated into three groups: a dominant R wave (R, qR, rR, rsR), Rs (Rs, Rsr), and rS. In general, the following hemodynamics for RV and LV systolic pressures are correlated with three patterns in V_1: qRS implies RV > LV; prominent R implies RV = LV; and rSr or RVH with incomplete RBBB implies RV < LV.

The left bundle branches into two fascicles, one lying anterior and superior and the other posterior and inferior. Thus, conduction delay in the anterior fascicle, left anterior hemiblock (LAHB), results in initial septal activation that proceeds inferiorly, anteriorly, and usually to the right; followed by activation of the inferior and apical areas with the vector oriented inferiorly, to the left, and anteriorly. The remainder of the QRS vector is then oriented posteriorly, superiorly, and to the left. The ECG pattern includes axis $\geq$ −45 degrees, qR in I, rS in III, small s in $V_5 + V_6$ reflecting the initial inferior activation and later, unopposed, LV anterolateral activation.

Left posterior fascicular block (left posterior hemiblock) (LPHB) is rare and usually associated with myocardial damage, and its pattern is nonspecific. Activation begins in midseptum, generating an initial vector directed to the left, anteriorly and superiorly. This is followed by activation of the anterior and anterolateral walls of the LV, with the QRS vector directed left and anteriorly. Finally, inferior and posterior walls are activated. The characteristic pattern includes axis +90 to 140 degrees; small R in I followed by deep S reflecting inferior, posterior, and rightward orientation of activation; QR in leads II, III, and aVF.

Wolff-Parkinson-White syndrome is characterized by a short P-R ($\leq$0.12 sec) interval, prolonged QRS ($\geq$0.12 sec) complex, and a slur on the upstroke of the QRS (delta wave), with secondary ST-segment and T-wave changes frequently present.

RBBB and LAHB is the most common combination of the left divisional and bundle branch blocks. The activation during the first 0.08 sec determines the axis and identifies LAHB. The delay of depolarization due to RBBB results in a final activation of the RV to the right and anteriorly.

ELECTROCARDIOGRAPHIC INTERPRETATIONS

104 *through* 129 (*Chapter 4; pp. 108–143 and 146–152*)

104. Artifact due to tremor
Sinus bradycardia with atrial premature complexes
Nonspecific ST- and T-wave abnormalities (Parkinson's disease)

105. Right-sided leads
Junctional rhythm (rate 50)
Normal axis
Acute inferior and right ventricular MI
Possible posterior MI

106. Sinus tachycardia
Marked Q-T interval shortening
Nonspecific ST- and T-wave abnormalities
(Patient with hypercalcemia)

107. Sinus rhythm with abnormal intraventricular conduction
Preexcitation syndrome pattern
(False-positive ETT due to WPW syndrome)

108. Normal sinus rhythm (rate 90)
Borderline right axis deviation
Left atrial abnormality
Right ventricular conduction delay (rsR′ in V_1 without prolonged QRS duration or voltage criteria for RVH)
Nonspecific ST-T wave abnormality in anterior leads
(This ECG is from a 23-year-old woman with a known secundum ASD)

109. Normal sinus rhythm
A second, atrial, nonconducted rhythm
Normal axis, low voltage in limb leads
Left atrial abnormality
Right bundle branch block
Nonspecific ST-T wave abnormality secondary to bundle branch block

110. Normal variant
Juvenile T-wave pattern

111. Normal sinus rhythm (without other abnormalities of rhythm or AV conduction)
Right bundle branch block (complete)
ST-T segment abnormalities secondary to the intraventricular conduction disturbance (Congenital right bundle branch block or atrial septal defect suggested)

112. Normal sinus rhythm (rate 85)
Right axis deviation (+110)
Biatrial enlargement
Right ventricular hypertrophy (R > S and qR pattern in V_1)
Nonspecific ST-T wave abnormality in anterior precordial leads
(The patient is a 35-year-old woman with critical MS)

113. Normal sinus rhythm (rate 96, axis indeterminate)
Borderline first-degree AV block
Right bundle branch block
Left anterior fascicular block
Left ventricular hypertrophy
Right ventricular hypertrophy (R′ > 15 mm in lead V_1), ST-T wave abnormality secondary to bundle branch block
Anterior MI, age indeterminate
(ECG is consistent with primary pulmonary disease and coronary artery disease)

114. Normal sinus rhythm (rate 65)
Left-axis deviation
Biventricular hypertrophy
Anterolateral Q waves consistent with pseudo-MI pattern

Anterolateral ST-T wave abnormality consistent with hypertrophy or ischemia

(The patient has familial hypertrophic cardiomyopathy)

115. Sinus tachycardia (rate 115)
Extreme right-axis deviation
Right bundle branch block
Left posterior fascicular block
Right atrial enlargement
Right ventricular hypertrophy
Diffuse ST-T wave abnormality consistent with hypertrophy and bundle branch block
(Tracing consistent with congenital left-to-right shunt or Ebstein's anomaly)

116. Sinus bradycardia
Ventricular pacing and ectopic atrial beats
Sinus rate 55 (normal intervals)
U waves present
Nonspecific inferior T-wave abnormality
Failure to sense and pseudofusion beat (pacemaker malfunction)

117. Normal sinus rhythm (rate 88)
Left-axis deviation
Preexcitation pattern resulting in pseudoinfarction pattern in inferior leads and anterolateral ST-T wave abnormality
(The patient is a 15-year-old boy with Wolff-Parkinson-White syndrome and a probable left posteroseptal bypass tract)

118. Sinus rhythm with aberrant intraventricular conduction due to the presence of a bypass tract
Preexcitation pattern
Right-axis deviation

119. Atrial flutter with variable 2:1 and 3:1 AV conduction (rate 140)
Vertical axis, low voltage throughout
Anterior MI age indeterminate
Anterolateral ST-segment elevation, consistent with acute injury or pericarditis
Inferior ST-segment depression, consistent with ischemia, tachycardia or reciprocal changes
(The patient presented with an evolving anterior MI)

120. Ventricular tachycardia (rate 130, axis indeterminate)
Right bundle branch block pattern
Retrograde P waves

121. Atrial fibrillation (rate 255)
Left-axis deviation
Preexcitation pattern

(Patient had Wolff-Parkinson-White syndrome and is conducting atrial fibrillation rapidly down her bypass tract, which is probably located in the left posteroseptal region)

122. Normal sinus rhythm (rate 65)
Right-axis deviation
Extensive old anterolateral MI
Inferior nonspecific ST-segment depression and T-wave abnormality consistent with ischemia, drug effect, or metabolic abnormality
Anterolateral ST-segment elevation and T-wave inversion consistent with aneurysm, pericarditis, or recent MI
(The patient had an anterior MI with a large anterior wall aneurysm complicating the event)

123. Right atrial abnormality
Normal sinus rhythm with first-degree AV block
Low voltage (limb leads only)
Right-axis deviation
Right bundle branch block (complete)
ST-T segment abnormalities secondary to the intraventricular conduction disturbance
(The patient had Ebstein's anomaly of the tricuspid valve; note in particular the abnormal P-wave morphology)

124. Atrial fibrillation with intermittent aberrant conduction of a left bundle branch type
Left-axis deviation
Poor precordial R-wave progression consistent with old anteroseptal/anterior myocardial infarction and/or intraventricular conduction defect
Possible old inferior myocardial infarction
Nonspecific ST- and T-wave abnormalities

125. Ventricular tachycardia

126. Sinus tachycardia
Ventricular premature complexes with fixed coupling
Fusion complexes
Anteroseptal Q-wave infarction of recent age
ST- and T-wave abnormalities suggesting myocardial ischemia, inferior leads
ST- and T-wave abnormalities suggesting myocardial injury, anteroseptal leads
(Coronary artery disease suggested)

127. Wandering atrial pacemaker
Left ventricular hypertrophy with accompanying ST- and T-wave abnormalities

128. Normal sinus rhythm with premature ventricular depolarizations and fusion beat (rate 90)
Left-axis deviation
Left anterior fascicular block
Left atrial enlargement
Left ventricular hypertrophy
Old anteroseptal MI
(This 75-year-old man has aortic stenosis and coronary artery disease)

129. Supraventricular tachycardia (rate 160, vertical axis)
Left ventricular hypertrophy by voltage
Diffuse nonspecific ST-T wave abnormalities, consistent with ischemia or tachycardia
(Patient is a 43-year-old woman with a history of SVT; she was successfully treated with IV adenosine)

Part II
Normal and Abnormal Circulatory Function

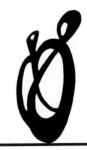

CHAPTERS 12 THROUGH 28

DIRECTIONS: Each question below contains five suggested responses. Select the ONE BEST response to each question.

130. True statements about paroxysmal supraventricular tachycardia (PSVT) due to reentry over a concealed accessory pathway include all of the following EXCEPT:

    A. In patients referred for electrophysiological evaluation of apparent PSVT, the prevalence of concealed accessory pathway is approximately 30 per cent
    B. Most accessory pathways that participate in concealed conduction are located between the RV and RA
    C. The PSVTs caused by retrograde conduction over an accessory pathway tend to be somewhat faster than those occurring in AV nodal reentry tachycardias
    D. Atrial fibrillation (AF) in patients with a concealed accessory pathway may be approached therapeutically as in AF patients without such a pathway
    E. Under some circumstances, anterograde conduction down a concealed accessory pathway may occur

131. True statements about the serum potassium in the management of heart failure include all of the following EXCEPT:

    A. Hypokalemia and hyperkalemia are both potential problems in patients with heart failure
    B. Potassium supplementation is usually indicated in patients receiving digitalis therapy
    C. Potassium therapy is especially indicated in geriatric patients with mild congestive heart failure
    D. Both hypokalemia and hyperkalemia may worsen digitalis-induced AV junctional delay

    E. Angiotensin-converting enzyme inhibitors may lead to a rise in serum potassium levels

132. True statements regarding implantable cardioverter defibrillators (ICD) include all of the following EXCEPT:

    A. ICD longevity is presently on the order of 4 to 5 years
    B. Present versions of the ICD have a lifetime total capacity of approximately 300 discharges
    C. Current ICDs use a "second-look" function to limit unnecessary discharges
    D. ICD placement significantly improves overall survival in sudden death patients
    E. Approximately 50 per cent of patients require antiarrhythmic drug therapy after ICD placement

133. Which of the following statements about the assessment of left ventricular diastolic function are true?

    A. The slope of the end-diastolic pressure-volume relation is the chamber stiffness
    B. The time constant of isovolumic relaxation, τ, is shortened by slowing the heart rate
    C. Pseudonormalization of the mitral inflow pattern by Doppler echocardiography is indistinguishable from normal mitral inflow
    D. The time constant of ventricular relaxation, τ, is affected by loading conditions
    E. In both normal and restrictive patterns of mitral inflow as assessed by Doppler echocardiography, the E/A ratio is >1

134. An increased resistance to pulmonary venous drainage may lead to secondary pulmonary hypertension. True statements about secondary pulmonary hypertension due to such a cause include all of the following EXCEPT:

A. Generation of RV systolic pressures ≥80 to 100 mm Hg requires RV hypertrophy
B. Vasodilatation and plexiform lesions are characteristic of the pulmonary response to acquired pulmonary venous hypertension
C. Pulmonary blood volume is one determinant of pulmonary artery pressure in patients with increased resistance to pulmonary venous drainage
D. Congenital pulmonary venous hypertension is pathologically different from acquired pulmonary venous hypertension
E. Considerable variability in pulmonary arterial vasoconstriction occurs in response to pulmonary venous hypertension

135. True statements regarding the impact of the implantable cardioverter defibrillator (ICD) on patient survival include all of the following EXCEPT:

A. Current evidence suggests that the ICD effectively decreases the incidence of sudden death
B. In the only randomized trial of the ICD published to date, the 5-year rate of sudden death in ICD recipients was markedly decreased in comparison with the drug treatment group
C. A 5-year rate of sudden death on the order of 5 per cent is observed in ICD recipients
D. Long-term survival is affected by the severity of underlying disease in ICD recipients
E. ICD therapy has not yet been directly compared with antiarrhythmic drug therapy with respect to surgical mortality

136. True statements about the use of Holter monitoring in the detection of cardiac arrhythmias include all of the following EXCEPT:

A. Wenckebach second-degree AV block may be seen in normal subjects
B. The frequency of PVCs after MI increases over the first several weeks
C. Holter monitoring has proven useful in the detection of potentially serious arrhythmias in patients with mitral valve prolapse
D. The predictive ability of Holter monitoring is comparable to that of EP testing for the determination of antiarrhythmic drug efficacy

E. In normal subjects, the cardiac rhythm detected by ambulatory monitoring shows little variation from one recording period to the next

137. All of the following statements about the auscultatory findings in mitral stenosis are correct EXCEPT:

A. The opening snap is an early diastolic sound
B. A long A_2-OS interval implies severe mitral stenosis
C. In atrial fibrillation, the A_2-OS interval varies with cycle length
D. The "snap" is generated by bowing of the anterior mitral leaflet
E. The presence of an opening snap implies a mobile mitral valve or anterior mitral leaflet

138. A 9-year-old girl is brought in for evaluation because of several episodes of fainting. During one episode, which occurred while she was reading a book with her mother, she turned blue and was resuscitated. Her past medical history is unremarkable except for congenital deafness. The family history is remarkable for a sister who died suddenly at the age of 3 years. The most likely diagnosis is:

A. sudden infant death syndrome
B. Jervell and Lange-Nielsen syndrome
C. Romano-Ward syndrome
D. Lown-Ganong-Levine syndrome
E. Barlow's syndrome

139. True statements about the Eisenmenger syndrome and pulmonary hypertension include all of the following EXCEPT:

A. The term Eisenmenger *syndrome* was first used to refer to patients with congenital cardiac lesions with severe pulmonary hypertension in whom reversal of a left-to-right shunt has occurred
B. Eisenmenger *complex* refers specifically to patients with ventricular septal defect, severe pulmonary hypertension, and a right-to-left shunt through the defect
C. Plexiform lesions of the muscular pulmonary arteries are a pathological indication of end-stage alterations in the pulmonary vasculature
D. In normal individuals, a doubling of pulmonary blood flow will only result in a 50 per cent increase in pulmonary artery pressure

E. The classification of Heath and Edwards of six grades of obstructive change in the pulmonary vasculature is widely employed to assess the potential reversibility of pulmonary vascular disease

140. Each of the following statements about the pathophysiology of cardiac and pulmonary dyspnea is true EXCEPT:

A. Since most bronchial capillaries drain by way of the pulmonary veins, congestion tends to develop in alveolar and bronchial vasculature simultaneously
B. Paroxysmal nocturnal dyspnea (PND) reflects the presence of interstitial edema, while pulmonary edema reflects the presence of alveolar edema
C. The difficulty in distinguishing between cardiac and pulmonary dyspnea may be compounded by their simultaneous presence in some patients
D. Sudden awakening at night occurs in patients with chronic obstructive pulmonary disease (COPD) and is commonly accompanied by sputum production
E. Acute cardiac asthma often occurs in patients with subclinical heart disease and less commonly leads to cyanosis than does acute bronchial asthma

141. True statements about the pulmonary vasculature include all of the following EXCEPT:

A. Acute hypoxemia leads to pulmonary vasoconstriction
B. Acidemia causes vasoconstriction of pulmonary arteries and arterioles
C. Beta-adrenoceptor stimulation elicits pulmonary vasoconstriction
D. Acetylcholine is a potent relaxant of pulmonary arteries and arterioles
E. While serotonin is a potent pulmonary vasoconstrictor in animals, it has little or no effect in humans

142. All the following characteristics are typical of hypertensive crisis EXCEPT:

A. diastolic blood pressure >140 mm Hg
B. retinal hemorrhages
C. normal mental status
D. proteinuria and azotemia
E. microangiopathic hemolytic anemia

143. True statements regarding beta blockage in heart failure include all of the following EXCEPT:

A. Beta blockade trials in heart failure have been based on the premise that long-term sympathetic nervous system hyperactivity may have deleterious consequences in heart failure
B. Metoprolol therapy has been shown to be clinically beneficial in heart failure
C. Down-regulation of beta-adrenergic receptors may account for the long-term benefit of beta blocker therapy in clinical studies
D. Beta blockers with intrinsic sympathomimetic activity (ISA) have been associated with an increased mortality as opposed to beta blockers with vasodilatory properties in patients with heart failure
E. Some clinical studies have provided clear evidence for the benefit of long-term beta blocker therapy in heart failure patients

144. A 63-year-old man who has been an insulin-requiring diabetic for 10 years presents to the office for initial management of hypertension (180/100). Urine and serum chemistries at this time are normal except for serum creatinine, 1.8 mg/dl, and blood urea nitrogen (BUN), 30 mg/dl. Because of gastroparesis you elect to initiate therapy with a potassium-sparing diuretic. When he returns in 2 weeks his serum potassium is 6.8 mEq/liter with no significant change in BUN or creatinine. The most likely explanation is:

A. consumption of tomatoes and bananas
B. a recent urinary tract infection
C. primary hypoaldosteronism
D. hyporeninemic hypoaldosteronism
E. tuberculous adrenal hypoplasia

145. Each of the following statements about cardiac transplantation is true EXCEPT:

A. Younger patients have better survival rates following cardiac transplantation
B. Use of the immunosuppressant agent cyclosporine has led to improvement in results of cardiac transplantation
C. The majority of patients who have received cardiac transplants have had end-stage heart disease due to coronary artery disease or cardiomyopathy
D. Patients with heart transplants have limited exercise capacity because of absence of autonomic neural control
E. Clinical signs of rejection include a fall in ECG voltage and the development of atrial arrhythmias

146. Each of the following statements about direct-current cardioversion of cardiac arrhythmias is true EXCEPT:

    A. In patients without clinical evidence of digitalis toxicity it is not necessary to withhold digitalis for 1 to 2 days before elective cardioversion
    B. In general, direct-current cardioversion of stable ventricular tachycardia requires greater energy levels than those required for atrial fibrillation
    C. Electrical cardioversion may be the therapy of choice for the treatment of rapid ventricular rates in patients with atrial fibrillation and the Wolff-Parkinson-White syndrome
    D. The occurrence of transient ventricular arrhythmias during attempted electrical cardioversion may be attenuated by administering a bolus of lidocaine before subsequent shocks
    E. Cardioversion of ventricular tachycardia by a chest "thump" may occasionally induce ventricular flutter of fibrillation

147. All of the following statements about cardiac hypertrophy in athletes are true EXCEPT:

    A. Isotonic exercise such as running and swimming increases left ventricular end-diastolic diameter
    B. Isometric exercise such as weight-lifting may cause an increase in left ventricular end-diastolic diameter
    C. Both isotonic and isometric exercise cause an increase in left ventricular mass
    D. Both isometric and isotonic exercise cause no change in left ventricular wall thickness
    E. Cardiac hypertrophy secondary to exercise usually disappears rapidly when training is discontinued

148. All of the following statements regarding the treatment of acute rejection in cardiac transplant recipients are true EXCEPT:

    A. Most episodes of acute rejection occur during the first 3 months after transplantation
    B. Episodes of early rejection are best treated by pulsed corticosteroid therapy
    C. OKT3 therapy is an effective treatment for rejection episodes that are resistant to steroid therapy
    D. The absence of a rejection episode in the first 3 months following transplantation

does not correlate with an overall lower incidence of late rejection
    E. Total lymphoid irradiation is a promising treatment for patients with repeated episodes of rejection

149. A 78-year-old man who lives in a nursing home is admitted via the emergency room because of fever and disorientation. His physical examination and ECG are normal except for sinus tachycardia and tachypnea. Laboratory results include an elevated white blood cell count, low platelet count, and prolonged prothrombin time. Urine sediment contains numerous polymorphonuclear leukocytes. A cardiology consultation is obtained for evaluation of the chest x-ray shown. The most likely explanation for the *accompanying chest x-ray* findings is:

    A. left ventricular failure
    B. pneumococcal pneumonia
    C. adult respiratory distress syndrome
    D. gram-negative pneumonia
    E. posterior wall MI

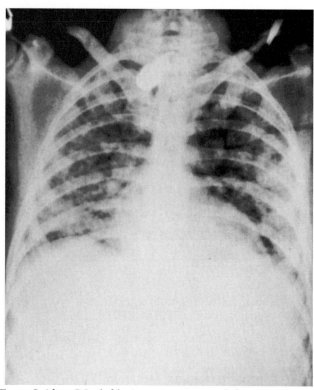

From Snider, G.L. (ed.): Acute respiratory failure. *In* Clinical Pulmonary Medicine, Boston, Little, Brown & Company, 1981, p. 378.

150. A pacemaker's pulse generator is connected electrically to the heart via an electrode system referred to as a lead. True statements with regard to unipolar and bipolar electrodes include all of the following EXCEPT:

   A. In bipolar systems both electrodes are located in the cardiac chamber
   B. Pacing thresholds for generation of stimuli are similar for unipolar and bipolar electrodes
   C. Unipolar electrodes are more susceptible to extracardiac interference from skeletal muscle potentials (myopotentials)
   D. The signal amplitudes of the electrograms generated by both types of electrodes are similar
   E. Electromagnetic interference causes oversensing and pacemaker malfunction more frequently with bipolar than with unipolar electrodes

151. The following statements about laboratory findings in heart failure are true EXCEPT:

   A. Serum electrolyte values are usually normal in patients with untreated heart failure of short duration
   B. Hyponatremia in heart failure may be due to a combination of dietary sodium restriction, diuretic therapy, and an elevated circulating vasopressin concentration
   C. Elevated serum aspartate aminotransferase (AST) levels may accompany congestive hepatomegaly due to heart failure
   D. Acute hepatic venous congestion due to heart failure may produce a syndrome that closely resembles viral hepatitis
   E. Elevations of pulmonary capillary pressure to 13 to 17 mm Hg are commonly responsible for pulmonary vascular redistribution and interstitial edema on the chest roentgenogram

152. All of the following statements about cardiac calcium channels are true EXCEPT:

   A. There is a great degree of structural homology between voltage-gated calcium and sodium channels
   B. Beta$_1$-adrenergic stimulation decreases the probability of open calcium channels
   C. The L, or long-lasting, calcium channel is thought to be involved in myocardial calcium-induced calcium release
   D. The T, or transient, calcium channel is thought to be important for the early electrical depolarization in the SA node

   E. A function of the beta-subunit of the calcium channel is to modify the calcium movement through the pore in the alpha-subunit

153. All of the following interventions may lower blood pressure EXCEPT:

   A. a diet that reduces caloric intake by 1000 calories per day
   B. reduction of dietary sodium to 2 gm/day
   C. a scheduled daily regimen of isometric exercise
   D. supplemental dietary calcium
   E. reduction of ethanol consumption to less than 1.0 oz/day

154. True statements regarding the evaluation and management of the heart *donor* for cardiac transplantation include all of the following EXCEPT:

   A. Nonspecific ST- and T-wave abnormalities are common on the donor electrocardiogram
   B. ABO compatibility and appropriate physical size are the two matching criteria currently used between donor and recipient
   C. Diabetes insipidus is a common problem in the donor
   D. Several serologies must be checked in the donor, including tests for HIV, Epstein-Barr virus, and toxoplasmosis
   E. In general, ischemic times of <6 hours for the donor heart are acceptable

155. Each of the following statements about procainamide is true EXCEPT:

   A. The plasma concentration of procainamide required to suppress PVCs in patients after acute myocardial infarction may be less than that required to prevent sustained ventricular tachycardia
   B. Procainamide, like quinidine, may accelerate the ventricular response in patients with atrial fibrillation or flutter
   C. Procainamide may block conduction in the accessory pathway of patients with the Wolff-Parkinson-White syndrome
   D. Toxic concentrations of procainamide may diminish myocardial performance
   E. Procainamide is the drug of choice for the control of the tachyarrhythmias in patients with bradycardia-tachycardia syndrome

156. All of the following are primary determinants of cardiac output EXCEPT:

    A. heart rate
    B. left ventricular preload
    C. left ventricular afterload
    D. myocardial contractile or inotropic state
    E. oxygen-carrying capacity of blood

157. Each of the following statements about exercise testing in the diagnosis of cardiac arrhythmias is true EXCEPT:

    A. Approximately one-third of normal subjects develop ventricular ectopy during exercise testing
    B. Nonsustained ventricular tachycardia of six beats or less can occur in normal patients and does not predict cardiovascular morbidity
    C. Patients with ischemic heart disease develop PVCs at lower heart rates than normal subjects
    D. Exercise testing should be avoided in patients with a history of serious ventricular arrhythmia
    E. Exercise testing is less sensitive than prolonged ambulatory monitoring in detecting ventricular ectopy

158. With respect to renovascular disease all of the following statements are true EXCEPT:

    A. Fewer than 2 per cent of adults with hypertension in a general practice have renovascular hypertension
    B. Atherosclerotic disease most commonly involves the proximal third of the main renal artery
    C. The most common form of fibroplastic renovascular disease in adults involves the media
    D. The incidence of renovascular hypertension is higher in blacks than whites
    E. Patients with severe, accelerated hypertension have the highest prevalence of renovascular disease

159. Each of the following statements about invasive electrophysiology study of the cardiac conduction system is true EXCEPT:

    A. Ventricular tachyarrhythmia is a common explanation for syncope or presyncope in patients with an intraventricular conduction disturbance
    B. The presence of an H-V interval equal to or greater than that recorded during normal sinus rhythm is consistent with the diagnosis of a ventricular tachycardia

    C. In patients with sinus node dysfunction, associated impaired AV conduction is commonly found
    D. Sinus node recovery time (SNRT) is defined as the difference between the spontaneous sinus node cycle length prior to pacing and the duration of the first spontaneous sinus response after termination of pacing
    E. Localization of accessory pathways by endocardial mapping in patients with the Wolff-Parkinson-White syndrome is an important prerequisite for ablative surgery

160. True statements about the use of adenosine in the management of cardiac arrhythmia include all of the following EXCEPT:

    A. Adenosine is useful in the treatment of patients with supraventricular tachycardia
    B. Intravenous bolus injections of adenosine at doses of 6 to 12 mg will terminate more than 90 per cent of supraventricular tachycardias
    C. IV verapamil remains the agent of choice to terminate acutely a supraventricular tachycardia
    D. Adenosine is useful in the diagnosis of wide QRS tachycardias
    E. Flushing, dyspnea, and chest pressure are all common side effects of adenosine therapy

161. Each of the following statements with respect to primary aldosteronism is true EXCEPT:

    A. The most common cause for primary aldosteronism is a solitary benign tumor
    B. Hypokalemia (<3.2 mEq/liter) is present in the majority of patients
    C. In patients with primary aldosteronism not receiving diuretics or supplemental potassium, urinary potassium will be >30 mEq/day
    D. Patients with primary aldosteronism usually have high plasma renin activity
    E. If a patient has high urinary potassium and low serum potassium but low serum aldosterone levels, licorice ingestion should be considered as a possible cause of the laboratory abnormalities

162. Comparison of left ventricular (LV) parameters in pressure- and volume-overloaded hearts reveals all of the following changes EXCEPT:

    A. LV systolic stress initially is greater in pressure overload

B. Eccentric hypertrophy is characteristic of volume overload

C. Concentric hypertrophy is characteristic of pressure overload

D. LV wall thickness is greater in pressure overload

E. LV peak systolic pressure is greater in volume overload

163. All of the following are correct statements with respect to management of hypertension in pregnancy EXCEPT:

A. Sodium restriction is an important component of therapy

B. Restriction of physical activity is advisable

C. Diuretics are usually contraindicated

D. Beta blockers may be useful

E. Methyldopa is frequently prescribed

164. Each of the following statements regarding recipient selection for cardiac transplantation is true EXCEPT:

A. Extension of the acceptable upper age limit for transplantation leads to an exponential increase in the number of potential recipients

B. The majority of patients undergoing transplantation have either primary cardiomyopathy or coronary artery disease

C. Chronic renal insufficiency is a contraindication to transplantation

D. Pretransplant evaluation usually includes endomyocardial biopsy

E. A strict upper-age limit of 55 years for transplant recipients is no longer considered appropriate

165. Each of the following statements about the clinical manifestations of digitalis toxicity is correct EXCEPT:

A. Digitalis overdose may lead to nausea and vomiting due to central nervous system mechanisms

B. Digitalis intoxication may result in malaise, disorientation, seizures, or other neurological symptoms

C. Digitalis may occasionally induce gynecomastia in men

D. Paroxysmal atrial tachycardia with AV block (PAT with block) is virtually pathognomonic of digitalis excess

E. Common arrhythmias due to digitalis toxicity include atrioventricular junctional escape rhythms and ventricular bigeminy or trigeminy

166. All of the following statements about shunt detection are true EXCEPT:

A. When "physiological" shunt is present, arterial oxygen saturation normalizes with administration of 100 per cent oxygen

B. Methods of shunt detection include oximetry, echocardiography, radionuclide, and magnetic resonance imaging

C. Among the sources of right atrial venous blood, the inferior vena cava has the lowest oxygen saturation

D. Although the sensitivity of oximetry for shunt detection is low, most clinically relevant left-to-right shunts can be detected using this method

E. The Flamm formula is used to estimate mixed venous oxygen saturation

167. True statements about the potassium-sparing diuretics in the management of heart failure include all of the following EXCEPT:

A. Amiloride is a direct inhibitor of collecting duct sodium conductance

B. Aldosterone antagonists lead to decreased protein synthesis in the aldosterone-responsive cells

C. When used alone, aldosterone antagonists are relatively ineffective in the therapy of heart failure

D. Patients with heart failure and chronic obstructive pulmonary disease may be particularly suited for therapy with potassium-sparing diuretics

E. Patients with renal insufficiency may be particularly prone to develop hyperkalemia from potassium-sparing diuretics

168. Each of the following statements about vasodilator agents used in heart failure is true EXCEPT:

A. The most important adverse effect of sodium nitroprusside is hypotension

B. Sublingual nitroglycerin may be used to effect a rapid reduction in left ventricular filling pressures

C. Chronic administration of a combination of hydralazine and isosorbide dinitrate has been shown to prolong survival in patients with heart failure

D. Hydralazine appears to be most effective in patients with normal heart size

E. Angiotensin-converting enzyme inhibitors lead to a decline in left and right ventricular filling pressures with little or no change in heart rate in patients with heart failure

169. All of the following statements regarding the risks of cardiac catheterization are true EXCEPT:

    A. Vascular complications are more common with a brachial artery approach than when the femoral artery approach is used
    B. Patients at highest risk for complications of cardiac catheterization are those with NYHA class IV symptoms of congestive heart failure and those with left main coronary artery stenoses >50 per cent
    C. The increased risk from cardiac catheterization in octogenarians is primarily due to peripheral vascular complications
    D. Nonionic contrast agents may be less thrombogenic than ionic contrast agents
    E. Minor complications occur in approximately 4 per cent of routine cardiac catheterizations

170. All of the following statements concerning measurement of cardiac output are true EXCEPT:

    A. Angiographic cardiac output measurement is preferred over Fick and thermodilution methods for calculation of stenotic valve areas in patients with severe aortic or mitral regurgitation
    B. There is a variability of up to 10 per cent in calculations of cardiac output by the Fick method
    C. When interpreting results of the indicator-dilution method, the area under the curve is directly related to the cardiac output
    D. Left-to-right shunts result in an early recirculation on indicator-dilution or thermodilution curves
    E. Thermodilution cardiac outputs may cause a falsely elevated cardiac output value in low-output states

171. All of the statements below concerning the effects of digitalis on myocardial contractility are true EXCEPT:

    A. The inotropic action of digitalis occurs in both normal and failing heart muscle
    B. The relative augmentation of the velocity of myocardial contraction by digitalis may be greater in failing than in normal myocardium
    C. Administration of cardiac glycosides in normal subjects leads to a rise in cardiac output
    D. Recent studies have documented sustained improvement in cardiac performance in patients with chronic congestive heart failure treated with digitalis

    E. Patient selection and the nature and extent of ventricular dysfunction are critical factors in the clinical response to digitalis therapy

172. True statements about the clinical use of lidocaine include all of the following EXCEPT:

    A. Lidocaine is generally ineffective against supraventricular tachyarrhythmias
    B. In patients with the Wolff-Parkinson-White syndrome, lidocaine may accelerate the ventricular response to atrial fibrillation
    C. The most common side effects of lidocaine are dose-related exacerbations of cardiac rhythm disturbances
    D. The use of lidocaine prophylactically in hospitalized patients with acute myocardial infarction remains a controversial subject
    E. In patients resuscitated from out-of-hospital ventricular fibrillatory arrests, lidocaine is comparable to bretylium in preventing recurrent episodes of ventricular tachyarrhythmia

173. Each of the following statements below concerning atrial fibrillation (AF) is true EXCEPT:

    A. AF is commonly seen in patients following cardiac surgery
    B. In patients with underlying cardiovascular disease, the development of chronic AF increases overall mortality
    C. Physical findings in patients with AF include variations in the intensity of S_1 and in the amplitude of a waves in the jugular venous pulse
    D. A greater frequency of right bundle branch block is noted in patients who develop AF in the year following acute myocardial infarction
    E. In the absence of underlying heart disease, subjects with AF have no increase in cardiovascular risk but do display a higher incidence of stroke than the general population

174. The frequency of various diagnoses in subjects with hypertension (HTN) in large series is best described as:

    A. essential HTN 95 per cent; chronic renal disease 4 per cent; renovascular disease 1 per cent
    B. essential HTN 90 per cent; chronic renal disease 1 per cent; renovascular disease 9 per cent

C. essential HTN 80 per cent; chronic renal disease 10 per cent; renovascular disease 10 per cent

D. essential HTN 80 per cent; chronic renal disease 15 per cent; renovascular disease 5 per cent

E. essential HTN 95 per cent; chronic renal disease 1 per cent; renovascular disease 1 per cent; Cushing's disease 1 per cent; coarctation of aorta 1 per cent; primary aldosteronism 1 per cent

175. True statements about the interaction of antiinflammatory drugs with loop diuretics in the treatment of congestive heart failure include all of the following EXCEPT:

A. The nonsteroidal antiinflammatory drugs (NSAIDs) may lead to sodium retention

B. The NSAIDs blunt the natriuretic response to all the loop diuretics

C. NSAIDs prevent the prostaglandin-induced increase in renal blood flow that is important to the efficacy of the loop diuretics

D. Low-dose aspirin also blunts the response to loop diuretics

E. The NSAIDs demonstrate different potencies in blunting the renal response to loop diuretics

176. True statements about the syndrome of circulatory shock include all of the following EXCEPT:

A. The clinical signs of shock reflect a decrease in blood flow to a variety of organs

B. ECG signs of myocardial ischemia may appear in patients with apparently normal hearts due to a reduction in regional coronary blood flow

C. Circulatory shock in the first 3 months of life is often due to gram-negative bacteremia

D. Increases in capillary hydrostatic pressure during circulatory shock lead to a depletion of plasma water and hemoconcentration

E. During circulatory shock, pulmonary blood flow is often protected at the expense of cerebral and renal perfusion

177. All of the following statements regarding quinidine are true EXCEPT:

A. Quinidine may be used to treat fetal arrhythmias because it can cross the placenta

B. Quinidine may cause significant hypotension because of its alpha-adrenoreceptor blocking effects

C. Quinidine is cleared from the circulation primarily by the kidneys

D. In patients with the Wolff-Parkinson-White syndrome quinidine may prevent reciprocating tachycardias and slow the ventricular response to atrial fibrillation

E. Quinidine therapy may cause a paradoxical increase in the ventricular response to atrial flutter or fibrillation

178. Each of the following statements about edema in heart failure is correct EXCEPT:

A. Edema in heart failure does not correlate well with the level of systemic venous pressure

B. Peripheral edema may be detected when extracellular fluid volume has increased by as little as 1 to 2 liters

C. Severe edema may cause rupture of the skin and extravasation of fluid

D. In patients with acute heart failure, edema may not be present initially

E. In patients with hemiplegia due to a cerebral vascular accident, edema is usually more apparent on the paralyzed side

179. True statements about the increased cardiac output that occurs during anemia include all of the following EXCEPT:

A. A decrease in blood viscosity contributes to the high cardiac output noted in anemia

B. Clinical evidence of impaired cardiac function may occur in patients without apparent underlying heart disease when the hematocrit falls below 25 per cent

C. Patients with sickle cell anemia may manifest heart failure with less severe degrees of anemia than those seen in patients with iron deficiency anemia

D. In patients with anemia, exercise may lead to an exaggerated increase in cardiac output

E. The rate of development of anemia plays an important role in the degree to which anemia affects cardiac output

180. Loop diuretics are used extensively in the treatment of heart failure. All of the following statements about loop diuretics are true EXCEPT:

A. Loop diuretics are among the most potent diuretic agents known and may induce natriuresis amounting to 20 per cent of the filtered sodium load

B. Loop diuretics are secreted into the tubular lumen by the organic acid secretory pathway and may therefore be competi-

tively inhibited by agents such as probenecid or indomethacin
C. Absolute bioavailability of loop diuretics
is reduced in patients with heart failure
D. Following the administration of an intravenous bolus of furosemide, the increase
in venous capacitance and decrease in
pulmonary capillary wedge pressure occur within minutes
E. Intravascular volume depletion and increasing doses of vasodilators may be underlying causes of diuretic resistance

181. Each of the following statements about high-
output heart failure is true EXCEPT:

A. Thyrotoxicosis, anemia, and pregnancy
are all examples of high-output states that
may lead to heart failure
B. The extremities of the patient with high-
output failure are usually warm and
flushed
C. Vasodilator therapy is usually helpful in
heart failure due to anemia
D. The pulse pressure in high-output failure
is normal or widened
E. Evidence of biventricular failure, sensory
and motor peripheral neuropathy, and
prolongation of the Q-T inverval is consistent with the diagnosis of thiamine deficiency (beriberi)

182. Each of the following statements about verapamil is true EXCEPT:

A. Verapamil exerts a direct myocardial depressant effect
B. Cardiac index may remain unchanged in
patients on verapamil because afterload
reduction produced by the drug counter-
acts its negative inotropic effect
C. Verapamil is helpful in slowing the rapid
ventricular response in patients with atrial
fibrillation and wide QRS complexes due
to Wolff-Parkinson-White syndrome
D. Verapamil is a useful drug for terminating
sustained AV nodal reentrant tachycardias

E. Verapamil has some alpha-adrenergic
blocking and antiplatelet effects

183. Each of the following statements about physical findings in heart failure is true EXCEPT:

A. Chronic marked elevation of systemic venous pressure may produce exophthalmos
or even visible systolic pulsation of the
eyes
B. Pallor and coldness of the extremities are
primarily due to elevation of adrenergic
nervous system activity
C. A positive abdominojugular reflux reflects
the combination of hepatic congestion and
the inability of the right side of the heart
to accept an increased venous return
D. The presence of hepatic tenderness reflects longstanding right-sided heart failure with chronic stretching of the liver
capsule
E. Protein-losing enteropathy may occur in
patients with visceral congestion and may
result in a reduced plasma oncotic pressure

184. Each of the following statements about the antiarrhythmic agent disopyramide is true EX-
CEPT:

A. It can accelerate or slow the sinus node
rate depending on serum concentration
and underlying sinus node disease
B. The mean elimination half-life of disopyramide is 8 to 9 hours, and is prolonged in
the presence of renal, hepatic, or heart
failure
C. It is effective in reducing the frequency of
spontaneous ventricular ectopy, and in
preventing the recurrence of ventricular
and preexcited supraventricular arrhythmia
D. It should not be combined with mexiletine, because of an opposing effect on repolarization
E. It is useful in the treatment of neurally mediated syncope

DIRECTIONS: Each question below contains suggested answers. For EACH of the alternatives, you are to respond either TRUE (T) or FALSE (F). In a given item, ALL, SOME, OR NONE OF THE ALTERNATIVES MAY BE CORRECT.

185. Digitalis is of potential benefit in which of the following conditions? For the following choices answer true (T) or false (F).

   A. Mitral stenosis with atrial fibrillation and normal right ventricular function
   B. Left ventricular hypertrophy, normal sinus rhythm, normal left ventricular ejection fraction, and elevated left ventricular end-diastolic pressure
   C. Hypertrophic obstructive cardiomyopathy with left ventricular ejection fraction of 70 per cent and normal sinus rhythm
   D. Mitral stenosis with normal sinus rhythm and normal right ventricular function
   E. Hypertrophic obstructive cardiomyopathy with left ventricular ejection fraction of 70 per cent and atrial fibrillation

186. Mark each statement regarding cardiac myocyte signal transduction as true (T) or false (F).

   A. Beta$_1$-adrenergic receptor activation leads to activation of adenylate cyclase and formation of cAMP
   B. Unlike the receptors of the sympathetic nervous system, the muscarinic receptor does not involve a three-protein sarcolemmal signaling system
   C. cGMP levels may be increased by acetylcholine or NO in myocytes and vascular tissue
   D. Phospholipase C activation is linked to alpha-adrenergic stimulation by a G protein
   E. The effects of cAMP are mediated by at least several different cAMP-binding proteins

187. Common features in the clinical presentation of renovascular hypertension secondary to fibromuscular hyperplasia, as opposed to atherosclerosis, include the following:

   A. age <50
   B. female gender
   C. coexisting cardiomegaly
   D. no family history of hypertension
   E. presence of carotid bruits

188. For each of the suggested answers, you are to respond either true (T) or false (F). Pulmonary function testing can help in the differentiation between cardiac and pulmonary dyspnea. In patients with cardiac dyspnea due to congestive heart failure, the following may be seen:

   A. Decreased pulmonary compliance
   B. Decreased pulmonary diffusion capacity at rest and during exercise
   C. Decreased functional residual capacity
   D. Decreased vital capacity
   E. Mild to moderate increase in airway resistance

189. For each of the suggested answers regarding cardiac arrhythmias and heart failure, you are to respond either true (T) or false (F).

   A. Tachyarrhythmias may precipitate heart failure by increasing myocardial oxygen demand, inducing ischemia, or reducing diastolic filling
   B. Asymptomatic ventricular ectopy is an independent marker of increased mortality, and warrants specific therapy
   C. Marked bradycardia may precipitate heart failure by reducing stroke volume
   D. AV dissociation may reduce cardiac output and precipitate heart failure especially in patients with decreased left ventricular compliance
   E. Abnormal intraventricular conduction may precipitate heart failure by impairing myocardial performance

190. For each of the suggested answers regarding treatment of digitalis intoxication, you are to respond either true (T) or false (F).

   A. Lidocaine and phenytoin are useful agents in treating arrhythmias due to digitalis excess
   B. Second- and third-degree AV block often respond to atropine
   C. Recurrence of digitalis toxicity can occur 24 to 48 hours following the administration of antidigoxin Fab antibodies
   D. Dialysis is very helpful in cases of massive overdose
   E. Direct-current cardioversion is safe in cases of digitalis-induced ventricular arrhythmias

191. For each of the suggested answers regarding the risks of hypertension, you are to respond either true (T) or false (F).

    A. If left untreated, 50 per cent of hypertensive patients will die of coronary artery disease or heart failure, and a third will die of stroke
    B. Hypertensive patients with low plasma renin activity have a lower incidence of heart attacks and strokes
    C. Impaired coronary artery blood flow reserve and thallium perfusion defects can be seen in the absence of fixed coronary obstruction in hypertensive patients
    D. Women suffer less cardiovascular morbidity as a consequence of hypertension than men
    E. The incidence of target organ damage is more closely correlated with diastolic blood pressure than with systolic pressure

192. True statements regarding hypomagnesemia in patients with congestive heart failure include which of the following?

    A. Both thiazide and loop diuretics may cause urinary magnesium wasting
    B. Chronic exposure to ethyl alcohol leads to increased renal magnesium losses
    C. Digitalis may lead to renal magnesium wasting
    D. A total daily urinary magnesium excretion of <1 mEq in the absence of diuretics is suggestive of magnesium depletion
    E. Elevated magnesium levels in congestive heart failure may predict as poor a prognosis as hypomagnesemia

193. For each of the suggested answers regarding procainamide, you are to respond either true (T) or false (F).

    A. Procainamide prolongs the action potential duration (APD) more than it prolongs the effective refractory period (ERP)
    B. Both procainamide and N-acetylprocainamide (NAPA), its major metabolite, can cause Q-T prolongation
    C. Though it has no alpha-blocking activity, procainamide can cause marked vasodilation and hypotension
    D. Procainamide can be effective in suppressing quinidine-resistant rhythms
    E. Maintenance doses of digoxin need to be reduced with coadministration of procainamide

194. For each of the suggested answers regarding risks and clinical features in patients with ventricular tachycardia (VT), you are to respond either true (T) or false (F).

    A. In patients with arrhythmogenic right ventricular dysplasia, VT exhibits a contour of left bundle branch block and right axis deviation
    B. Ventricular arrhythmias in patients with mitral valve prolapse are not associated with increased risk for sudden cardiac death
    C. Ventricular arrhythmias in patients with cardiomyopathy and low ejection fraction are associated with increased risk of sudden cardiac death
    D. Drug-induced or aggravated cardiac arrhythmias can be seen in as many as 5 to 10 per cent of patients on antiarrhythmic drug therapy
    E. Patients with a history of repaired tetralogy of Fallot are at increased risk for the development of ventricular arrhythmias

195. For each of the suggested answers regarding use of amiodarone in the treatment of patients with cardiac arrhythmias, you are to respond either true (T) or false (F).

    A. Intravenous amiodarone may exert a negative inotropic action and must be given with great caution to patients with LV dysfunction
    B. Amiodarone's efficacy in general equals or exceeds that of other antiarrhythmic agents in suppressing ventricular arrhythmias
    C. Pulmonary toxicity from amiodarone occurs in approximately 5 to 15 per cent of patients treated with maintenance doses and is usually not fatal
    D. Amiodarone maintenance therapy is more likely to cause hyperthyroidism than hypothyroidism
    E. When used in the management of patients with heart failure, amiodarone can be expected to lower overall mortality, independent of the presence of nonsustained ventricular tachycardia

196. For each of the suggested answers regarding cor triatriatum, you are to respond either true (T) or false (F).

    A. Pulmonary hypertension secondary to pulmonary venous obstruction may occur
    B. A membrane separates the left atrial appendage from the anterior subchamber of the left atrium
    C. The posterior subchamber receives pulmonary venous flow
    D. When this disorder causes pulmonary hypertension, pressure in the anterior subchamber can be markedly elevated

E. This anomaly always involves the left atrium

---

197. Atrioventricular block exists when the atrial impulse is conducted with delay or is not conducted at all to the ventricle. True statements about second-degree AV block include:

A. Type I AV block is associated with a benign clinical course in all age groups
B. Type II AV block in inferior MI is not associated with an increase in mortality
C. Type I AV block with a normal QRS complex occurs at the level of the AV node or in the His bundle
D. Type II AV block in association with bundle branch block occurs at the level of the AV node or the His bundle
E. 2:1 AV block may be either type I or type II second-degree AV block and is more likely to be type I if the QRS complex is normal

---

198. Correct statements with regard to the contractile proteins of cardiac cells include:

A. The thick filaments are composed of aggregates of myosin filaments
B. The thin filaments are composed largely of actin molecules
C. Troponin C is a regulatory protein which binds Ca^{++}
D. Troponin C normally interacts with actomyosin to inhibit the Mg^{++}-stimulated ATPase
E. When a cardiac cell is depolarized, intracellular Ca^{++} concentration falls from 10^{-5} M to 10^{-7} M with release of Ca^{++} from troponin C

---

199. A 74-year-old man with a long history of left ventricular failure secondary to several myocardial infarctions comes to the emergency room acutely short of breath 2 hours after eating a large holiday meal. Physical examination and chest x-ray are consistent with acute pulmonary edema. ECG shows a narrow complex junctional tachycardia at a rate of 130/min with 1-mm ST-segment depression in leads V_4 through V_6. Blood pressure is 170/

100; respirations, 32. His current medical treatment includes nitrates, calcium channel antagonists, digoxin, and chlorothiazide. Appropriate initial therapy in the emergency room would include:

A. nasal O_2
B. morphine sulfate
C. intravenous furosemide
D. intravenous digoxin
E. sublingual nitroglycerin

---

200. For each of the suggested answers regarding receptors and signaling systems in the heart, you are to respond either true (T) or false (F).

A. Glucagon and thyroid hormone can couple to the adenylate cyclase system independently of myocardial beta-receptors
B. Vagal stimulation has more potent negative inotropic effect in the absence of beta-adrenergic stimulation
C. Adenosine inhibits sinus and AV nodal activity by stimulating acetylcholine-sensitive K^+ channels
D. Especially when heart failure is due to dilated cardiomyopathy, there is marked (50 to 70 per cent) down-regulation of $beta_1$-receptors
E. Epinephrine is more potent than norepinephrine in stimulating $beta_1$-receptors

---

201. A 60-year-old man had a pacemaker inserted 5 years ago because of sinus bradycardia with poor LV function following an anterior MI. As part of his exercise program he has been using a rowing machine. Recently, he has had several episodes of near-syncope which occurred only while rowing. An ambulatory ECG (Holter monitor) revealed an abnormal rhythm during a near-syncopal event while rowing. The ECG *shown below* indicates:

A. There is evidence for a dual chamber pacing system
B. There is inappropriate inhibition of ventricular pacing
C. There is undersensing of atrial activity
D. There is lack of capture of the ventricles
E. There is lack of capture of the atria

From Schuller, H., and Fahraeus, T.: Pacemaker Electrocardiograms: An Introduction to Practical Analysis. Sweden, Siemens-Elema, 1983, p. 141.

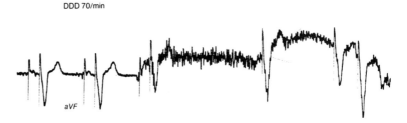

25 mm/s

DDD 70/min

aVF

202. True statements about digoxin include:

    A. The half-life of digoxin in subjects with normal renal function is about 36 to 48 hours
    B. In patients with normal renal function who have not previously taken digitalis, institution of daily maintenance therapy without a loading dose leads to a steady-state plateau concentration of the drug in about 7 days
    C. Dialysis is a relatively effective way of removing digoxin from the body
    D. Obese patients taking digoxin who undergo dramatic weight loss must have their digoxin dosage decreased to avoid toxicity
    E. Patients taking digoxin who subsequently begin quinidine therapy often require a decrease in digoxin dosage to avoid toxicity

203. For each of the suggested answers, you are to respond either true (T) or false (F). The following physical examination findings can be seen in both moderately severe anemia and chronic aortic regurgitation:

    A. Duroziez's sign
    B. Quincke's pulse
    C. A systolic murmur at the left sternal border
    D. Hill's sign
    E. A mid-diastolic murmur

204. For each of the suggested answers regarding electrical therapy of cardiac arrhythmias, you are to respond either true (T) or false (F).

    A. Direct-current cardioversion is successful in terminating up to 95 per cent of reentrant arrhythmias
    B. Direct-current cardioversion can be safely used to terminate digitalis-induced reentrant arrhythmias
    C. Synchronized shocks delivered late in the QRS complex are more effective and less likely to induce acceleration of the arrhythmia than shocks delivered near the QRS onset
    D. When properly synchronized, direct-current shock does not result in ventricular fibrillation
    E. Elevation of myocardial enzymes following cardioversion is not uncommon

205. A 50-year-old woman visits the office complaining of episodes characterized by hot flushes, palpitations, sweats, and a sense of apprehension. Her blood pressure reaches 210/100 mm Hg and in the interim periods is 150/85. Correct statements about this patient's condition include:

    A. 90 per cent of these patients have a solitary tumor in the adrenal cortex
    B. It is likely that a 24-hour urine assay for total metanephrines will be elevated
    C. Multiple adrenal tumors are more likely in patients with type II multiple endocrine neoplasia (Sipple's syndrome)
    D. Abdominal ultrasound is the best noninvasive diagnostic test
    E. Urinary metanephrine secretion is increased following an intravenous pyelogram (IVP) with Renografin

206. True statements about cardiac physical findings in patients with congestive heart failure include:

    A. Heart failure due to restrictive cardiomyopathy is usually accompanied by signs of cardiomegaly
    B. Pulsus alternans occurs most commonly in heart failure due to concomitant mitral regurgitation
    C. Pulsus alternans results from variation of the stroke volume due to incomplete recovery of contracting myocardial cells
    D. A low-grade fever that is due to cutaneous vasoconstriction and impaired heat loss may occur in severe heart failure
    E. Cheyne-Stokes respiration is a cyclic respiratory pattern that results from a combination of a change in the sensitivity of the respiratory center and the presence of left ventricular failure

207. Correct statements regarding the association of oral contraceptive pills and hypertension include:

    A. The likelihood of developing hypertension is increased by significant alcohol consumption
    B. The incidence of hypertension is about 2.5 times greater in pill users than in nonusers
    C. The likelihood of developing hypertension is unaffected by the age of the user
    D. The mechanism for contraceptive-induced hypertension probably involves renin-aldosterone—mediated volume expansion
    E. Cigarette smoking more than doubles the cardiovascular complications associated with use of oral contraceptives

208. All of the following statements regarding pulmonary edema are true EXCEPT:

    A. Pulmonary edema can complicate pulmonary embolism
    B. Pulmonary edema can be associated with bronchoconstriction
    C. When it follows rapid lung expansion after treatment of pneumothorax, pulmonary edema is usually unilateral and causes minimal symptoms
    D. High-altitude pulmonary edema is more common in younger persons
    E. Sympatholytic agents are useful in the prevention and treatment of neurogenic pulmonary edema

209. True statements with regard to distribution of blood flow and intravascular pressure in the upright lung include:

    A. Pulmonary artery pressure is greater than alveolar pressure at the lung apices
    B. Pulmonary venous pressure exceeds alveolar pressure at the lung bases
    C. Alveolar pressure increases from the lung base to the lung apex
    D. Pulmonary vascular redistribution occurs when there is a relative reduction in perfusion of the bases with a relative increase in apical perfusion

210. Which of the following are considered complications of cyclosporine therapy in the cardiac transplant recipient?

    A. Renal dysfunction
    B. Bone marrow suppression
    C. Hepatotoxicity
    D. Neurological effects
    E. Hirsutism

211. True statements regarding renovascular hypertension include all of the following EXCEPT:

    A. Renovascular hypertension is the most common form of secondary hypertension
    B. The most common cause of renal artery stenosis is fibromuscular dysplasia
    C. The best initial tests in patients with clinical features suggestive of renovascular hypertension are radioisotope renography and plasma renin measurements after an oral captopril challenge
    D. Angioplasty of the renal arteries is more successful in cases of stenosis due to atherosclerosis

212. True statements with respect to the association of sudden cardiac death (SCD) and premature ventricular contractions (PVCs) include:

    A. PVCs in the absence of heart disease are, in general, prognostically benign
    B. In patients who have survived MI, >10 PVCs/hr are associated with an increased risk of SCD
    C. Left ventricular dysfunction after MI increases the risk of SCD associated with the presence of PVCs
    D. Treatment with flecainide, encainide, or moricizine of increased numbers of PVCs after MI has been shown recently to decrease significantly the incidence of SCD

213. Features of the systemic lupus erythematosus (SLE) –like syndrome that may be induced by procainamide include:

    A. the development of antinuclear antibodies in 20 to 30 per cent of patients on chronic procainamide therapy
    B. the development of clinical symptoms of SLE in 20 to 30 per cent of patients on chronic procainamide therapy
    C. a similar occurrence of SLE syndrome due to the N-acetylprocainamide (NAPA) metabolite of the drug
    D. a response to steroids in some patients

214. A 32-year-old man who is a chronic intravenous drug abuser is admitted to the hospital in respiratory distress. Despite conservative therapy there is progressive deterioration of systemic oxygenation, and mechanical ventilation is instituted. During the next 24 hours further impairment of oxygenation occurs despite an increased oxygen concentration (FIO_2) of 100 per cent. Therefore, positive end-expiratory pressure (PEEP) at 10 mm Hg is initiated. Possible complications secondary to PEEP in this setting may include:

    A. decreased cardiac output
    B. augmented venous return with right ventricular failure
    C. barotrauma with pneumothorax
    D. enhanced oxygen toxicity to pulmonary alveoli

215. True statements concerning the symptoms and signs of heart failure in the neonate and infant include:

    A. Excessive diaphoresis may be a manifestation of heart failure during the first year of life

B. Atelectasis may be precipitated by obstruction of the airways from enlargement of the main pulmonary artery
C. Hepatomegaly may be seen commonly in both left and right heart failure
D. Ascites and peripheral edema are common sequelae of right heart failure

216. True statements regarding sudden cardiac death include all of the following EXCEPT:

A. It represents ~25 per cent of all cardiovascular deaths in the United States
B. A previous myocardial infarction can be identified in as many as 75 per cent of patients who die suddenly
C. The presence of ventricular ectopy is the most powerful predictor of sudden cardiac death in patients with underlying coronary artery disease
D. The most common cardiac mechanism is ventricular fibrillation, followed by bradyarrhythmias or asystole
E. The outcome in patients in whom ventricular fibrillation is the initial rhythm is worse than in those presenting with sustained ventricular tachycardia

217. All of the following are class II indications for permanent cardiac pacing EXCEPT:

A. First-degree AV block with PR interval >0.5 sec
B. Persistent infra-His block following myocardial infarction
C. Persistent advanced or complete AV block at the AV node following acute MI
D. Intermittent complete AV block in the absence of reversible causes, regardless of symptoms
E. Symptomatic first-degree AV block improved by temporary pacing

218. Patients with the electrocardiogram *shown below* could also exhibit:

A. a gradual increase in atrial rate with the administration of digitalis

B. an irregular atrial rate
C. precipitation of the arrhythmia by hypokalemia
D. an absence of underlying cardiac disease in 50 per cent of cases

219. Which of the following statements are true regarding rate-adaptive pacemakers?

A. They are designated by the letter A (adaptive) in the fourth position of the pacemaker code
B. Recent advances in technology allow rate change due to emotional stress
C. The magnitude and rate of change of the sensor-driven response are programmable
D. Accelerometer-based systems respond to changes in motion and thus are less susceptible than conventional sensors to environmental noise
E. They are not useful in the presence of atrial chronotropic incompetence

220. Correct statements about patients with unexplained syncope or palpitations include:

A. A careful, accurately documented history and physical examination are the most important tests to perform in this population
B. In those patients with syncope of noncardiovascular causes, the 1- to 2-year mortality rate is <15 per cent
C. When a putative cause for unexplained syncope is found by electrophysiological study, subsequent therapy prevents recurrence of symptoms in about 80 per cent of patients
D. Electrophysiological induction of a sustained tachycardia in patients who do not develop spontaneous arrhythmia on noninvasive evaluations suggests that the induced rhythm is clinically significant and responsible for their symptoms

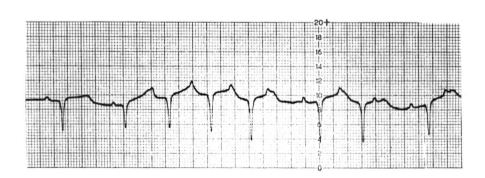

221. Lidocaine is a widely used pharmacological agent for the treatment of cardiac arrhythmias. Correct statements about lidocaine include:

    A. Lidocaine has little effect on the electrophysiological properties of atrial myocardial cells or on conduction in accessory pathways
    B. In the absence of severe left ventricular dysfunction, clinically significant adverse hemodynamic effects from lidocaine are rarely noted
    C. The elimination half-life of lidocaine in patients after relatively uncomplicated myocardial infarction is two to four times that in normal subjects
    D. Patients treated with an initial bolus of lidocaine followed by a maintenance infusion may experience transient excessive plasma concentrations of the drug 30 to 120 minutes after therapy is begun

222. Regulation of the intracellular concentration of Ca^{++} in myocardial cells is determined by the following mechanisms:

    A. Phospholamban, a Ca^{++}-stimulated Mg^{++}-ATPase, transports Ca^{++} into the sarcoplasmic reticulum (SR)
    B. Voltage-dependent Ca^{++} channels increase Ca^{++} influx in response to membrane depolarization
    C. A bidirectional Na^+-Ca^{++} exchange carrier transports Ca^{++} in exchange for Na^+
    D. Receptor-operated channels in response to beta-adrenoceptor agonists increase Ca^{++} efflux

223. For each of the suggested answers, you are to respond either true (T) or false (F). For equivalent total and effective stroke volumes, left ventricular end-diastolic pressure and volume are greater in:

    A. Mitral regurgitation as opposed to aortic regurgitation
    B. Ventricular septal defect as opposed to patent ductus arteriosus
    C. Ventricular septal defect as opposed to aortic regurgitation
    D. Mitral regurgitation as opposed to tetralogy of Fallot

224. In response to an excessive hemodynamic burden, the heart utilizes the following mechanisms to maintain cardiac output:

    A. the Frank-Starling mechanism
    B. increased catecholamine release from adrenergic nerves and adrenal medulla

    C. myocardial hypertrophy
    D. decreased venous return

225. Which of the following statements regarding atherosclerosis in the coronary arteries of the transplanted heart (allograft vasculopathy) are true?

    A. The incidence of graft atherosclerosis is between 20 and 50 per cent 5 years after transplantation
    B. The introduction of cyclosporine has led to a significant reduction in the occurrence of allograft vasculopathy
    C. CMV infection may contribute significantly to allograft vasculopathy
    D. Diffuse allograft vasculopathy often requires retransplantation
    E. The use of statins (HMG Co-A reductase inhibitors) is associated with reduction in cardiac rejection and in the incidence of allograft vasculopathy

226. A 59-year-old woman with left ventricular dysfunction presents in mild congestive heart failure despite adhering to her regimen of digoxin and furosemide. You initiate outpatient therapy with oral captopril (12.5 mg). About 30 minutes after taking her first dose, while getting dressed, she has a syncopal event. Likely explanations include:

    A. an episode of tachyarrhythmia
    B. failure of baroreceptor-mediated increase in heart rate on standing up to dress
    C. abnormalities in regulation of peripheral vascular resistance
    D. decreased circulating renin levels with decreased angiotensin II levels

227. For each of the suggested answers, you are to respond either true (T) or false (F). The following disorder(s) is/are known to be associated with an increased risk for pulmonary hypertension:

    A. Hepatic cirrhosis
    B. HIV infection
    C. Hyperthyroidism
    D. Vitamin B_1 deficiency
    E. Osler-Weber-Rendu disease

228. In patients with marked left ventricular dysfunction, which of the following statements is/are true regarding pulsus alternans:

    A. It is usually associated with electrical alternans
    B. It is more readily detected in the femoral as compared to radial arteries

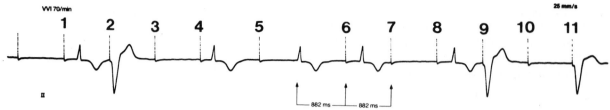

From Schuller, H., and Fahraeus, T.: Pacemaker Electrocardiograms: An Introduction to Practical Analysis. Sweden, Siemens-Elema, 1983, p. 77.

C. It can be appreciated with sphygmomanometry
D. It can be elicited by the assumption of erect posture
E. The strong and weak beats are almost always concordant on both sides of the circulation (i.e., both ventricles)

229. For each of the suggested answers, you are to respond either true (T) or false (F). In patients with asymptomatic systolic left ventricular dysfunction, the SOLVD prevention trial showed that angiotensin-converting enzyme (ACE) inhibitors:

A. Improve symptoms
B. Reduce LV dilation
C. Have no effect on overall mortality
D. Reduce mortality due to heart failure
E. Reduce time to hospitalization for heart failure

230. The electrocardiogram illustrated *above* shows a pacemaker malfunction. The pacemaker is a VVI set at a rate of 70/min. True statements with respect to the malfunction include:

A. There is pacing at an altered rate from initial programming
B. There is intermittent undersensing
C. There is intermittent oversensing
D. There is intermittent loss of capture

231. Clinical features consistent with preeclampsia (as opposed to chronic hypertension) in a pregnant patient include:

A. younger age (<20 years)
B. proteinuria
C. primigravida status
D. systolic blood pressure <160 mm Hg

232. Clinical features of the Wolff-Parkinson-White (WPW) syndrome include:

A. an absence of heart disease in most adults
B. a decrease in the frequency of paroxysmal tachycardia with increasing age
C. an association with Ebstein's anomaly
D. the majority of tachycardias presenting as atrial fibrillation

233. True statements about the adverse effects of quinidine include:

A. Quinidine may produce syncope in up to 2 per cent of patients
B. The most common side effects of chronic oral quinidine therapy are central nervous system disturbances
C. Potential therapies for quinidine-induced torsades de pointes include overdrive pacing and intravenous isoproterenol or magnesium
D. The mechanism of thrombocytopenia due to quinidine is nonspecific bone marrow suppression

234. For each of the suggested answers, you are to respond either true (T) or false (F). Randomized controlled trials evaluating the use of angiotensin-converting enzyme (ACE) inhibitors in heart failure have demonstrated that these agents reduce mortality in patients with:

A. Mild to moderate symptomatic heart failure
B. Severe symptomatic heart failure
C. Asymptomatic left ventricular dysfunction
D. Asymptomatic left ventricular dysfunction following myocardial infarction
E. Symptomatic heart failure following myocardial infarction

235. The following physiological changes will exacerbate pulmonary edema:

A. Increased pulmonary venous pressure

B. Increased pulmonary capillary pressure secondary to increased pulmonary arterial pressure
C. Rapid removal of unilateral pneumothorax
D. Increased plasma oncotic pressure

236. For each of the suggested answers, you are to respond either true (T) or false (F). Thiazide diuretics may cause many side effects, including:
    A. Hypomagnesemia
    B. Hypouricemia
    C. Hypercalcemia
    D. Hypercholesterolemia
    E. Hyponatremia

DIRECTIONS: The questions below consist of lettered headings followed by a set of numbered items. For each numbered item select the ONE lettered heading with which it is MOST closely associated. Each lettered heading may be used ONCE, MORE THAN ONCE, OR NOT AT ALL.

For each rhythm disturbance, match the appropriate description.

    A. Sinus arrest
    B. Sinoatrial exit block
    C. Ventriculophasic sinus arrhythmia
    D. Wandering pacemaker
    E. Sinus arrhythmia

237. During complete AV block, P-P cycles that contain a QRS complex are shorter than P-P cycles without an intervening QRS complex

238. A pause in sinus rhythm for which the P-P interval does not equal a multiple of the sinus P-P interval

239. Both Wenckebach type I and type II forms of this arrhythmia are noted

240. Presumed to be secondary to augmented vagal tone, this arrhythmia is considered a normal phenomenon, particularly in the very young and the athlete

For each description, match the appropriate cardiopulmonary exercise parameter

    A. $\dot{V}O_{2\,max}$
    B. Anaerobic threshold
    C. $\dot{V}CO_2/\dot{V}O_2$
    D. $\dot{V}d/\dot{V}t$

241. The best measure(s) of exercise capacity and exercise cardiac output

242. Highly reproducible when measured days or weeks apart

243. Not altered by underlying pulmonary disease

244. Influenced by type of foods consumed

For each statement or definition, match the appropriate physiological principle or reflex.

    A. Bainbridge reflex
    B. Force-frequency relation
    C. Laplace's law
    D. Anrep effect
    E. Cushing reflex

245. Increased heart rate causes increased rate of force development and developed force

246. Ventricular wall stress is inversely related to wall thickness and directly related to the cross-sectional ventricular diameter

247. Abrupt increase in systolic BP causes increased cardiac contractility

248. Decreased cerebral blood flow causes bradycardia and an increase in peripheral vascular resistance

For each condition capable of precipitating high-output cardiac failure, match the appropriate phrase.

    A. Hyperthyroidism
    B. Beriberi
    C. Arteriovenous fistula
    D. Carcinoid syndrome
    E. Osler-Weber-Rendu syndrome

249. Branham's sign

250. Hepatomegaly and abdominal bruits

251. Means-Lerman scratch

252. Parasthesias and painful glossitis

For each disease state match the appropriate left ventricular volume data.

	End-diastolic Volume (ml/m²)	Stroke Volume (ml/m²)	Mass (gm/m²)
A.	70	45	92
B.	84	44	172
C.	193	92	200
D.	199	37	145
E.	70	40	80

253. Aortic valve stenosis with peak systolic gradient >30 mm Hg

254. Myocardial disease (primary dilated cardiomyopathy)

255. Aortic regurgitation with regurgitant flow >30 ml per beat

256. Mitral valve regurgitation with regurgitant flow >20 ml per beat

---

For each clinical condition, match the most appropriate pacemaker modality.

 A. VAT
 B. VVIR
 C. DDD
 D. DDDR
 E. AAIR

257. A 58-year-old male with tachycardia-bradycardia syndrome who develops symptomatic sinus bradycardia with beta-blocker therapy (which was given for inappropriate sinus tachycardia)

258. A 70-year-old woman with atrial fibrillation who complains of dizziness, and is found on examination to have a ventricular rate of 30/min

259. A 62-year-old male with complete heart block following aortic valve surgery

260. A 45-year-old man with symptomatic sino-atrial exit block and junctional escape rhythm

For each phase of the cardiac action potential, match the appropriate physiological description:

 A. Phase 1
 B. Phase 2
 C. Phase 3
 D. Phase 4
 E. Phase 0

261. The phase determined primarily by intracellular potassium concentration

262. Mediated by I_{Ca} in the normal sinus and atrioventricular nodes

263. There is inactivation of I_{Ca-L} and activation of the delayed rectifier channel

264. The phase that is particularly well defined in Purkinje fibers

---

For each drug, match the appropriate effect.

 A. Prolongation of the PR interval
 B. Widening of the QRS complex
 C. Prolongation of the QT interval
 D. Increased serum digoxin levels
 E. Antiadrenergic effect
 F. None of the above

265. Flecainide

266. Lidocaine

267. Aminodarone

268. Sotalol

For each of the contractile proteins, match the characteristic property(ies).

 A. A mutant gene is responsible for hypertrophic cardiomyopathy
 B. Interaction with calcium ions is essential for contraction
 C. Attached to the Z lines
 D. Supports myosin and provides elasticity
 E. Major component of the I band

269. Actin

270. Myosin heavy chains

271. Troponin C

272. Titin

DIRECTIONS: The questions below consist of four lettered headings followed by a set of numbered items. For each numbered item select

A if the item is associated with (A) *only*
B if the item is associated with (B) *only*
C if the item is associated with *both* (A) and (B)
D if the item is associated with *neither* (A) nor (B)

Each lettered heading may be used ONCE, MORE THAN ONCE, OR NOT AT ALL.

A. Primary pulmonary hypertension
B. Eisenmenger syndrome
C. Both
D. Neither

273. An occult ventricular septal defect may be present

274. An operative procedure may relieve the pulmonary hypertension

275. "Onion skinning" or intimal thickening of the smaller pulmonary arteries with fibrosis is frequently seen

276. "Plexiform lesions" of the muscular pulmonary arteries and arterioles are frequently seen

277. "Silent" mitral stenosis is part of the initial differential diagnosis

A. Atrial flutter
B. Atrial fibrillation
C. Both
D. Neither

278. Associated with irregular heart beat

279. Associated with constant intensity of S_1

280. Requires relatively low energy for cardioversion

281. Can be cured with radiofrequency ablation

A. Relatively cardioselective
B. Intrinsic sympathomimetic activity (ISA)
C. Both
D. Neither

282. Nadolol

283. Propranolol

284. Acebutolol

285. Pindolol

Part II
Normal and Abnormal Circulatory Function

Chapters 12 through 28

ANSWERS

130-B *(Braunwald, pp. 665–667)*

The surface ECG is uninformative in patients with an accessory pathway that conducts unidirectionally from the ventricle to the atrium while sinus rhythm is present. However, when a PVST occurs due to this mechanism, one clue to the possibility of concealed retrograde conduction over an accessory pathway may be the occurrence of a normal QRS complex and retrograde P waves that occur after completion of the QRS complex (either in the ST segment or early in the T wave).[1] In patients with apparent PSVT referred for electrophysiological study, the incidence of concealed accessory pathway participation in a reentry mechanism is estimated to be approximately 30 per cent. Most such accessory pathways are located between the LV and LA and participate in the tachycardia by retrograde conduction of an impulse conducted in an anterograde manner over the AV node—His bundle pathway, resulting in an AV-reciprocating tachycardia.[2]

Treatment usually involves the use of agents that produce transient degrees of AV nodal block, such as verapamil, digitalis, and propranolol. Antiarrhythmic agents capable of prolonging activation time or refractory period in the accessory pathway may be useful in the prevention of such reciprocating tachycardias. The presence of AF in patients with a concealed accessory pathway may be approached in a manner identical to that of AF in patients without such a pathway because anterograde AV conduction in both instances occurs in an orthodromic manner (over the AV node). Under some circumstances, such as vagal or catecholamine stimulation, anterograde conduction down the accessory pathway may be provoked.

REFERENCES

1. Ross, D.L., and Uther, J.B.: Diagnosis of concealed accessory pathways in supraventricular tachycardia. PACE 7:1069, 1984.

2. Kuck, K.H., Friday, K.J., and Kunze, K.P.: Sites of conduction block in accessory atrioventricular pathways: Basis for concealed accessory pathways. Circulation 82:407, 1990.

131-C *(Braunwald, p. 479)*

Hypokalemia is a frequent consequence of the widespread use of diuretics in the management of heart failure.[1] A longstanding controversy exists regarding whether diuretic-induced hypokalemia needs to be treated with oral potassium supplementation. Several generalizations may be made regarding this controversy. Potassium is often helpful in the treatment of ventricular arrhythmias due to digoxin; therefore, it is appropriate to administer potassium supplements or a potassium-sparing diuretic to patients receiving cardiac glycosides. One caveat to this exists: since both hypokalemia and hyperkalemia may worsen digitalis-induced AV block, patients with digitalis-induced AV block and normal serum potassium levels must be carefully evaluated as to potassium therapy, because hyperkalemia may worsen AV-junctional conduction delays in this setting. The use of diuretics that inhibit aldosterone synthesis, angiotension-converting enzyme inhibitors, or beta blockers may result in a rise in serum potassium levels, as may excessive potassium supplementation or use of potassium-sparing diuretics by themselves.

Thus, specific factors influencing potassium homeostasis for each patient must be carefully considered before any therapeutic interventions are initiated. For example, the risk of inducing hyperkalemia may increase in the presence of reduced renal function, a common finding in geriatric patients.[2] It is therefore considered prudent to avoid potassium supplementation in older patients with mild congestive heart failure or isolated hypertension treated with a diuretic alone. In contrast, clinical and experimental evidence supports the use of potassium supplementation in some patients with essential hypertension, including blacks and elderly patients with poor dietary potassium intake and normal renal function.

REFERENCES

1. Dykner, T.: Relation of cardiovascular disease to potassium and magnesium deficiencies. Am. J. Cardiol. *65*:44K, 1990.
2. Chakko, S.C., Frutchley, J., and Gheorgiade, M.: Life-threatening hyperkalemia in severe heart failure. Am. Heart J. *117*:1083, 1989.

132-D *(Braunwald, pp. 732–734; Table 23–9)*

ICDs have undergone enormous changes in the past decade. From the first ICDs, which were large units placed in the abdomen and linked to thoracotomy-placed pericardial patches, to the newer, smaller devices which are placed pectorally and are linked to transvenous leads, obviating the need for thoracotomy. Present versions of ICDs are capable of backup pacing, antitachycardia pacing (ATP), low-energy cardioversion and defibrillation. Therapy utilizes a tiered approach, starting with ATP, and progressing to defibrillation as needed. Multiple aspects of each type of therapy are programmable. This approach significantly limits the number of shocks needed for therapy, since many episodes may be terminated by ATP depending on the characteristics of the VT. Current units have a lifetime range of 4 to 5 years, and a total capacity of about 300 discharges.

A source of unnecessary shocks in early devices was spontaneous termination of the arrhythmia while the ICD was charging. Such unnecessary shocks may induce arrhythmias should they occur at a vulnerable period in the cardiac cycle. To prevent unnecessary shocks, newer devices are "committed." Uncommitted devices utilize a second look after the capacitors have charged for a shock. The second look determines whether the arrhythmia is still present after the device has charged. The device has the ability to abort the shock if the arrhythmia has spontaneously terminated.

About 50 per cent of patients with ICDs require antiarrhythmic drug therapy to reduce the incidence of arrhythmias and limit the number of ICD detections and shocks. ICD function should be carefully assessed while on antiarrhythmic drugs which may affect the defibrillation threshold. While it is generally believed that ICDs decrease the incidence of sudden cardiac death to <1 to 2 per cent per year, the impact of ICDs on total survival is unknown, since there are no controlled randomized trials comparing ICDs to other types of therapy reported to date.[1]

REFERENCE

1. Kim, S.G.: Impact of implantable cardioverter-defibrillator therapy on patient survival. Cardiol. Rev. *2*:113, 1994.

133 A-T, B-F, C-F, D-T, E-T *(Braunwald, pp. 434–436)*

Measurement of indices of left ventricular diastolic function can be divided into three groups: assessment of passive left ventricular relaxation via pressure-volume curves, measurement of isovolumic relaxation time, and assessment of the pattern of left ventricular filling by Doppler echocardiography or adionuclide angiography.

The characteristics of passive left ventricular filling can be assessed by constructing a pressure-volume curve. The position of the pressure-volume curve is an indication of the distensibility of the left ventricle. A more upward located curve indicates a less distensible chamber. The slope of the pressure-volume curve is the chamber *stiffness*.

Another assessment of left ventricular function is the measurement of the time course of isovolumic left ventricular pressure decline. This can be quantified by the time constant of the exponential decline in pressure, or τ; τ is increased by factors that hinder ventricular relaxation, such as ischemia, and τ is decreased by factors that facilitate ventricular relaxation, such as increased heart rate. Loading conditions may also affect τ.

A common method of evaluating left ventricular diastolic function is examination of the mitral inflow pattern by Doppler echocardiography. Normally, the majority of ventricular diastolic filling occurs early and a smaller component of filling occurs late with atrial contraction. By Doppler this is seen as a rapid early filling wave (E wave) and a somewhat slower atrial filling wave (A wave). The normal E/A ratio is slightly more than 1. When impaired ventricular relaxation occurs, the ratio is reversed, with the E/A ratio becoming <1. When impaired ventricular relaxation becomes more severe, left atrial pressure rises to compensate for elevated left ventricular diastolic pressure. This results in restoration of the normal E/A ratio, known as a *pseudonormalization* pattern.[1] Pseudonormalization may be differentiated from normal mitral inflow by a characteristically more rapid early diastolic flow deceleration. Another pattern of mitral inflow that is associated with severe ventricular diastolic dysfunction is the *restrictive* pattern.[1,2] This is characterized by an E/A ratio much greater than 1 (usually >2), with a very short early diastolic flow deceleration time. The restrictive pattern reflects very high left atrial pressures and increased left ventricular stiffness.

REFERENCES

1. Appleton, C.P.: Doppler assessment of left ventricular diastolic function: The refinements continue. J. Am. Coll. Cardiol. *21*:1607, 1993.
2. Appleton, C.P., and Hatle, L.K.: The natural history of left ventricular filling abnormalities: Assessment by two-dimensional and Doppler echocardiography. Echocardiography *9*:437, 1992.

134-B *(Braunwald, pp. 796–797; Fig. 25–15)*

Pulmonary arterial hypertension due to increased resistance to pulmonary venous drainage may result from diseases affecting the LV or pericardium, left-sided valvular disease, and a variety of rare entities. The severity of pulmonary hypertension that develops depends in part on the performance capabilities of the RV. Systolic pressures of 80 to 100 mm Hg can be generated only by a hypertrophied RV that is normally perfused. If RV failure occurs with relatively low pulmonary vascular pressures, marked pulmonary hypertension cannot develop despite an increase in pulmonary vascular resistance.

In the human there is marked variability in pulmonary arterial vasoconstriction in response to pulmonary venous hypertension. While the precise mechanisms involved in elevating pulmonary vascular resistance are not well defined, pulmonary blood volume is an identified determinant of pulmonary artery pressure in patients with increased resistance to pulmonary venous drainage. Pulmonary blood volume in turn is determined by the balance between flow into and out of the pulmonary vascular bed and is therefore influenced by both right and left ventricular output as well as by the relative distensibility of the pulmonary vasculature and the left side of the heart.

Regardless of the etiology, structural changes occur in the pulmonary vascular bed in response to chronic pulmonary venous hypertension. The anatomical changes that occur in the pulmonary arteries in pulmonary hypertension secondary to increased resistance to pulmonary venous drainage depend on whether the pulmonary venous hypertension is acquired or congenital. When it is congenital, the elastic tissue in the main pulmonary artery is of the fetal variety (long, uniform, unbranched, and parallel elastic fibers). In contrast, acquired pulmonary hypertension is characterized by elastic tissue in the pulmonary trunk of the adult variety (short, irregular, and branched elastic fibers). Small pulmonary arteries, arterioles, and venules undergo a variety of structural alterations, including medial hypertrophy, intimal fibrosis, and rarely necrotizing arteritis. However, vasodilatation and plexiform lesions are not seen in response to chronic pulmonary venous hypertension. Rather, these lesions characterize the "irreversible" forms of pulmonary arterial hypertension.

135-B   (Braunwald, p. 735)

Because the ICD is a new form of therapy, direct comparisons with traditional therapies such as antiarrhythmic drugs have not yet been completed. No randomized trials concerning the efficacy of the ICD have been published and the device has not been compared with other forms of therapy in terms of patient selection, morbidity, surgical complications and mortality, or patient survival.[1] However, the ICD is generally considered to be effective in reducing the incidence of sudden death, and, using historical controls, the 5-year rate of sudden death with the ICD is on the order of 5 per cent. This compares quite favorably to the 20 per cent 5-year rate of sudden death in similar patients re-

fractory to drug therapy and has been used as evidence that the ICD is currently the most effective therapy for sudden death prevention in high-risk patients. However, it must be remembered that not all appropriate ICD shocks are able to prevent sudden death, and the patient population that receives ICDs has a higher risk of sudden death due to MI, congestive heart failure, and asystole than most other populations.[2]

REFERENCES

1. Furman, S.: Implantable cardioverter defibrillator statistics. PACE 13:1, 1990.
2. Manolis, A.S., Rastegar, H., and Estes, N.A.M. III: Automatic implantable cardioverter defibrillator. Current status. JAMA 262:1362, 1989.

136-E   (Braunwald, pp. 578–579)

Prolonged Holter monitoring of patients engaged in normal daily activity has proven extremely useful as a noninvasive method to document and quantitate underlying cardiac arrhythmias. While significant rhythm disturbances are relatively uncommon in healthy persons, a variety of arrhythmias, including sinus bradycardia (with rates as low as 35 beats/min), sinus arrhythmia, sinoatrial exit block, Wenckebach second-degree AV block (especially during sleep), and junctional escape complexes may be seen in normal persons. In addition, the prevalence of arrhythmias in normal subjects increases with increasing age. Persons with ischemic heart disease, especially those recovering from acute myocardial infarction, exhibit PVCs when long-term recordings of the heart rhythm are obtained. The frequency of PVCs progresses over the first several weeks following infarction and decreases about 6 months after infarction. While controversy still exists regarding the significance of ventricular ectopy in this population, it is generally acknowledged that more complex forms and increased frequency of ventricular ectopy are correlated with an increased risk of sudden cardiac death.

Long-term ECG recordings have been useful for the detection of underlying rhythm disturbances in patients with hypertrophic cardiomyopathy[1] and mitral valve prolapse[2] as well as in patients who have unexplained syncope or transient cerebrovascular symptoms.[3] In both normal subjects and in patients with underlying rhythm disturbances, the cardiac rhythm may vary dramatically from one long-term recording period to the next.[4] Therefore, in order to help establish efficacy, it is important to show that an antiarrhythmic agent effects a large reduction in the frequency of ventricular ectopy. Both Holter monitoring and EP studies have been used to establish the efficacy of antiarrhythmic drug therapy. There is no significant difference in the efficacy of drug therapy as guided by either of these two methods.[5]

REFERENCES

1. Maron, B.J., Savage, D.D., Wolfson, J.K., and Epstein, S.E.: Prognostic significance of 24-hour ambulatory electrocardiographic monitoring in patients with hypertrophic cardiomyopathy: A perspective study. Am. J. Cardiol. *48*:252, 1981.
2. Mason, D.T., Lee, G., Chan, M.C., and DeMaria, A.N.: Arrhythmias in patients with mitral valve prolapse: Types, evaluation and therapy. Med. Clin. North Am. *68*:1039, 1984.
3. Mikolich, J.R., Jacobs, W.C., and Fletcher, G.F.: Cardiac arrhythmias in patients with acute cerebrovascular accidents. JAMA *246*:1314, 1981.
4. Pratt, C.M., Slymen, D.J., Wierman, A.M., et al.: Analysis of the spontaneous variability of ventricular arrhythmias: Consecutive ambulatory electrocardiographic recordings of ventricular tachycardia. Am. J. Cardiol. *56*:67, 1985.
5. Mason, J.W.: A comparison of electrophysiologic testing with Holter monitoring to predict antiarrhythmic drug efficacy for ventricular tachyarrhythmias: Electrophysiologic study versus electrocardiographic monitoring. N. Engl. J. Med. *329*:445, 1993.

137-B   *(Braunwald, pp. 1010–1011)*

In mitral stenosis, the opening snap is an early diastolic sound caused by the rapid movement of the anterior mitral valve leaflet toward the left ventricle in response to high left atrial pressures. The presence of an opening snap implies a mobile anterior mitral leaflet. The first heart sound is quite loud in mitral stenosis. The increased intensity of the first heart sound in mitral stenosis is due to abrupt systolic movement of the anterior mitral leaflet which was recessed into the left ventricle during diastole.

The timing of the A_2-OS interval has important implications for the severity of mitral stenosis. When mitral stenosis is severe, and left atrial pressure is high, left atrial and left ventricular pressures equilibrate earlier in diastole, resulting in a shorter A_2-OS interval. The A_2-OS interval varies in atrial fibrillation with cycle length. When left atrial pressure is higher, which occurs after short cycles because less left atrial emptying can occur, the A_2-OS interval is shorter.

138-B   *(Braunwald, pp. 685–686)*

This child appears to have a disease that is familial and associated with sudden death. The prolonged Q-T interval syndrome is a functional abnormality that is associated with lethal arrhythmias. Two hereditary varieties have been reported: those with autosomal recessive inheritance and associated deafness (the Jervell and Lange-Nielsen syndrome) and those with autosomal dominant inheritance *without* deafness (the Romano-Ward syndrome). Since this patient was born with deafness, it is likely that she has the Jervell and Lange-Nielsen syndrome. Although it is unclear which patients with prolonged Q-T intervals are most likely to develop ventricular arrhythmias, particularly torsades de pointes, patients at higher risk appear to be those characterized by deafness, female gender, and a history of syncope.[1]

A variety of other acquired causes of prolonged Q-T syndrome exist, including reactions to antiarrhythmic and psychotropic drugs, electrolyte abnormalities, hypothermia, central nervous system injury, and excessive weight loss associated with use of liquid protein diets.

The sudden infant death syndrome, by definition, occurs between birth and 6 months of age, more commonly in males. Although it is unclear whether or not the primary abnormality is neurological, cardiac, or pulmonary (sleep apnea), this syndrome has an incidence of close to 2 per 1000 live births.[2] The Lown-Ganong-Levine syndrome is a syndrome associated with a short P-R interval that appears to be caused by the presence of an anomalous pathway for conduction from the atria to the ventricle but is not associated with an increased incidence of sudden death. Barlow's syndrome, one of the eponyms for mitral valve prolapse, is associated with cardiac arrhythmias, but the incidence of sudden cardiac death is low.[3]

REFERENCES

1. Moss, A.J., Schwartz, P.J., Crampton, R.S., et al.: The long Q-T syndrome: A prospective international study. Circulation *71*:17, 1985.
2. Schwartz, P.J.: The quest for the mechanisms of the sudden infant death syndrome: Doubts and progress. Circulation *75*:677, 1987.
3. Pocock, W.A., Bosman, C.K., Chesler, E., et al.: Sudden death in primary mitral valve prolapse. Am. Heart J. *107*:378, 1984.

139-D   *(Braunwald, pp. 799–800)*

Patients described originally by Eisenmenger had ventricular septal defect as the specific cause of the shunt; therefore, such patients are diagnosed as having Eisenmenger *complex*. The term Eisenmenger *syndrome* was first used by Wood to describe patients with congenital cardiac lesions with severe pulmonary hypertension in whom a reversal of a left-to-right shunt had occurred. In normal individuals, when pulmonary blood flow is doubled, the pulmonary vascular resistance is halved, resulting in no change in pulmonary artery pressure. Pulmonary artery pressure does not rise until pulmonary blood flow increases by four- to sixfold.

The degree of reversibility of pulmonary vascular obstructive disease that exists in a given patient is determined primarily by the underlying pathology in the pulmonary vasculature. Heath and Edwards constructed a classification of structural change composed of six grades[1] that is widely used to describe the underlying pulmonary vascular pathology. Grade 1 is characterized by hypertrophy of the media of small muscular pulmonary arteries and arterioles; grade 2 by intimal cellular proliferation; and grade 3 by advanced medial thickening with hypertrophy and hyperplasia that, together with progressive intimal proliferation in concentric fibrosis, may begin to result in obliteration of arterioles and small arteries. These first three grades of the Heath-Edwards classification appear to represent a chronological progression and may be reversible.

Grade 4 is marked by the development of "plexiform" lesions; grade 5 by complex plexiform, angiomatous, and cavernous lesions as well as hyalinization of the intima; and grade 6 by the presence of necrotizing arteritis. Some evidence exists for the idea that grade 6 may appear before grades 4 and 5, but in any case grades 4 to 6 represent changes that are end-stage and that signify a particularly poor prognosis. The presence of anatomical changes in the pulmonary vasculature of grades 4 to 6 is generally considered to be a *contraindication* to surgical closure of any intracardiac communication because the right-to-left communication is closed, the irreversible nature of the pulmonary lesions merely increases the load on an already overburdened RV.

REFERENCE

1. Heath, D., and Edwards, J.E.: The pathology of hypertensive pulmonary vascular disease. A description of six grades of structural changes in the pulmonary arteries with special reference to congenital cardiac septal defects. Circulation *18*:533, 1958.

140-E *(Braunwald, pp. 450–451; Table 15–5)*

The differentiation of pulmonary and cardiac causes of dyspnea may not always be straightforward. The sensation of dyspnea is a clinical expression of pulmonary venous and capillary congestion. The sudden onset of dyspnea and wheezing at night (PND) occurs as a result of the development of interstitial edema, which precipitates respiratory distress or cardiac asthma. Pulmonary edema, on the other hand, is a manifestation of alveolar edema caused by elevated left-sided cardiac pressures and the resultant transudation of fluid into the alveolar spaces. Since most bronchial capillaries drain via the pulmonary veins (which empty into the left atrium), bronchial and alveolar congestion tends to occur at the same time. When patients having COPD awaken at night with excessive sputum production, the condition may be relieved by coughing. Acute cardiac asthma (PND) usually occurs in patients with clinically *evident* heart disease. The presence of diaphoresis and "bubblier" airway sounds and the *more common* occurrence of cyanosis all help differentiate cardiac asthma from bronchial asthma.

141-C *(Braunwald, pp. 781–783)*

A variety of substances are capable of exerting substantial effects upon the tone of the pulmonary vasculature. Acute hypoxia is a well-established cause of pulmonary vasoconstriction, and this mechanism in part allows for self-regulation of the ventilation-perfusion characteristics of the lung. In addition to the effects of alveolar oxygen tension

upon pulmonary arteriolar tone, a decrease in oxygen tension in the mixed venous blood that flows through the small pulmonary arteries and arterioles may also lead to pulmonary arterial vasoconstriction.[1] Acidemia appears to lead to vasoconstriction as well; therefore, two of the most potent stimuli for *vasodilatation* in the systemic arteriolar bed lead to *vasoconstriction* of pulmonary arteries and arterioles.

While controversy exists concerning the effects of alpha-adrenoceptor agonists on the pulmonary vascular bed, beta-adrenoceptor stimulation with isoproterenol has been shown consistently to cause pulmonary vasodilatation. Acetylcholine is also a potent relaxant of pulmonary arteries and arterioles. In patients with elevated pulmonary vascular resistance with a major reversible component, this drug is capable of transiently lowering resistance. Histamine is a vasodilator in the systemic circulation but is primarily a vasoconstrictor in the pulmonary vascular bed. While serotonin is a potent pulmonary vasoconstrictor in animals, it has little or no effect in humans. In patients with malignant carcinoid syndrome of the bowel and hepatic metastases, for example, large quantities of systemic serotonin release may lead to endocardial and valvular changes on the right side of the heart but do not lead to pulmonary hypertension.

REFERENCE

1. Silove, E.D., Inoue, T., and Grover, R.F.: Comparison of hypoxia, pH, and sympathomimetic drugs on bovine pulmonary vasculature. J. Appl. Physiol. *24*:355, 1968.

142-C *(Braunwald, pp. 832–834; Table 26–15 and 26–16)*

When a sudden rise in blood pressure (typically diastolic blood pressure >140 mm Hg) causes acute damage to retinal vessels (hemorrhages, exudates, or papilledema), accelerated malignant hypertension is present. Hypertensive encephalopathy is frequently present and is manifested by headache, irritability, confusion, somnolence, stupor, focal neurological deficits, seizures, and eventually coma. It should be noted, however, that encephalopathy is not always present in malignant hypertension. Young black men are particularly prone to malignant hypertension with severe target organ damage but few symptoms of encephalopathy. In previously normotensive persons, encephalopathy may occur at considerably lower blood pressure than in someone who was previously hypertensive.

Other clinical features include renal insufficiency with proteinuria, hematuria, azotemia, and occasionally oliguric renal failure; microangiopathic hemolytic anemia with red cell fragmentation and intravascular coagulation; congestive heart failure; and nausea and vomiting. The pathogenesis of hypertensive encephalopathy is thought to be failure of cerebral autoregulation with dilatation of cerebral arterioles leading to excessive cerebral blood flow and damage to the arteriolar wall with increased vascular permeability.[1,2]

REFERENCES

1. Kincaid-Smith, P.: Understanding malignant hypertension. Aust. N.Z. J. Med. *11*:64, 1981.
2. Strandgaard, S., and Paulson, O.B.: Cerebral blood flow and its pathophysiology in hypertension. Am. J. Hypertens. *2*: 486, 1989.

143-C *(Braunwald, pp. 486–488; Table 16–7)*

Up-regulation of beta-adrenoceptors in myocardial tissue of heart failure patients tested with metoprolol has been documented,[1] and the idea that sympathetic nervous system hyperactivity may lead to long-term negative consequences in heart failure patients has been used as justification for a number of clinical trials.[2] It is not yet firmly established that the long-term benefit reported in some studies of beta blocker therapy in heart failure is due to the observed increases in beta-adrenoceptor density. However, this is currently considered a reasonable explanation.[3]

Trials of beta blockade in heart failure have yielded conflicting results; some have shown a clear benefit of long-term beta blockade, while others (of shorter duration) have shown no benefit at all.[4,5] Long-term metoprolol therapy in patients with heart failure due to dilated cardiomyopathy has been shown to lead to an improved contractile response to catecholamine stimulation, and an improvement in resting cardiac output.[1] A trial of a beta blocker with ISA, Xamoterol, reported excess mortality among patients with severe heart failure receiving the drug.[6,7] In contrast, beta blockers with alpha-blocking activity such as labetalol, carvedilol, and bucindolol have all been well tolerated in small trials of patients with both idiopathic and ischemic cardiomyopathies. Because of potential exacerbation of heart failure, beta blockers must be used with extreme caution in patients with heart failure, particularly those with marked depression in left ventricular function.

REFERENCES

1. Heilbrunn, S.M., Shah, P., Bristow, M.R., et al.: Increased beta receptor density and improved hemodynamic response to catecholamine stimulation during long-term metoprolol therapy in heart failure from dilated cardiomyopathy. Circulation *79*:483, 1989.
2. Packer, M., et al: Role of the sympathetic nervous system in heart failure. Basic mechanisms and clinical directions. Circulation *82*(Suppl. 1):1, 1990.
3. Packer, M.: Pathophysiologic mechanisms underlying the effects of beta-adrenergic agonists and antagonists on functional capacity and survival in chronic heart failure. Circulation *82*:I-77, 1990.
4. Eichhorn, E.J., Bedetto, J.B., Malloy, C.R., et al.: Effect of beta adrenergic blockade on myocardial function and energetics in congestive heart failure. Circulation *32*:473, 1990.

5. Ikram, H., and Fitzpatrick, D.: Double-blind trial of chronic oral beta blockade in congestive cardiomyopathy. Lancet *2*:490, 1981.
6. The German and Austrian Xamoterol Study Group: Double-blind placebo-controlled comparison of digoxin and Xamoterol in chronic heart failure. Lancet *1*:489, 1988.
7. The Xamoterol in Severe Heart Failure Study Group: Xamoterol in severe heart failure. Lancet *336*:1, 1990.

144-D *(Braunwald, p. 823)*

Diabetics with mild chronic renal disease are particularly prone to develop the syndrome of hyporeninemic hypoaldosteronism because they are affected by a combination of low renin production and impaired insulin secretion, both of which increase the serum potassium concentration. Thus, supplemental potassium and potassium-sparing diuretics must be used with caution in such patients. Calcium channel blockers have also been reported to impair the adrenal secretion of aldosterone. Although tomatoes and bananas are rich sources of potassium, it would be unusual for a normal diet to cause such a marked rise in potassium. Urinary tract infections may increase potassium in the setting of worsened renal function (which was not observed in this patient). It is likely that either primary hypoaldosteronism or adrenal hypoplasia would have been detected by the finding of an elevated potassium concentration during the initial visit.[1]

REFERENCE

1. Gordon, R.D.: Syndrome of hypertension and hyperkalemia with normal glomerular filtration rate. Hypertension *8*:93, 1986.

145-D *(Braunwald, pp. 515–516; Fig. 18–2)*

Cardiac transplantation has also been performed since 1967; recent improvement in results is due to the potency and effectiveness of the immunosuppressant cyclosporine.[1] Important positive factors in considering a candidate for heart transplantation include psychological stability, a history of compliance with medical therapy, and younger age. Contraindications to cardiac transplantation include pulmonary hypertension or parenchymal pulmonary disease, insulin-dependent diabetes, coexistent liver or renal disease, psychological instability or substance abuse, active infection or duodenal ulcer, and clinically evident cerebral or vascular disease.

The transplanted heart is denervated but exhibits normal contractility and contractile reserve. It therefore responds to exercise by first increasing stroke volume, after which elevated levels of catecholamines lead to a reflex tachycardia. This mechanism allows near-normal circulatory response, excellent exercise tolerance, and successful rehabilitation in a large majority of long-term survivors. Acute rejection is monitored by right ventricular endomyocardial biopsy, which is carried out routinely at weekly intervals for the first 3 weeks postoperatively. The appearance of myocardial edema may be reflected in a fall in electrocardiographic QRS voltage; atrial arrhythmias and an S_3 gallop are other signs of rejection. Patients who survive for 3 months after transplantation have a greater than 80 per cent 2-year survival rate.

The difficulty in maintaining an adequate supply of donor hearts continues to be the limiting factor in the number of transplants performed. At present, most of the recipients of heart transplants have had coronary artery disease or cardiomyopathies.[2]

REFERENCES

1. Baumgartner, W.A., Reitz, B.A., and Achuff, S.A.: Heart and Heart-Lung Transplantation. Philadelphia, W.B. Saunders Co., 1990.
2. Kriett, J.M., and Kaye, M.P.: The Registry of the International Society for Heart Transplantation: Seventh Official Report—1990. J. Heart Transplant. 9:323, 1990.

146-B   (Braunwald, pp. 619–620)

Electrical cardioversion has proven to be an excellent method for termination of a variety of tachyarrhythmias, especially those presumed secondary to a reentry mechanism. In nonemergency situations, the procedure is well tolerated and may be performed on patients receiving digitalis therapy without stopping the digitalis prior to elective cardioversion, provided that no clinical evidence of digitalis toxicity exists.[1] Maintenance therapy with quinidine 1 to 2 days before electrical cardioversion in patients with atrial fibrillation produces reversion to sinus rhythm in 10 to 15 per cent and may help prevent recurrence of atrial fibrillation once sinus rhythm is restored in a number of these patients. The use of electrical cardioversion required a clinical assessment of the likelihood of establishing and maintaining sinus rhythm and the potential risks of other forms of therapy. Emergent use of direct current cardioversion is warranted for any tachycardia that produces congestive heart failure, angina, or hypotension and does not respond quickly to medical management. Rapid ventricular responses in patients with Wolff-Parkinson-White syndrome and atrial fibrillation may be best approached by using electrical cardioversion. Electrical cardioversion should be avoided, however, in patients with digitalis-induced tachyarrhythmias.

Since myocardial damage is directly related to the amount of energy employed for electrical cardioversion, it is important to use the lowest energy required to terminate the arrhythmia. Subsequent shocks should be titrated up to the energy necessary for successful cardioversion. Supraventricular arrhythmias may be interrupted with energies as low as 25 to 50 joules. An exception to this is atrial fibrillation, which may require a starting energy of 50 to 100 joules. Starting energies for cardioversion of stable ventricular tachycardia should be in the range of 25 to 50 joules. Ventricular fibrillation usually requires 200 to 400 joules for successful cardioversion.

On occasion, the initial attempt at cardioversion will precipitate transient ventricular arrhythmias; these may be suppressed by administration of a bolus of lidocaine before subsequent cardioversion attempts.[2] Cardioversion restores sinus rhythm in 70 to 95 per cent of patients, depending upon the underlying tachyarrhythmia present initially. In patients with chronic atrial fibrillation, however, the majority revert to atrial fibrillation within the first 12 months after cardioversion, limiting the effectiveness of cardioversion in the therapy of this disorder.

Complications from carefully performed direct-current cardioversion are uncommon, although occasionally even a properly synchronized shock may lead to ventricular fibrillation. Embolic episodes may occur in 1 to 3 per cent of patients converted to sinus rhythm and form the basis for the widespread clinical practice of prior anticoagulation for 3 weeks in patients at high risk for emboli and with no contraindictions to anticoagulant therapy. However, few controlled studies regarding the use of anticoagulants in the prevention of cardioversion-induced embolic events have been published. While cardioversion of ventricular tachycardia may be achieved by a chest "thump" the thump cannot be timed well to the cardiac cycle and may, on rare occasions, precipitate ventricular flutter or fibrillation.[3] This technique must therefore be applied cautiously and only in emergency clinical settings.

REFERENCES

1. Mann, D.L., Maisel, A.S., Atwood, J.E., et al.: Absence of cardioversion-induced ventricular arrhythmias in patients with therapeutic digoxin levels. J. Am. Coll. Cardiol. 5: 882, 1985.
2. Waldecker, B., Brugada, P., Zehender, M., et al.: Dysrhythmias after direct-current cardioversion. Am. J. Cardiol. 57: 120, 1986.
3. Cotoi, S.: Precordial thump and termination of cardiac reentrant tachyarrhythmias. Am. Heart J. 101:675, 1981.

147-D   (Braunwald, pp. 399–400)

Isotonic exercise resembles volume overload and causes a predominant increase in left ventricular (LV) end-diastolic volume, while isometric exercise resembles pressure overload and causes a predominant increase in wall thickness. However, both types of exercise increase LV wall thickness, mass, and stroke volume with little change in ejection fraction or resting cardiac output.[1] Furthermore, these changes are physiological adaptations that disappear when the increased exercise demands are reduced.

REFERENCE

1. Huston, T.P., Puffer, J.C., and Rodney, W.M.: The athletic heart syndrome. N. Engl. J. Med. 313:24, 1985.

148-D *(Braunwald, pp. 522–523; Fig. 18–6)*

Treatment of acute rejection following cardiac transplantation requires achieving a careful balance between effective immunosuppression and excessive immunosuppression; the latter carries the possibility of multiple opportunistic infections and other complications. Most acute rejection episodes occur within the first 3 months after transplantation. Among patients treated with the standard triple-drug regimen that includes cyclosporine, azathioprine, and prednisone, the vast majority will demonstrate at least one episode of rejection during the first 3 months. Patients with a good donor-recipient match who do not experience an acute rejection episode in the first 3 months have a lower incidence of late rejection.

Treatment of rejection is dictated by the time of its occurrence following transplantation (see Braunwald, Fig. 18–6, p. 522). Episodes occurring during the first 3 months following transplantation or that are moderate to severe in nature are currently treated by pulsed therapy with methylprednisolone. A number of centers are testing the possibility of using oral regimens in this setting, and such an approach may prove efficacious in time subsets of patients with rejection. When steroid therapy is ineffective in reversing rejection, the use of OKT3 monoclonal antibody therapy is the most frequent approach for rescue therapy and has proven to be an effective treatment for most resistant rejection episodes.[1] Increased doses of oral cyclosporine dosing may also be used in this setting. Some workers have also advocated the addition of methotrexate to the treatment regimen for resistant rejection. Total lymphoid irradiation as an alternative therapy for patients who do not respond to these conventional therapies has recently been advocated.[2] Preliminary studies suggest that this approach is effective in preventing further rejection and has minimal side effects, suggesting that it may be a more widely used approach in the future.

REFERENCES

1. O'Connell, J.B., Renlund, D.G., Gay, W.A., Jr., et al.: Efficacy of OKT3 retreatment for refractory cardiac allograft rejection. Transplantation *47*:788, 1989.
2. Hunt, S., Strober, S., Hoppe, R., et al.: Use of total lymphoid irridiation for therapy of intractable cardiac allograft rejection (abstr.). J. Heart Transplant. *8*:104, 1989.

149-C *(Braunwald, p. 465)*

Many medical and surgical conditions are associated with a chest x-ray pattern consistent with pulmonary edema, as in the accompanying x-ray. The physical examination of this hypothetical patient was essentially normal, without dramatic chest examination findings, jugular venous distention, or a third heart sound. This suggests that in this patient the edema was primarily caused not by an alteration in the Starling forces across pulmonary capillaries but rather by abnormal permeability of the alveolar capillary membrane. This situation is described by the term adult respiratory distress syndrome (ARDS).[1,2] Among the conditions that have been associated with ARDS are infectious pneumonia, inhaled toxins, circulating foreign substances including bacterial endotoxins, aspiration of gastric contents, acute radiation pneumonitis, release of endogenous vasoactive substances such as histamine, disseminated intravascular coagulation, immunological events including hypersensitivity pneumonitis and production of leukoagglutinins, shock lung in association with nonthoracic trauma, and acute hemorrhagic pancreatitis.

In the patient described there appear to be at least two pathological processes predisposing to ARDS—possible gram-negative septicemia due to a urinary tract infection, which would be common in a nursing home patient, as well as incipient disseminated intravascular coagulation manifested by the low platelet count and prolonged prothrombin time.

Although there are many theories proposed for the development of ARDS, a current model is that chemotactic factors, either circulating or in the tissues, cause movement of polymorphonuclear leukocytes to the lung where they adhere to damaged endothelium.[3] This interaction results in the release of many vasoactive substances, including arachidonic acid metabolites, oxygen radicals, proteases, kinins, and histamines. These factors combine to cause an increase in alveolar capillary permeability as well as to augment blood flow to the lung, the combination of which results in transudation of fluid and pulmonary edema. This theory is particularly attractive, since chemotoxins can arrive either from distal sources or can be derived from macrophages of the alveolar wall. This may explain the presence of ARDS in systemic illnesses such as gram-negative septicemia, hemorrhagic pancreatitis, and disseminated intravascular coagulation.

Bronchoalveolar lavage fluid from patients with ARDS demonstrates a predominance of neutrophils, leukocyte elastase, and partially inactivated alpha$_1$-antitrypsin (an antiprotease normally present in the lung). However, at this time, clinical therapeutic modalities specifically targeted at the neutrophil interactions in the lung are not available.

REFERENCES

1. Jardin, F., Eveleight, M.C., Gurdjian, F., et al.: Venous admixture in human septic shock. Comparative effects of blood volume expansion, dopamine infusion and isoprotererol infusion on mismatching of ventilation and pulmonary blood flow in peritonitis. Circulation *60*:155, 1979.
2. Vincent, J.L., Weil, M.H., Puri, V., and Carlson, R.W.: Circulatory shock assessed with purulent peritonitis. Am. J. Surg. *142*:262, 1981.
3. Rinaldo, J.E., Dauber, G.H., Christman, J., and Rogers, R.M.: Neutrophil alveolitis endotoxemia. Am. Rev. Respir. Dis. *130*:1065, 1984.

150-E *(Braunwald, p. 728)*

In bipolar lead systems the positive and negative electrodes are in an intracardiac position about 2.5 cm apart, while in unipolar systems only the cathode (negative) electrode is in the heart and a large area anode (positive) electrode, usually the metal housing of the pulse generator, is at a remote location. Since the tips of both types of electrodes are placed in intimate contact with the endocardium (or epicardium/myocardium), the thresholds for depolarization are similar. Although many 12-lead ECGs show larger depolarization spikes with unipolar electrodes, there is no statistical difference in signal amplitude generated by unipolar and bipolar electrodes. The amplitude of the pacemaker spike depends on the quality and settings of the ECG recorder and the pulse energy; the latter is the product of voltage and pulse duration.

However, there is a significant difference between unipolar and bipolar electrodes in terms of their susceptibility to electromagnetic interference (EMI) from power lines, radio and television transmitters, and skeletal muscle potentials. Because of the large separation between electrodes in the unipolar configuration, there is enhanced EMI detection. Thus, when myopotentials cause inappropriate triggering or inhibition of a pacemaker employing a unipolar electrode, switching to a bipolar lead system may solve the problem.

151-E *(Braunwald, pp. 456–457)*

A variety of laboratory abnormalities may be noted in patients with congestive heart failure. Alterations in serum electrolyte values usually occur after patients have begun treatment or in more longstanding, severe cases of heart failure. Hyponatremia may be seen for a variety of reasons. Included among these are prolonged or rigid sodium restriction, intensive diuretic therapy, a decrease in the ability to excrete water from reductions in renal blood flow and glomerular filtration rate,[1] and elevations in the concentration of circulating vasopressin.[2] Hypokalemia may result from aggressive diuretic therapy. Conversely, hyperkalemia may occasionally occur in patients with severe heart failure who have marked reductions in glomerular filtration rate. Such patients may be particularly prone to hyperkalemia if they are also receiving potassium-sparing diuretics.

Congestive hepatomegaly due to "backward" failure and cardiac cirrhosis from longstanding heart failure is often accompanied by impaired hepatic function, which may be reflected in abnormal values of the liver enzymes.[3] In acute hepatic venous congestion, severe jaundice may result, with bilirubin levels as high as 15 to 20 mg/dl, dramatic elevations of serum AST levels, and prolongation of the prothrombin time. While the clinical and laboratory profile of such an event may resemble viral hepatitis, the diagnosis of hepatic congestion due to heart failure is confirmed by the rapid normalization of these hepatic laboratory values with successful treatment of heart failure. It should be noted that in patients with longstanding heart failure and secondary severe hepatic damage, albumin synthesis may be impaired. Rarely, more severe sequelae may occur, including hepatic hypoglycemia, fulminant hepatic failure, and even hepatic coma.

The size and shape of the cardiac silhouette on the chest roentgenogram are two features of particular clinical relevance in the patient with congestive heart failure. Increases in cardiothoracic ratio and heart volume on the plain chest x-ray film are specific but not sensitive indicators of elevated left ventricular end-diastolic volume. Elevations in pulmonary capillary pressure are reflected in the appearance of the vasculature on the plain chest film. With minimal elevations (i.e., ~13 to 17 mm Hg), early equalization in the size of the vessels in the apices and bases is first discernible. It is not until greater pressure elevations occur (~18 to 20 mm Hg) that actual pulmonary vascular redistribution occurs. When pressure exceeds 20 to 25 mm Hg, frank interstitial pulmonary edema is usually observed.

REFERENCES

1. Cody, R.J., Ljungman, S., Covit, A.B., et al.: Regulation of glomerular filtration rate in chronic congestive heart failure patients. Kidney Int. *34*:361, 1988.
2. Szatalowicz, V.L., Arnold, P.E., Chaimovitz, C., et al.: Radioimmunoassay of plasma arginine vasopressin in hyponatremic patients with congestive heart failure. N. Engl. J. Med. *305*:263, 1981.
3. Kaplan, M.M.: Liver dysfunction secondary to congestive heart failure. Pract. Cardiol. *6*:39, 1980.

152-B *(Braunwald, pp. 369–370; Fig. 12–13)*

The calcium and sodium voltage-gated channels are structurally similar. Both are thought to contain four membrane-spanning alpha domains, as well as a beta-subunit that may regulate ion conductance through the channel pore. Each alpha-subunit contains six helices. The voltage sensor region of the calcium channel is contained within the positively charged S4 helical segment of each alpha-subunit. The alpha-subunits are folded in such a way that the S5 and S6 domains of each of the four alpha-subunits are in close proximity to the others, forming the functional pore of the ion channel.

Beta₁-adrenergic stimulation *increases* the open probability of voltage-gated calcium channels. Beta₁ stimulation increases levels of intracellular cAMP, leading to phosphorylation of the alpha-subunit of the voltage-gated calcium channel. The phosphorylation of the alpha-subunits results in a conformation change in the pore region of the channel, increasing the open probability.[1] The L type calcium channels are found in myocytes and are principally involved in calcium-induced calcium release. L channels may open for either short bursts or prolonged periods. The T channels open for short bursts and at a more negative membrane potential.[2] They may be important in early depolarization in cells of the SA node. It is not known if T channels are also present in ventricular cells.

REFERENCES

1. Tomaselli, G.F., Backx, P.H., and Marban, E: Molecular basis of permeation in voltage-gated ion channels. Circ. Res. *72*:491–496, 1993.
2. Flockerzi, V., and Hofmann, F.: Molecular structure of the cardiac calcium channel. *In* Sperelakis, E. (ed.): Physiology and Pathophysiology of the Heart. 3rd ed. Boston, Kluwer Academic Publishers, 1995, pp. 91–99.

153-C   *(Braunwald, pp. 844–846; Figs. 27–5 and 27–6)*

Many patients with mild hypertension (diastolic blood pressure <95 mm Hg) may benefit significantly from nondrug therapy. In several studies, weight loss has resulted in significant decreases in blood pressure; in one study an average of 8-kg weight reduction was associated with a 13 mm Hg decrease in diastolic blood pressure.[1] The effectiveness of decreasing sodium intake depends on the severity of pretreatment hypertension, with patients who have systolic blood pressure <190 registering 20 mm Hg decreases and those with systolic blood pressure of 160 mm Hg averaging 10 mm Hg decreases.[2] Furthermore, activation of counterregulatory mechanisms such as the renin-angiotensin system limits the overall effect of lowering sodium intake. Daily *isotonic* (but not isometric) exercise is associated with a 5 to 10 mm Hg reduction in blood pressure, as well as decreased cardiovascular mortality.[3]

Although increased vascular smooth muscle calcium may represent a common pathway for hypertension, paradoxically, hypertensive patients have a lower calcium intake and higher urinary calcium excretion than normotensive individuals.[4] Furthermore, about half of hypertensives have lowering of their blood pressure acutely in response to supplemental calcium.[5] Thus, reduction of dietary calcium is unlikely to be beneficial, and calcium supplementation may even lower blood pressure. Alcohol consumption of about 1 oz/day is associated with decreased cardiac mortality, but excessive alcohol intake exerts a pressor effect, so that alcohol abuse is the most common cause of reversible hypertension.[6,7]

REFERENCES

1. MacMahon, S.W., MacDonald, G.J., Bernstein, L., et al.: Comparison of weight reduction with metoprolol in treatment of hypertension in young overweight patients. Lancet *1*:1233, 1985.
2. MacGreggor, G.A.: Sodium is more important than calcium in essential hypertension. Hypertension *7*:628, 1985.
3. Jennings, G., Nelson, L., Nestel, P., et al.: The effects of changes in physical activity on major cardiovascular risk

factors, hemodynamics, sympathetic function and glucose utilization in man: A controlled study of four levels of activity. Circulation *73*:30, 1986.
4. McCarron, D.A.: Is calcium more important than sodium in the pathogenesis of essential hypertension? Hypertension *7*:607, 1985.
5. McCarron, D.A., and Morris, C.D.: Blood pressure response to oral calcium in persons with mild to moderate hypertension. Ann. Intern. Med. *103*:825, 1985.
6. Jackson, R., Stewart, A., Beaglehole, R., and Scragg, R.: Alcohol consumption and blood pressure. Am. J. Epidemiol. *122*:1037, 1985.
7. Alderman, M.H.: Non-pharmacological treatment of hypertension. Lancet *344*:307, 1994.

154-D   *(Braunwald, pp. 517–519)*

The availability of donor organs has proven to be the limiting factor for the number of cardiac transplantations that may be performed. A number of specific characteristics of cardiac donors are sought and carefully evaluated. In recent years, the upper age limit for the donor has been extended in many centers from the traditional limit of 35 years to higher than 55 years. Complete evaluation of potential donors includes both a thorough history and physical examination as well as a 12-lead electrocardiogram and an echocardiogram. Nonspecific ST- and T-wave abnormalities are common on the electrocardiogram due to increases in intracranial pressure following the specific neurological event that leads to death, as well as to the hypothermia commonly employed while the donor is being maintained. At the present time, ABO compatibility and appropriate size matching are the two criteria used to ensure compatibility between donor and recipient. When transplantation is performed without an ABO match, a significant increase in the number of acute rejection episodes occurs.[1]

Neurological events leading to brain death usually result in some degree of instability in the donor due to diabetes insipidus and altered fluid balance. Therefore, donors are frequently maintained with central venous pressure and fluid monitoring as well as with administration of vasopressin and fluid replacement as appropriate. If hypotension ensues, vasopressors are often used to maintain donor blood pressure while awaiting the harvesting of the donor heart. Thorough donor evaluation also includes serological testing. Currently, tests for HIV, hepatitis B antigen, cytomegalovirus and toxoplasmosis are performed. However, a routine screening for EBV is not currently considered necessary. HIV-positive status is a clear contraindication to transplantation, and in some centers the presence of CMV antibody excludes a donor for any CMV-negative recipient. Procurement of donor hearts from distant locations is routine. The average amount of ischemic time for the donor heart is 3 to 4 hours. Although there is thought to be a relationship between duration of donor ischemic time and survival, most centers do not report any relation with up to 6 hours of ischemic time.[2]

REFERENCES

1. Cooper, D.K.C., Human, P.A., Rose, A.G., et al.: Can cardiac allografts and xenografts be transplanted against the ABO blood group barrier? Transplant Proc. *21*:549, 1989.
2. Kaye, M.P.: The Registry of the International Society for Heart Transplantation: Fourth Official Report—1987. J. Heart Transplant. *6*:63, 1987.

155-E (Braunwald, pp. 603–604)

Procainamide is widely used to treat both supraventricular and ventricular arrhythmias. In electrophysiological studies, the intravenous response to procainamide predicts the response to the drug when given orally.[1] These studies have proven to be useful for evaluating the efficacy of this agent in appropriate patients. In patients with acute myocardial infarction, plasma concentrations of procainamide required to suppress PVCs may be less than the concentrations required to prevent spontaneous episodes of sustained ventricular tachycardia.[2] Procainamide may be used in the conversion of atrial fibrillation to sinus rhythm; however, as with quinidine, the prior use of digitalis, propranolol, or verapamil to slow atrial rate is recommended. This is because accelerated conduction through the AV node due to procainamide use, without prior slowing of the atrial rate, may lead to 1:1 conduction and an increase in the ventricular rate. Procainamide may block conduction in the accessory pathway of patients with WPW syndrome and thus may be useful in the treatment of tachyarrhythmias in these patients.

Multiple noncardiac side effects of procainamide have been reported, including skin rashes, myalgias, digital vasculitis, Raynauld's phenomenon, gastrointestinal side effects, and central nervous system toxicity. Higher doses of the drug may depress myocardial contractility and diminish myocardial performance, with resultant hypotension. In the presence of sinus node disease, procainamide tends to prolong the corrected sinus node recovery time and may therefore worsen symptoms in patients with the bradycardia-tachycardia syndrome.[3]

REFERENCES

1. Marchlinski, F.E., Buxton, A.E., Vassallo, J.A., et al.: Comparative electrophysiologic effects of intravenous and oral procainamide in patients with sustained ventricular arrhythmias. J. Am. Coll. Cardiol. *4*:1247, 1984.
2. Myerburg, R.J., Kessler, K.M., Kiem, I., et al.: Relationship between plasma levels of procainamide, suppression of premature ventricular complexes and prevention of recurrent ventricular tachycardia. Circulation *64*:280, 1981.
3. Goldberg, D., Reiffel, J.A., Davis, J.C., et al.: Electrophysiologic effects of procainamide on sinus node function in patients with and without sinus disease. Am. Heart J. *103*:75, 1982.

156-E (Braunwald, pp. 394–397)

The four determinants of ventricular performance of cardiac output are (1) heart rate, which can also affect contractility; (2) preload, which is closely related to left ventricular end-diastolic volume; (3) afterload, which is closely related to aortic impedance (i.e., the sum of the external factors that oppose ventricular ejection); and (4) contractility, which is a fundamental property of cardiac muscle and reflects the level of activation of cross-bridge formation. The oxygen-carrying capacity of blood, under normal conditions, is not rate limiting for cardiac performance. Anemia raises cardiac output presumably by reducing afterload (secondary to vasodilation) and increasing preload.

157-D (Braunwald, pp. 577–578)

Exercise testing has proven to be a useful diagnostic tool in the evaluation of patients with a history of cardiac arrhythmias. About one-third of normal subjects develop ventricular ectopy in response to exercise testing. A reading of up to six beats of nonsustained ventricular tachycardia, which does not indicate any increased risk of cardiovascular morbidity or mortality, may occur in such subjects.[1] Similarly, supraventricular premature beats are more common during exercise and do not necessarily suggest the presence of underlying heart disease. Patients with coronary artery disease develop PVCs at lower heart rates than do normal subjects, and they may demonstrate such ventricular ectopy more frequently during the early recovery period. Controversy still exists about whether exercise-induced ventricular arrhythmias in patients with coronary artery disease predict a higher cardiovascular risk.

Exercise testing is useful and relatively safe in patients who have had previously identified serious ventricular arrhythmias. Only a small percentage of such patients require immediate intervention for induced arrhythmias during the exercise testing protocol.[2] While stress testing is more sensitive than the standard 12-lead resting ECG for the detection of ventricular ectopy, it is not as sensitive as prolonged ambulatory monitoring. However, the use of the combination of ambulatory monitoring and stress testing to uncover arrhythmias may be a prudent course in selected patients, because each technique may identify arrhythmias that the other technique fails to uncover.

REFERENCES

1. Fleg, J.L., and Lakatta, E.G.: Prevalence and prognosis of exercise-induced nonsustained ventricular tachycardia in apparently healthy volunteers. Am. J. Cardiol. *54*:762, 1984.
2. Young, D.Z., Lampert, S., Graboys, T.B., and Lown, B.: Safety of maximal exercise testing in patients at high risk for ventricular arrhythmias. Circulation *70*:184, 1984.

158-D (Braunwald, pp. 825–827; Tables 26–10 and 26–11)

Although renovascular disease is the second most common cause of secondary hypertension (after chronic renal disease), it is still quite rare.[1] The most common cause (60 per cent of cases) of renovascular hypertension is atherosclerosis affecting the proximal 2 cm of the renal artery and occurs most frequently in elderly males.[2] Nonatherosclerotic renal artery stenoses involve all layers of the vessel, most frequently the media. In children and young adults, intimal and fibromuscular hyperplasia is common. Among blacks, renovascular hypertension is less common than in Caucasians, although chronic renal disease is more common.[3] The greatest prevalence of renovascular disease (20 per cent) occurs in patients with severe hypertension.[4]

REFERENCES

1. Sinclair, A.M., Isles, C.G., Brown, I., et al.: Secondary hypertension in a blood pressure clinic. Arch. Intern. Med. *147*:1289, 1987.
2. Novick, A.C.: The case for surgical therapy. *In* Narins, R.G. (ed.): Controversies in Nephrology and Hypertension. New York, Churchill Livingstone, 1984, p. 181.
3. Keith, T.A., III: Renovascular hypertension in black patients. Hypertension *4*:438, 1982.
4. Working Group on Renovascular Hypertension: Detection, evaluation, and treatment of renovascular hypertension. Final Report. Arch. Intern. Med. *147*:820, 1987.

159-B   *(Braunwald, pp. 641–643, 678–679)*

Invasive electrophysiological (EP) studies have proven to be safe and useful in the diagnostic evaluation of patients with underlying disturbances of cardiac rhythm and conduction. In patients with an intraventricular conduction disturbance, EP study may be used to evaluate the length of the H-V interval. H-V intervals >55 msec are associated with organic heart disease, a greater likelihood of developing trifascicular block, and higher mortality. In patients with intraventricular conduction defects and syncope or presyncope, ventricular tachyarrhythmias are often found to be responsible.[1]

The technique of overdrive suppression may be used to evaluate sinus node function. The SNRT is measured by subtracting the spontaneous sinus node cycle length before pacing from the length of the first spontaneous sinus response after termination of pacing. Normal values are generally <525 msec, and prolongation of SNRT has been found in patients suspected of having sinus node dysfunction. Since many patients with impaired sinus node function also exhibit abnormal AV conduction, it is important also to evaluate AV nodal and His-Purkinje function in this population.[2]

In patients with tachycardias, EP studies may be used to differentiate between supraventricular tachycardia with aberrant intraventricular conduction and a ventricular origin of the tachycardia. Supraventricular tachycardia is recognized electrophysiologically by the presence of an H-V interval equal to or greater than that recorded during normal sinus rhythm. In contrast, only two situations result in an H-V interval that is consistently shorter than normal: ventricular tachycardia when retrograde activation of the His bundle from a site originating in the ventricle leads to a short H-V interval, and atrioventricular conduction that occurs over an accessory pathway.[2] Localizing the site of origin and the pathway involved in the maintenance of tachycardia due to Wolff-Parkinson-White syndrome or its variants by endocardial mapping has proven to be an important part of the preoperative evaluation of patients considered for ablative surgery. Patients with this syndrome who are at risk for the development of serious supraventricular or ventricular tachycardias or sudden cardiac death may be first identified by EP testing.[3]

REFERENCES

1. Dhingra, R.C., Palileo, E., Strasberg, B., et al.: Significance of the HV interval in 517 patients with chronic bifascicular block. Circulation *64*:1265, 1981.
2. Zipes, D.P., Akhtar, M., Denes, P., et al.: ACC/AHA guidelines for clinical intracardiac electrophysiologic studies. J. Am. Coll. Cardiol. *14*:1827, 1989 and Circulation *80*:1925, 1989.
3. Gallagher, J.J.: Accessory pathway tachycardia: Techniques of electrophysiologic study and mechanisms. Circulation *75*:III-31, 1987.

160-C   *(Braunwald, pp. 618–619)*

Adenosine is an endogenous nucleoside that has recently been approved for the treatment of supraventricular tachycardias. The agent interacts with specific adenosine receptors on the surface of cardiac cells and results ultimately in transient prolongation of the A-H interval and a transient AV nodal block of varying degrees. The drug is given as a bolus intravenous injection at doses of 6 to 12 mg, which consistently lead to transient sinus slowing, or AV nodal block.[1] Adenosine is now probably the drug of choice for acute termination of supraventricular tachycardias.[2] In addition to achieving termination of 92 per cent of supraventricular tachycardias within 30 sec, adenosine does not have the negative inotropic effects of verapamil; this allows more widespread use in the acute setting.

Adenosine may be helpful in the differentiation of wide QRS tachycardia.[3] In this setting, the drug may terminate supraventricular tachycardias with aberrancy or reveal an underlying atrial mechanism, although it does not block conduction over accessory pathways or terminate most ventricular tachycardias. Therefore, the drug may also be of use in differentiating conduction over the AV node versus an accessory pathway during ablative procedures designed to interrupt accessory pathways.[4] Interestingly, patients with heart transplants exhibit a supersensitive response to adenosine.[5] Transient side effects are common with adenosine, occurring in up to 40 per cent of patients. The most common side effects are dyspnea, chest pressure, and flushing, all of which are fleeting and generally resolve within a minute.

REFERENCES

1. Belardinelli, L., Linden, J., Berne, R.M.: The cardiac effects of adenosine. Prog. Cardiovasc. Dis. *32*:73, 1989.
2. DiMarco, J.P., Miles, W., Akhtar, M., et al.: Adenosine for paroxysmal supraventricular tachycardia: Dose ranging and comparison with verapamil. Assessment in placebo controlled, multicenter trials. Ann. Intern. Med. *113*:104, 1990.
3. Sharma, A.D., Klein, G.J., and Yee, R.: Intravenous adenosine triphosphate during wide QRS complex tachycardia. Safety, therapeutic efficacy and diagnostic utility. Am. J. Med. *88*:337, 1990.
4. Rinne, C., Sharma, A.D., Klein, G.J., et al.: Comparative effects of adenosine triphosphate on accessory pathway and arterioventricular nodal conduction. Am. Heart J. *115*: 1042, 1988.
5. Ellenbogen, K.A., Thames, M.D., DiMarco, J.P., et al.: Electrophysiological effects of adenosine in the transplanted human heart: Evidence of super sensitivity. Circulation *81*:821, 1990.

161-D   (Braunwald, pp. 827–829)

Primary aldosteronism is rare in unselected hypertensive patients but should be considered in hypertensive patients presenting with hypokalemia.[1] Although solitary benign tumors are the most common etiology, up to 25 per cent of patients may have bilateral adrenal hyperplasia.[2] Typically, patients with excessive aldosterone have urinary potassium excretion >30 mEq/day. Hypertensive patients with hypokalemia and low urine potassium may have gastrointestinal losses or may have had prior diuretic therapy. In primary aldosteronism plasma renin activity is low owing to feedback inhibition by high levels of circulating aldosterone. A high renin state with urinary potassium >30 mEq/day suggests renovascular hypertension, or a salt-wasting renal disease. If renin and aldosterone are both low, and elevated urinary potassium coexists with hypokalemia, ingestion of exogenous mineralocorticoids such as licorice (glycyrrhizinic acid) should be considered.[3]

REFERENCES

1. Young, W.F., Jr., Hogan, M.J., Klee, G.G., et al.: Primary aldosteronism: Diagnosis and treatment. Mayo Clin. Proc. *65*:96, 1990.
2. Banks, W.B., Kastin, A.J., Biglieri, E.D., and Ruiz, A.E.: Primary adrenal hyperplasia: A new subset of primary hyperaldosteronism. J. Clin. Endocrinol. Metab. *58*:783, 1984.
3. Coreda, J.M., Trono, D., and Schifferli, J.: Liquorice intoxication caused by alcohol-free pastis. Lancet *12*:1442, 1983.

162-E   (Braunwald, pp. 399–400)

Myocardial hypertrophy appears to develop in a manner that maintains systolic stress within normal limits. When the primary stimulus is pressure overload, the increase in systolic wall stress leads to addition of new myofibrils in parallel, wall thickening, and concentric hypertrophy. When the primary stimulus is volume overload, there initially is increased diastolic wall stress with addition of new myofibrils in series and ventricular di-

latation, which results in a small increase in systolic stress (by the Laplace relationship) and a small increase in wall thickness. Thus, in states of volume overload, chamber enlargement (eccentric hypertrophy) predominates, while in pressure overload, wall thickness (concentric hypertrophy) predominates.

163-A   (Braunwald, pp. 830–832)

Diagnosis of susceptibility to pregnancy-associated hypertension is performed by the "rollover" test at the 28th week. This test involves measuring blood pressure first in the left lateral recumbent position and then in the supine position. A rise in the diastolic blood pressure of >20 mm Hg within 2 to 5 minutes is considered positive.[1] Patients with a positive test should be told to restrict their activity. Neither diuretics nor sodium restriction is an effective therapy.[2] Because pregnancy-induced hypertension is usually associated with decreased uteroplacental flow, reduction in intravascular volume is contraindicated. Methyldopa is useful in the chronic management of hypertension, while hydralazine is often chosen for acute parenteral use.[3] Beta blockers, especially metoprolol, have also been shown to be safe and effective antihypertensive therapy,[4] though recently atenolol has been associated with intrauterine growth retardation.[5]

REFERENCES

1. O'Brien, W.F.: Predicting preeclampsia. Obstet. Gynecol. *75*: 445, 1990.
2. Collins, R., Yusuf, S., and Peto, R.: Overview of randomized trials of diuretics in pregnancy. Br. Med. J. *290*:17, 1985.
3. Cockburn, J., Ounsted, M., Moar, V.A., and Redman, C.W.B.: Final report of study on hypertension during pregnancy. The effects of specific treatment on the growth and development of the children. Lancet *1*:647, 1982.
4. Plouin, P.F., Breart, G., Llado, J., et al.: A randomized comparison of early with conservative use of antihypertensive drugs in the management of pregnancy-induced hypertension. Br. J. Obstet. Gynaecol. *97*:134, 1990.
5. Butters, L., Kennedy, S., and Rubin, P.C.: Atenolol in essential hypertension during pregnancy. Br. Med. J. *301*:587, 1990.

164-C   (Braunwald, pp. 515–517; Table 18–1)

One of the most difficult facets of cardiac transplantation is the development of appropriate guidelines for selecting recipients. More than 85 per cent of all transplantations have occurred since 1985, and selection criteria have been in a constant state of evolution during this time. The upper age limit for transplantation is a case in point. The initial Stanford University criteria used an upper age limit of 50 years. As results improved, this was extended to 55 years, and current experience indicates that even a strict chronological age criterion of 55 is no longer appropriate.[1] An exponential rise in the number of potential recipients occurs as the age limit is extended. Definitions of appropriate upper age limits for transplantation recipients therefore is a central and complicated issue. Most transplantation candidates come from one of two diagnostic categories: cardiomyopathy or coronary artery disease. Valvular heart disease, retransplantation, or congenital heart disease each make up <5 per cent of the underlying diseases in potential transplant recipients (see Braunwald, Fig. 18–2, p. 516).

Careful evaluation of a potential transplant recipient includes thorough consideration of all conventional medical or surgical therapeutic options, a comprehensive psychosocial evaluation, exclusion of any potentially treatable causes of cardiomyopathy and reversible forms of heart failure, and identification of any clear contraindications to transplantation. Most centers include an endomyocardial biopsy in the evaluation of the transplant patient in order to rule out potentially treatable causes of cardiomyopathy, such as active myocarditis or sarcoidosis. Pulmonary vascular disease must be carefully identified and evaluated. Although the optimal method of measuring pulmonary vascular resistance is still controversial, most centers use the pulmonary vascular resistance index or transpulmonary pressure gradient to quantitate this variable.[2] Specific contraindications to heart transplantation currently include insulin-dependent diabetes mellitus, advanced age, and irreversible hepatic or renal dysfunction. Patients with involvement of organs that are themselves subject to transplantation may be candidates for dual organ transplantation. This includes heart-lung, heart-kidney, and heart-liver transplantation.

REFERENCES

1. Loeb, M., Schueler, S., Warnecke, H., et al.: The effect of older age on the outcome of heart transplantation. J. Heart Transplant. 7:258, 1988.
2. Renlund, G.D., Gilbert, E.M., O'Connell, J.B., et al.: Age-associated decline in cardiac allograft rejection. Am. J. Med. 83:391, 1987.

165-D (Braunwald, p. 484)

Digitalis toxicity is an extremely common adverse drug reaction encountered in clinical practice and may occur in between 5 and 15 per cent of hospitalized patients receiving these drugs. While a variety of clinical manifestations may occur with digitalis toxicity, gastrointestinal symptoms, neurological symptoms, and cardiac rhythm disturbances are among the most frequent.[1] Early digitalis intoxication may be manifested by anorexia, which then may be followed by nausea and vomiting resulting from central nervous system mechanisms.[2] A variety of neurological symptoms may result from excess digitalis. These include visual symptoms such as scotomas, halos, and changes in color perception, as well as headache, fatigue, malaise, neuralgic pain, disorientation, delirium, and even seizures. With both gastrointestinal and neurolog-

ical symptoms it may be difficult to determine whether digitalis excess is the causative factor or whether the associated illness leads to these disturbances.

Cardiac toxicity from digitalis may be manifested by essentially any known rhythm disturbance.[3] Among the most common of these are atrioventricular junctional escape rhythms, ventricular bigeminy or trigeminy, nonparoxysmal junctional tachycardia, unifocal or multifocal ectopic ventricular beats, and ventricular tachycardia. Rhythms that combine features of increased automaticity of ectopic pacemakers with impaired conduction, such as PAT with block, strongly suggest digitalis toxicity (see also Question and Answer 218, p. 121 this book). However, PAT with block may frequently result from underlying heart disease rather than digitalis excess. A demonstration of a reversion to normal rhythm when the drug is withheld may at times help clarify this dilemma. Other less common manifestations of digitalis toxicity include allergic skin lesions, sexual dysfunction, and occasionally gynecomastia.[4]

REFERENCES

1. Wellens, H.J.J.: The electrocardiogram in digitalis intoxication. In Yu, P.N., and Goodwin, J.F. (eds.): Progress in Cardiology. Vol. 5. Philadelphia, Lea & Febiger, 1976, p. 271.
2. Borison, H.L., and Wang, S.C.: Physiology and pharmacology of vomiting. Pharmacol. Rev. 5:193, 1953.
3. Friedman, P.L., and Antman, E.M.: Electrocardiographic manifestations of digitalis toxicity. In Smith, T.W. (ed.): Digitalis Glycosides. Orlando, Grune & Stratton, 1985, pp. 241–275.
4. LeWinn, E.B.: Gynecomastia during digitalis therapy: Report of eight additional cases with liver-function studies. N. Engl. J. Med. 248:316, 1953.

166-C (Braunwald, pp. 196–198)

Detection and quantification of shunts within the cardiac chambers or great vessels can be accomplished by cardiac catheterization, echocardiography, radionuclide, and magnetic resonance imaging. Shunt evaluation by cardiac catheterization involves utilizing oximetry in multiple locations and calculation of pulmonary and systemic blood flow. Comparison of pulmonary and systemic blood flows helps to establish the presence and magnitude of shunt, whereas oximetry in multiple locations helps to localize the site of shunting. During right heart catheterization, screening oxygen saturations are obtained from the superior vena cava and pulmonary artery. A screening pulmonary artery saturation of >80 per cent or a "step-up" of >8 per cent suggests a left-to-right shunt, whereas an unexplained systemic arterial saturation of <95 per cent suggests a right-to-left shunt. "Physiological" shunting, such as hypoventilation, pulmonary edema, and cardiogenic shock, should be correctable with the administration of 100 per cent oxygen. Failure to correct with 100 per cent oxygen suggest an anatomical shunt.

A shortcoming of oximetric shunt detection is its lack of sensitivity. Despite the lack of sensitivity, most clinically relevant shunts can be detected using this method. When performing an oximetry run, multiple sites in the inferior vena cava, superior vena cava, and right atrium must be sampled. The oxygen saturation from these sites may vary widely. The inferior vena cava, because of the relatively low renal oxygen consumption for its blood flow, usually has the *highest* oxygen saturation. Conversely, the coronary sinus delivers venous blood with a very low oxygen saturation. The Flamm formula, the most common formula for estimating mixed venous oxygen content, states that mixed venous oxygen content is equal to 3(SVC oxygen content) + 1(IVC oxygen content) ÷ 4.[1]

REFERENCE

1. Flamm, M.D., Cohn, K.E., and Hancock, E.W.: Measurement of systemic cardiac output at rest and exercise in patients with atrial septal defect. Am. J. Cardiol. *23*:258, 1969.

167-B *(Braunwald, p. 478; Table 16–3)*

The two classes of potassium-sparing diuretics are (1) the aldosterone antagonists such as spironolactone and (2) the direct inhibitors of collecting duct sodium conductance, amiloride and triamterene (see Braunwald, Table 16–3, p. 477). Aldosterone antagonists actually lead to an *increase* in the synthesis of new cation-transporting proteins following binding to a cytoplasmic receptor in aldosterone-responsive cells.[1] These agents are not very effective in the treatment of heart failure when used alone, although in conditions such as ascites, in which aldosterone levels are high, single-diuretic therapy with spironolactone is often efficacious. Amiloride and triamterene, by reducing sodium conductance of the apical membrane, inhibit sodium uptake and thus effect a natriuresis.[2] Because these agents lead to decreased renal natriuresis.[2] Because these agents lead to decreased renal potassium secretion, they may cause hyperkalemia, especially in patients with underlying renal insufficiency. Potassium-sparing diuretics used in combination with loop diuretics are widely used in the therapy of both hypertension and congestive heart failure. These agents confer several advantages, including protection of patients from potassium and magnesium depletion, and possible beneficial effects on peripheral vascular tone.[3]

REFERENCES

1. Fanestil, D.D.: Mechanism of action of aldosterone blockers. Semin. Nephrol. *8*:249, 1988.
2. Kleyman, T.R., and Cragoe, E.J., Jr.: The mechanism of action of amiloride. Semin. Nephrol. *8*:242, 1988.
3. LaGrue, G., Anaquer, J.C., and Meyer-Heine, A.: Peripheral action of spironolactone: Improvement in arterial elasticity. Am. J. Cardiol. *65*:9K, 1990.

168-D *(Braunwald, pp. 471–476)*

A number of vasodilator agents have been used to treat congestive heart failure. Sodium nitroprusside is a short-acting, balanced vasodilator with direct relaxing effects on vascular smooth muscle in both arteries and veins. The most important adverse effect of the agent, hypotension, is thus an extension of its therapeutic actions. Other, less common, side effects are toxicity from its metabolic by-products hydrocyanic acid and cyanide. Cyanide is metabolized in the liver to thiocyanate, which is excreted by the kidneys. Hepatic or renal failure and hepatic congestion can lead to toxicity from hydrocyanic acid or cyanide. Hydrocyanic acid toxicity may cause abdominal pain, mental status changes, or convulsions. Cyanide toxicity should be suspected if there is a fall in cardiac output or onset of metabolic acidosis (due to lactic acid accumulation) during nitroprusside therapy.

A variety of nitrate formulations have all found application in the treatment of congestive heart failure.[1] Sublingual nitroglycerin has been shown to initiate a rapid decrease in LV filling pressure. In patients in whom LV filling pressure is elevated, a decline of approximately 40 per cent occurs in 5 to 10 minutes following administration of the drug. The effect is maximal in 8 to 10 minutes and persists for up to 30 minutes.

Hydralazine is an orally effective agent that acts directly on arteriolar smooth muscle. Patients with marked cardiomegaly and elevations of systemic vascular resistance appear to respond most favorably to this agent. An important multicenter trial, the VheFT-1 study,[2] demonstrated that 300 mg of hydralazine daily combined with isosorbide dinitrate results in improved survival compared with placebo or prazosin in patients with heart failure. This was the first demonstration of a beneficial effect of vasodilator agents on survival. Hydralazine may also be able to modify favorably the natural history of minimally symptomatic aortic regurgitation.[3]

In many patients with congestive heart failure, the renin-angiotensin-aldosterone system is highly active. Angiotensin-converting enzyme (ACE) inhibitors have found wide application in the management of heart failure in recent years, particularly after the SOLVD trials proved a survival benefit from ACE inhibitors in patients with heart failure.[4] These agents usually diminish both left and right ventricular filling pressures and lead to a rise in cardiac output. However, they have little or no effect on heart rate or arterial blood pressure.[5] In addition to improving hemodynamics in response to other therapeutic agents, ACE inhibitors often enhance the sense of well-being in patients with congestive heart failure.

REFERENCES

1. Cohn, J.N.: Nitrates for congestive heart failure. Am. J. Cardiol. *56*:19A, 1985.

2. Cohn, J.N., Archibald, D.G., Ziesche, S., et al.: Effect of vasodilator therapy on mortality in chronic congestive heart failure. Results of a Veterans Administration Cooperative Study. N. Engl. J. Med. 314:1547, 1986.
3. Greenberg, B., Massie, B., Bristow, J.D., et al.: Long-term vasodilator therapy of chronic aortic insufficiency. A randomized double-blind, placebo-controlled clinical trial. Circulation 78:92, 1988.
4. SOLVD Investigators: Effect of enalapril on survival in patients with reduced left ventricular ejection fractions and congestive heart failure. N. Engl. J. Med. 325:293, 1991.
5. Creager, M.A., Halperin, J.L., Bernard, D.B., et al.: Acute regional circulatory and renal hemodynamic effects of converting enzyme inhibition in patients with congestive heart failure. Circulation 64:483, 1981.

169-D (Braunwald, pp. 179–180)

Although generally a safe procedure, cardiac catheterization has well-defined risks that are more prevalent in certain patient populations. The overall risk of death from cardiac catheterization is from 0.14 to 0.75 per cent of patients.[1-4] Patients at highest risk of death from cardiac catheterization include patients with significant left main coronary artery disease, NYHA class III or IV symptoms of heart failure, advanced age, severe aortic valve disease, and three-vessel coronary artery disease (see Braunwald, Table 6–2, p. 179).[2] Minor complications, including transient hypotension or brief episodes of angina, occur in approximately 4 per cent of patients. The increased risk of cardiac catheterization in octogenarians is primarily due to peripheral vascular complications. In addition to advanced age, risk factors for vascular complications include congestive heart failure and larger body surface area. There is a slightly higher risk of complications when the brachial artery approach is used. Nonionic contrast agents are associated with fewer hemodynamic and arrhythmic side effects. Nonionic contrast agents may be *more* thrombogenic than ionic contrast agents. The inherent thrombogenicity or nonionic contrast agents may be related to the formulation of "thin" fibrin in the thrombus.[5]

REFERENCES

1. Braunwald, E., and Swan, H.J.C.: Cooperative study on cardiac catheterization. Circulation 37(Suppl. III):1, 1968.
2. Kennedy, J.W.: Complication associated with cardiac catheterization and angiography. Cathet. Cardiovasc. Diagn. 8:13, 1982.
3. Johnson, L.W., Lozner, E.C., Johnson, S., et al.: Coronary arteriography 1984–1987: A report of the Registry of the Society for Cardiac Angiography and Interventions. Results and complications. Cathet. Cardiovasc. Diagn. 17:5, 1989.
4. Davis, K., Kennedy, J.W., Kemp, H.G., et al.: Complications of coronary arteriography from the collaborative study of coronary artery surgery (CASS). Circulation 59:1105, 1979.
5. Granger, C.B., Gabriel, D.A., Reece, N.S., et al.: Fibrin modification by ionic and non-ionic contrast media during cardiac catheterization. Am. J. Cardiol. 69:8217, 1992.

170-C (Braunwald, pp. 189–192)

Several methods, including indicator-dilution, thermodilution, Fick, and angiography, can be used to measure cardiac output. Thermodilution and Fick methods are now the most frequently used. The thermodilution method, based on the principles of the indicator-dilution technique developed in the late nineteenth century, utilizes the temperature change on a cold saline or dextrose injectate as a function of cardiac output. When the cardiac output is high, the injectate is rapidly dispersed and the area under the curve is small. Therefore, the area under the thermodilution curve is *inversely* related to the cardiac output valve.

Although the thermodilution method is easily and widely used, it is subject to pitfalls. Thermodilution cardiac output is inaccurate in the presence of tricuspid regurgitation. In low-output states, the low-temperature injectate disperses into surrounding cardiac tissue causing a small area under the curve and therefore a falsely elevated value for cardiac output. When measuring cardiac output using the thermodilution technique, it is important to examine the curve generated to minimize sources of error. Examination of thermodilution curves may also provide clues about cardiac pathology. Patients who have left-to-right shunts may have early recirculation on the thermodilution curve.

The Fick principle states that the rate of blood flow in a given period of time is equal to the amount of an indicator entering the blood in that period of time divided by the difference in concentration of the indicator at points proximal and distal to the point of entry of the indicator.[1] This is accomplished in the cardiac catheterization laboratory using oxygen as the indicator. Oxygen consumption is measured while the arterial and mixed venous oxygen saturations are measured. Inaccuracy in oxygen consumption values leads to variability in the cardiac output measurements by as much as 10 per cent. The Fick method is, however, more accurate than thermodilution in low-output states.

Cardiac output may also be calculated angiographically by measuring stroke volume from tracings of end-diastolic and end-systolic images. The cardiac output is determined by multiplying the angiographic stroke volume by the heart rate. Sources of error in this method result from inaccuracy in determining cardiac volumes. However, angiographic cardiac output is preferred over thermodilution and Fick methods for calculation of stenotic orifice areas in the presence of aortic or mitral regurgitation because these latter methods grossly underestimate flow across the diseased valve, since they measure only forward flow.

REFERENCE

1. Winniford, M.D., and Lambert, C.R.: Blood flow measurement. In Pepine, C.J., Hill, J.A., and Lambert, C.R. (eds.): Diagnostic and Therapeutic Cardiac Catheterization. 2nd ed. Baltimore, Williams & Wilkins, 1994, p. 322.

171-C *(Braunwald, pp. 480–482)*

The beneficial effects of digitalis in congestive heart failure derive in part from the positive inotropic effect on the myocardium that the drug displays. This inotropic action of digitalis has been demonstrated in both normal and failing heart muscle. Experimental studies of the velocity of contraction of heart muscle at varying loads have demonstrated an augmentation of the velocity of muscle shortening at any given load by digitalis. The absolute increase in tension development induced by digitalis in normal myocardium is at least as great as that induced in failing myocardium. However, because the failing myocardium has a lower peak tension, the *relative* augmentation of tension in failing myocardium may be greater.

It should be noted that administration of cardiac glycosides in normal subjects results in little or no change in cardiac output. It has been demonstrated that digitalis augments the contractile state of the nonfailing myocardial tissue, but compensatory adjustments in preload, afterload, and heart rate prevent any obvious increase in cardiac output in the normal heart.[1]

A number of studies using both noninvasive and invasive techniques have demonstrated sustained improvement in cardiac performance in patients with chronic congestive heart failure. Both patient selection and the degree of ventricular dysfunction help determine whether or not a clinical response will be achieved. In general, studies of patients with depressed left ventricular ejection fractions and an audible S_3 gallop sound have demonstrated a benefit from digoxin therapy.[2] The role of digitalis therapy in minimally symptomatic or treated patients with congestive heart failure is less well defined.[3,4]

REFERENCES

1. Braunwald, E.: Effects of digitalis on the normal and the failing heart. J. Am. Coll. Cardiol. *5*:51A, 1985.
2. Lee, D.C.S., Johnson, R.A., Bigham, J.B., et al.: Heart failure in outpatients. A randomized trial of digoxin versus placebo. N. Engl. J. Med. *306*:699, 1982.
3. Fleg, J.L., Gottlieb, S.H., and Lakatta, E.G.: Is digoxin really important in treatment of compensated heart failure? Am. J. Med. *73*:244, 1982.
4. Gheorghiade, M., and Beller, G.A.: Effects of discontinuing maintenance digoxin therapy in patients with ischemic heart disease and congestive heart failure in sinus rhythm. Am. J. Cardiol. *51*:1243, 1983.

172-C *(Braunwald, pp. 605–607)*

Lidocaine has found wide clinical application in the treatment of ventricular arrhythmias due to the ease and rapidity of parenteral administration of the drug and a low incidence of complications and side effects. The drug, however, is generally ineffective against arrhythmias of supraventricular origin. In addition, in patients with the Wolff-Parkinson-White syndrome with a short effective refractory period of the accessory pathway, lidocaine has no significant effect and may even accelerate the ventricular response during atrial fibrillation.[1]

Lidocaine has been used clinically primarily in patients with acute myocardial infarction or recurrent ventricular tachyarrhythmias. In patients resuscitated from out-of-hospital ventricular fibrillation, lidocaine and bretylium are comparable for prevention of recurrent episodes of ventricular tachyarrhythmias. The use of lidocaine in a prophylactic manner to prevent ventricular arrhythmias in patients hospitalized with acute myocardial infarction remains a controversial issue, though most data suggest that prophylactic lidocaine is probably *not* indicated for all patients.[2] Thus, the choice of patients appropriate for prophylactic lidocaine therapy is primarily a clinical one, with factors such as age, the presence of hepatic dysfunction, and the elapsed time since the onset of chest pain all contributing to the decision to employ this agent.

REFERENCES

1. Akhtar, M., Filbert, C.K., and Shenasa, M.: Effect of lidocaine on atrioventricular response via the accessory pathway in patients with Wolf-Parkinson-White syndrome. Circulation *63*:435, 1981.
2. Yusuf, S., Wittes, J., and Friedman, L.: Overview of results of randomized clinical trials in heart disease. 1. Treatments following myocardial infarction. JAMA *260*:2088, 1988.

173-C *(Braunwald, pp. 654–656)*

Atrial fibrillation (AF) is characterized by total disorganization of atrial depolarization without effective atrial contractions. This disorganization results in the absence of P waves on the ECG and an irregular ventricular response between 100 and 160 beats/min (in the untreated patient with normal AV conduction). When the ventricular rate is quite rapid or quite slow, an apparent regularization of the ventricular response may occur.

Physical findings in patients with AF may include a slight variation in the intensity of S_1, an *absence* of *a* waves in the jugular venous pulse, and an irregularly irregular ventricular rhythm. As the ventricular rate increases, a pulse *deficit* may appear. During this, the apical rate is notably faster than the rate palpated at the wrist because some early ventricular depolarizations are not associated with normal opening of the aortic valve.

Although intermittent AF may occur in patients without cardiac disease, the chronic form of the arrhythmia is usually associated with underlying heart disease. AF is commonly found in populations with hypertensive cardiovascular disease, rheumatic heart disease, and atrial septal defect, as well as with cardiomyopathies and coronary artery disease, and after cardiac surgery.[1] In patients without obvious cardiovascular disease and paroxysms of AF, no increase in mortality rates has been noted. However, the development of chronic AF in patients with known cardiovascular disease results in a doubling of overall mortality.[2]

In individuals with "lone" AF (without obvious structural heart disease), no increase in the risk of cardiac events is noted. Patients who are younger than 65 and have no risk factors have a 1 per cent yearly risk of stroke. It therefore appears that patients with lone AF who are younger than 60 do not require anticoagulation, whereas those with lone AF between 60 and 75 years of age (risk of stroke about 2 per cent) can be adequately anticoagulated with aspirin. AF may develop in the peri-infarction setting as well as in the year following MI. Patients developing AF at the time of an acute MI tend to be older and to have a higher pulmonary capillary wedge pressure. Those developing AF in the first year following MI in general have a more severe infarction, a higher total mortality, and a greater frequency of ventricular tachyarrhythmias and right bundle branch block.[3]

REFERENCES

1. Ormerod, O.J., McGregor, C.G., Stone, D.L., et al.: Arrhythmias after coronary bypass surgery. Br. Heart J. *51*:618, 1984.
2. Kannel, W.B., Abbott, R.D., Savage, D.D., and McNamara, P.M.: Epidemiologic features of chronic atrial fibrillation. The Framingham study. N. Engl. J. Med. *306*:1018, 1982.
3. Hunt, D., Sloman, G., and Penington, C.: Effects of atrial fibrillation on prognosis of acute myocardial infarction. Br. Heart J. *40*:303, 1978.

174-A   (Braunwald, pp. 811–812; Table 26–5)

In an unselected general practice the overwhelming majority of patients with hypertension have essential hypertension, as shown in many studies.[1,2] This is true even in a series in which patients have pressures above 175/110 mm Hg were studied.[3] Chronic renal disease is the second most common cause of hypertension; the third most common cause, renovascular disease, is rare (≤1 per cent). Other forms of secondary hypertension such as co-arctation of the aorta, pheochromocytoma, Cushing's disease, and primary aldosteronism have an incidence much less than 1 per cent.

REFERENCES

1. Rudnick, K.V., Sackett, D.L., et al.: Hypertension in family practice. Can. Med. Assoc. J. *3*:492, 1977.
2. Danielson, M., and Dammstrom, B.: The prevalence of secondary and curable hypertension. Acta Med. Scand. *209*:451, 1981.
3. Berglund, G., et al.: Prevalence of primary and secondary hypertension. Studies in a random population sample. Br. Med. J. *2*:554, 1976.

175-D   (Braunwald, p. 479)

The NSAIDs, including aspirin, inhibit the renal cyclooxygenase and therefore prevent the prostaglandin-induced increase in renal blood flow that usually sustains diuretic-induced natriuresis.[1]

These agents are capable of decreasing glomerular filtration and causing sodium retention when given alone and are especially prone to cause these side effects in patients with diminished renal perfusion. Low-dose aspirin, which is used commonly in cardiovascular patients, has no apparent effect on the enhanced urinary prostaglandin production that accompanies increased renal blood flow and therefore does not interfere with natriuresis following furosemide therapy.[2] Some NSAIDs are especially potent in reducing an interaction with loop diuretics. For example, indomethacin both inhibits the renal cyclooxygenase and competitively inhibits furosemide and hydrochlorothiazide excretion into the proximal tubule. In contrast, sulindac is not excreted into the tubule in its active form and has a lesser effect on both the natriuresis and antihypertensive effects of loop diuretics.[3]

REFERENCES

1. Webster, J.: Interactions of NSAIDs with diuretics and beta blockers. Mechanisms and clinical implications. Drugs *30*:32, 1985.
2. Wilson, T.W., McCauley, F.A., and Wells, H.D.: Effects of low-dose aspirin on responses to furosemide. J. Clin. Pharmacol. *26*:1100, 1986.
3. Koopmans, P.O., Thien, T.H., Thomas, C.M., et al.: The effect of sulindac and indomethacin on antihypertensive and diuretic action of hydrochlorothiazide in patients with mild to moderate essential hypertension. Br. J. Clin. Pharmacol. *21*:417, 1986.

176-E   (Braunwald, pp. 408–410)

Circulatory shock is characterized by a marked reduction in blood flow to vital organs. In general, cerebral and coronary blood flow are protected at the expense of splanchnic and renal perfusion. Although coronary and cerebral blood flow are initially protected, if the process of shock continues, clinical signs of hypoperfusion of these organs will appear. A decrease in mental alertness may then be noted and electrocardiographic abnormalities including ischemic ST- and T-wave changes may appear, even in patients with clinically normal hearts.[1] Perfusion of the kidneys, the gastrointestinal tract, and the skin is less well maintained than are coronary and cerebral blood flow. In patients with septic shock, pulmonary arteriovenous shunts may appear, and further ventilation/perfusion mismatch may develop as therapeutic agents are used in attempts to reverse the condition.[2]

The pathophysiology of circulatory shock may vary on the basis of the underlying etiology. In addition, age and sex differences may contribute to the pathophysiology of the syndrome. Circulatory shock during the first 3 months of life is frequently associated with bacteremia due to gram-negative bacilli. During the syndrome of shock, large increases in sympathetic activity lead to arterial vasoconstriction and to an even larger increase in postcapillary venular constriction. This results in an increase in capillary hydrostatic pressure and a net loss of plasma water, with resultant decreases in intravascular volume and hemoconcentration.

REFERENCES

1. Terradellas, J.B., Bellot, J.F., Saris, A.B., et al.: Acute and transient ST-segment elevation during bacterial shock in seven patients without apparent heart disease. Chest 81: 444, 1982.
2. Jardin, F., Eveleigh, M.C., Guarjian, F., et al.: Venous admixture in human septic shock. Comparative effects of blood volume expansion, dopamine infusion and isoproterenol infusion on mismatching of ventilation and pulmonary blood flow in peritonitis. Circulation 60:155, 1979.

177-C   (Braunwald, pp. 601–603)

Quinidine is an alkaloid that is isolated from the bark of the cinchona tree. The agent suppresses automaticity in normal Purkinje fibers by decreasing the slope of phase IV diastolic depolarization and shifting resting threshold voltage toward zero. Quinidine can produce early afterdepolarizations, which may be responsible for the known ability of the drug to provide torsades de pointes.[1] Quinidine is capable of exerting a significant anticholinergic effect as well as an alpha-adrenoceptor blocking effect that may lead to reflex sympathetic stimulation. Therefore, quinidine decreases peripheral vascular resistance and may lead to significant hypotension in certain clinical settings. Both the liver and the kidneys clear quinidine, with hepatic metabolism being the more important. The elimination of half-life of quinidine is 5 to 8 hours after oral administration, but drugs that induce hepatic enzymes, such as phenobarbital and phenytoin, may shorten this half-life.

Quinidine may be used in the treatment and prevention of a variety of supraventricular and ventricular arrhythmias. AV-nodal reentry tachyardias are inhibited by quinidine, in part by depression of conduction of the retrograde fast pathway.[2] In patients with the Wolff-Parkinson-White syndrome, quinidine may prevent reciprocating tachycardias and slow the ventricular response to atrial flutter or fibrillation by prolonging the effective refractory period of the accessory pathway. While quinidine may be useful in the termination or subsequent suppression of atrial fibrillation or flutter, because of the vagolytic effect of the drug on AV-nodal conduction quinidine may occasionally convert a 2:1 AV response in atrial flutter to a 1:1 response, unless the atrial rate is slowed prior to the administration of quinidine by another agent such as propranolol or verapamil. Because it crosses the placenta, quinidine has been found useful in the treatment of fetal arrhythmias.[3]

REFERENCES

1. El-Sherif, N., Bekheit, S.S., and Hankin, R.: Quinidine-induced long QTU interval and torsades de pointes: Role of bradycardia-dependent early afterdepolarizations. J. Am. Coll. Cardiol. 14:252, 1989.
2. Wu, D., Hung, J.S., Kuo, C.T., et al.: Effects of quinidine on atrioventricular nodal reentrant paroxysmal tachycardia. Circulation 64:823, 1981.
3. Guntheroth, W.G., Cyr, D.R., Mack, L.A., et al.: Hydrops from reciprocating atrioventricular tachycardia in 27-week fetus requiring quinidine for conversion. Obstet. Gynecol. 66(Suppl 3):29S, 1985.

178-B   (Braunwald, pp. 453–455)

While edema is a common and important physical finding in congestive heart failure, its presence does not correlate well with the level of systemic venous pressure. The excess volume of extracellular fluid volume is a more important determinant of edema. Thus in adults, a minimum of 5 liters of excess extracellular fluid volume usually must accumulate before peripheral edema is manifested. In patients with chronic LV failure and a low cardiac output, peripheral edema may develop in the presence of normal or minimally elevated systemic venous pressure because of a gradual but persistent accumulation of extracellular fluid volume.

Edema generally accumulates in dependent portions of the body such as the ankles or feet of ambulatory patients or the sarcum of bedridden patients. As heart failure progresses, edema becomes more severe and may become massive and generalized (anasarca). In rare instances, especially when edema develops suddenly and severely, frank rupture of the skin with extravasation of fluid may result. Edema is usually more marked on the paralyzed side of patients with hemiplegia; unilateral edemia may also result from unilateral venous obstruction.

179-B   (Braunwald, p. 460)

Anemia is one of the most common conditions that is associated with a sustained increase in cardiac output. While an increase in cardiac output occurs consistently when the hematocrit falls below 25 per cent, the occurrence of heart failure at this level of anemia usually implies the presence of underlying heart disease. In patients with severe anemia (hematocrit <15 per cent) clinical evidence of heart failure may occur even in the absence of underlying heart disease. In addition, patients with sickle cell anemia may develop signs of heart failure at less severe levels of anemia for a variety of reasons, including impaired systemic cardiac oxygenation due to microthrombi and a loss of the hemodynamic benefits of reduced viscosity, which is not seen in this particular form of anemia.[1,2]

The rate of development of anemia plays an important role in determining whether increases in cardiac output occur to any significant degree. When anemia is secondary to rapid blood loss, maintenance of blood volume is not possible and a clinical picture of hypovolemic shock ensues. However, when anemia develops more slowly, cardiac output is augmented primarily through an increase in stroke volume that is associated with cardiac dilatation and hypertrophy. Heart rate usually remains in the normal range. The augmentation of cardiac output that occurs during exercise in patients with anemia tends to be excessive.[3] Such a response may occur in patients with only mild anemia who have normal resting cardiac output.[4]

REFERENCES

1. Varat, M.A., Adolph, R.J., and Fowler, N.O.: Cardiovascular effects of anemia. Am. Heart J. *83*:415, 1972.
2. Denenberg, B.S., Criner, G., Jones, R., and Spann, J.F.: Cardiac function in sickle cell anemia. Am. J. Cardiol. *51*: 1674, 1983.
3. Sproule, B.J., Mitchell, J.H., and Miller, W.F.: Cardiopulmonary physiological responses to heavy exercise in patients with anemia. J. Clin. Invest. *39*:378, 1960.
4. Graettinger, J.S., Parsons, R.L., and Campbell, J.A.: A correlation of clinical and hemodynamic studies in patients with mild and severe anemia with and without congestive failure. Ann. Intern. Med. *58*:617, 1963.

180-C *(Braunwald, pp. 476–477)*

The loop diuretics, including ethacrynic acid, furosemide, and bumetanide, are capable of inducing vigorous natriuresis by blocking the sodium transport system in the ascending limb of Henle's loop. Each of these drugs is secreted into the renal tubular lumen by the organic acid pathway; therefore, their pharmacological actions may be delayed or diminished by exogenous competitive inhibitors of this pathway such as probenecid and indomethacin. The absorption of loop diuretics is highly variable even among normal subjects; furosemide, for instance, has an average bioavailability of 60 per cent that is markedly decreased if the drug is given with meals. In addition, the presence of heart failure may lead to delayed intestinal absorption and delivery of the drug to its tubular site of action. However, the absolute bioavailability of the drug is not decreased.

Following the administration of an intravenous bolus of furosemide (0.5 to 1.0 mg/kg), there is an increase in venous capacitance due to venodilation with resultant decrease in pulmonary capillary wedge pressure within minutes. This accounts for the rapid improvement of symptoms even before a diuretic response is seen. Finally, the apparent resistance to diuretics in patients who showed a diuretic response initially is usually multifactorial and may be due to intravascular volume depletion, increasing doses of vasodilators (with possible exception of ACE inhibitors which may enhance the response to diuretics), coadministration of certain medications like nonsteroidal antiinflammatory drugs, or dietary indiscretion (especially high intake of sodium).

181-C *(Braunwald, pp. 460–462; Table 15–7)*

Several conditions that are characterized by chronically increased cardiac output may cause heart failure, especially in the presence of underlying heart disease. These include pregnancy, anemia, hyperthyroidism, beriberi disease, Paget's disease, large arteriovenous fistulae, and multiple myeloma. In these conditions, stroke volume and cardiac output are increased and, coupled with peripheral vasodilatation, result in the typical findings of high-output failure: widened pulse pressure and warm, flushed extremities. Because of the marked vasodilatation that occurs in this condition (especially in association with severe anemia), vasodilating agents may be of little or no benefit. Patients with thiamine deficiency who manifest "wet beriberi" have evidence of biventricular failure with pulmonary congestion and peripheral edema, sensory and motor neuropathy, and may have additional physical findings of other nutritional deficiency or alcoholism.

182-C *(Braunwald, pp. 616–618)*

The calcium antagonist verapamil prolongs conduction time through the AV node by blocking the slow inward (calcium) current in cardiac fibers. Because the drug interferes with excitation-contraction, it inhibits contraction of vascular smooth muscle and leads to dilatation of coronary and peripheral vascular beds. In addition, verapamil exerts a direct negative inotropic action on isolated cardiac muscle. In patients with impaired left ventricular function, verapamil may exert accentuated hemodynamic depressant effects, especially if administered simultaneously with a beta blocker. Within 3 to 5 minutes after intravenous injection of verapamil, mean arterial pressure decreases and left ventricular end-diastolic pressure rises. The resultant reduction of afterload due to the agent's vasodilatory effects minimizes its negative inotropic action so that the net result is little or no change in the cardiac index.

Intravenous verapamil is one of the treatments of choice for terminating sustained sinus-nodal or AV-nodal reentry tachycardias, as well as reciprocating tachycardias associated with Wolff-Parkinson-White syndrome when one of the reentrant pathways is the AV node. However, reflex sympathetic stimulation induced by verapamil may increase the ventricular response over the accessory pathway to atrial fibrillation in patients with the Wolff-Parkinson-White syndrome[1]; therefore, the drug is contraindicated in this situation. Verapamil is able to terminate between 60 and 80 per cent of paroxysmal supraventricular tachycardias within several minutes and probably is the next agent to choose if IV adenosine does not terminate such tachycardias.[2]

In patients with atrial fibrillation, verapamil decreases the ventricular response by increasing the effective refractory period of the AV node and may convert a small percentage of episodes to sinus rhythm, especially if the atrial flutter or fibrillation is of recent onset.[3] However, in patients with chronic atrial fibrillation, quinidine appears to be more effective than verapamil in the establishment and maintenance of sinus rhythm.

Side effects in patients on verapamil are more likely if preexisting LV dysfunction or beta blocker therapy is present. In addition, hemodynamic collapse has been noted in response to verapamil in infants. Therefore, the drug should be used extremely cautiously in patients <1 year of age. Contraindications to the use of verapamil include marked sinus node dysfunction, second- or third-degree AV block, and hypotension, as well as the clinical conditions just mentioned. In patients taking digoxin, verapamil may increase the serum digitalis level by decreasing excretion of digoxin. Appropriate caution is warranted.

Verapamil has other effects in addition to its slow calcium channel blocking effect.[4] It has some sodium channel and alpha-adrenergic blocking activity, and it has a mild antiaggregatory effect on platelets.[5] Verapamil has no beta-adrenergic blocking activity.

REFERENCES

1. Gulamhusein, S., Ko, P., Carruthers, S.G., and Klein, G.J.: Acceleration of the ventricular response during atrial fibrillation in the Wolff-Parkinson-White syndrome after verapamil. Circulation 65:348, 1982.
2. Belhassen, B., Glick, A., and Laniado, S.: Comparative clinical and electrophysiologic effects of adenosine triphosphate and verapamil on paroxysmal reciprocating junctional tachycardia. Circulation 77:795, 1988.
3. Waxman, H.L., Myerburg, R.J., Appel, R., and Sung, R.J.: Verapamil for control of ventricular rate in paroxysmal supraventricular tachycardia and atrial fibrillation or flutter: A double-blind randomized cross-over study. Ann. Intern. Med. 94:1, 1981.
4. Weir, M.R., and Zachariah, P.K.: Verapamil. In Messerli, F.H. (ed.): Cardiovascular Drug Therapy. 2nd ed. Philadelphia, W.B. Saunders Co., 1996.
5. Chierchia, S., Crea, F., Bernini, W., et al.: Antiplatelet effects of verapamil in man. Am. J. Cardiol. 47:399, 1981.

183-D   *(Braunwald, pp. 453–455)*

A variety of physical findings appear in patients with heart failure. Elevation of systemic venous pressure for long periods of time may produce several signs in patients, including protrusion of the eyes and severe tricuspid regurgitation. This may result in a visible systolic pulsation of the eyes.[1] In attempts to compensate and support the circulation in the presence of reduced cardiac output, increased activity of the adrenergic activity system is noted in patients with heart failure. This adrenergic activity is responsible for peripheral vasoconstriction, which leads to both pallor and coldness of the extremities as well as cyanosis of the digits in severe cases.

In patients with right heart failure the resting jugular venous pressure may not appear abnormal but may be seen to be elevated when the abdomen is compressed by palpation over the liver. This sign is known as abdominojugular reflux. Since a positive test usually reflects both hepatic congestion and failure of the right side of the heart to transport the increased venous return of this condition appropriately, a positive test may be helpful in differentiating hepatomegaly due to heart failure from other causes.

If hepatomegaly occurs rapidly with a relatively acute onset of heart failure, stretching of the liver capsule occurs; this may lead to tenderness in the right upper quadrant. However, in chronic heart failure, this tenderness is less likely to be present, although the liver itself usually remains large. Accumulation of ascitic fluid in the peritoneal cavity may occur in patients with increased hepatic venous pressure. The ascitic fluid has an elevated protein content relative to a pure transudate, suggesting that increased capillary permeability plays a role in this process. Longstanding, severe heart failure may be accompanied by a protein-losing enteropathy caused by visceral congestion.[2] The resultant reduction in plasma oncotic pressure may exacerbate the underlying tendency to form ascites.

REFERENCES

1. Earnest, D.L., and Hurst, J.W.: Exophthalmos, stare and increase in intraocular pressure and systolic protrusion of the eyeballs due to congestive heart failure. Am. J. Cardiol. 26:351, 1970.
2. Strober, W., Cohen, L.S., Waldmann, T.A., and Braunwald, E.: Tricuspid regurgitation: A newly recognized cause of protein-losing enteropathy, lymphocytopenia, and immunologic deficiency. Am. J. Med. 44:842, 1968.

184-D   *(Braunwald, pp. 604–605)*

Disopyramide is one of the class Ia antiarrhythmic agents that has multiple effects in addition to its sodium channel activity. One of its more important effects is muscarinic blocking activity, which can result in acceleration of the sinus node and facilitation of AV conduction. However, when given in high doses or in patients with underlying SA node dysfunction (e.g., sick sinus syndrome), disopyramide can cause sinus node slowing or sinus arrest. The drug's elimination half-life can be prolonged in the presence of renal or hepatic failure. In addition, disopyramide can cause decompensation in patients with heart failure due to its marked negative inotropic activity. Because this agent lengthens conduction time and prolongs the refractory period in atrial, ventricular, nodal, and accessory pathway tissues, it is very effective in suppressing initiation and propagation of a wide variety of atrial and ventricular arrhythmias. In those patients with minimal or no response to therapy, combination with a class Ib agent (e.g., mexiletine) can result in enhanced effectiveness, while avoiding further prolongation of the Q-T interval secondary to disopyramide.[1] Finally, disopyramide has been effective in treating certain patients with neurally mediated syncope who have minimal or no response to beta blockers.

REFERENCE

1. Awaji, T., and Hashimoto, K.: Antiarrhythmic effects of combined application of class I antiarrhythmic drugs; addition

of low-dose mexiletine-enhanced antiarrhythmic effects of disopyramide and aprindine in various-rate canine ventricular tachycardias. J. Cardiovasc. Pharmacol. 21:960–966, 1993.

185 A-T, B-F, C-F, D-F, E-T   (Braunwald, pp. 499–500)

Digitalis preparations are of benefit in improving symptoms of heart failure in patients with systolic dysfunction.[1,2] Digitalis increases myocardial contractility, resulting in improvement in cardiac output and diuresis. Reduced filling pressures relieve symptoms of pulmonary congestion and peripheral edema.

In isolated mitral stenosis, left ventricular function is preserved and elevated left atrial pressures are a result of obstruction to left atrial outflow rather than elevated left ventricular end-diastolic pressure. Because left ventricular function is preserved, digitalis is not useful in improving symptoms of pulmonary congestion. An exception is in patients who have mitral stenosis with atrial fibrillation. In mitral stenosis with atrial fibrillation, rapid ventricular rates greatly reduce diastolic filling time, resulting in decreased cardiac output. Reducing the ventricular rate to 60 to 70 beats/min with digitalis may improve symptoms. Another indication for digitalis in patients with mitral stenosis is right ventricular systolic dysfunction.

Patients with left ventricular hypertrophy and normal systolic function may have signs of heart failure due to diastolic dysfunction and elevated filling pressures. There is no evidence that patients with left ventricular hypertrophy and normal ejection fraction benefit from digitalis. In patients with hypertrophic obstructive cardiomyopathy and normal or supranormal ejection fraction, digitalis may potentially worsen outflow obstruction by increasing contractility. In both left ventricular hypertrophy and hypertrophic obstructive cardiomyopathy, atrial fibrillation may worsen symptoms of heart failure due to rapid ventricular rates and loss of atrial systole. In this situation, and when ventricular systolic dysfunction develops, digitalis may be of clinical benefit for rate control.

REFERENCES

1. Uretsky, B.F., Young, J.B., Shahidi, F.E., et al.: Randomized study assessing the effect of digoxin withdrawal in patients with mild to moderate chronic congestive heart failure: Results of the PROVED trial. J. Am. Coll. Cardiol. 22: 955, 1993.
2. Packer, M., Gheorghiade, M., Young, J.B., et al.: Withdrawal of digoxin from patients with chronic heart failure treated with angiotensin-converting enzyme inhibitors. N. Engl. J. Med.329:1, 1992.

186 A-T, B-F, C-T, D-T, E-F   (Braunwald, pp. 372–376; Figs. 12–17 through 12–20)

Beta$_1$-receptor stimulation by agonist leads to formation of cAMP, the second-messenger molecule, via a series of three proteins known collectively as the beta-adrenergic system.[1] The beta-adrenergic system includes the adrenergic receptor, a G protein and the effector enzyme, adenylate cyclase. When the agonist, or first-messenger molecule, binds to the beta-adrenergic receptor, activation of a stimulatory G protein occurs. G proteins are heterotrimeric GTPases that link the receptor molecule to the second messenger system. A subunit of the G protein dissociates from the receptor–G-protein complex and interacts with adenylate cyclase, increasing its activity. The increase of adenylate cyclase activity results in augmented formation of cAMP.

The parasympathetic nervous system, as in the beta-adrenergic system, likely involves a three-protein signaling mechanism. The signaling mechanism includes the extracellular messenger, acetylcholine, the muscarinic receptor, and a sarcolemmal G-protein system. Muscarinic stimulation in the heart results in a negative chronotropic effect.

In vascular smooth muscle cells, NO leads to increases in intracellular cGMP by activating the soluble guanylate cyclase. The increase in vascular smooth muscle cGMP leads to vasodilatation. In the myocyte, NO leads to an enhanced response to acetylcholine and decreases the positive inotropic effect of beta-receptor stimulation.[2] This raises the possibility that NO and cGMP may play a modulatory role in the myocyte response to autonomic stimulation.

Alpha-adrenergic receptors in vascular smooth muscle and in ventricular myocytes are linked to phospholipase C by a G protein. Although the events are not as clearly elucidated as those for the linkage between the beta-adrenergic receptor and its G protein, alpha-receptor stimulation by agonist leads to G protein activation. The G protein then causes activation of phospholipase C.[3] Phospholipase C activation leads to formation of inositol triphosphate (IP3) and diacylglycerol (DAG) from phosphatidylinositol bisphosphate. IP3 is a second messenger itself, whereas DAG participates in the activation of protein kinase C.

The effects of cAMP appear to be primarily mediated by cAMP-dependent protein kinases (A-kinase).[4] A-kinase is an enzyme which activates other proteins by phosphorylating them. A-kinase has both regulatory and catalytic subunits. Upon binding the cAMP, the catalytic subunit is released from the complex. The active kinase (catalytic subunit) then catalyzes the donation of a phosphate group from ATP to a target protein, thereby activating the target protein.

REFERENCES

1. Spinale, F.G., Tempel, G.E., Mukherjee, R., et al.: Cellular and molecular alterations in the beta-adrenergic system with cardiomyopathy induced by tachycardia. Cardiovasc. Res. 28:1243–1250, 1994.
2. Balligand, J.L., Kelly, R.A., Marsden, P.A., et al.: Control of cardiac muscle cell function by an endogenous nitric ox-

ide signaling system. Proc. Natl. Acad. Sci. U.S.A.: *90:* 347–351, 1993.
3. Deckmyn, H., Ven Geet, C., and Vermylen, J.: Dual regulation of phospholipase C activity by G-proteins. NIPS *8:*61–63, 1993.
4. Shabb, J.B., and Corbin, J.D.: Protein phosphorylation in the heart. *In* Fozzard, H.A., et al.: The Heart and Cardiovascular System. 2nd ed. New York, Raven Press, 1992, pp. 1539–1562.

187 A-T, B-T, C-F, D-T, E-F *(Braunwald, pp. 825–827)*

The Cooperative Study on Renovascular Hypertension[1] delineated two major forms of renovascular disease—atherosclerosis and fibromuscular hyperplasia. Atherosclerotic patients were older, had higher systolic blood pressure, and had greater target organ damage. Patients with fibromuscular hyperplasia were younger, were more often female, had no family history of hypertension, and had less evidence of target organ damage.

REFERENCE

1. Simon, N., Franklin, S.S., Bleifer, K.W., and Maxwell, M.H.P.: Clinical characteristics of renovascular hypertension. JAMA *220:*1209, 1972.

188 A-T, B-T, C-F, D-T, E-T *(Braunwald, p. 451)*

Pulmonary function testing can be very helpful in the differentiation between cardiac and pulmonary dyspnea. Patients with congestive heart failure generally exhibit a restrictive ventilatory defect primarily due to increased interstitial fluid, and characterized by reduction in diffusion and vital capacities, and decrease in pulmonary compliance. Ventilation/perfusion mismatching results in a widened A-a gradient and increased ratio of dead space to tidal volume (Vd/Vt). Other alterations in pulmonary function tests include reduction in total lung capacity, and mild reduction of PCO_2 and PO_2. Residual volume and functional residual capacity are usually normal in congestive heart failure. Airway resistance in congestive heart failure may be increased due to edema of the airways and air trapping secondary to reduction in compliance, which results in premature closure of dependent airways.

189 A-T, B-F, C-F, D-T, E-T *(Braunwald, p. 449)*

Both supraventricular and ventricular tachycardias can precipitate heart failure in patients with underlying heart disease. They can also cause hemodynamic instability in patients without underlying heart disease, and longstanding tachyarrhythmias also may lead to dilated cardiomyopathy and left ventricular dysfunction. Increases in myocardial oxygen demand, induction of ischemia, AV dissociation, and reduction in diastolic filling are all mechanisms by which tachyarrhythmias can cause or precipitate heart failure. The last two mechanisms are especially relevant in patients with noncompliant left ventricles (e.g., LVH or re-

strictive cardiomyopathy). Severe bradycardia, on the other hand, can cause heart failure by reducing cardiac output, which offsets any increase in stroke volume due to increased diastolic filling time. In patients with left ventricular dysfunction, asymptomatic ventricular ectopy is a marker for increased risk of sudden death. However, treatment directed towards this abnormality has not been shown to improve survival, and the CAST trial showed further that treatment of asymptomatic ventricular ectopy following myocardial infarction is associated with increased mortality.[1]

REFERENCE

1. Echt, D.S., Liebson, P.R., Mitchell, L.B., et al.: Mortality and morbidity in patients receiving encainide, flecainide, or placebo. The Cardiac Arrhythmia Suppression Trial. N. Engl. J. Med. *324:*781–788, 1991.

190 A-T, B-T, C-T, D-F, E-F *(Braunwald, p. 484)*

Disturbances of cardiac rhythm are important and potentially life-threatening complications of digitalis toxicity. Maintaining a high level of suspicion is very important for early detection of digitalis toxicity. Digitalis toxicity can cause a wide variety of ventricular and supraventricular arrhythmias, including sinus bradycardia, sinus exit block and arrest, junctional and ventricular ectopy, and tachycardia. Lidocaine and phenytoin may be helpful in managing ventricular arrhythmias in this situation, and vagally mediated AV block often responds to therapeutic doses of atropine. Direct-current cardioversion, on the other hand, can precipitate serious ventricular arrhythmias in patients with overt digitalis toxicity, and elective cardioversion is contraindicated in this setting. Because of significant binding to plasma proteins and its large volume of distribution, digoxin is not efficiently removed by dialysis. However, in cases of life-threatening overdose, antidigoxin immunotherapy can be life saving.[1,2] Doses of Fab are administered on the basis of estimated dose of digoxin administered, or total body burden. Although rare, recurrence of toxicity can occur, usually 24 to 48 hours later in patients with normal renal function and later in those with renal failure.

REFERENCES

1. Cambridge, D., Morgan, C.R., and Allen, G.: Digoxin and digoxin derivative induced arrhythmias: In vitro binding and in vivo abolition of arrhythmias by digoxin immune Fab (DIGIBIND). Cardiovasc. Res. *26:*906–911, 1992.
2. Antman, E.M., Wenger, T.L., Butler, V.P., Jr., et al.: Treatment of 150 cases of life-threatening digitalis intoxication with digoxin-specific Fab antibody fragments. Final report of a multicenter study. Circulation *81:*1744–1752, 1990.

191 A-T, B-F, C-T, D-T, E-F *(Braunwald, pp. 812–813)*

Despite the widely recognized morbidity and mortality associated with hypertension, this disease remains inadequately diagnosed and treated. If left untreated, about 50 per cent of patients will die from cardiac events such as myocardial infarction and congestive heart failure. Thirty-three per cent of such patients will suffer a fatal cerebrovascular accident, either thrombotic or hemorrhagic, and another 10 to 15 per cent will die from complications related to renal failure. Contrary to earlier suggestions and with few exceptions, patients with low plasma renin activity (PRA) are no less likely to develop vascular complications than patients with high PRA.[1] In addition to accelerating atherosclerosis, hypertension is associated with evidence of endothelial dysfunction and abnormal vascular tone.[2] Impaired coronary flow reserve and abnormal defects on thallium scintigraphy can be seen in patients with longstanding hypertension, even in the absence of fixed coronary disease.[3] Males and blacks in general have increased morbidity from hypertension independent of other risk factors, and systolic blood pressure is more closely linked to cardiac risks than is diastolic pressure, consistent with the increased morbidity in patients with isolated systolic hypertension and the therapeutic benefit of treating this disorder.

REFERENCES

1. Kurtz, A.: Renin and hypertension. Nephrol. Dial. Transplant. 10:1521–1523, 1995.
2. Panza, J.A., Garcia, C.E., Kilcoyne, C.M., et al.: Impaired endothelium-dependent vasodilation in patients with essential hypertension. Evidence that nitric oxide abnormality is not localized to a single signal transduction pathway. Circulation 91:1732–1738, 1995.
3. Iriarte, M.M., Caso, R., Murga, N., et al.: Microvascular angina in systemic hypertension: Diagnosis and treatment with enalapril. Am. J. Cardiol. 76:31D–34D, 1995.

192 A-T, B-T, C-T, D-T, E-T *(Braunwald, p. 479)*

In recent years, the deleterious effects of magnesium depletion on cardiovascular morbidity and mortality have been recognized.[1] Magnesium homeostasis is only partially reflected in the serum magnesium level because such a large percentage of the cation is bound to intracellular buffers and bone. However, serial measurements of serum magnesium in individual patients give a reasonable assessment of ongoing magnesium metabolism, as do markedly depressed or elevated absolute magnesium levels. The potassium-sparing diuretics do not lead to urinary magnesium wasting, but both thiazide and loop diuretics cause this complication.[2] Hypomagnesemia is also encountered in patients with poor dietary intake and may be associated with chronic exposure to alcohol, as well as some aminoglycoside antibiotics, and cisplatinum therapy. While digitalis toxicity may be exacerbated by decreased magnesium levels, digitalis preparations may actually potentiate renal magnesium wasting.[3] Therefore, serial magnesium in patients receiving digitalis should be monitored. Diagnosis of hypomagnesemia requires an index of suspicion and a low normal or low serum magnesium level either initially or during serial determinations. A total daily magnesium excretion <1 mEg/day, in the absence of diuretics, is strongly suggestive of magnesium depletion. In at least one study of congestive heart failure patients, a magnesium level >2.1 mEq/liter was equally predictive of a poor prognosis, as was hypomagnesemia.[4] These patients had increased BUN levels, consistent with decreased renal function and/or relative intravascular volume depletion.

REFERENCES

1. Iseri, L.T.: Role of magnesium in cardiac tachyarrhythmias. Am. J. Cardiol. 65:47K, 1990.
2. Kelepourus, E., and Agus, Z.S.: Effects of diuretics on calcium and phosphate transport. Semin. Nephrol. 8:273, 1988.
3. Gottlieb, S.S.: Importance of magnesium in congestive heart failure. Am. J. Cardiol. 63:39G, 1989.
4. Ralston, M.A., Murnane, M.R., Unverferth, D.V., and Leier, C.V.: Serum and tissue magnesium concentrations in patients with heart failure and serious ventricular arrhythmias. Ann. Intern. Med. 113:841, 1990.

193 A-F, B-T, C-T, D-T, E-F *(Braunwald, pp. 603–604)*

Procainamide is a class Ia antiarrhythmic agent that shares many electrophysiological effects with quinidine. Procainamide predominantly blocks inactivated I_{Na} channels, but also blocks I_K and $I_{K \, ATP}$ channels. Procainamide usually prolongs ERP more than APD, blocking early responses and preventing reentrant arrhythmias. Procainamide is acetylated in the liver to *N*-acetylprocainamide (NAPA), its major metabolite, which is then excreted by the kidneys. NAPA has class III antiarrhythmic effects, prolonging both repolarization and the Q-T interval. When administered intravenously, procainamide can cause marked hypotension due to its vasodilatory activity, which is thought to be mediated by centrally inhibiting sympathetic nerve activity.[1] Procainamide has no apparent alpha-adrenergic blocking activity. It can be effective in controlling ventricular arrhythmias not suppressed by quinidine and, unlike quinidine, procainamide does not alter serum levels of digoxin.

REFERENCE

1. Rea, R.F., Hamdan, M., Schomer, S.J., and Geraets, D.R.: Inhibitory effects of procainamide on sympathetic nerve activity in humans. Circ. Res. 69:501–509, 1991.

194 A-T, B-T, C-T, D-T, E-T *(Braunwald, pp. 677–683)*

Ventricular arrhythmias including ventricular tachycardia (VT) have been identified in association with a variety of clinical conditions. Arrhythmogenic right ventricular (RV) dysplasia, a localized cardiomyopathy with hypokinetic areas involving the wall of the RV, is associated with increased risk for VT. Characteristics of this VT include a left bundle branch morphology, often with right axis deviation and inverted T waves in the right precordial leads. RV dysplasia may be first diagnosed during evaluation of children and young adults with ventricular arrhythmias, shows a male predominance, and is best identified by echocardiography or RV angiography. Patients with mitral valve prolapse can display both symptomatic and asymptomatic ventricular arrhythmias. However, there is no clear correlation between sudden death and underlying ventricular ectopy in these patients.[1] This is clearly different from patients with both dilated and hypertrophic cardiomyopathies, who may exhibit increased incidence of ventricular arrhythmias, that are associated with an increased risk of sudden death.[2]

One very important variety of ventricular arrhythmias is the drug-aggravated arrhythmia (proarrhythmia), which can be seen in as many as 5 to 10 per cent of patients on antiarrhythmic therapy. Drug-induced ventricular arrhythmia is more common in patients with underlying cardiac disease and/or LV dysfunction. In patients who have undergone repair of tetralogy of Fallot, sustained VT may emerge years after the operation, and may be due to reentry at the repair site on the RV outflow tract.[3,4]

REFERENCES

1. Hauer, R.N.W., and Wilde, A.A.W.: Mitral valve prolapse. *In* Zipes, D.P., and Jalife, J. (eds.): Cardiac Electrophysiology: From Cell to Bedside. 2nd ed. Philadelphia, W.B. Saunders Co., 1994, p. 833.
2. Mulrow, J.P., Healy, M.J., and McKenna, W.J.: Variability of ventricular arrhythmias in hypertrophic cardiomyopathy and implications for treatment. Am. J. Cardiol. 58:615–618, 1986.
3. Vaksmann, G., Fournier, A., Davignon, A., et al.: Frequency and prognosis of arrhythmias after operative "correction" of tetralogy of Fallot. Am. J. Cardiol. 66:346–349, 1990.
4. Cullen, S., Celermajer, D.S., Franklin, R.C., et al.: Prognostic significance of ventricular arrhythmia after repair of tetralogy of Fallot: A 12-year prospective study. J. Am. Coll. Cardiol. 23:1151–1155, 1994.

195 A-T, B-T, C-F, D-F, E-T   *(Braunwald, pp. 610–613)*

Amiodarone was originally introduced as a smooth muscle relaxant and coronary vasodilator for the treatment of angina. Oral administration of the drug in ordinary doses does not depress left ventricular ejection fraction; however, the intravenous form of amiodarone may exert some negative inotropic action and must be given cautiously to patients with depressed ejection fractions.[1] The use of amiodarone clinically is complex, in part due to the slow and variable achievement of plasma concentrations of the drug capable of suppressing arrhythmias. The onset of action following oral administration ranges from 2 days to 1 to 3 weeks. The elimination half-life of amiodarone is biphasic,

with a 50 per cent reduction in plasma concentration in the first 2 weeks after stopping therapy and a subsequent terminal half-life of between 26 and 107 days. To achieve steady-state amiodarone concentrations without an initial loading dose takes approximately 9 months. In addition, marked interpatient variability of the pharmacokinetics described above complicates therapy with this agent.

Although optimal dosing of amiodarone has not been clearly defined, the usual approach begins with daily doses of 800 to 1600 mg, tapering over 1 to 2 weeks to an eventual maintenance dose of 400 mg/day.

Amiodarone has been used to suppress a wide variety of both supraventricular and ventricular tachyarrhythmias. In general, the drug's efficacy is equal to or greater than that of other antiarrhythmic agents and is in the range of 60 to 80 per cent for most supraventricular tachyarrhythmias and 40 to 60 per cent for ventricular tachyarrhythmias.[2] However, because of amiodarone's long half-life, its interactions with other antiarrhythmic drugs, and an extensive list of side effects, therapy with this agent is usually a late or last resort. Side effects from amiodarone occur in approximately 75 per cent of patients maintained on 400 mg/day. Discontinuation of the drug is required in up to 20 per cent of patients.[3]

The most serious noncardiac side effect of amiodarone is its pulmonary toxicity, which occurs in between 5 and 15 per cent of patients after 1 year of treatment and is an absolute contraindication for continuation of the drug. The toxicity is marked by dyspnea and nonproductive cough as well as fever, with a positive gallium scan and radiographic evidence of pulmonary infiltrates often noted. The mortality due to this pulmonary process approaches 10 per cent, especially in patients with unrecognized pulmonary involvement that is allowed to continue. All patients on amiodarone therapy should therefore be monitored with chest x-rays at 3-month intervals during the first year and then twice annually.

Amiodarone blocks the conversion of thyroxine (T_4) to triiodothyronine (T_3). This effect results in a slight increase in T_4, reverse T_3, and TSH with clinical hypothyroidism appearing in 2 to 4 per cent of patients.[4] In 1 to 2 per cent of patients, hyperthroidism may appear and is characterized by an increase in T_3 levels.

A recent study attempted to define the role of amiodarone in the management of heart failure. The Grupo de Estudio de la Sobrevida en la Insuficiencia Cardiaca en Argentina (GESICA) trial randomized patients with symptomatic heart failure on optimal standard therapy to 300 mg/day of amiodarone or to standard treatment. Patients receiving amiodarone had lower all-cause mortality (33.5 per cent versus 41.4 per cent, risk reduction 28 per cent, p = 0.024) and lower risk of death or hospitalization for worsening heart failure (risk reduction 31 per cent, p = 0.0024). There was a non-significant trend towards reduction in sudden death and death due to progressive heart failure. The reduction in all-cause mortality and hospital admissions was present in all subgroups examined, regardless of the presence of nonsustained ventricular tachycardia.

REFERENCES

1. Kosinski, E.J., Albin, J.B., Young, E., et al.: Hemodynamic effects of intravenous amiodarone. J. Am. Coll. Cardiol. 4: 565, 1984.
2. Amiodarone vs Sotalol Study Group: Multicentre randomized trial of sotalol vs amiodarone for chronic malignant ventricular tachyarrhythmias. Eur. Heart J. 10:685, 1989.
3. Herre, J.M., Sauve, M.J., Malone, P., et al.: Long-term results of amiodarone therapy in patients with recurrent sustained ventricular tachycardia or ventricular fibrillation. J. Am. Coll. Cardiol. 13:442, 1989.
4. Borowski, G.D., Garofano, C.D., Rose, L.I., et al.: Effect of longterm amiodarone therapy on thyroid hormone levels and thyroid function. Am. J. Med. 78:443, 1985.
5. Mason, J.W.: Amiodarone. N. Engl. J. Med. 316:455, 1987.
6. Doval, H.C., Nul, D.R., Grancelli, H.O., et al.: Randomized trial of low-dose amiodarone in severe congestive heart failure. Grupo de Estudio de la Sobrevida en la Insuficiencia Cardiaca en Argentina (GESICA). Lancet 344:493–498, 1994.

196 A-T, B-F, C-T, D-F, E-T   (Braunwald, p. 923)

Cor triatriatum is a congenital malformation of the left atrium characterized by partitioning of the atrial cavity into two subchambers by a membrane. The posterior subchamber receives blood flow from the pulmonary venous system and the anterior subchamber empties into the LV cavity through the mitral valve. When the opening of the membrane is small, severe pulmonary venous and later arterial hypertension can result.[1] Pressure in the anterior subchamber, distal to the site of pulmonary venous obstruction, is often normal. Diagnosis can be confirmed by echocardiography and detailed features of anatomy and physiological significance of the obstructing membrane can be defined using transesophageal echocardiography.[2] An important echocardiographic feature that distinguishes cor triatriatum from the entity of submitral membrane is the relation of the left atrial appendage to the membrane. In cor triatriatum the left atrial appendage is part of the anterior subchamber, while in submitral membrane the appendage is part of the posterior subchamber.[3,4] Operative correction of this malformation may be curative.[4]

REFERENCES

1. Magidson, A.: Cor triatriatum. Severe pulmonary arterial hypertension and pulmonary venous hypertension in a child. Am. J. Cardiol. 9:603, 1962.
2. Vuocolo, L.M., Stoddard, M.F., and Longaker, R.A.: Transesophageal two-dimensional and Doppler echocardiographic diagnosis of cor triatriatum in the adult. Am. Heart J. 124:791–793, 1992.
3. Horowitz, M.D., Zager, W., Bilsker, M., et al.: Cor triatriatum in adults. Am. Heart J. 126:472–474, 1993.
4. Van Son, J.A., Danielson, G.K., Schaff, H.V., et al.: Cor triatriatum: Diagnosis, operative approach, and late results. Mayo Clin. Proc. 68:854–859, 1993.

197 A-F, B-F, C-F, D-F, E-T   (Braunwald, pp. 688–691; Figs. 22–48, 22–51 through 22–53)

Type I second-degree AV block is characterized by progressive P-R prolongation culminating in a nonconducted P wave while type II second-degree AV block is characterized by a constant P-R interval prior to a blocked P wave. Clinically, type I AV block with a normal QRS complex is a generally benign rhythm. However, in older age groups type I AV block has been associated with a more serious, symptomatic presentation.[1] Type I second-degree AV block in acute myocardial infarction usually accompanies inferior infarction, especially if an RV infarction is present. When higher degrees of AV block such as type II second-degree block occur in patients with acute inferior myocardial infarction, an association is seen with greater myocardial damage and a higher mortality rate.[2]

The surface ECG allows a reasonably reliable differentiation of the site of block in instances of second-degree AV block. Type I AV block with a normal QRS complex almost always occurs at the level of the AV node *proximal* to the His bundle. In contrast, type II AV block, especially when it occurs in association with bundle branch block, may be localized to the His-Purkinje system. Type I AV block in a patient with a bundle branch block may be due to block either in the AV node or more distally in the His-Purkinje system. In patients with 2:1 AV block it is difficult to distinguish between Type I and Type II forms of second-degree block. However, if the QRS complex is normal, Mobitz type I is the more likely diagnosis and longer rhythm strips may reveal transition from 2:1 to, for example, 3:2 block with typical P-R interval prolongation prior to block.

REFERENCES

1. Shaw, D.B., Kekwick, C.A., Veale, D., et al.: Survival in second degree atrioventricular block. Br. Heart J. 53:587, 1985.
2. Strasberg, R., Pinchas, A., Arditti, A., et al.: Left and right ventricular function in inferior acute myocardial infarction and significance of advanced atrioventricular block. Am. J. Cardiol. 54:985, 1984.

198 A-T, B-T, C-T, D-T, E-F   (Braunwald, pp. 361–366; Fig. 12–4)

The contractile apparatus of cardiac tissue consists of partially overlapping rod-like filaments that are fixed in length both at rest and during contraction. The thicker filaments, which are composed of myosin molecules, are created by an orderly aggregation of approximately 300 longitudinally stacked molecules from myosin proteins held parallel and in register by a centrally located connection termed the "M" line. The structure formed by these aggregates can form cross bridges and interact with actin filaments. Myosin by itself has the ability to split the ATP, which is due to its activity as an ATPase, inhibited by magnesium and activated by calcium. When myosin combines with actin it becomes enzymatically much more active in its ability to split ATP. Myosin can be separated into three isoenzyme components—V_1, V_2, and V_3, which have different heavy chain compositions. It has been shown that hypertrophied heart muscle has a greater proportion of the V_3 isoenzyme. The thin filament, which is a double alpha helix, contains two strands of actin. These actin molecules interact with myosin to form actomyosin, which is the primary contractile protein of the cardiac cell.

The proteins that regulate the activity of actomyosin are called troponin and tropomyosin. Tropomyosin is a rod-like protein forming a continuing strand through the center of the thin filament. Troponin consists of three separate proteins and is located at intervals along the thin filament. Troponin can be separated into three components: (1) troponin C, a calcium-sensitizing factor that binds calcium; (2) troponin I, an inhibitory factor that inhibits magnesium-stimulated ATPase of actomyosin; and (3) troponin T, which serves to allow attachment of the troponin complex to actin and tropomyosin.[1]

Under normal conditions when intracellular calcium is low, troponin C has no effect on the ability of troponin I to inhibit actin-myosin binding. However, calcium can rise in the cell with a depolarization, during which the calcium concentration *increases* from 10^{-7} M to 10^{-5} M. When this occurs, troponin C binds calcium and inhibits the binding of troponin I to actin, which triggers the interaction between actin and myosin. The formation of actomyosin results in hydrolysis of ATP by myosin. The actin rods are drawn toward the center of the sarcomere. Once such a stroke is completed, another ATP is bound and attaches to the actin site and the cycle is repeated, the myosin head attaching to a different actin monomer. Thus, shortening of cardiac muscle involves a relative change in the position of the two sets of filaments; actin filaments are displaced by the force-generating process at many cross-bridge sites and pulled in toward the center of the sarcomere. The force that is developed is related to the quantity of calcium that is bound to troponin C, which in turn is related to the intracellular calcium concentration. Finally, removal of calcium from troponin results in relaxation.[2]

REFERENCES

1. Tao, T., Gong, B.J., and Leavis, P.C.: Calcium-induced movement of troponin I relative to actin in skeletal muscle thin filaments. Science *247*:1339, 1990.
2. Eisenberg, E., and Hill, J.L.: Muscle contraction and free energy transduction in biological systems. Science *277*:999, 1985.

199 A-T, B-T, C-T, D-F, E-T   *(Braunwald, pp. 474–477, 480–482, 485–486)*

The initial treatment of acute pulmonary edema is multifaceted. Important measures include the following:

1. Administration of oxygen to improve oxygenation of arterial blood.

2. Placing the patient in a sitting position to improve oxygenation and diminish venous return.

3. Administration of morphine sulfate to reduce patient distress and to diminish central sympathetic output responsible for venous and arterial constriction. This peripheral vasoconstriction increases venus return and elevates blood pressure, actions that are detrimental in this setting.

4. Administration of a diuretic, such as furosemide, preferably in an intravenous form. The fact that even before diuresis occurs there is an improvement in respiratory function suggests that the initial effect of furosemide is not on renal function but on venous dilation.[1]

5. Reduction of preload. This can be accomplished by applying rotating tourniquets, by sitting, and by administration of furosemide and nitrates.

6. Use of vasodilators. As in this patient, cardiogenic pulmonary edema frequently is a consequence of elevations of arterial and left ventricular end-diastolic pressures and systemic vascular resistance. Therefore, vasodilators would be appropriate initial therapy. In this patient nitroglycerine would be of particular value, since myocardial ischemia may be present. It should be noted that administration of vasodilators is contraindicated, while administration of a positive inotropic agent may be useful, in patients with pulmonary edema who are hypotensive.

7. Phlebotomy, which in the past has been advocated as an appropriate intervention, is not widely used because it is time-consuming and also cumbersome in an acutely ill patient.

8. Administration of digitalis is frequently a useful means of slowing heart rate and improving ventricular function. However, in patients such as the one described, who are known to be taking digoxin chronically, the issue of digitalis toxicity must be raised. In particular, this patient presents with a narrow complex junctional tachycardia, which may be seen in digitalis intoxication. Other findings suggestive of digitalis intoxication include nausea, vomiting, paroxysmal atrial tachycardia with atrioventricular block, frequent premature ventricular contractions, ventricular tachycardia, and hyperkalemia.

9. Use of aminophylline. This drug is particularly useful when bronchospasm complicates pulmonary edema because it dilates bronchioles and is also a mild positive inotropic agent. However, in patients with severe congestive heart failure, metabolism of theophylline is impaired and careful monitoring of blood levels is critical to avoid intoxication.

REFERENCE

1. Wilson, J.R., Reichek, N., Dunkman, W.B., and Goldberg, S.: Effect of diuresis on the performance of the failing left ventricle in man. Am. J. Med. 70:234, 1981.

200 A-T, B-F, C-T, D-T, E-F *(Braunwald, pp. 372–376)*

Adenylate cyclase is the enzyme system that generates cyclic AMP (cAMP) in response to beta-adrenergic stimulation, and cAMP then acts as a second messenger. Adenosine, on the other hand, acting through A_1-receptors, inhibits adenylate cyclase, and stimulates acetylcholine-sensitive K^+ channels (therefore inhibiting sinus and AV nodal activity). A few hormones, such as glucagon and thyroid hormone, have the ability to couple to myocardial adenylate cyclase independently of beta receptors. These hormones therefore can have a positive inotropic effect. Bypassing beta receptors can be useful in cases of beta blocker overdose, where glucagon, for example, may be useful.[1]

Cardiac beta-adrenergic receptors are chiefly of the $beta_1$-subtype. The receptor site is highly stereospecific, and isoproterenol is the optimal agonist for this receptor. Epinephrine and norepinephrine are equipotent but have less agonist activity than isoproterenol on $beta_1$-receptors. However, epinephrine is a more potent agonist than norepinephrine for $beta_2$-receptors. In patients with heart failure, there is marked (50 to 70 per cent) down-regulation of $beta_1$-receptors (especially those with dilated cardiomyopathy), uncoupling of $beta_2$-receptors from adenylate cyclase, decreased adenylate cyclase activity, and increased levels of inhibitory G_i proteins.[2,3] Down-regulation of $beta_1$-receptors is thought to be related in part to chronically increased circulating catecholamine levels, but there may be other poorly understood mechanisms that also result in decreased myocardial $beta_1$-receptors.[2]

In contract to the adrenergic system, vagal stimulation has a negative inotropic effect. This is thought to be mediated through slowing of the heart rate, inhibition of the formation of cAMP, and stimulation of the cGMP system. In animal as well as human experiments, it has been observed that this negative inotropic effect is more pronounced in the presence of beta-adrenergic stimulation. This is thought to reflect the importance of inhibition of the G_s subunit of the receptor system (which normally stimulates cAMP production).[4]

REFERENCES

1. Critchley, J.A., and Ungar, A.: The management of acute poisoning due to beta-adrenoceptor antagonists. Med. Toxicol. Adverse Drug Exp. 4:32–45, 1989.
2. Englehardt, S., Bohm, M., Erdmann, E., and Lohse, M.J.: Analysis of beta-adrenergic receptor mRNA levels in human ventricular biopsy specimens by quantitative polymerase chain reactions: Progressive reduction of beta 1-adrenergic receptor mRNA in heart failure. J. Am. Coll. Cardiol. 27:146–154, 1996.
3. Beau, S.L., Tolley, T.K., and Saffitz, J.E.: Heterogenous transmural distribution of beta-adrenergic receptor subtypes in failing human hearts. Circulation 88:2501–2509, 1993.
4. Matsuda, J.J., Lee, H.C., and Shibata, E.F.: Acetylcholine reversal of isoproterenol-stimulated sodium currents in rabbit ventricular myocytes. Circ. Res. 72:517–525, 1993.

201 A-T, B-T, C-F, D-F, E-F *(Braunwald, pp. 727–728)*

Most dual-chamber pacemakers operate with unipolar leads, as in this case. The metal capsule of the generator then serves as the indifferent electrode. This can result in oversensing, in which skeletal muscle potentials generated by contraction of the major pectoralis muscles result in inappropriate inhibition (AAI, VVI, DVI, DDI, VDD, or DDD) or triggering (AAT, VVT, VDD, VAT, or DDD) of stimuli. Whether sensing of myopotentials in the VVD or DDD mode occurs via the atrial or via the ventricular amplifier depends on the configuration, amplitude, and timing of the interference signals. In the illustrated example the occurrence of total inhibition during arm movements indicates sensing via the ventricular amplifier.

The first two PQRST complexes show appropriate dual-chamber atrial and ventricular sensing and pacing at a rate of 70/min. There is no evidence for lack of capture (all pacing stimuli cause myocardial depolarizations) or undersensing (since there are no native atrial or ventricular complexes).

After the third PQRST complex there is a 4-sec period during which no pacemaker activity is observed. This complete lack of pacemaker activity indicates that the ventricular lead has sensed the erratic electrical activity generated by the arm and chest muscles and has been inappropriately inhibited.

In the cases of suspected oversensing, placing the pacemaker in an asynchronous mode (with application of a magnet) will abolish the symptoms caused by pacemaker malfunction and aid in the diagnosis. Conversion of the lead system to bipolar function frequently eliminates sensing of myopotentials.

202 A-T, B-T, C-F, D-F, E-T *(Braunwald, pp. 482–484)*

Digoxin has become the most widely used digitalis glycoside preparation in clinical practice. An understanding of digoxin pharmacokinetics is important in avoiding the serious side effects that may result from the drug's narrow toxic/therapeutic ratio. In patients with normal renal function, about one-third of body stores are lost daily via renal excretion, with a resultant half-life of about 36 to 48 hours. The excretion of digoxin is proportional to glomerular filtration rate and therefore creatinine clearance. When patients use digitalis on a daily basis, a steady state is achieved in which daily excretion via the renal route is matched by the daily dosage intake. For patients not previously taking digitalis, initiating a daily maintenance dose of digitalis without a loading dose leads to this steady state after approximately four to five half-lives, or about 7 days in subjects with normal renal function.[1] Digoxin is highly bound to tissue, making it resistant to removal from the body by dialysis, exchange transfusion, and cardiopulmonary bypass.[2] Studies of digoxin metabolism in obesity[3] reveal that serum digoxin levels and pharmacokinetics remain essentially unchanged before and after weight loss in massively obese subjects. This implies that lean body mass should be used as a basis for the calculation of digoxin dosage.

In the late 1970's the clinically important interaction between digoxin and quinidine was described.[4] Investigators noted that initiation of quinidine therapy in patients taking digoxin resulted in an appropriate doubling of the serum digoxin concentration and that this increase was not uncommonly associated with the rhythm disturbances of digoxin toxicity. Subsequent reports have identified interactions between digoxin and other drugs used in cardiovascular therapy, such as verapamil and amiodarone.

REFERENCES

1. Marcus, F.L., Burkhalter, L., Cuccia, C., et al.: Administration of tritiated digoxin with and without a loading dose: A metabolic study. Circulation *34*:865, 1966.
2. Coltart, D.J., Chamberlain, D.A., Howard, M.R., et al.: The effect of cardiopulmonary bypass on plasma digoxin concentrations. Br. Heart J. *33*:334, 1971.
3. Ewy, G.A., Groves, B.M., Ball, M.F., et al.: Digoxin metabolism in obesity. Circulation *44*:810, 1971.
4. Leahey, E.B., Jr., Reiffel, J.A., Drusin, R.E., et al.: Interaction between quinidine and digoxin. JAMA *240*:533, 1978.

203 A-T, B-T, C-T, D-F, E-F   *(Braunwald, p. 460)*

Anemia is one of the causes of hyperdynamic circulation and may result in heart failure in patients with underlying heart disease. To compensate for reduction in oxygen-carrying capacity of the blood, cardiac output must increase, which places a state of volume overload on the left ventricle. This is similar in many respects to the situation in chronic aortic regurgitation where the regurgitant blood also results in a volume overload of the left ventricle. The increased blood flow with peripheral vasodilatation characteristic in both conditions leads to the various physical examination findings including "pistol shot" sounds, and systolic murmur over the femoral arteries (Duroziez's sign), subungual capillary pulsation (Quincke's pulse), and systolic flow murmurs over the precordium.

A mid-diastolic flow murmur also can be heard in patients with anemia or aortic regurgitation due to augmented blood flow across mitral and tricuspid valves. In patients with chronic aortic regurgitation, a mid-diastolic murmur can sometimes be heard in the apical region due to rapid antegrade flow across a mitral orifice that is narrowed by the rapidly rising left ventricular end-diastolic pressure and/or by the regurgitant jet (Austin-Flint murmur). Hill's sign refers to popliteal cuff systolic pressure exceeding brachial cuff pressure by more than 60 mm Hg. This sign is seen in chronic aortic regurgitation and may be helpful in assessing its severity, but it is not seen in patients with anemia.[1]

REFERENCE

1. Talley, J.D.: The correlation of clinical findings and severity of aortic insufficiency: Hill's sign. Heart Dis. Stroke *2*: 468—470, 1993.

204 A-T, B-F, C-T, D-F, E-F   *(Braunwald, pp. 619–621)*

Electrical direct-current (DC) cardioversion effectively terminates up to 95 per cent of reentrant arrhythmias through a combination of mechanisms, including depolarization of all excitable myocardium, and prolonging refractoriness. Because of increased potential for inducing fatal postshock ventricular arrhythmias, cardioversion of digitalis-induced rhythms is contraindicated. However, it is not necessary to withhold digitalis for elective cardioversion in patients without clinical evidence of toxicity.[1] A synchronized shock is used for almost all cardioversions with the exception of ventricular flutter and fibrillation. Recent data suggest that synchronized shocks delivered late in the QRS complex are more effective and less likely to induce acceleration of the arrhythmia than shocks delivered near the QRS onset.[2] However, even when properly synchronized, there remains a finite risk of inducing ventricular fibrillation. The minimum effective energy for cardioversion should be used to minimize cardiac damage. Although CPK elevation is frequently seen after cardioversion, elevation of the MB fraction is uncommon.[3]

REFERENCES

1. Leja, F.S., Euler, D.E., and Scanlon, P.J.: Digoxin and the susceptibility of the canine heart to countershock-induced arrhythmia. Am. J. Cardiol. *55*:1070–1075, 1985.
2. Li, H.G., Yee, R., Mehra, R., et al.: Effect of shock timing on efficacy and safety of internal cardioversion for ventricular tachycardia. J. Am. Coll. Cardiol. *24*:703, 1994.
3. Mattana, J., and Singhal, P.C.: Determinants of elevated creatine kinase activity and creatine kinase MB-fraction following cardiopulmonary resuscitation. Chest *101*:1386–1392, 1992.

205 A-F, B-T, C-T, D-F, E-F   *(Braunwald, pp. 829–830)*

This patient presents with the classic symptoms of epinephrine excess as would be found in association with a pheochromocytoma. About 90 per cent of pheochromocytomas arise in the adrenal *medulla*, while 10 per cent are bilateral and another 10 per cent are malignant. Multiple adrenal tumors are common in patients with familial pheochromocytoma and in association with multiple endocrine neoplasia type II, medullary carcinoma of the thyroid (Sipple's syndrome), or mucosal ganglioneuromas (type III). If the predominant substance released is epinephrine (formed only in the adrenal medulla), the symptoms include systolic hypertension, tachycardia, sweating, flushing, and apprehension. If norepinephrine is primarily secreted, as is the case for some adrenal medullary tumors and most extraadrenal tumors, symptoms include both systolic and diastolic hypertension (increased vasoconstriction) and, less frequently, tachycardia, palpitations, and anxiety.

The easiest and most reliable test for tumor localization is abdominal CT scan, while laboratory confirmation is typically made by measurement of urinary metanephrines or vanillylmandelic acid.[1] Interference with urinary secretion of metabolites is common, with *increases* in patients taking sympathomimetic drugs, monoamine oxidase inhibitors, or labetalol[2] and *decreases* after administration of x-ray contrast media containing methylglucamine (e.g., Renografin, Hypaque).

REFERENCES

1. Manu, P., and Hunge, L.A.: Biochemical screening for pheochromocytoma: Superiority of urinary metanephrine measurements. Am. J. Epidemiol. *120*:788, 1984.
2. Bouloux, P.M.G., and Perrett, D.: Interference of labetalol metabolites in the determination of plasma catecholamines by HPLC with electrochemical detection. Clin. Chim. Acta *150*:111, 1985.

206 A-F, B-F, C-T, D-T, E-T (Braunwald, p. 455)

While cardiomegaly is a nonspecific, common finding in chronic heart failure in the majority of patients, there are several notable situations in which its presence is an exception. In circumstances in which heart failure develops before the heart has had a chance to enlarge, cardiomegaly is often absent. Such circumstances include the sudden development of arrhythmias, rupture of a valve or valve apparatus, and acute myocardial infarction. In addition, heart failure due to chronic constrictive pericarditis or restrictive cardiomyopathy is usually not associated with cardiomegaly.

Pulsus alternans is characterized by a regular rhythm with alternation of strong and weak contractions in which the weak beat is equally spaced from or slightly closer to the preceding strong beat. It usually occurs in patients who have a protodiastolic gallop sound, who have advanced myocardial disease, and who have not yet received treatment. Pulsus alternans most commonly occurs in heart failure caused by increased resistance to left ventricular ejection such as in systemic hypertension or AS. It is also seen in coronary atherosclerosis and dilated cardiomyopathies. The mechanism of pulsus alternans is thought to be a depletion in the number of contracting myocardial cells in alternating cardiac cycles, caused by incomplete recovery, which results in an alternation in stroke volume.[1]

The presence of fever in congestive heart failure should always alert the physician to the possibility of underlying infection, pulmonary infarction, or infective endocarditis. In severe heart failure, low-grade fever may be seen as a consequence of cutaneous vasoconstriction and impairment of heat loss due to the marked elevation of adrenergic nervous system activity.

The mechanism of Cheyne-Stokes respirations in congestive heart failure results from the complex interaction between left ventricular failure and the sensitivity of the medullary respiratory center. Left ventricular dysfunction leads to a prolongation of the circulation time from the lung to the brain and results in a sluggish response of the respiratory center. During apnea, arterial P_{O_2} falls and P_{CO_2} rises. This combination excites the depressed respiratory center and leads to hyperventilation, a reduction of P_{CO_2}, and another period of apnea. While the principal cause of Cheyne-Stokes respiration is cerebral lesions as in stroke or cerebral arteriosclerosis, the alterations in circulation time mentioned are capable of exaggerating and making more clinically evident a Cheyne-Stokes pattern of respiration.

REFERENCE

1. Gleason, W.B., and Braunwald, E.: Studies on Starling's law of the heart. VI. Relationships between left ventricular end-diastolic volume and stroke volume in man with observations on the mechanisms of pulsus alternans. Circulation *25*:841, 1962.

207 A-T, B-T, C-F, D-T, E-T (Braunwald, pp. 823–824)

The use of oral contraceptive pills may be the most common cause of secondary hypertension, resulting in a 5 per cent incidence of hypertension over 5 years of use.[1] The likelihood of developing hypertension is increased by alcohol consumption, age >35 years, and obesity and is probably related to the estrogen content of the agent.[2] The excess annual death rate attributable to oral contraceptive use among nonsmokers is 1 per 77,000, while for women 35 to 44 who smoke this rate is 1 per 2000. Since estrogen increases the hepatic production of renin substrate, one probable mechanism for hypertension induced by oral contraceptives is activation of the renin-angiotensin systems with sodium retention and volume expansion.

REFERENCES

1. Royal Collage of General Practitioners' Oral Contraception Study: Further analyses of mortality in oral contraceptive users. Lancet *1*:541, 1981.
2. Tsai, C.C., Williamson, O., Kirkland, B.H., et al: Low-dose oral contraception and blood pressure in women with a past history of elevated blood pressure. Am. J. Obstet. Gynecol. *151*:28, 1985.

208 A-T, B-T, C-T, D-T, E-F   *(Braunwald, pp. 465–466)*

Pulmonary edema associated with acute pulmonary embolism is a well-described syndrome. In this setting, pulmonary edema is thought to result from both LV dysfunction secondary to hypoxia and from encroachment of the intraventricular septum on the LV cavity (reversed Bernheim effect). There is also some evidence to suggest that increased permeability of the alveolar-capillary membrane contributes to this syndrome. Acute pulmonary edema can present with bronchoconstriction, and differentiation from acute bronchial asthma can be aided by demonstrating the presence of a third heart sound, electrocardiographic changes suggestive of an underlying cardiac etiology, or the presence of cardiomegaly and alveolar infiltrates on a chest x-ray. Pulmonary edema can follow rapid expansion of the lung following a pneumothorax. Usually the pneumothorax has been present for several hours to days, and the resulting edema is usually unilateral, with minimal clinical findings.

Normal persons who ascend rapidly to high altitudes (usually above 2500 m or 8000 ft) and then engage in a strenuous activity soon after their ascent can be at risk for developing high-altitude pulmonary edema. Young patients in their teens or early twenties are at higher risk than older patients. Rapid reversal of this syndrome can be achieved by either returning patients to a lower altitude or by the administration of oxygen. Neurogenic pulmonary edema, which can complicate certain CNS disorders such as head trauma, seizures, and intracranial bleeding, is thought to be secondary to transient sympathetic hyperactivity. Sympatholytic agents prevent this syndrome, but appear to have no place in its treatment, since pulmonary capillary pressures usually have normalized by the time the syndrome is diagnosed.

209 A-F, B-T, C-F, D-T   *(Braunwald, p. 463; Fig. 15–8)*

There is a gravity-dependent distribution of blood in the lungs. Since blood is more dense than gas-containing lung tissue, effects of gravity are much greater on the distribution of blood flow than on the distribution of tissue forces in the lung. Thus, from apex to base the effect of perfusion pressure on the pulmonary circulation increases by 1 cm H_2O per cm of vertical distance, whereas the pleural pressure increases by only 0.25 cm H_2O per cm of vertical distance. Pulmonary capillaries are exposed to alveolar pressure that does not vary from apex to base. However, pulmonary arteries and veins are exposed to pleural pressure that does vary from apex to base.

On the basis of these concepts, the upright lung can be divided into three zones (see Fig. 15–8, p. 463). In zone 1 (at the apex), pulmonary arterial pressure is less than alveolar pressure so that there is essentially no flow. In zone 2, arterial pressure exceeds alveolar pressure, which in turn exceeds venous pressure. Here, the pressure which controls blood flow is determined by the difference between upstream (arterial) and chamber (alveolar) pressures. It is in this zone that large increases in blood flow occur as the lung is studied from apex to base. In zone 3, venous pressure exceeds alveolar pressure, which results in distention of the capillaries. Mean intravascular pressures are greatest in this zone so that small elevations in venous pressure can cause edema formation most rapidly in this zone. It is only in this zone that calculations of pulmonary vascular resistance and measurement of pulmonary capillary wedge pressure have relevance. Furthermore, it is in this zone that elevation of pulmonary capillary wedge pressure causes vascular redistribution.

True vascular redistribution reflects a relative reduction of perfusion of the bases with a relative increase in apical perfusion. This phenomenon is probably due to compression of vessels at the lung bases as a result of greater formation of edema. This leads to hypoxemia, pulmonary arteriolar vasoconstriction, and increased pressure, which in turn cause blood flow redistribution to more apical segments.

210 A-T, B-F, C-T, D-T, E-T   *(Braunwald, p. 524)*

The widespread use of cyclosporine to achieve immunosuppression in cardiac transplant recipients has led to the identification of a number of complications of cyclosporine therapy. The most clinically evident effects of cyclosporine involve renal dysfunction. Most patients receiving the drug develop a reduction in creatinine clearance, an increase in fluid retention and edema, and significant hypertension.[1] Recent evidence suggests that some of the increase in blood pressure may be due to local vasoconstrictor effects following increases in platelet aggregation and thromboxane generation, which result from the cyclosporine therapy. Some transplant groups advocate omission of cyclosporine from the early posttransplant regime until serum creatinine has normalized and the patient has reestablished normal hemodynamics following cardiopulmonary bypass.[2] Abnormalities in liver function are also a consequence of cyclosporine therapy. Like many of the cyclosporine-associated side effects, hepatic dysfunction appears to be dose related; treatment is best approached by decreasing the daily dose of cyclosporine. Fine tremors, paresthesias, and occasionally seizures are all part of the neurotoxic response to cyclosporine therapy. Many patients who receive cyclosporine also develop hypertrichosis (hirsutism). Gingival hyperplasia is also associated with cyclosporine therapy and has been reported to occur much more frequently in patients treated simultaneously with nifedipine.[3] Bone marrow suppression is the major morbidity of long-term azathioprine administration and is not associated with cyclosporine therapy.

REFERENCES

1. Myers, B.D., Ross, J., Newton, L.: Cyclosporine-associated chronic nephropathy. N. Engl. J. Med. *311*:699, 1984.
2. Renlund, G.D., O'Connell, J.B., Gilbert, E.M., et al.: A prospective comparison of murine monoclonal CD-3 antibody-based and equine antithymocyte globulin-based rejection prophylaxis in cardiac transplantation: Decreased rejection and less corticosteroid use with OKT3. Transplantation *47*:599, 1989.
3. Slavin, J., and Taylor, J.: Cyclosporine, nifedipine and gingival hyperplasia. Lancet *2*:739, 1987.

211 A-T, B-F, C-T, D-F   (Braunwald, pp. 825–827)

Renovascular hypertension is the most common form of secondary hypertension. The most common etiology is renal artery stenosis due to either atherosclerosis (~65 per cent) or fibromuscular dysplasia (~34 per cent). Atherosclerotic disease is seen mainly in older men, while fibromuscular dysplasia is a disease of younger women. The latter usually affects the distal two-thirds of the renal arteries and its branches. Diagnosis is suspected initially on clinical grounds, such as the presence of severe and refractory hypertension in a young patient, abdominal bruits, and elevation of serum creatinine whether spontaneously or following therapy with angiotensin-converting enzyme inhibitors. The best initial tests in patients with such clinical features are radioisotope renography and plasma renin measurements after an oral captopril challenge.[1] In some centers, renal artery duplex sonography is utilized as an initial screening test. This is followed by renal arteriography in those with positive results. Although medical therapy has been traditionally the first line of management, angioplasty of the renal arteries is being performed more frequently as the initial procedure, particularly in patients who are poor surgical candidates. Angioplasty is more successful (60 to 70 per cent) in cases of fibromuscular dysplasia, where the likelihood of restenosis is less than with atherosclerotic renal artery stenosis.

REFERENCE

1. Frederickson, E.D., Wilcox, C.S., Bucci, C.M., et al.: A prospective evaluation of a simplified captopril test for the detection of renovascular hypertension. Arch. Intern. Med. *150*:569, 1990.

212 A-T, B-T, C-T, D-F   (Braunwald, pp. 676–677)

Most forms of PVCs are prognostically benign in patients who have no known heart disease.[1] However, in patients who have had a prior MI, the occurrence of PVCs—particularly if they are frequent and of certain forms—is associated with a high risk of sudden cardiac death.[2] Although there is a great deal of controversy over which classification system and which kinds of PVCs are most frequently associated with SCD, in general increased frequency (usually defined as ≥10 PVCs per hour), certain forms of PVCs (multiform, bigeminy, short-coupling intervals [R-on-T phenomenon]), and runs of three or more ectopic beats are associated with increased risk of SCD.

LV dysfunction has been shown to be a major factor for increased risk in association with PVCs following MI.[3] Furthermore, it appears that the increased risk of SCD following MI persists for at least up to 3 years following MI as long as frequent and complex forms of PVCs are present. The Cardiac Arrhythmia Suppression Trial (CAST) showed that encainide and flecainide[4] increased mortality in post-MI patients treated to suppress PVCs. The moricizine arm of this study has also recently been stopped because of the lack of any beneficial effect. Thus it presently is not clear which therapy, if any, is appropriate in the post-MI patient with increases in ventricular ectopy.

REFERENCES

1. Kennedy, H.L., Whitlock, J.A., Sprague, M.K., et al.: Long-term follow-up of asymptomatic healthy subjects with frequent and complex ventricular ectopy. N. Engl. J. Med. *312*:193, 1985.
2. Ruberman, W., Weinblatt, E., Goldberg, J.D., et al.: Ventricular premature beats and mortality after myocardial infarction. N. Engl. J. Med. *297*:750, 1977.
3. Bigger, J.T., Fleiss, J.L., Kleiger, R., et al.: The relationships among ventricular arrhythmias, left ventricular dysfunction and mortality in the 2 years after myocardial infarction. Circulation *69*:250, 1984.
4. The Cardiac Arrhythmia Suppression Trial (CAST) Investigators: Effect of encainide and flecainide on mortality in a randomized trial of arrhythmia suppression after myocardial infarction. N. Engl. J. Med. *321*:406, 1989.

213 A-F, B-T, C-F, D-T   (Braunwald, p. 604)

The systemic lupus erythematosus (SLE) –like syndrome induced by procainamide therapy occurs in approximately 20 to 30 per cent of patients taking the drug on a chronic basis despite the development of antinuclear antibodies in between 60 and 70 per cent of all patients receiving this drug. The syndrome, which is reversible when procainamide therapy is stopped, is characterized by a variety of symptoms including arthralgias, pleuropericarditis, fever, hepatomegaly, and less commonly a hemorrhagic pericardial effusion with tamponade. Formation of NAPA, which occurs by acetylation of the aromatic amino group on procainamide, appears to prevent the development of the SLE-like syndrome, implicating this amino group in the pathophysiology of the syndrome.[1] It is not necessary to discontinue the drug upon the development of positive serological tests. However, the development of symptoms or a positive anti-DNA antibody is a contraindication to procainamide therapy, except in patients whose life-threatening arrhythmia is controlled only by procainamide. In this latter group, the concomitant use of steroids may eliminate the clinical manifestations of the SLE-like syndrome.

REFERENCE

1. Kluger, J., Drayer, D.E., Reidenberg, M.M., and Lahita, R.: Acetylprocainamide therapy in patients with previous procainamide-induced lupus syndrome. Ann. Intern. Med. 95:18, 1981.

214 A-T, B-F, C-T, D-F   (Braunwald, p. 303)

In the case of respiratory failure in which hypoxemia is present without hypercapnia, the role of mechanical ventilation is to increase the mean lung volume during the respiratory cycle; this opens more alveoli for gas exchange. If hypoxemia is not corrected by mechanical ventilation, increasing concentrations of inspired O_2 are required, as in this case. When the FIO_2 exceeds 60 per cent for more than 24 hours, pulmonary alveolar damage due to O_2 toxicity develops. Therefore, positive end-expiratory pressure (PEEP) is utilized because it allows equivalent levels of arterial oxygenation at lower concentrations of FIO_2 by increasing end-expiratory lung volume.

Several common complications of PEEP should be considered. The first is that the high intrathoracic pressure and increased lung volumes which occur impede venous return and prevent appropriate functioning of the right ventricle, with resulting reductions in cardiac output. This is manifested by the development of cool extremities and decreased urine output. Therefore, it is important to monitor cardiac function with a Swan-Ganz catheter and/or thermodilution techniques upon institution of PEEP. The appropriate PEEP setting is achieved when the pulmonary capillary wedge pressure is minimized while cardiac output is maintained.

The predominant mechanism for decreased cardiac output secondary to PEEP is believed to be increased intrathoracic pressure with impaired venous return. This causes inadequate right ventricular output, which results in decreased left ventricular output. Displacement of the interventricular septum toward the left ventricle impairs left ventricular diastolic filling directly. Barotrauma, another complication of mechanical ventilation, is worsened by PEEP. The development of pneumomediastinum, pneumothorax, and subcutaneous emphysema is not uncommon during PEEP.

215 A-T, B-T, C-T, D-F   (Braunwald, pp. 884–885; Table 29–3)

The clinical expression of congestive heart failure in neonates and infants is somewhat different from that in adults or older children. Growth retardation, feeding difficulties, tachypnea, and excessive sweating may all be manifestations of heart failure in the first year of life. Other common signs of heart failure in this group include recurrent pul-

monary infections, tachycardia, and tachypnea (from the reduction in tidal volume precipitated by interstitial edema), nasal flaring and rib retraction with breathing, and poor peripheral perfusion with cool limbs. Left atrial or pulmonary artery enlargement may actually impinge on adjacent airways, leading to emphysematous expansion of the left lung or even atelectasis. While hepatomegaly is seen frequently in either right or left heart failure, the ascites and peripheral edema that are often seen in adults with heart failure are much less common in infants. Interestingly, facial edema is more common than peripheral edema in this age group. A further physical finding of systemic venous congestion is the prominence of veins on the dorsum of the hands. This may be a valuable clue in an infant, in whom jugular venous distention is not easily observed because of a short neck.

216 A-F, B-T, C-F, D-T, E-T   (Braunwald, pp. 743, 746–747)

Estimates for the annual incidence of sudden cardiac death (SCD) in the United States range from 300,000 to nearly 400,000 cases, which represent at least 50 per cent of all cardiac deaths.[1] The majority of patients who present with SCD have underlying coronary artery disease and up to 75 per cent have had a previous myocardial infarct. However, other myocardial, congenital, and valvular pathologies can cause and contribute significantly to the incidence of SCD. Of the premorbid clinical predictors of risk of SCD, ejection fraction (EF) is the most powerful, with an EF <30 per cent being the single most powerful predictor for future development of SCD. Ventricular ectopy is a less powerful but independent predictor of SCD, especially when frequent or complex. Most frequently the presenting rhythm in SCD patients is ventricular fibrillation, while bradyarrhythmias and asystole are less common. The latter two rhythms each carry a worse prognosis than sustained ventricular tachycardia, which carries a better prognosis when it is the presenting rhythm in SCD patients. By comparison, ventricular fibrillation has an intermediate prognosis.

REFERENCE

1. Gilman, J.K., Jalal, S., and Naccarelli, G.V.: Predicting and preventing sudden death from cardiac causes. Circulation 90:1083–1092, 1994.

217 A-F, B-F, C-T, D-F, E-T   (Braunwald, pp. 707–709; Table 23–2)

A recent report from the ACC/AHA Joint Committee on Pacemaker Implantation defined three classes of indications for permanent cardiac pacing.[1] Class I indications are conditions for which there is general agreement that permanent pacemakers should be implanted. Class II indications are conditions for which pacemakers are used frequently but opinion diverges on whether they are necessary. Class III indications are conditions for which there is general agreement that permanent pacing is unnecessary. Several factors may influence the decision to place a permanent pacemaker. In general, the presence of symptoms is the most important reason for a condition to be defined as a class I indication (with the exception of first-degree AV block, or isolated bundle branch block). Asymptomatic first-degree AV block is considered a class III indication regardless of the length of the PR interval. Symptomatic first-degree AV block improved by temporary pacing is a class II indication. Infranodal second-degree AV block not induced by pacing is a class I indication for permanent pacing; when induced by pacing, it is a class II indication. Persistent advanced or complete AV block at the AV node level following acute MI is considered a class II indication. Persistent or intermittent complete AV block regardless of symptoms, in the absence of reversible causes, is a class I indication.

REFERENCE

1. Dreifus, L.S., Fisch, C., Griffin, J.C., et al.: Guidelines for implantation of cardiac pacemakers and antiarrhythmia devices: A report of the American College of Cardiology/ American Heart Association Task Force on Assessment of Diagnostic and Therapeutic procedures (Committee on Pacemaker Implantation). J. Am. Coll. Cardiol. 18:1, 1991.

218 A-T, B-T, C-T, D-F   (Braunwald, pp. 656–658)

The electrocardiogram illustrated shows atrial tachycardia with block (or paroxysmal atrial tachycardia with block; PAT with block). In this condition an atrial rate of 130 to 200 beats/min with a ventricular response less than or equal to the atrial rate is noted. Digitalis toxicity accounts for this rhythm in 50 to 75 per cent of cases, and in such instances the atrial rate may show a gradual increase as digitalis dosing is continued. Other signs of digitalis excess are often present, including frequent premature ventricular complexes and noncardiac signs of digitalis toxicity.

In nearly half of all patients with PAT with block, the atrial rate is irregular and demonstrates a characteristic isoelectric interval between each P wave, in contrast to the morphology of atrial flutter waves. Most instances of PAT with block occur in patients with significant organic heart disease. Etiologies other than digitalis toxicity include ischemic heart disease, MI, and cor pulmonale. In patients taking digitalis, potassium depletion may precipitate the arrhythmia, and the oral administration of potassium and the withholding of digitalis often will allow reversal to normal sinus rhythm. Because PAT with block is seen primarily in patients with serious underlying heart disease, its onset may lead to significant clinical deterioration. Thus it must be carefully sought in cardiac patients receiving digitalis treatment.

219 A-F, B-F, C-T, D-T, E-F   (Braunwald, pp. 723–725)

Rate-adaptive or responsive pacemakers are pulse-generator systems with the ability to change their output rate in response to a biological parameter that directly or indirectly reflects the subject's activity. They are designated by the letter R in the fourth position of the pacemaker code. They are currently indicated in the management of patients with chronotropic incompetence (practically defined as inability to achieve a heart rate exceeding 70 per cent of the maximum predicted rate or the inability to reach a heart rate of 100 beats/min on exercise). Currently approved devices respond to activity, minute ventilation, or temperature. Newer systems will respond to hemodynamic (e.g., RV pressure), electrical (e.g., Q-T interval), or chemical parameters (e.g., O_2 saturation and H^+ ion concentration in central venous blood). Rate-adaptive pacemakers do not respond to mental exercise or emotional stress. Such devices recognize the onset and end of exercise quite precisely, which may be important for older patients who do primarily short bursts of physical exertion. The magnitude and rate of change of the sensor-driven response are programmable, and should be adjusted based on heart rate response to low and high levels of activity. Activity-sensing pacemakers are the most commonly used systems. They are limited, however, by the fact that they can respond to external vibrations such as riding in a vehicle. New accelerometer-based systems respond to changes in motion and thus are less susceptible than conventional sensors to environmental noise.

220 A-T, B-T, C-T, D-T   (Braunwald, pp. 872–874)

A careful, accurate history and thorough physical examination are most important in the evaluation of syncope of unknown cause.[1] In patients with syncope of unknown cause, the overall 1-year mortality approaches 6 per cent. In patients with noncardiovascular causes, 1-year mortality is between 1 and 12 per cent, but in those with identified cardiovascular causes, mortality approaches 20 to 30 per cent.[2] The three most common arrhythmic causes of syncope are sinus node dysfunction, tachyarrhythmias, and AV block. While electrophysiological (EP) studies have proven useful for identifying each of these disturbances, of the three, tachyarrhythmias are most reliably initiated in the electrophysiology laboratory.

When an abnormality is found on EP testing that may explain syncope, subsequent therapy directed at this abnormality prevents recurrence of syncope in about 80 per cent of patients.[3] However, the ability of EP testing to uncover a cause for syncope varies widely and is lowest in patients with no recognizable structural heart disease. The induction of a sustained supraventricular or monomorphic ventricular tachycardia in patients who have not displayed spontaneous development of such tachycardias on noninvasive evaluation is relatively uncommon but highly suggestive that the induced tachyarrhythmia is clinically relevant.

REFERENCES

1. Lipsitz, L.A.: Syncope in the elderly. Ann. Intern. Med. *90:* 92, 1983.
2. Kapoor, W.: Evaluation and outcome of patients with syncope. Medicine *69:*160, 1990.
3. DiMarco, J.P., Garan, H., and Ruskin, J.N.: Approach to the patient with recurrent syncope of unknown causes. Mod. Concepts Cardiovasc. Dis. *52:*11, 1983.

221 A-T, B-T, C-T, D-F   *(Braunwald, pp. 605–607)*

Lidocaine has proven to be an extremely effective agent in the therapy of ventricular arrhythmias of diverse etiologies. The drug has a fairly wide toxic/therapeutic ratio, with a low incidence of hemodynamic complications that are rarely seen unless left ventricular function is severely impaired. While lidocaine reduces the action potential duration and the effective refractory period of Purkinje fibers and ventricular muscle, it has little effect on atrial fibers and does not affect conduction in accessory pathways.

Metabolism of lidocaine is largely hepatic and thus depends on hepatic blood flow. The elimination half-life of the substance averages 1 to 2 hours in normal subjects but is more than 4 hours in patients after relatively uncomplicated MI and is 10 hours or longer in patients who sustain MI complicated by cardiac failure or cardiogenic shock. In addition, hepatic disease or decreased hepatic blood flow, as in congestive heart failure, decreases the rate of lidocaine metabolism. Thus, there are a variety of clinical situations requiring that maintenance doses of lidocaine be reduced by one-third to one-half of normal. Patients treated with an initial bolus of lidocaine followed by a maintenance infusion may experience transient *subtherapeutic* plasma concentrations at 30 to 120 minutes after therapy is begun (see Braunwald, Fig. 21–4, p. 606). Therefore, a second bolus of lidocaine of approximately one-half the initial dose 20 to 40 minutes following onset of therapy is recommended.

222 A-T, B-T, C-T, D-F   *(Braunwald, pp. 366–372)*

Since the classic experiments of Ringer in 1882, it has been appreciated that cardiac contraction depends on the presence of intracellular Ca^{++}. In fact, the magnitude of cardiac contraction has been shown to be proportional to the intracellular Ca^{++} concentration. It has also been observed that depolarization of the plasma membrane associated with the upstroke of the action potential opens voltage-dependent channels that bring Ca^{++} into the cell. Ca^{++} that passes into the cell through these channels does not actually appear to activate the contractile system directly but rather is stored in membrane sites within the cells, specifically the T system and the sarcoplasmic reticulum (SR). The Ca^{++} that actually activates the contractile system appears to be stored in the cisternae of the SR and released upon membrane depolarization. This process is termed Ca^{++}-induced Ca^{++} release. According to this concept, the depolarization of the cell membrane causes release of Ca^{++} from the terminal cisternae of the SR into the cytoplasm. Ca^{++} binding by troponin results in activation of the contractile elements, and relaxation is brought about by the active uptake of Ca^{++} into another area of the SR. There it is stored only to be released during the subsequent contraction.

Several mechanisms have been identified for regulation of intracellular Ca^{++} concentration in cardiac cells.[2] Included in these are:

1. Inward movement of Ca^{++} along its concentration gradient across the sarcolemma via Ca^{++} channels to generate the "slow" inward current. Beta-adrenergic agonists increase myocardial contractility in part by increasing Ca^{++} *influx* into cardiac cells by opening receptor-activated channels.
2. A bidirectional Na^+-Ca^{++} exchange system that mediates movement of Ca^{++} across the sarcolemma along a concentration gradient provided by Na^+. In general, Ca^{++} is pumped out in exchange for Na^+. However, when cardiac glycosides inhibit the Na^+, K^+-ATPase with elevation of intracellular Na^+, then Ca^{++} may enter the cell, bringing about a positive inotropic effect.
3. A sarcolemmal Ca^{++}-ATPase that extrudes Ca^{++} from the cell.
4. A Ca^{++}-stimulated magnesium-ATPase in the membrane of the SR which transports Ca^{++} into the SR.[3]
5. Uptake of Ca^{++} in other structures such as mitochondria.
6. A buffering of intracellular Ca^{++} by proteins such as calmodulin, troponin C, and the myosin light chains.

REFERENCES

1. Fabiato, A.: Stimulated calcium current can both cause calcium loading in and trigger calcium release from the sarcoplasmic reticulum of a skinned canine cardiac Purkinje cell. J. Gen. Physiol. *85:*291, 1985.
2. Braunwald, E.: Mechanisms of actions of calcium channel blocking agents. N. Engl. J. Med. *307:*1618, 1982.
3. Mercadier, J.-J., Lompre, A.-M., Duc, P., et al.: Altered sarcoplasmic reticulum Ca^{++}-ATPase gene expression in the human ventricle during end-stage heart failure. J. Clin. Invest. *85:*305, 1990.

223 A-F, B-F, C-F, D-F   *(Braunwald, pp. 428–429)*

LV afterload, which reflects the impedance resistance) to ejection, is a fundamental determinant of LV performance. In mitral regurgitation (MR) and ventricular septal defect (VSD), LV afterload is low. In both aortic regurgitation (AR) and patent ductus arteriosus (PDA), there is a decrease in aortic impedance as documented by the fall in diastolic pressure. However, the net decrease in impedance to ventricular ejection is considerably smaller than in VSD or MR. Furthermore, the myocardial oxygen requirements are much lower in MR and VSD, allowing for greater myocardial reserve at any workload. Thus, LV end-diastolic pressure and volume are greater for AR and PDA. The decrease in impedance in cases of VSD can be muted if high RV pressures are present, such as in cases of tetralogy of Fallot or following the development of Eisenmenger syndrome. In these cases, the decrease in impedance is clearly greater for MR, and thus the left ventricular end-diastolic pressure and volume will be lower for this lesion.

REFERENCES

1. Urschel, C.W., Covell, J.W., Sonnenblick, E.H., et al.: Myocardial mechanics is aortic and mitral valvular regurgitation: The concept of instantaneous impedance as a determinant of the performance of the intact heart. J. Clin. Invest. *47*:867, 1968.
2. Urschel, C.W., Covell, J.W., Graham, T.P., et al.: Effects of acute valvular regurgitation on the oxygen consumption of the canine heart. Circ. Res. *23*:33, 1968.

224 A-T, B-T, C-T, D-F *(Braunwald, p. 394–396)*

The three fundamental mechanisms by which the left ventricle compensates for decreased contractile function or increased contractile burden are:

1. The Frank-Starling mechanism, by which an increase in preload lengthens resting sarcomeres to enhance their performance via increased activation;
2. An increase in neurohumoral adrenergic responses which results in increased inotropy; and
3. Myocardial hypertrophy with or without chamber dilation.

Venous return in congestive heart failure is often maintained by coexisting venoconstriction.

225 A-T, B-F, C-T, D-T, E-T *(Braunwald, pp. 525–526)*

The development of atherosclerosis in the coronary arteries of the transplanted heart is the major long-term problem following cardiac transplantation. The incidence of this complication is between 20 and 50 per cent 5 years after the surgical procedure.[1] Unfortunately, the use of cyclosporine has not led to any significant decline in the incidence of this problem. The etiology of graft atherosclerosis is likely to be multifactorial and probably involves a complex immune mechanism. In one comprehensive study of patients treated with prednisone and azathioprine, the only significant and clinical parameters identified as risk factors for

graft atherosclerosis were donor age over 35, HLA incompatibility, and elevated serum triglyceride concentrations.[2] In reports from centers using cyclosporine, however, lipid levels and donor age were not correlated with atherosclerosis, although this complication was correlated with two or more rejection episodes.[1] CMV infection may play a role in graft atherosclerosis. In one comprehensive report, the incidence of graft rejection was markedly increased in patients with known CMV infections, as was graft atherosclerosis as assessed by angiographic or autopsy criteria.[3] Most transplantation centers use preventive measures to attempt to modify known risk factors for atherosclerosis in transplant recipients. Symptoms of angina pectoris are usually undetectable in patients with cardiac allograft procedures, because the donor heart is essentially denervated. Diffuse graft atherosclerosis often requires retransplantation. The results of a second procedure are not as favorable as the primary procedure, with a 1-year patient survival rate of 44 per cent in one report[4] (compared to a 1-year survival rate of approximately 85 per cent in primary transplants).

The value of HMG Co-A reductase inhibitors was recently evaluated in a randomized trial.[5] Forty-seven patients received pravastatin early following transplantation, and 50 did not. Those who received pravastatin had less frequent cardiac rejection accompanied by hemodynamic compromise (3 versus 14 patients, p = 0.005), better survival (94 per cent versus 78 per cent, p = 0.025), and a lower incidence of coronary vasculopathy in the transplant as determined by angiography and at autopsy (3 versus 10 patients, p = 0.049).

REFERENCES

1. Billingham, M.E.: Cardiac transplant atherosclerosis. Transplant Proc. *19*(Suppl. 5):19, 1987.
2. Belber, C.P., Hunt, S.A., Schwinn, D.A., et al.: Complications in long-term survivors of cardiac transplantations. Transplant Proc. *13*:207, 1981.
3. Grattan, M.T., Moreno-Cabral, C.E., Sternes, V.A., et al.: Cytomegalovirus infection is associated with cardiac allograft rejection and atherosclerosis. JAMA *261*:3561, 1989.
4. Dein, J.R., Oyer, P.E., Stinson, E.B., et al.: Cardiac retransplantation in the cyclosporine era. Ann. Thorac. Surg. *48*:350, 1989.
5. Kobashigawa, J.A., Katznelson, S., Lakas, H., et al.: Effect of pravastatin on outcomes after cardiac transplantation. N. Engl. J. Med. *333*:621–627, 1995.

226 A-F, B-T, C-T, D-F *(Braunwald, p. 497)*

The importance of the adrenergic nervous system in heart failure is shown by the nearly universal worsening of symptoms upon administration of adrenoceptor blocking agents. On one hand there is an enhanced adrenoceptor state that may be responsible for vasoconstriction and that may cause cardiac arrhythmias. On the other hand, there is diminished adrenoceptor control in heart failure, including blunted increases in heart rate, vascular resistance, and arterial pressure during tilting.[1] In low–cardiac output states there also usually is activation of the renin-angiotensin-aldosterone axis with elevations of circulating renin and angiotensin II. Therefore, although administration of an angiotensin-converting enzyme inhibitor will benefit the patient by decreasing afterload, it may also increase the risks of development of orthostatic hypotensive events.

To avoid hypotensive episodes such as occurred in this patient, several precautions should be observed. First, patients with elevated blood urea nitrogen values, low blood pressure, and signs of volume depletion who are taking high diuretic doses should be considered at increased risk. In patients with heart failure captopril should be initiated under close supervision, and in those at increased risk of hypotension, as outlined, it should be begun with a small dose (6.25 mg). If well tolerated, the dosage can be increased at weekly intervals, based on clinical response and blood pressure, to a maximum of 50 mg t.i.d. Following the first dose and each upward adjustment of dosage, the patient should be particularly cautious when assuming the erect posture.

REFERENCE

1. Hubo, S.T., and Cody, R.J.: Circulatory aorto-regulation in chronic congestive heart failure. Responses to head-up tilt in 41 patients. Am. J. Cardiol. *52*:512, 1983.

227 A-T, B-T, C-T, D-T, E-F *(Braunwald, pp. 786–787)*

A number of conditions have recently been identified as risk factors associated with primary or unexplained pulmonary hypertension. Pulmonary abnormalities are frequently seen in patients with liver cirrhosis and portal hypertension, and include intrapulmonary shunting and hypoxemia, portal-pulmonary shunting, and pulmonary hypertension. The risk in this population was recently shown to be at least five times the risk of primary pulmonary hypertension in subjects without cirrhosis.[1,2] Potential mechanisms include recurrent small emboli and increased circulating levels of vasoactive substances and cytokines that are normally cleared by the liver or generated in response to the metabolic damage induced by cirrhosis. A recent report suggested that hyperdynamic circulation with increased cardiac output in patients with liver failure causes elevation in pulmonary arterial pressures without elevation in pulmonary vascular resistance. Other causes of hyperdynamic circulation and increased cardiac output can also cause pulmonary hypertension, including hyperthyroidism and beriberi (vitamin B_1 deficiency).[3]

Recently, several series and case reports have raised the possibility that HIV infection can cause pulmonary hypertension by mechanisms unrelated to immune deficiency or intravenous drug abuse.[4]

A possible role for vasoactive substances or cytokines has been suggested in HIV-associated pulmonary hypertension. Osler-Weber-Rendu disease is characterized by multiple visceral arteriovenous communications, but pulmonary hypertension is not associated with this disease.

REFERENCES

1. Castro, M., Krowka, M.J., Schroeder, D.R., et al.: Frequency and clinical implications of increased pulmonary artery pressures in liver transplant patients. Mayo Clin. Proc. *71*: 543–551, 1996.
2. Raffy, O., Sleiman, C., Vachiery, F., et al.: Refractory hypoxemia during liver cirrhosis. Hepatopulmonary syndrome or "primary" pulmonary hypertension? Am. J. Respir. Crit. Care Med. *153*:1169–1171, 1996.
3. Okura, H., and Takatsu, Y.: High-output heart failure as a cause of pulmonary hypertension. Intern. Med. *33*:363–365, 1994.
4. Mette, S.A., Palevsky, H.I., Pietra, G.G., et al.: Primary pulmonary hypertension in association with human immunodeficiency virus infection. A possible viral etiology for some forms of hypertensive pulmonary arteriopathy. Am. Rev. Respir. Dis. *145*:1196–1200, 1992.

228 A-F, B-T, C-T, D-T, E-T *(Braunwald, p. 455)*

Pulsus alternans is a sign of marked left ventricular dysfunction characterized by alternating strong and weak ventricular contractions, which result in alternating intensity of peripheral pulses and sometimes heart sounds and murmurs. It is thought to be due to alternation in stroke volume secondary to a deletion in the number of contracting cells in every other cardiac cycle, presumably owing to incomplete myocyte recovery. Therefore, pulsus alternans is rarely accompanied by electrical alternans, which is usually due to alternating position of the heart within a fluid-filled pericardium (i.e., a large pericardial effusion). Alternans is more detectable in the femoral than in the brachial, radial, or carotid arteries, and can be detected with sphygmomanometry. It can be elicited with maneuvers that decrease venus return such as the assumption of erect posture and is reduced with exercise and recumbency. Alternans is almost always concordant in the two ventricles.

229 A-F, B-T, C-T, D-F, E-F *(Braunwald, p. 493)*

Despite the use of ACE inhibitors, mortality from heart failure continues to be high. Recent efforts to reduce this high mortality have focused on the possibility that ACE inhibitors may be beneficial in patients with low ejection fractions but without overt symptoms of heart failure. The SOLVD prevention trial randomized 4228 patients with EF ≤35 per cent to enalapril versus placebo.[1] After an average follow-up of 37.4 months, patients randomized to enalapril had no significant reduction in all-cause or cardiac mortality. However, there was a significant reduction in the risk of development of heart failure symptoms and prolongation of time to first hospitalization for heart failure. There was also a significant reduction in the combined endpoint of death or hospitalization for heart failure (which was mainly driven by a reduction in the latter). A substudy from SOLVD showed further that chronic ACE inhibition can reduce or even reverse LV dilatation in this population.[2]

REFERENCES

1. The SOLVD Investigators: Effect of enalapril on mortality and the development of heart failure in asymptomatic patients with reduced ventricular ejection fractions. N. Engl. J. Med. *327*:685–691, 1992.
2. Konstam, M.A., Kronenberg, M.W., Rousseau, M.F., et al.: Effect of the angiotensin converting enzyme inhibitor enalapril on the long-term progression of left ventricular dilatation in patients with asymptomatic systolic dysfunction. Circulation *88*:2277–2281, 1993.

230 A-F, B-T, C-F, D-T   *(Braunwald, p. 727)*

The electrocardiogram illustrates a combination of intermittent failure to pace with loss of capture (pacer spikes 1, 3–8, and 10) and intermittent undersensing (pacer spike 7). Failure to pace occurs when the pacemaker fails to deliver a stimulus when it should or when it delivers a stimulus that fails to depolarize the myocardium at a time when the tissue is excitable. Failure to deliver a stimulus may be due to (1) improper lead connection to the generator, (2) broken lead wires, (3) failure of a component of the pulse generator, (4) power-source depletion, or (5) oversensing. Delivery of an ineffective stimulus with loss of capture may result from (1) lead dislodgement or an unstable tip, as in this case; (2) defective lead insulation or wire breakage; (3) increased stimulation threshold due to infarct, drugs, or fibrosis; and (4) inappropriate pacemaker stimulus strength.

Failure to sense may be due to lead dislodgement (the most common cause). Inadequate amplitude or wave slope of the intracardiac electrogram may be caused by fibrosis, infarct, drugs, electrolyte disturbances, inappropriate programming sensitivity, lead breakage or insulation defect, or component failure.

Oversensing occurs when a pacemaker senses signals other than the signals it is designed to detect. Common causes include sensed T waves if unusually large or delayed, sensed atrial activity, and sensed skeletal muscle potential with inappropriate inhibition.

Pacing at an altered rate may be caused by oversensing with rate slowing due to inhibition or rate acceleration due to triggering; built-in rate reduction, which indicates power source depletion; and component failure.

231 A-T, B-T, C-T, D-T   *(Braunwald, pp. 830–832)*

Pregnancy-induced hypertension is defined as hypertension developing after the 20th week of gestation. If proteinuria or edema accompanies the hy-

pertension, preeclampsia is present. The development of convulsions heralds eclampsia. Features of preeclampsia include age <20, primigravid state, sudden weight gain (>2 lb/week) or edema, and increasing plasma uric acid. The absolute level of blood pressure is usually lower than in the chronic hypertensive (<160 mm Hg), especially since blood pressure falls during the course of normal pregnancy.[1] However, the blood pressures of women who develop preeclampsia are found to be higher during the first half of pregnancy compared with those who remain normotensive throughout.[1]

REFERENCE

1. Mountquin, J.M., Rainville, C., Giroux, L., et al.: A prospective study of blood pressure in pregnancy. Prediction of preeclampsia. Am. J. Obstet. Gynecol. *151*:191, 1985.

232 A-T, B-F, C-T, D-F   *(Braunwald, pp. 673–674)*

Electrocardiographic evidence of the WPW syndrome is present in approximately 0.25 per cent of healthy individuals. Three basic features characterize the ECG abnormalities of the syndrome: the presence of a P-R interval less than 120 msec during sinus rhythm, a QRS duration greater than 120 msec with a slurred, slowly rising onset of the QRS in some leads (the delta wave); and secondary ST-T wave changes generally directed opposite to the major QRS vector.[1]

While the prevalence of WPW decreases with age, the frequency of paroxysmal tachycardia associated with the syndrome apparently increases with age. Most such tachycardias are reciprocating arrhythmias (80 per cent), with 15 to 30 per cent presenting as atrial fibrillation and 5 per cent as atrial flutter. Although most adults with the WPW syndrome have normal hearts, a number of cardiac defects are occasionally associated with this syndrome, including Ebstein's anomaly.[2] In patients with Ebstein's anomaly, multiple accessory pathways are often present and are located on the right side of the heart, with preexcitation localized to the atrialized ventricle. These patients often have reciprocating tachycardia with a long V-A interval and RBBB morphology of the QRS complex.

REFERENCES

1. Willens, J.L., Robles de Medina, E.O., Bernard, R., et al.: Criteria for intraventricular conduction disturbances and preexcitation. J. Am. Coll. Cardiol. *5*:1261, 1985.
2. Smith, W.M., Gallagher, J.J., Kerr, C.R., et al.: The electrophysiologic basis and management of symptomatic recurrent tachycardia in patients with Ebstein's anomaly of the tricuspid valve. Am. J. Cardiol. *49*:1223, 1982.

233 A-T, B-F, C-T, D-F   *(Braunwald, pp. 602–603)*

Gastrointestinal symptoms, which include nausea, vomiting, anorexia, diarrhea, and abdominal pain, are the most common side effects of chronic oral quinidine therapy. *Cinchonism* is the term used to describe the less common central nervous system toxic side effects of the drug. These are manifested as tinnitus, hearing loss, visual disturbances, and alternations in mental status including confusion, delirium, and even psychosis. Allergic reactions to the drug may occur and include rash or fever as well as an immune-mediated thrombocytopenia. This arises from the presence of antibodies to quinidine-platelet complexes capable of causing platelet agglutination and lysis. In between 0.5 and 2 per cent of patients, quinidine may produce syncope, which is usually the result of a self-terminating episode of polymorphic ventricular tachycardia with a long Q-T interval as an antecedent, known as torsades de pointes.[1] Quinidine prolongs the Q-T interval in most patients, and relatively marked prolongation of this interval is a general characteristic of quinidine therapy. Therapy for quinidine syncope includes immediate discontinuation of the drug, the use of atrial or ventricular pacing to suppress the tachyarrhythmia, isoproterenol infusion to pharmacologically increase the heart rate, and the use of intravenous magnesium to suppress the rhythm.[2] In addition, concomitant hypokalemia must be corrected and other antiarrhythmic agents with similar mechanisms of action (such as disopyramide) must be avoided in patients with quinidine syncope.

REFERENCES

1. Roden, D.M., Woolsey, R.L., and Primm, K.: Incidence and clinical features of the quinidine-associated long QT syndrome: Implications for patient care. Am. Heart J. *111*: 1088, 1986.
2. Tzivoni, D., Keren, A., Cohen, A.M., et al.: Magnesium therapy for torsades de pointes. Am. J. Cardiol. *53*:538, 1984.

234 A-T, B-T, C-F, D-T, E-T   (Braunwald, pp. 495–496)

Several randomized controlled trials have proven the benefit of ACE inhibitors in different subsets of patients with LV systolic dysfunction. The CONSENSUS trial showed that ACE inhibition in patients with severe symptomatic heart failure significantly reduce all-cause mortality and death due to heart failure.[1] The SOLVD treatment trial showed that such benefit can also be expected in those patients with class II and III symptomatic heart failure.[2] However, the SOLVD prevention trial showed subsequently that treatment of patients with asymptomatic LV dysfunction does not lead to a reduction in mortality.[3] Instead, chronic ACE inhibition in these asymptomatic patients reduced the risk of development of symptomatic heart failure and prolonged time to first hospitalization for heart failure. The SAVE trial showed that administration of captopril to patients with reduced LV systolic function (EF ≤ 40 per cent) 3 to 14 days following acute myocardial infarction reduced mortality, recurrent coronary events, and death due to heart failure.[4] Similarly, the AIRE study, which was similar to SAVE in design except that it randomized patients with manifest heart failure following acute myocardial infarction, showed a significant reduction in mortality that was apparent within 30 days of treatment.[5] Together, these trials, and several other smaller studies, establish the value of ACE inhibition in patients with LV systolic dysfunction.

REFERENCES

1. The CONSENSUS Trial Study Group: Effect of enalapril on mortality in severe congestive heart failure. Results of the Cooperative North Scandinavian Enalapril Survival Study (CONSENSUS). N. Engl. J. Med. *316*:1429–1435, 1987.
2. The SOLVD Investigators: Effect of enalapril on survival in patients with reduced left ventricular ejection fractions and congestive heart failure. N. Engl. J. Med. *325*:293–302, 1991.
3. The SOLVD Investigators: Effect of enalapril on mortality and the development of heart failure in asymptomatic patients with reduced left ventricular ejection fractions. N. Engl. J. Med. *327*:685–691, 1992.
4. Pfeffer, M.A., Braunwald, E., Moye, L.A., et al.: Effect of captopril on mortality and morbidity in patients with left ventricular dysfunction after myocardial infarction. Results of the survival and ventricular enlargement study. N. Engl. J. Med. *327*:669–677, 1992.
5. AIRE (Acute Infarction Ramipril Efficacy) Study Investigators: Effect of ramipril on mortality and morbidity of survivors of acute myocardial infarction with clinical evidence of heart failure. Lancet *342*:821–828, 1993.

235 A-T, B-T, C-T, D-F   (Braunwald, pp. 462–464)

In the lung there is normally a continuous exchange of liquid, colloid, and solutes between the vascular bed and interstitium. An imbalance of the forces resulting in net influx of liquids, colloids, and solutes from the vasculature to the interstitial space results in pulmonary edema. The classic Starling equation can be applied to the lung as well as to the systemic circulation, and it states that the net rate of transudation (flow of liquid from blood vessels to interstitial space) is equal to the hydrostatic force minus the colloid osmotic force. Thus, the classification of pulmonary edema can be made on the basis of whether there are imbalances of the Starling forces or alterations in alveolar capillary membrane permeability, lymphatic insufficiency, or other unknown mechanisms such as neurogenic pulmonary edema.

With regard to imbalance of the Starling forces, three major mechanisms exist: (1) increased pulmonary capillary pressure secondary to increased pulmonary venous pressure without left ventricular failure (as in mitral stenosis or with left ventricular failure as in acute MI) or increased pulmonary capillary pressure secondary to increased pulmonary arterial pressure as occurs in so-called overperfusion pulmonary edema, which exists experimentally (although questionably clinically); (2) decreased plasma oncotic pressure, as occurs with hypoalbuminemia secondary to nephrotic syndrome, hepatic disease, or protein-losing enteropathy; and (3) increased negative interstitial pressure as occurs with rapid removal of a pneumothorax with a large applied negative unilateral pressure. Theoretically, increased interstitial oncotic pressure could also generate pulmonary edema; however, no clinical example of this has been documented. Nonetheless, the appearance of increased concentrations of macromolecules in the liquid phase of the interstitium or in the alveoli probably does serve to perpetuate the process of edema formation. Increased plasma oncotic pressure would decrease the transudative forces and theoretically decrease flow from the blood vessel to the lung.

236 A-T, B-F, C-T, D-T, E-T   (Braunwald, pp. 479–480)

Thiazide diuretics remain the most frequently prescribed first-line agents for the treatment of hypertension, and are also used in cases of chronic congestive heart failure (CHF). They have a number of important and potentially life-threatening side effects that are not uncommon. The most common side effect is hypokalemia; serum potassium falls an average 0.67 mmol/liter after institution of continuous daily thiazide therapy.[1] Hypomagnesemia is usually mild but may prevent the restoration of intracellular deficit of potassium.[2] Therefore, it should be corrected. Hyperuricemia is present in one-third of untreated hypertensives, and appears in another third during therapy with thiazides. This is probably caused by increased proximal tubular reabsorption of urate. Thiazides may increase the total blood cholesterol by an average of 15 to 20 mg/dl in a dose-related fashion.[3] Low-density lipoproteins (LDL) and triglycerides also increase. There also may be a rise in serum calcium (usually <0.5 mg/dl) due to thiazides, which is probably secondary to increased proximal tubular reabsorption.[4] Hyponatremia may sometimes occur with thiazide therapy, especially in the elderly. This is multifactorial and is probably related to increased antidiuretic hormone levels combined with increased free water intake due to thirst.

REFERENCES

1. Morgan, D.B., and Davidson, C.: Hypokalemia and diuretics: An analysis of publications. Br. Med. J. 280:905, 1980.
2. Whang, R., Flink, E.B., Dyckner, T., et al.: Magnesium depletion as a cause of refractory potassium repletion. Arch. Intern. Med. 145:1686, 1985.
3. Johnson, B.F., Saunders, R., Hickler, R., et al.: The effects of thiazide diuretics upon plasma lipoproteins. J. Hypertension 4:235, 1986.
4. Stier, C.T., Jr., and Itskovitz, H.D.: Renal calcium metabolism and diuretics. Annu. Rev. Pharmacol. Toxicol. 26:101, 1986.

237-C, 238-A, 239-B, 240-D   (Braunwald, pp. 646–647, 649; Figs. 22–4, 22–5 and 22–7)

Ventriculophasic sinus arrhythmia is the term applied to phasic variations in the underlying sinus rhythm P-P interval caused by the occurrence of ventricular contractions. Changes in the P-P interval may be due to the influence of the autonomic nervous system upon sinus discharge rate in response to changes in ventricular stroke volume. The most common example of ventriculophasic sinus arrhythmia occurs when complete AV block is present. In some cases of complete AV block, P-P cycles that contain a QRS complex may be shorter than P-P cycles without a QRS complex. The occurrence of a premature ventricular complex during normal sinus rhythm may be followed by a compensatory pause; lengthening of the subsequent P-P cycle is another example of a ventriculophasic sinus arrhythmia.

The general term sinus arrhythmia is applied to instances of phasic variation in sinus cycle length that are found frequently and are considered a normal event. In sinus arrhythmia, P wave morphology does not change and the P-R interval exceeds 120 m/sec and is also unchanged. Sinus arrhythmia appears in two basic forms: a respiratory form in which the P-P interval shortens during inspiration as a result of the reflex inhibition of vagal tone in a cyclic manner and a nonrespiratory form that is characterized by a phasic variation in P-P interval that cannot be related to the underlying respiratory events. Sinus arrhythmia commonly occurs in the young, especially in the respiratory form. The nonrespiratory form of sinus arrhythmia may be seen in instances of increased vagal tone, such as after digitalis therapy.[1]

Sinus arrest or sinus pause (see Braunwald, Fig. 22–4, p. 646) is characterized by a pause in the sinus rhythm for which the P-P interval limiting the pause does not equal a multiple of the basic underlying sinus P-P interval. The mechanism of this arrhythmia is believed to be a transient loss of spontaneous sinus-nodal automaticity and may be produced by excessive vagal tone, involvement of the sinus node during acute MI, degenerative fibrotic changes, and digitalis-induced effects. While brief episodes of sinus arrest may not require treatment, patients with chronic forms of sinus node disease with recurrent symptomatic sinus bradycardia or sinus arrest often require permanent pacing.

Sinoatrial (SA) exit block is also characterized by a pause during normal sinus rhythm, but in this arrhythmia the duration of the pause is a multiple of the basic P-P interval. The mechanism of SA exit block involves failure of a sinus impulse to emerge from the sinus node and depolarize the atria.[2] Two types of SA exit block, analogous to AV-nodal blocks, are recognized. Type I (Wenckebach) second-degree SA exit block is marked by the progressive shortening of sequential P-P intervals prior to the pause and by a pause duration that is less than 2 P-P cycles (see Braunwald, Fig. 22–5A, p. 647). Type II second-degree SA exit block is marked by a constant P-P interval, and a pause without P waves that is equal to approximately two, three, or even four times the normal P-P cycle (see Braunwald, Fig. 22–5B, p. 647). While in theory both first-degree and third-degree SA exit block may occur, their diagnosis with routine surface electrocardiography is not possible.

A variant of sinus arrhythmia known as wandering pacemaker occurs when the dominant pacemaker focus shifts from the sinus node to a latent pacemaker with a degree of automaticity close to but slightly less than that of the sinus node. The shift from the sinus focus to the ectopic focus occurs gradually over the duration of several beats, and is characterized by a gradual shortening of the P-R interval and a change in the P wave contour as the focus shifts (see Braunwald, Fig. 22–7, p. 648). Wandering pacemaker is considered to be a normal occurrence secondary to augmented vagal tone and may be seen particularly in young individuals and athletes.

REFERENCES

1. Hrushesky, W.J., Fader, D., Schmitt, O., and Gilbertson, V.: The respiratory sinus arrhythmia: The measure of cardiac age. Science 224:1001, 1984.
2. Asseman, P., Berzin, B., Desry, D., et al.: Persistent sinus nodal electrograms during abnormally prolonged post pacing atrial pauses in sick sinus syndrome in humans. Sinoatrial block versus overdrive suppression. Circulation 68:33, 1983.

241-A, 242-A & B, 243-C, 244-C *(Braunwald, pp. 439–441)*

The best measure of cardiovascular performance is maximal exercise cardiac output. This measurement requires arterial and venous sampling during and at peak exercise and is considered impractical. Instead, exercise physiologists and cardiologists use maximal O_2 consumption at peak exercise ($\dot{V}O_{2max}$) as an indirect measure of cardiac output. $\dot{V}O_{2max}$ (also called aerobic capacity) is thus considered the best measure of exercise cardiac output, because it is a function of both the maximal cardiac output and the maximal extraction of O_2 by the tissues.[1] $\dot{V}O_{2max}$ is defined as the value achieved when $\dot{V}O_2$ remains stable despite further increases in exercise intensity. It is highly reproducible and can be obtained noninvasively during exercise.

Several other measurements can be made during cardiopulmonary exercise that are considered of great diagnostic value. Anaerobic threshold, defined as the $\dot{V}O_2$ at which CO_2 production ($\dot{V}CO_2$) starts to increase in a nonlinear fashion (leading to an increase in $\dot{V}CO_2/\dot{V}O_2$), indicates inadequate supply of O_2 to the tissues.[2] This parameter is also highly reproducible. Normal values for $\dot{V}O_{2max}$ and anaerobic threshold decline after 20 years of age and are higher in men than women. Impairment of cardiac or pulmonary function can result in reduced $\dot{V}O_{2max}$. Patients with underlying pulmonary disease can be distinguished by the presence of exercise-induced arterial desaturation and abnormal pulmonary function testing. Another measurement that can be obtained during cardiopulmonary exercise or with pulmonary function testing is the respiratory quotient (R) or $\dot{V}CO_2/\dot{V}O_2$. This reflects the production of CO_2 relative to the production of O_2 and is normally 0.8 at rest on a balanced diet. Carbohydrate metabolism results in higher production of CO_2, and can increase the respiratory quotient. R also increases significantly at the onset of anaerobic threshold, but it is not significantly altered by underlying pulmonary disease.

REFERENCES

1. Wasserman, K.: Measures of functional capacity in patients with heart failure. Circulation 81(Suppl. 2):1, 1990.
2. Wasserman, K., Beaver, W.L., and Whipp, B.J.: Gas exchange theory and the lactic acidosis (anaerobic) threshold. Circulation 81(Suppl. 2):14, 1990.

245-B, 246-C, 247-D, 248-E *(Braunwald, pp. 379–381, 646)*

There are many physiological mechanisms that regulate myocardial contractility. Increases in heart rate cause increases in the rate of force development and developed force and also shorten the time to peak tension with accelerated relaxation. This response is called the *force-frequency relation*. The positive inotropic action presumably reflects an increase in intracellular calcium resulting from the increased number of depolarizations. There does not appear to be a shift of the ventricular function curve (i.e., the relation between ventricular end-diastolic pressure and stroke work with a decrease in heart rate). Instead, there appears to be an increase in stroke power at any given level of filling pressure consistent with an increase in myocardial contractility. It is likely that, under normal conditions in the conscious state, venous return to the heart is reflexly and metabolically stabilized so that varying heart rate between 60 and 160 beats/min has little effect on cardiac output despite the force-frequency relation.[1] However, if the diastolic volume of the heart is maintained by increasing venous return such as would occur during exercise, then there is an increase in cardiac output. Also, it is likely that tachycardia plays a major role in increasing cardiac output under conditions of exercise. In contrast, when the heart is paced at a very rapid rate by electrical stimulation of the atrium such as during a pacing test, there is much less inotropic effect because the reflexes that maintain an increase in venous return are absent and also the diastolic filling time permitted is much less. This effect obviously has important implications for ventricular pacing with implanted pacemakers and illustrates the importance of the development of rate-responsive ventricular pacemakers that can respond to appropriate physiological needs.[2]

Laplace's law states that the average circumferential wall stress (force per unit of cross-sectional area of wall) is related directly to the product of intraventricular pressure and internal radius and inversely to wall thickness. Thus, as the ventricle hypertrophies (wall thickness increases) there is a decrease in circumferential wall stress. As the heart dilates (increase in the radius), there is an increase in average circumferential wall stress. Therefore, concentric hypertrophy (such as with stenotic valvular disease) maintains normal wall stress while eccentric hypertrophy (such as with regurgitant valvular disease) increases wall stress. The normal right ventricle is more compliant than the left ventricle, not because of any intrinsic difference in muscle stiffness but because it has a small radius and hence less wall stress.

The *Anrep effect* is the name given to "homeometric autoregulation," by which is meant a positive inotropic effect following an abrupt elevation of systolic aortic and left ventricular pressure. This effect occurs during the first minutes after aortic pressure is abruptly elevated and appears to be related to recovery from transient subendocardial ischemia.

The *Cushing reflex* is a common manifestation of cerebral ischemia and consists of an increase in peripheral vascular resistance, constriction of the capacitance vessels, and bradycardia. The Cushing effect is particularly common during stroke and intracerebral hemorrhage, during which the rise in blood pressure and bradycardia can be dramatic. These phenomena are to be differentiated from the other effects of the chemoreceptor responses. One of these is hyperventilation, which by itself causes reflex phenomena. It should be noted that the chemoreceptors in the aortic arch and carotid bodies are stimulated by reductions in arterial PO_2 and pH, by elevations of arterial PCO_2, by hemorrhage, and by sympathetic efferents. Among the variety of effects mediated by the chemoreceptors are bradycardia, vasoconstriction, positive inotropy, and hyperventilation.[3]

An increase in heart rate following expansion of blood volume is called the *Bainbridge reflex*. With volume loading it has been shown that heart rate increases in proportion to cardiac output even though the elevation of arterial pressure would tend to oppose the increase by activation of the carotid sinus reflex. On the other hand, volume depletion causes tachycardia as well, presumably as a consequence of reflex activation, with reduced stimulation of arterial blood pressure receptors.[4]

REFERENCES

1. Vatner, S.F., and Braunwald, E.: Cardiovascular control mechanisms in the conscious state. N. Engl. J. Med. *293*: 970, 1975.
2. Narahara, K.A., and Blettel, M.L.: Effect of rate on left ventricular volumes and ejection fraction during chronic ventricular pacing. Circulation *67*:323, 1983.
3. Fujii, I., and Vatner, S.F.: Sympathetic mechanisms regulating myocardial contractility in conscious animals. *In* Fozzard, H.A., et al. (eds.): The Heart and Cardiovascular System. New York, Raven Press, 1986, pp. 1119–1132.
4. Vatner, S.F., and Boettcher, D.H.: Regulation of cardiac output by stroke volume and heart rate in conscious dogs. Circ. Res. *42*:557, 1978.

249-C, 250-E, 251-A, 252-B *(Braunwald, pp. 460–462)*

Each of the conditions listed is associated with sustained increases in cardiac output that may precipitate heart failure in the appropriate clinical setting. Hyperthyroidism leads to an increase in cardiac output by a variety of mechanisms, including (1) vasodilation due to augmented metabolic rate; (2) increased heat production (both of these contribute to the decreased systemic vascular resistance in this condition); (3) increases in blood volume and mean circulatory filling pressure; (4) direct effects of thyroid hormone on myocardial contractility; and (5) effects of the sympathoadrenal system on a variety of cardiovascular functions. Clinical findings in hyperthyroidism include constitutional changes such as nervousness, diaphoresis, heat intolerance, and fatigue as well as cardiovascular manifestations such as palpitations, atrial fibrillation with a relatively rapid ventricular response, and sinus tachycardia with a hyperkinetic heart action. Examination of the heart may therefore reveal tachycardia, widened pulse pressure, brisk arterial pulsations, and a variety of findings associated with the hyperkinetic state. These may include a prominent S_1, the presence of an S_3 and/or S_4, and a midsystolic murmur along the left sternal border secondary to increased flow. When a particularly hyperdynamic cardiac effect is seen, this murmur may have an unusual scratching component known as the *Means-Lerman scratch*. This is thought to be caused by the rubbing together of normal pleural and pericardial surfaces. The ECG in thyrotoxicosis often reveals widespread, nonspecific ST- and T-wave abnormalities with terminal T-wave inversion and shortening of the Q-T interval in approximately 25 per cent of patients.[1] Treatment of hyperthyroidism is directed at the specific endocrine abnormality. However, control of the cardiac manifestations of the disorder may be achieved by use of antiadrenergic agents[2] in an adjunctive manner, although these are capable of controlling symptomatology only and do not reduce the elevated metabolic rate. Furthermore, the use of beta-adrenoreceptor blockade may be difficult and even contraindicated in patients with thyrotoxic heart disease and heart failure.

Systemic arteriovenous fistulas may be acquired as a result of trauma or they may be congenital. The increase in cardiac output that such lesions create is related to the size of the communication and the resultant reduction in the systemic vascular resistance that it promotes. In general, systemic AV fistulas lead to a widened pulse pressure, brisk arterial pulsations, and mild tachycardia. *Branham's sign*, defined as the slowing of heart rate after manual compression of the fistula,[3] is commonly present. The maneuver may also raise arterial and lower venous pressure. Congenital AV fistulas most frequently involve vessels of the lower extremities and on physical examination may reveal varices, swelling, increases in limb length, and warmth. Treatment is difficult in part because surgical excision is often not feasible technically. Acquired AV fistulas occur most often due to traumatic injuries such as stab or gunshot wounds or as a consequence of surgical procedures such as nephrectomy, laminectomy, cholecystectomy, and percutaneous vascular catheterizations. In addition, high-output congestive heart failure may be precipitated by the AV shunts that are intentionally placed to provide access for chronic hemodialysis. In general, surgical repair of AV fistulas is the recommended treatment.

Osler-Weber-Rendu disease or hereditary hemorrhagic telangiectasis is a specific inherited condition that may be associated with AV fistulas, especially in the liver and the lungs. The disease may produce a hyperkinetic circulation with abdominal bruits and hepatomegaly due to intrahepatic arteriovenous connections.[4] Because these connections may lead to the presence of oxygenated blood in the inferior vena cava and right atrium, Osler-Weber-Rendu disease may be a factor in the misdiagnosis of atrial septal defect in selected patients.[5]

Beriberi heart disease is a rare condition caused by severe thiamine deficiency that is found most frequently in the Far East. The absence of thiamine as a coenzyme for transketolase in the pentose phosphate pathway of glucose metabolism accounts for the basic pathophysiology in this condition. Elevation in cardiac output in beriberi heart disease is presumed to be due to a reduction in systemic vascular resistance and an augmentation of venous return. This occurs as a result of lesions created in the sympathetic nervous system nuclei by the absence of thiamine. Patients with beriberi may present with findings of the high-output state, severe generalized malnutrition, and vitamin deficiency. Evidence is noted of peripheral neuropathy with paresthesias of the extremities, decreased or absent knee and ankle jerks, anemia, hyperkeratinized skin lesions, and painful glossitis. The presence of edema characterizes "wet beriberi" and differentiates this condition from the "dry" form. Beriberi heart disease is characterized by biventricular failure, an S_3 and an apical systolic murmur, and a hyperkinetic state with wide pulse pressure. The ECG demonstrates low voltage, Q-T interval prolongation, and inversion of T waves. It should be emphasized that, especially in Western society, alcoholic cardiomyopathy may contribute to or overlap with this clinical picture because of the tendency for alcoholics to become vitamin defi-

cient from a low intake of vitamin B_1 and high carbohydrate ingestion. "Shoshin" beriberi is a fulminant form of the disease that may lead to severe illness or death within 48 hours.[6] Treatment of all forms of beriberi involves the administration of thiamine first intravenously and subsequently orally, as well as digitalis and diuretics to treat concomitant congestive heart failure.

The carcinoid syndrome is an uncommon disease which results from the release of serotonin and other vasoactive substances by carcinoid tumors. Physical findings may include cutaneous flushing, telangiectasia, diarrhea, and bronchial constriction due to release of humoral mediators. The syndrome may be accompanied by an elevation in cardiac output with a reduction in arterial–mixed venous oxygen difference.[7] This results from a reduction in systemic vascular resistance due either to mediator release and/or to shunting of blood to the carcinoid tumors themselves.

REFERENCES

1. Hoffman, I., and Lowrey, R.D.: The electrocardiogram in thyrotoxicosis. Am. J. Cardiol. *8*:893, 1960.
2. Grossman, W., Robin, N.L., Johnson, L.W., et al.: Effects of beta blockade on the peripheral manifestations of thyrotoxicosis. Ann. Intern. Med. *74*:875, 1971.
3. Branham, H.H.: Aneurysmal varix of the femoral artery and vein following a gunshot wound. Int. J. Surg. *3*:250, 1890.
4. Baranda, M.M., Perez, M., DeAndres, J., et al.: High-output congestive heart failure as first manifestation of Osler-Weber-Rendu disease. J. Vasc. Dis. *35*:568, 1984.
5. Radtke, W.E., Smith, H.C., Fulton, R.E., and Adson, M.A.: Misdiagnosis of atrial septal defect in patients with hereditary telangiectasia (Osler-Weber-Rendu disease) and hepatic arteriovenous fistulas. Am. Heart J. *95*:235, 1978.
6. Jeffrey, F.E., and Abelmann, W.H.: Recovery of proved Shoshin beriberi. Am. J. Med. *50*:123, 1971.
7. Schwaber, J.R., and Lukas, D.S.: Hyperkinemia and cardiac failure in the carcinoid syndrome. Am. J. Med. *32*:846, 1962.

253-B, 254-D, 255-C, 256-C *(Braunwald, pp. 424–426)*

Patient A has values typical of those in normal human subjects. Left ventricular mass increases in response to chronic pressure or volume overload or secondary to primary myocardial disease. With predominant pressure overload, as in aortic stenosis, there is an increase in mass with little change in chamber volume (concentric hypertrophy) (Patient B). In contrast, hypertrophy due to volume overload (as in aortic or mitral regurgitation), or due to primary myocardial disease, is caused by ventricular dilatation with only a small increase in wall thickness (eccentric hypertrophy). In regurgitant disease (Patient C) there is usually a nearly normal ejection fraction in the compensated state, while in cardiomyopathy there is impaired systolic function (Patient D). In mitral regurgitation there may be a paradoxically elevated ejection fraction caused by the decreased afterload afforded by the left atrium.

257-D, 258-B, 259-C, 260-E *(Braunwald, pp. 725–726; Fig. 23–18)*

Pacemakers are categorized with a five-lettered code. The first letter refers to the chamber paced, the second letter to the chamber sensed, the third letter to the response to any sensed stimulus, the fourth to programmability and rate modulation, and the fifth letter, which is infrequently used, to whether the pacemaker has antiarrhythmic function. In general, dual-chamber pacemakers are more expensive than single-chamber pacemakers and should be used only in patients who require sensing and/or pacing of both the atria and ventricles. Similarly, rate-modulating pacemakers are used in patients with chronotropic incompetence due to abnormal or absent sinus node function.

In the 58-year-old male with tachycardia-bradycardia syndrome who developed symptomatic sinus bradycardia with beta blocker therapy, the most appropriate pacemaker mode would be DDDR. Ventricular pacing is necessary here because there is a risk of AV block due to beta blockers, and the rate-modulating function is important because of the abnormal sinus node function. Use of a non–rate-responsive (DDD) pacemaker in this patient would most likely result in lower rate pacing most of the time with inappropriate response to physical activity.

In the 70-year-old woman with atrial fibrillation who complains of dizziness and is found on examination to have a ventricular rate of 30/min, VVIR pacing is most appropriate. Atrial sensing or pacing is not possible due to atrial fibrillation, and the rate-modulating function is necessary because of the evident chronotropic dysfunction.

In the 62-year-old male with complete heart block following aortic valve surgery, there is no indication of sinus node disease and DDD pacing will be sufficient.

In the 45-year-old man with symptomatic sinoatrial exit block and junctional escape rhythm, loss of sinus mechanism requires atrial pacing and rate modulation. There is no evidence of AV block and ventricular pacing is necessary, so the AAIR pacing mode is preferred. The above examples are all consistent with class I (definite) indications for pacing, as recommended by the guidelines published in 1991 by the ACC/AHA Joint Committee on Pacemaker Implantation.[1]

REFERENCE

1. Dreifus, L.S., Fisch, C., Griffin, J.C., et al.: Guidelines for implantation of cardiac pacemakers and antiarrhythmia devices: A report of the American College of Cardiology/American Heart Association Task Force on Assessment of Diagnostic and Therapeutic Procedures (Committee on Pacemaker Implantation). J. Am. Coll. Cardiol. *18*:1, 1996.

261-D, 262-E, 263-C, 264-A *(Braunwald, pp. 555, 557, 559–563)*

During diastole, the cell membrane is permeable to K^+ and impermeable to Na^+, and the Na-K pump transfers Na^+ out of the cell and against its electrochemical gradient. For these reasons the major determinant of the resting membrane potential during diastole (phase 4) is K^+. The arrival of a stimulus to the cardiac cell results in a sudden increase in membrane conductance to Na^+, which causes the upstroke (phase 0) of the action potential. Action potential in the normal SA and AV nodes is characterized by a very slow upstroke with reduced $\dot{V}_{max}$. This is called a "slow response," and is mediated by a slow inward, predominantly Ca^{++} current called I_{Ca}. Following phase 0, the membrane repolarizes rapidly due to inactivation of Na^+ currents and inward movement of Cl^- down its concentration gradient. This phase (phase 1) is particularly well defined and separated from phase 2 in the cardiac Purkinje fibers. Following the plateau phase (phase 2), which is characterized by increased I_{Ca-L}, phase 3 results from inactivation of those channels and activation of the delayed rectifier current (I_K). Phase 3 results in rapid repolarization leading into phase 4.

265-A & B, 266-F, 267-B, C, D & E, 268-C & E *(Braunwald, pp. 605–613, 615–616)*

Antiarrhythmic agents produce their effects by blocking sodium, potassium, or calcium channels or beta-adrenergic receptors. These effects translate into changes seen on the surface electrocardiogram, because of the dependence of ECG complexes on ionic movements. Therefore, agents that prolong AV nodal conduction cause prolongation of the PR interval. Drugs with beta blocking or calcium channel blocking activity, including agents that belong to other classes of antiarrhythmic agents, also can prolong the PR interval. Agents that block fast sodium channels with intermediate (class Ia) or slow (class Ic) onset and offset kinetics can reduce $\dot{V}_{max}$ and result in reduction in action potential amplitude and prolongation of its duration. This translates to widening of the QRS complex on the surface ECG. Drugs that prolong repolarization by blocking I_K cause prolongation of the Q-T interval. These include agents in classes Ia, III, and the calcium channel blocker bepridil which has sodium and potassium channel activity.

Flecainide, which is a slow sodium channel blocker, widens the QRS. It also prolongs the PR interval, but the mechanism of this effect is unclear. Flecainide causes minimal or no prolongation of the Q-T interval, probably due to marked widening of the QRS complex. Amiodarone, on the other hand, blocks sodium and potassium channels and causes widening of the QRS complex and the Q-T interval. It also has a beta blocking effect which may uncommonly cause prolongation of the PR interval. Amiodarone increases serum digoxin levels by reducing its clearance. Lidocaine blocks fast sodium channels with rapid onset and offset. It does not reduce $\dot{V}_{max}$, and has no effect on the PR, QRS, or Q-T intervals, except for occasional shortening of the latter. Lidocaine has no beta blocking effect and does not alter serum digoxin levels. Sotalol is a nonspecific beta blocker which prolongs repolarization in the atria and ventricles by blocking I_K. Sotalol has no effect on sodium channels and only inconsistently prolongs the PR interval. It does not alter serum digoxin levels.

269-C & E, 270-A, 271-B, 272-C & D   (Braunwald, pp. 361–363)

The major function of the cardiac myocyte is in the contraction-relaxation cycle. To perform its function, the myocyte depends on an assembly of contractile proteins and supporting proteins. The two chief contractile proteins are the thin actin filament and the thick myosin filament. The thin filaments are composed of two actin units which are carried on a backbone of the heavier tropomyosin. The actin filaments are attached to the Z line and form the major component of the I band. Myosin, on the other hand, is the major component of the A band. It is composed of two light chains and two heavy chains. The terminal part of the heavy chains forms the myosin head. Myosin heavy chain isoforms help regulate myosin ATPase activity, which is located on the myosin head. A mutant gene for the B-myosin heavy chain is thought to be responsible for one of the familial forms of human hypertrophic cardiomyopathy.[1] Myosin molecules are supported by a newly discovered protein called titin. This is the largest protein molecule yet described, and extends from the Z lines, stopping just short of the M line. It provides elasticity and supports the myosin molecule by tethering it to the Z line.

At regular intervals on the actin molecule is a trimolecular complex of proteins called the troponin complex. Of these three, it is troponin-C that responds to the calcium ions that are released in large amounts from the sarcoplasmic reticulum to start the cross-bridge cycle.

REFERENCE

1. Geisterfer-Lowrance, A.A., Kass, S., Tanigawa, G., et al.: A molecular basis for familial hypertrophic cardiomyopathy: A beta cardiac myosin heavy chain gene missense mutation. Cell 62:999–1006, 1990.

273-B, 274-D, 275-A, 276-C, 277-C   (Braunwald, pp. 783–786, 791, 795–796, 799–800)

Distinguishing between causes of pulmonary hypertension may be difficult on both clinical and pathological grounds. The term "Eisenmenger syndrome" was popularized by Dr. Paul Wood in reference to patients with congenital cardiac lesions and severe pulmonary hypertension in whom reversal of a left-to-right shunt had occurred across an existing pulmonary-systemic communication. In the patients described originally by Eisenmen-

ger, a ventricular septal defect was present. However, any right-to-left shunt that undergoes reversal due to increasing pulmonary pressures is referred to as Eisenmenger syndrome. In this syndrome, the progressive pathophysiological process that leads to obliterative changes in the pulmonary vasculature involves a variety of anatomical changes. These begin with hypertrophy of small muscular pulmonary arteries, progress through dilation and so-called "plexiform lesions" of the muscular pulmonary arteries and arterioles, and end in complex lesions with accompanying necrotizing arteritis.[1] (See Answer 139, p. 91, this book.) Once the pulmonary vascular resistance increases to equal or greater than systemic resistance, resulting in a predominantly right-to-left shunt and end-stage changes of the pulmonary vessels, surgical closure of the intracardiac communication is contraindicated. This is because of the sudden increase in the load on the already overburdened RV which may be precipitated by such an intervention and which may lead to a more rapid death.

Primary pulmonary hypertension is by definition idiopathic, or unexplained. While controversy exists regarding the precise pathophysiology of this syndrome, most patients considered to have primary pulmonary hypertension have no evidence of an associated tendency toward thromboembolism, congenital or immunological abnormalities, collagen vascular disease, or drug ingestion.[2] Patients with primary pulmonary hypertension do appear to have increased pulmonary vascular reactivity and a more marked vasospastic or constrictive tendency. There are several common pathological findings in primary pulmonary hypertension, including intimal thickening of smaller pulmonary arteries and arterioles with accompanying fibrosis, which is referred to as "onion skinning." In addition, plexiform lesions similar to those seen in patients with Eisenmenger syndrome may develop. Dilated, thin-walled branches of muscular pulmonary arteries may lead to the lesions that are responsible for the phrase "plexogenic pulmonary arteriopathy," which is frequently used to characterize the pathological changes in primary pulmonary hypertension. The finding of such lesions on lung biopsy mandates exclusion of any intracardiac shunts as an explanation for their presence.

The differential diagnosis for elevated pulmonary pressures includes silent mitral stenosis for both of the lesions noted. In some instances, the characteristic diastolic murmur of mitral stenosis is not appreciated, and echocardiographic visualization of the mitral valve with exclusion of the presence of any transvalvular pressure gradient is necessary to exclude this disorder. Other conditions to be considered in the differential diagnosis include cor triatriatum, which must be recognized by appropriate hemodynamic studies and angiographic visualization of the left atrial membrane; pulmonary embolism; and pulmonary venus obstruction. Other diagnoses to be excluded include pulmonary parenchymal disease, collagen vascular disease, and pulmonary venoocclusive disease.

REFERENCES

1. Yamaki, S., and Wagenvoort, C.A.: Comparison of primary plexogenic arteriopathy in adults and children. A morphometric study in 40 patients. Br. Heart J. *54*:428, 1985.
2. Newman, J.H., and Ross, J.C.: Primary pulmonary hypertension: A look at the future. J. Am. Coll. Cardiol. *14*:551, 1989.

278-C, 279-A, 280-A, 281-A   *(Braunwald, pp. 652–656)*

Both atrial flutter and atrial fibrillation can produce an irregular heart beat. Atrial flutter frequently conducts to the ventricles with 2:1 block at the AV node. Less commonly, due to agents that block AV nodal conduction or due to AV nodal disease, there is an alternating ratio of block resulting in a regularly irregular heart beat. In atrial fibrillation, regular heart beats are uncommon and should raise the suspicion of digitalis toxicity with accelerated junctional rhythm. Typically, the first heart sound in atrial fibrillation is of variable intensity. In atrial flutter, if the AV conduction ratio is constant, S_1 is of constant intensity. Atrial flutter generally requires low energy for cardioversion, typically in the range of 50 joules, while atrial fibrillation tends to require higher energy (around 100 joules). Radiofrequency ablation of atrial flutter near the ostium of the coronary sinus was associated with 75 to 90 per cent success rate in a recent study.[1] Radiofrequency is not used in the treatment of atrial fibrillation at the present time.

REFERENCE

1. Saxon, L.A., Kalman, J.M., Olgin, J.E., et al.: Results of radiofrequency catheter ablation for atrial flutter. Am. J. Cardiol. *77*:1014–1016, 1996.

282-D, 283-D, 284-C, 285-B   *(Braunwald, p. 611; Table 21–8)*

The wide variety of beta blockers available reflects their popularity, which is in part due to their relative effectiveness with few serious side effects. They can be classified on the basis of cardioselectivity, intrinsic sympathomimetic activity (ISA), and lipid solubility, although all are equally effective at lowering blood pressure.

Acebutolol, atenolol, and metoprolol are relatively more selective for cardiac beta$_1$ receptors than beta$_2$ adrenoreceptors present in bronchi, vascular smooth muscle, and other areas. However, it should be noted that at the doses usually prescribed, cardioselective effects may be lost.

Pindolol, acebutolol, alprenolol, and oxprenolol have ISA, which means that they possess partial agonist activity but still block the effects of endogenous catecholamines on adrenoreceptors. Thus, these drugs cause relatively smaller decreases in heart rate and cardiac output and smaller increases or no changes in serum lipids.[1,2] These drugs may be useful in patients with bradycardia and/or peripheral vascular disease.

The lipid solubility of a beta blocker determines the relative degree of clearance by hepatic uptake (high lipid solubility) and renal excretion (low lipid solubility). The least lipid-soluble drugs—atenolol and nadolol—share two theoretical advantages: longer serum half-lives due to decreased hepatic metabolism and fewer central nervous side effects due to lower brain concentrations.

REFERENCES

1. Choong, C.Y.P., Roubin, G.S., Harris, P.J., et al.: A comparison of the effects of beta blockers with and without intrinsic sympathomimetic activity on hemodynamics and left ventricular function at rest and during exercise in patients with coronary artery disease. J. Cardiovasc. Pharmacol. *8*:441, 1986.
2. Johnson, B.F., Weiner, B., Marwaha, R., and Johnson, J.: The influence of pindolol and hydrochlorothiazide on blood pressure, and plasma renin and plasma lipid levels. J. Clin. Pharmacol. *26*:258, 1986.

Part III
Diseases of the Heart, Pericardium, Aorta, and Pulmonary Vascular Bed

CHAPTERS 29 THROUGH 47

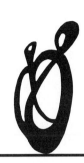

DIRECTIONS: Each question below contains five suggested responses. Select the ONE BEST response to each question.

286. Which of the following is true regarding atrial septal defect (ASD)?

A. Children with ASD tend to be somewhat physically underdeveloped
B. Atrial arrhythmias are common
C. The first heart sound can exhibit wide fixed splitting similar to the second heart sound
D. Left axis deviation on the ECG suggests the presence of sinus venosus ASD
E. Operative repair is not indicated in patients with shunt ratios <2.5:1.0

287. An 80-year-old man presents with syncope. During his evaluation, a cardiac murmur is detected and an echocardiographic study obtained. A continuous-wave Doppler recording through the aortic valve is shown *on the right.* True statements about this case include all of the following EXCEPT:

A. Dyspnea is a more common presenting complaint than syncope in this disorder
B. Some patients with this disorder and angina will not have significant coronary arterial obstruction on angiographic examination
C. Syncope in this disorder commonly occurs without significant change in systemic vascular tone
D. Syncope may also have been due to an arrhythmia in this patient
E. Gastrointestinal bleeding may be associated with this disorder

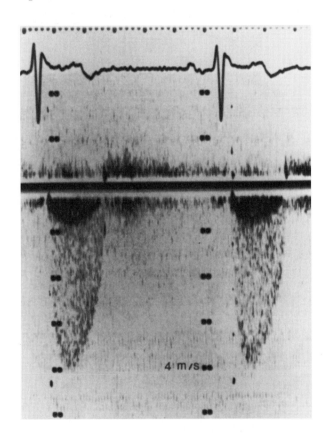

288. A 45-year-old man comes to the office because of recurrent chest discomfort and shortness of breath. He rides his bicycle daily to and from work and this past winter noticed occasional episodes of discomfort during bicycling. An exercise tolerance test (ETT) was performed for 12 minutes with a standard Bruce protocol without the development of significant symptoms or ECG findings. He was

placed on a beta blocker, but his symptoms have persisted. You perform a repeat ETT, which again is negative, except for upsloping ST-segment depressions present at 85 per cent of maximal predicted heart rate. You would recommend next:

A. switching medications to nifedipine
B. no further workup
C. echocardiography
D. stress thallium-201 scintigraphy
E. coronary arteriography

---

289. All of the following statements are true regarding the Scandinavian Simvastatin Survival Study (4S) trial EXCEPT:

A. Simvastatin lowered triglycerides by 10 to 15 per cent only
B. Randomization to simvastatin was associated with 30 per cent reduction in all-cause mortality
C. Reduction in all-cause mortality by simvastatin was seen in those older than 60 years
D. Reduction in coronary risk was most profound in the patients with total serum cholesterol in the highest quartile at baseline

---

290. A 44-year-old farmer develops fever, chills, and a cough. He is treated by his local physician with tetracycline for 1 week and feels improved. However, a week later he again develops a low-grade fever associated with myalgias. Over the next few days he has several episodes of palpitation and chest tightness which are worse with exertion. He is referred to you for further evaluation. On examination he has a temperature of 99.5°F, pulse 90/min, respirations 16/min, blood pressure 130/85. His lungs are clear. There is no jugular venous distention and the carotid upstrokes are normal. The LV impulse is not displaced; S_1 and S_2 are normal. There is a grade II/VI midsystolic murmur that increases with handgrip. A midsystolic click is also present. The rest of the examination is unremarkable. His chest x-ray and ECG are normal. Laboratory findings include Hgb 14.2 mg/dl; WBC 15,000/mm^3 with 80 per cent polys, 3 per cent bands, 17 per cent lymphs; Na 140 mEq/liter, Cl 100, K 5.0, HCO_3 25; urinalysis: clear, pH 6.6, 1+ protein, no WBC, 2 to 3 RBC/hpf. What would you order now?

A. Exercise testing
B. Exercise thallium testing
C. Ambulatory Holter monitor
D. Blood cultures
E. 1-week course of erythromycin

---

291. True statements regarding the macrophage in the pathogenesis of atherosclerosis include all of the following EXCEPT:

A. Macrophages demonstrate both a contractile and a synthetic state
B. Macrophages are the principal cells in the initial lesion of atherosclerosis, the fatty streak
C. Macrophages are derived from circulating monocytes
D. Macrophages are capable of taking up oxidized LDL
E. Hypercholesterolemia increases the adhesion of circulating monocytes to the endothelium

---

292. True statements about the clinical history in patients with acute myocardial infarction (AMI) include all of the following EXCEPT:

A. Approximately one-third of these patients may present with symptoms of unstable angina that have been present for longer than 24 hours
B. The duration of analgesic requirement after hospital admission is positively correlated with the likelihood of AMI being confirmed
C. The pain associated with AMI probably represents pain caused by infarcted myocardial tissue
D. Nausea and vomiting occur in more than half of patients with transmural MI
E. Between 20 and 60 per cent of nonfatal myocardial infarctions are unrecognized by the patient and are discovered on routine electrocardiographic examination

---

293. Each of the following statements regarding the use of percutaneous transluminal coronary angioplasty (PTCA) as a primary therapy in acute myocardial infarction (AMI) is true EXCEPT:

A. PTCA can be performed relatively safely during AMI
B. The primary success rate for PTCA during AMI is approximately 90 per cent
C. The PAMI trial showed that patients randomized to primary PTCA had a lower incidence of death or reinfarction by hospital discharge and at 6-month follow-up
D. When performed in experienced centers, hospital length of stay and follow-up costs are significantly less than for patients treated with thrombolysis
E. Primary PTCA is associated with worse outcome compared with thrombolysis for AMI patients presenting in cardiogenic shock

294. True statements about effusive-constrictive pericarditis include all of the following EXCEPT:

   A. In effusive-constrictive pericarditis, removal of pericardial fluid by aspiration does not lead to a normal right atrial pressure
   B. Idiopathic or presumed viral pericarditis is a common cause of effusive-constrictive pericarditis
   C. Physical findings in effusive-constrictive pericarditis resemble chronic constrictive pericarditis more than cardiac tamponade
   D. The diagnosis of effusive-constrictive pericarditis is made by careful hemodynamic monitoring before and after pericardiocentesis
   E. Treatment of effusive-constrictive pericarditis consists of total parietal and visceral pericardiectomy

295. The following statements regarding myocardial stunning are true EXCEPT:

   A. It is a state of depressed myocardial function due to chronic hypoperfusion
   B. Stunning can be global or regional
   C. Stunning can follow cardiopulmonary bypass
   D. Oxygen free radicals and excess intracellular calcium likely contribute to stunning
   E. Stunning affects both systolic and diastolic function

296. True statements regarding the effects of concurrent medications on hyperlipidemias include all of the following EXCEPT:

   A. Angiotensin-converting enzyme inhibitors may lead to alterations in the lipoprotein profile
   B. Estrogen therapy tends to increase triglyceride levels
   C. Alpha-adrenergic blockers do not adversely affect lipids
   D. Calcium antagonists tend to have a neutral effect on lipids
   E. Noncardioselective beta blockers may lead to an increase in VLDL levels

297. True statements about the electrocardiogram in congenital heart disease include all of the following EXCEPT:

   A. T-wave inversions may be seen in normal neonatal electrocardiograms
   B. By the time the infant is 72 hours of age the T waves should be inverted in V_1 to V_3
   C. The presence of right ventricular hypertrophy suggests single ventricle or inversion of the ventricles

   D. An electrocardiographic pattern of myocardial infarction may indicate an anomalous origin of a coronary artery
   E. T-wave inversion in the lateral precordial leads may be observed in subendocardial ischemia

298. All of the following statements are true with regards to abrupt closure following coronary angioplasty EXCEPT:

   A. It is expected to occur in 10 per cent of patients
   B. Most cases occur before the patient has left the catheterization laboratory
   C. Most episodes commonly result from extensive disruption of the medial layer with subsequent thrombosis
   D. Mortality associated with abrupt closure approaches 25 per cent
   E. Initial management typically consists of repeat prolonged baloon dilatation

299. True statements about the progression of atherosclerosis in venous aortocoronary artery bypass grafts include all of the following EXCEPT:

   A. Between 12 and 20 per cent of vein grafts are occluded by the end of the first year following surgery
   B. At 10 years, the overall occlusion rate for a saphenous vein graft approaches 50 per cent
   C. The atherosclerotic process that occurs in venous grafts is histologically different from that which occurs in native arterial vessels
   D. Progression of disease in native coronary arteries occurs at a rate of 18 to 38 per cent over the first decade after operation
   E. The annual rate of saphenous vein graft occlusion after the first year is only on the order of 2 per cent

300. All of the following statements regarding ventricular septal defect (VSD) are true EXCEPT:

   A. It is the most common form of congenital heart disease in infants and children
   B. The most common VSD occurs in the membranous septum
   C. Spontaneous VSD closure occurs in 45 per cent of patients by the age of 3 years
   D. Spontaneous closure occurs primarily by continued growth of the muscular septum
   E. Complete heart block following surgical repair is uncommon

301. Each of the following statements about coarctation of the aorta is true EXCEPT:

    A. Coarctation of the aorta usually occurs just proximal to the left subclavian artery
    B. Coarctation is frequently associated with a bicuspid aortic valve
    C. The most common symptoms of coarctation are headaches, intermittent claudication, and leg fatigue
    D. Simultaneous palpation of the upper and lower extremity pulses may reveal the diagnosis
    E. A suprasternal thrill is common in this condition

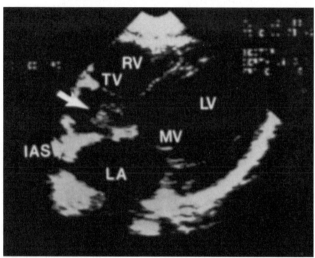

RV = right ventricle, TV = tricuspid valve, LV = left ventricle, MV = mitral valve, LA = left atrium. (From Panadis, I.P., et al.: Am. Heart J. 107:745, 1984.)

302. The two-dimensional echocardiogram illustrated above most likely demonstrates the presence of:

    A. a right atrial myxoma
    B. a left atrial myxoma
    C. a rhabdomyoma
    D. a lymphosarcoma
    E. a pericardial cyst

303. True statements regarding genetic forms of hypertriglyceridemia include all of the following EXCEPT:

    A. Type IV hyperlipoproteinemia (HLP) is usually first manifested in adulthood
    B. Two main genetic forms of type IV HLP exist: primary (familial) endogenous hypertriglyceridemia and familial combined hyperlipidemia
    C. The presence of chylomicrons excludes type V HLP
    D. In familial endogenous hypertriglyceridemia, triglyceride levels are usually not markedly elevated
    E. Type V HLP is less common in women

304. The following statements regarding antiplatelets and anticoagulants in the treatment of unstable angina are correct EXCEPT:

    A. Aspirin reduces the incidence of myocardial infarction and death from cardiac causes by 50 per cent
    B. Heparin therapy is superior to aspirin in preventing recurrent episodes of unstable angina
    C. The combination of aspirin and heparin is superior to heparin alone in that a "rebound" unstable angina is less likely to occur after discontinuation of heparin
    D. When aspirin is contraindicated, ticlopidine is an acceptable alternative with similar beneficial influence on outcome
    E. Low doses of aspirin (<160 mg/day) have no beneficial effect on mortality and reinfarction

305. True statements about atrial infarction include all of the following EXCEPT:

    A. Atrial infarction occurs in <20 per cent of autopsy-proven cases of MI
    B. Atrial infarction is seen more commonly in the right atrium
    C. Atrial infarction may lead to rupture of the atrial wall
    D. Atrial arrhythmias are relatively uncommon in atrial infarction
    E. Atrial infarction may often be seen in conjunction with left ventricular infarction

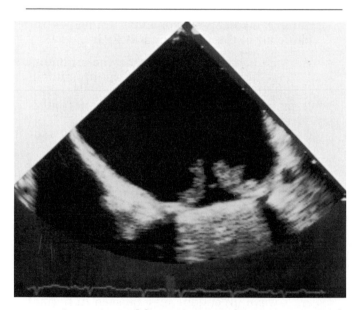

306. A 42-year-old woman underwent a mitral valve replacement with a St. Jude prosthesis. She was maintained on warfarin therapy and was documented to have adequate anticoagulation. Two years after the operation she had recurrent transient ischemic attacks; a

workup was performed. Transthoracic echocardiogram proved unrevealing. A transesophageal echocardiogram was next performed and the image displayed on the previous page was obtained. True statements about this case include each of the following EXCEPT:

A. Two large thrombi are seen on the left atrial surface of the St. Jude valve
B. *Streptococcus viridans* is the most likely organism to be cultured in this setting
C. Methicillin resistance is present in the majority of patients with this complication
D. The prosthetic mitral valve appears to be seated in a normal position
E. Transesophageal echocardiography is consistently more sensitive than transthoracic studies for establishing this diagnosis

307. True statements about the percutaneous treatment of valvular stenosis include all of the following EXCEPT:

A. Balloon valvuloplasty has essentially replaced surgical repair for valvular pulmonic stenosis
B. In general, rheumatic mitral stenosis does not allow for successful balloon valvuloplasty repair
C. The development of moderate or severe mitral regurgitation following balloon mitral valvuloplasty for mitral stenosis is rare
D. In patients without left atrial thrombus, there appears to be no evidence of systemic embolization due to mitral valvuloplasty
E. In general, application of balloon valvuloplasty to aortic stenosis leads to a smaller improvement in orifice area than that obtained with valve replacement

308. All of the following statements are true regarding sporadic cardiac myxomas EXCEPT:

A. They comprise up to 50 per cent of cardiac tumors
B. They are more common in females
C. They are the commonest cause of cardiac tumor–related emboli
D. Location of the tumor on the right side of the heart is more often associated with malignant type of myxomas
E. Following resection of the initial myxoma, a recurrence or a second myxoma is expected in about 10 per cent of cases

309. A 3-month-old infant is referred to you because of failure to thrive and cardiomegaly. Gestation and delivery were normal. The physical examination shows evidence of congestive heart failure and poor skeletal muscle tone. Chest x-ray shows cardiomegaly and mild pulmonary edema. ECG reveals tall broad QRS complexes consistent with left ventricular hypertrophy and a P-R interval of 0.08 sec. The most likely diagnosis is:

A. endocardial fibroelastosis
B. coarctation of the aorta
C. Shone syndrome
D. Type II glycogen storage disease (Pompe disease)
E. Friedreich's ataxia

310. All of the following statements regarding nicotinic acid are correct EXCEPT:

A. It acts primarily by reducing hepatic synthesis of VLDL, and reduction of free fatty acid release from tissues
B. It reduces LDL by 10 to 25 per cent and triglycerides by 20 to 50 per cent
C. It reduces serum levels of Lp(a)
D. Hepatic toxicity can be reduced by the use of sustained-release forms
E. Preadministration of aspirin can reduce flushing

311. All of the following statements regarding coronary collateral circulation are correct EXCEPT:

A. After coronary occlusion, preexisting collaterals open instantly
B. A mature collateral vessel may reach 1 mm in luminal diameter and become a three-layered structure
C. Exercise significantly increases collateral density in patients with coronary stenosis
D. Collaterals dilate in response to nitrates and beta-adrenergic agents
E. The presence of angiographically visible collaterals is associated with reduced fibrosis and better contractile function in the area of the myocardium which they supply

312. All of the following are true statements about the pathophysiology of cardiac tamponade EXCEPT:

A. Cardiac tamponade occurs when the intrapericardial pressure is equal to the RA and RV diastolic pressures
B. In the presence of hypovolemia, the rise of the RA and intrapericardial pressures is less obvious; therefore, cardiac tamponade may be more difficult to detect
C. Equalization of intrapericardial and ventricular filling pressures may lead initially to a small increase in stroke volume

D. Sinus bradycardia may occur during severe cardiac tamponade

E. Hemodynamic deterioration during tamponade is dependent upon atrial compression during diastole

---

313. True statements about the apoproteins in lipoprotein metabolism include all of the following EXCEPT:

A. Apo A-I is a major protein in HDL
B. Combined A-I/C-III deficiency is a genetic disorder associated with premature atherosclerosis
C. Apo B-48, synthesized by the small intestine, and apo B-100, secreted by the liver, are synthesized by two distinct genes
D. Apo B-100 is the major apoprotein in LDL
E. Type III hyperlipoproteinemia is a disorder of apoprotein E

---

314. A 67-year-old woman, a Russian immigrant, comes to your office complaining of rapid heartbeat, fatigue, weight loss, and swelling of her ankles. She also complains of a sensation of fullness in her neck. She has been in apparent good health for all of her life until the last 6 months. She is taking no medications except furosemide. Examination discloses clear lungs, an irregular pulse, prominent jugular veins, a nearly pansystolic murmur that exhibits respiratory variation in intensity, and marked peripheral edema. There are no cardiac heaves or lifts. She also tells you that she has recurrent episodes of flushing and diarrhea. A likely cause of her illness is:

A. subacute bacterial endocarditis
B. carcinoid syndrome
C. Ebstein's anomaly
D. chronic pulmonary emboli disease
E. Marfan syndrome

---

315. All of the following statements regarding left ventricular free wall rupture are correct EXCEPT:

A. Rupture occurs in about 1 to 2 per cent of patients dying in the hospital of acute myocardial infarction
B. Rupture incidence is reduced by early use of thrombolytic therapy
C. Free wall rupture is more frequent in the elderly and in women
D. Rupture usually involves the anterior or lateral walls in the distribution of the left anterior descending artery
E. Rupture commonly occurs in patients without prior myocardial infarction

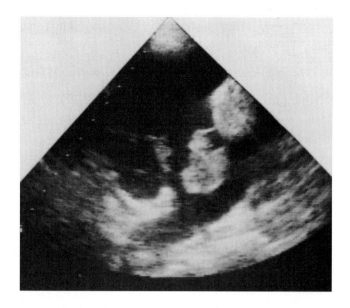

316. A 32-year-old woman with a history of intravenous drug abuse presents to the emergency room with fatigue and intermittent night sweats. Physical examination reveals a temperature of 38.4°C, scattered rhonchi and wheezes in the lung fields, tachycardia without obvious murmurs, and needle tracks. Chest x-ray reveals several small infiltrates in the left lung field. A transthoracic echocardiogram is obtained and a right heart inflow view from this study is displayed above. Each of the following statements about this case is true EXCEPT:

A. The vegetation displayed occupies the most common endocardial site of infection observed in IV drug abusers
B. The site of involvement displayed is associated with a higher mortality than other endocardial sites
C. The most likely organism associated with the region displayed is *S. aureus*
D. Fungi are isolated from such lesions in approximately 5 per cent of cases
E. The majority of patients with this presentation are noted to have pneumonia or multiple septic emboli on chest x-ray

---

317. All of the following statements regarding blunt cardiac trauma are true EXCEPT:

A. Cardiac trauma most commonly occurs as a result of a motor vehicle accident
B. Clinical manifestations of cardiac trauma are usually apparent soon after the accident
C. Myocardial contusion usually is asymptomatic
D. CK-MB levels are not very helpful in the diagnosis of cardiac trauma in those patients with severe skeletal muscle injury

E. Cardiac rupture most commonly involves the right ventricle

318. All of the following statements regarding cardiac involvement in human immunodeficiency virus (HIV) infection are true EXCEPT:

A. Symptomatic cardiac involvement occurs in about 10 per cent of cases
B. The most common manifestation is congestive heart failure (CHF)
C. Cardiac tamponade is frequent in the presence of an effusion
D. HIV may be isolated from myocardial cells in affected patients
E. Response to therapy is variable

319. True statements about hypertriglyceridemia as a risk factor for coronary artery disease include all of the following EXCEPT:

A. Data from the Framingham Study suggest that triglyceride elevation is an independent cardiac risk factor in women
B. In the Cholesterol-Lowering Atherosclerosis Study (CLAS), triglyceride levels were predictive of progression of atherosclerotic disease
C. Hypertriglyceridemia may be associated with chronic renal failure or diabetes mellitus
D. Triglyceride levels of 250 mg/dl or greater are considered high risk
E. Excess alcohol consumption and cigarette use are both associated with increased triglyceride levels

320. True statements about the clinical findings in patients with atrial septal defect (ASD) include all of the following EXCEPT:

A. A midsystolic ejection murmur and a diastolic rumbling murmur at the lower left sternal border may both be features of the cardiac examination in ASD
B. Patients with ostium primum defects usually show RV hypertrophy, a small rSR' pattern in the right precordial levels, and normal axis on the ECG
C. P-R interval prolongation may be seen with any of the types of ASD
D. Echocardiographic features of ASD include RV and pulmonary arterial dilatation as well as paradoxical septal motion
E. In children with a large left-to-right shunt, catheterization often reveals normal right-sided pressures

321. In hypertrophic cardiomyopathy, all of the following statements are correct regarding the effect of hemodynamic interventions on outflow murmur and gradient EXCEPT:

A. The murmur and gradient are increased with amyl nitrite
B. The murmur and gradient are increased with Mueller maneuver
C. The murmur and gradient are decreased with phenylephrine
D. The murmur and gradient are decreased with beta-adrenergic blockers
E. The murmur and gradient are increased with tachycardia

322. Which of the following is NOT true regarding Lp(a):

A. It is an independent risk factor for coronary artery disease
B. One part of Lp(a) is structurally identical to LDL and another is similar to plasminogen
C. More than 90 per cent of the variation in Lp(a) is attributable to variation in the gene for apo(a)
D. Levels of Lp(a) can be reduced by both nicotinic acid and estrogen
E. A decrease in Lp(a) level is associated with a reduction in coronary events

323. True statements about right ventricular infarction (RVI) include all of the following EXCEPT:

A. RVI may be accompanied by Kussmaul's sign
B. ST-segment elevation in lead V_4 is commonly present in RVI
C. Echocardiography may help distinguish RVI from pericardial effusion and tamponade
D. Marked hypotensive responses to small doses of nitroglycerin may suggest the possibility of RVI
E. Sequential atrioventricular pacing may be of benefit in selected patients with RVI

324. Each of the following statements regarding internal mammary artery (IMA) bypass grafts is true EXCEPT:

A. Placement of an IMA graft often involves surgical entry into the pleural space
B. Endothelium-dependent relaxation is more pronounced in saphenous vein grafts than it is in IMA grafts

C. The diameter of an IMA graft is usually closer to that of the native coronary vessel than a saphenous vein graft

D. Recent studies have confirmed the original suggestion that IMA grafts have improved 10-year survivals compared with those for saphenous veins

E. Multiple IMA grafts have a similar operative mortality and morbidity to single IMA grafts

---

325. True statements about the surgical management of abdominal aortic aneurysm (AAA) include all of the following EXCEPT:

A. All such aneurysms >6 cm in diameter should be treated by elective surgical repair

B. The usual surgical repair consists of resection of the aneurysm with insertion of a synthetic prosthesis

C. Marked hypotension following release of the aortic crossclamp continues to be a cause of perioperative morbidity

D. Approximately half of the perioperative deaths following AAA repair are due to myocardial infarction

E. The operative risk in the lowest-risk patients who undergo elective AAA repair is approximately 2 to 5 per cent

---

326. All of the following features suggest acute as opposed to chronic mitral regurgitation (MR) EXCEPT:

A. no cardiomegaly on chest x-ray

B. a normal ECG

C. a systolic murmur that radiates to the neck

D. a systolic murmur that clearly ends before S_2

E. normal jugular venous pressure

---

327. True statements about the clinical manifestations of cardiac tamponade include all of the following EXCEPT:

A. Patients in whom cardiac tamponade develops slowly usually complain of dyspnea

B. Patients with rapid development of severe cardiac tamponade due to intrapericardial hemorrhage commonly demonstrate pulsus paradoxus

C. Jugular venous distention is a common physical finding in patients with cardiac tamponade

D. Massive pulmonary embolism may be difficult to distinguish from cardiac tamponade

E. Tamponade may be present in a patient in whom the physical examination is normal except for a moderate elevation of jugular venous pressure

---

328. All of the following features of post-myocardial infarction (post-MI) pericarditis are true EXCEPT:

A. Thrombolytic therapy increases the incidence of early post-MI pericarditis and reduces that of Dressler syndrome

B. Post-MI pericarditis is more common following Q-wave MI

C. A pericardial friction rub can be detected as early as 12 hours after the infarction

D. The use of heparin is not associated with an increased risk of pericarditis

E. Diagnostic ECG changes include persistently positive T waves and premature normalization of initially inverted T waves

---

329. All of the following statements regarding the management of aortic dissection are correct EXCEPT:

A. Mortality of untreated aortic dissection exceeds 25 per cent in the first 24 hours

B. Surgery is clearly superior to medical therapy in the management of proximal dissection

C. Medical therapy is recommended for chronic uncomplicated aortic dissection regardless of its location

D. Aortic valve replacement should be performed when there is significant aortic regurgitation in patients with proximal aortic dissection

E. Labetalol can be used safely in dissection patients to lower arterial pressure

---

330. All of the following statements regarding radiation pericarditis are correct EXCEPT:

A. When the whole pericardium is included in the radiation field, the risk of pericarditis is about 20 per cent

B. It occurs more commonly late (months) after therapy

C. In its early stages, radiation pericarditis is commonly associated with large pericardial effusions

D. Up to 20 per cent of patients with delayed pericardial injury will progress to chronic pericarditis that will require pericardiectomy

E. Operative mortality for pericardiectomy in these patients can be up to 20 per cent

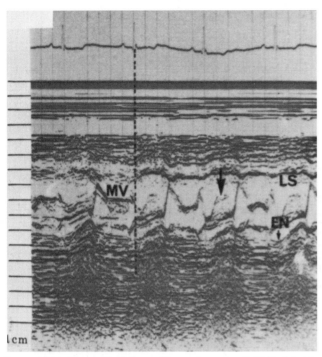

From Feigenbaum, H.: Echocardiography, 4th ed. Philadelphia, Lea & Febiger, 1986, p. 526.

331. The M-mode echocardiogram illustrated above would most likely be observed in a patient with which disease?

A. Hypertrophic cardiomyopathy
B. Marfan syndrome
C. Mitral stenosis
D. Ruptured papillary muscle
E. Aortic regurgitation

332. Each of the following statements regarding the choice of thrombolytic agents in acute myocardial infarction (MI) is true EXCEPT:

A. Anisoylated plasminogen streptokinase activator complex (APSAC) does not appear to be more fibrin clot-selective than streptokinase itself
B. The appropriate dosage of tissue-plasminogen activator (t-PA) in acute myocardial infarction is 100 mg total, with 60 mg delivered in the first hour
C. Trials using early angiography suggest that the patency rate of the infarct-related vessel is approximately equivalent between streptokinase and t-PA
D. The GISSI-II trial showed no significant difference in the mortality rates between streptokinase and t-PA
E. Repeat dosing is possible with t-PA but not with streptokinase or APSAC

333. Each of the following statements about congenital valvular aortic stenosis (AS) is true EXCEPT:

A. This anomaly occurs more frequently in males than in females
B. Most children with congenital AS grow and develop normally and are asymptomatic
C. The presence of left ventricular hypertrophy with "strain" on the ECG in childhood usually indicates severe AS
D. Any child with clinical evidence of AS should undergo cardiac catheterization
E. Antibiotic prophylaxis for endocarditis is indicated in all patients with this disorder, regardless of the severity of obstruction

334. True statements about Holter monitoring in patients with unstable angina include all of the following EXCEPT:

A. Patients with unstable angina usually demonstrate silent ischemia on Holter monitoring
B. Up to 90 per cent of ischemic episodes in patients with unstable angina are silent
C. Ischemia on Holter monitoring independently predicts unfavorable postdischarge outcomes
D. In patients with unstable angina, silent ECG changes on Holter monitoring are not correlated with ventricular dysfunction
E. Unstable angina patients who respond to therapy may have persistent silent ischemia shown by Holter monitoring

335. True statements about congenital heart disease in infancy and childhood include all of the following EXCEPT:

A. Children with congenital heart disease are more commonly male
B. Patent ductus arteriosus is found more commonly in females
C. Approximately one-third of infants with both cardiac and extracardiac congenital anomalies have an established syndrome
D. The rubella syndrome may be accompanied by patent ductus arteriosus or pulmonic valvular stenosis
E. Maternal systemic lupus erythematosus may lead to congenital cardiac defects in ventricular septal defect and pulmonic stenosis

336. All of the following statements regarding streptococcal and enterococcal endocarditis are correct EXCEPT:

A. In cases of pneumococcal endocarditis, concurrent pneumonia or meningitis is common
B. The majority of cases of enterococcal endocarditis occur in elderly males
C. Group B streptococcal endocarditis is characterized by large vegetations and a high incidence of systemic embolism
D. Patients with uncomplicated *Streptococcus viridans* or *bovis* endocarditis can be adequately treated with a 2-week course of penicillin plus gentamicin
E. Endocarditis caused by penicillin-resistant enterococci can be adequately treated with high doses of vancomycin intravenously for 4 to 6 weeks

337. A 60-year-old man comes to the coronary care unit with severe chest pain. His ECG reveals 2-mm ST-segment elevations in leads II, III, and aV$_f$. The initial cardiac examination is unremarkable. On the second day a faint late systolic murmur is heard, and by the third day this murmur has increased to grade 3/6. The patient has mild dyspnea, and a chest x-ray shows pulmonary vascular redistribution. The *most* likely explanation for the murmur is:

A. ruptured posterior papillary muscle
B. ruptured anterior papillary muscle
C. infarcted posterior papillary muscle
D. infarcted anterior papillary muscle
E. ruptured chordae tendineae

338. True statements about abdominal aortic aneurysms (AAA) include all of the following EXCEPT:

A. The majority of AAA are asymptomatic
B. Aneurysms may be sensitive and even tender to palpation
C. Careful physical examination is among the most accurate of noninvasive methods for evaluating AAA
D. Half of all aneurysms >6 cm in diameter rupture within 1 year
E. Recent studies suggest that aneurysms expand by approximately 0.4 to 0.5 cm in diameter each year

339. A 50-year-old man with longstanding hypertension and chronic aortic regurgitation presented to his physician with daily fevers and new dyspnea. He had previously been asymptomatic. Physical examination revealed bilat-

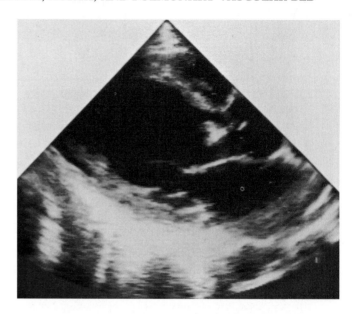

eral crackles in the lung fields, the patient's usual murmur of aortic regurgitation, and bilateral pitting edema of the ankles. The electrocardiogram revealed sinus rhythm and intermittent unifocal ventricular premature beats. A transthoracic echocardiogram was obtained, and a parasternal long-axis view from that study is illustrated *above*. True statements about this patient include all of the following EXCEPT:

A. The left ventricle is dilated due to chronic aortic insufficiency
B. The posterior mitral valve leaflet is prolapsing into the left atrium
C. The aortic valve appears heavily calcified and stenotic
D. Mild dilatation of the ascending aortic root is present
E. A vegetation is clearly demonstrated

340. The following statements are true regarding use and management of prosthetic cardiac valves EXCEPT:

A. Because of a better hemodynamic profile, the St. Jude valve is especially useful in children
B. Bioprosthetic valves are preferred in the tricuspid position
C. In the mitral position, perivalvular regurgitation is more common with mechanical valves than with bioprosthetic valves
D. Warfarin anticoagulation with INR maintained in the range of 2.5 to 3.5 is recommended for all mechanical valves in the mitral and aortic positions
E. Bioprosthetic valves tend to have better durability when implanted in younger patients

341. True statements about pericardial effusion and pericarditis in the setting of acute MI (AMI) include all of the following EXCEPT:

A. Pericardial effusions occur to some degree in approximately 50 per cent of patients with AMI
B. Pericarditis usually occurs between the second and fourth days following AMI
C. The Dressler syndrome usually occurs 2 to 10 weeks after infarction
D. The Dressler syndrome has become less common in recent years
E. Tamponade due to pericarditis in the setting of AMI is quite uncommon

342. True statements concerning the diastolic murmur of mitral stenosis (MS) include all of the following EXCEPT:

A. The intensity of the murmur is closely related to the severity of stenosis
B. In severe stenosis the murmur is holodiastolic
C. A myxoma in the left atrium may sound identical to MS
D. The duration of the murmur is a rough guide to the severity of stenosis
E. The murmur is reduced during inspiration and during the strain of the Valsalva maneuver

343. Each of the following statements regarding patients with chest pain and normal coronary arteriograms is true EXCEPT:

A. The prognosis is usually excellent in syndrome X
B. The majority of patients with chest pain and normal coronary arteriograms have typical angina pectoris
C. Approximately 20 per cent of patients of this type have a positive exercise test
D. Esophageal studies may be appropriate in this group
E. The presence of a left bundle branch block in patients of this type is correlated with a worse prognosis

344. All of the following statements regarding the physical examination in aortic regurgitation (AR) are true EXCEPT:

A. Hill's sign is more frequently seen in acute AR
B. The severity of regurgitation correlates better with the duration rather than severity of the murmur

C. A musical murmur ("cooing dove" murmur) usually signifies eversion or perforation of a cusp
D. Murmurs auscultated on the right side of the sternum suggest dilation of the ascending aorta
E. Austin Flint murmur intensity is reduced by amyl nitrite inhalation

345. True statements about bacterial pericarditis include all of the following EXCEPT:

A. Uremic pericarditis with a preexisting pericardial effusion may predispose to the development of purulent bacterial pericarditis
B. Direct extension into the pericardium of bacterial pneumonia accounts for the majority of cases of purulent pericarditis
C. Bacterial pericarditis is most often an acute fulminant illness that develops over a few days
D. Long-term survival after purulent bacterial pericarditis remains poor despite the availability of antibacterial therapy
E. High concentrations of antibiotics may be achieved in pericardial fluid

346. A 16-year-old boy requests a physical examination before competing in high school athletics. His mother states that a cousin died suddenly during a basketball game and she recalls that there was something wrong with his heart. The boy has no symptoms. His vital signs are heart rate 64/min, respirations 12/min, and blood pressure 120/75. His cardiac examination is remarkable for a grade 2/6 systolic ejection murmur along the left sternal border, which decreases with squatting and increases with sudden standing. An ECG shows evidence of left-ventricular hypertrophy and a chest x-ray shows an increased cardiothoracic ratio. You would recommend:

A. no competitive sports
B. noncontact competitive sports
C. noncontact competitive sports with beta blocker therapy
D. high-intensity competitive sports
E. high-intensity competitive sports with beta blocker therapy

347. All of the following statements regarding creatine kinase (CK) in acute myocardial infarction (AMI) are true EXCEPT:

A. It increases beyond the normal range within 4 to 6 hours following the onset of AMI

B. It peaks earlier in patients who have had reperfusion with thrombolytic agents, mechanical intervention, or spontaneously
C. CK-MB is not found in normal skeletal muscle
D. Patients suspected of having AMI with elevated CK-MB but normal total CK have a somewhat worse prognosis than those with normal CK-MB
E. Measurement of CK isoforms may permit diagnosis of AMI within 2 hours

---

348. True statements about atrial septal defect (ASD) include all of the following EXCEPT:

A. Sinus venosus type ASD is frequently associated with anomalous pulmonary venous connections
B. An incomplete seal of the foramen ovale occurs in approximately 25 per cent of adults
C. Approximately 10 to 20 per cent of patients with ostium secundum ASD have associated mitral valve prolapse
D. Children with ASD often experience easy fatigability and exertional dyspnea
E. Atrial arrhythmias are uncommon in children with ASD

---

349. All of the following statements regarding intracoronary stenting are true EXCEPT:

A. Stents are indicated in the treatment of threatened closure
B. Approved stents are made of stainless steel
C. Despite anticoagulation with warfarin, subacute stent thrombosis occurs in 2 to 5 per cent of patients
D. Smaller stents carry a higher risk of thrombosis than larger stents
E. Stents reduce restenosis by reducing neointimal hyperplasia

---

350. Changes in left ventricular function and hemodynamics in isolated moderately severe aortic stenosis (AS) include all of the following EXCEPT:

A. normal cardiac output at rest
B. elevated left ventricular end-diastolic pressure
C. elevated left ventricular end-diastolic volume
D. increased *a* waves in the left atrial pressure pulse
E. normal left ventricular stroke volume

---

351. All of the following are absolute indications for surgical intervention in prosthetic valve endocarditis EXCEPT:

A. fungal etiology
B. congestive heart failure
C. vegetations observed on echocardiography
D. new heart block in aortic valve endocarditis
E. positive blood cultures despite 2 weeks of appropriate antibiotic therapy

---

352. True statements regarding the management of patients with Prinzmetal's (variant) angina include all of the following EXCEPT:

A. Long-acting nitrate preparations are useful in preventing attacks of Prinzmetal's angina
B. Calcium channel antagonists are particularly effective in the treatment and prevention of coronary artery spasm in this syndrome
C. The selective alpha-adrenoreceptor blocker prazosin may be contraindicated in treatment of Prinzmetal's angina
D. Aspirin may be contraindicated in Prinzmetal's angina
E. Patients with variant angina and single-vessel disease occasionally benefit from PTCA

---

353. True statements with regard to the calcium channel antagonists include all the following EXCEPT:

A. Verapamil is the most likely to cause constipation and gastrointestinal symptoms
B. Nicardipine may be useful as an intravenous calcium antagonist
C. Verapamil is the most likely to cause flushing and headache
D. Nifedipine is the least likely to cause decreased heart rate and/or AV block in patients with conduction system disease
E. Amlodipine has an especially long duration of action compared with the other calcium antagonists

---

354. All of the following statements regarding coronary atherectomy are true EXCEPT:

A. Directional atherectomy (DCA) has an overall success rate of 85 to 90 per cent
B. Acute procedural ischemic complications (including death or myocardial infarction) are more likely to occur with DCA
C. DCA is associated with a significantly reduced restenosis rate when compared with PTCA

D. Rotational atherectomy is particularly effective in heavily calcified lesions

---

355. True statements about tuberculous pericarditis include all of the following EXCEPT:

A. Tuberculous pericarditis usually develops by retrograde spread from adjacent lymph nodes or by early hematogenous spread from the primary infection
B. The tuberculous pericardial effusion usually develops slowly
C. Acute pericardial chest pain is not commonly found in tuberculous pericarditis
D. It is often difficult to establish a definitive bacteriological diagnosis of tuberculous pericarditis
E. Initial therapy for tuberculous pericarditis should include a standard three-drug regimen as well as corticosteroids to reduce pericardial inflammation

---

356. A 32-year-old woman complains of dizzy spells and one syncopal episode. She had been asymptomatic until the previous summer when she developed mild arthritis and a knee effusion. Her orthopedist found no evidence of infection and thought that she might have injured herself while on vacation in Nantucket, Massachusetts.

On examination, she appeared healthy and no abnormalities were found except for a resting pulse of 48/min. ECG was normal except for a P-R interval of 0.24 sec. A 24-hour ambulatory Holter ECG showed many episodes of Mobitz type II second-degree AV block. Although her erythrocyte sedimentation rate was elevated to 77 mm/hr, the antinuclear antibody titer was negative. The most likely diagnosis is:

A. subacute rheumatic fever
B. Lyme disease
C. systemic lupus erythematosus
D. *Trichinella spiralis* infection
E. hemochromatosis

---

357. Each of the following statements regarding balloon mitral valvuloplasty is true EXCEPT:

A. The balloon flotation catheter is usually positioned near the apex of the left ventricle in this procedure
B. The overall mortality for balloon mitral valvuloplasty is 1 to 2 per cent
C. Echocardiography prior to valvuloplasty is helpful in predicting both early and late hemodynamic success rates

D. Balloon mitral valvuloplasty occasionally leads to an iatrogenic atrial septal defect
E. Valvular thickening is considered an unfavorable factor in mitral valvuloplasty procedures, while subvalvular thickening is not

---

358. All of the following are commonly associated with myocardial contusion EXCEPT:

A. congestive heart failure
B. ECG findings of pericarditis
C. elevated CPK-MB isoenzyme
D. positive uptake of technetium pyrophosphate
E. sinus node dysfunction

---

359. All of the following statements regarding prosthetic valve endocarditis (PVE) are true EXCEPT:

A. PVE episodes account for <5 per cent of all cases of endocarditis
B. The highest risk of PVE is during the initial 6 months following surgery
C. Mechanical valves have a higher risk of PVE in the first few months after surgery, while bioprosthetic valves have a higher risk of PVE beyond 12 months
D. The most common organisms causing PVE 1 year after surgery are streptococci
E. Optimal therapy for non–methicillin-resistant staphylococcal PVE should include gentamicin, rifampin, and nafcillin for at least 6 weeks

---

360. True statements about conduction disturbances in acute myocardial infarction (AMI) include all of the following EXCEPT:

A. Most patients with first-degree AV block and AMI have an intranodal conduction disturbance
B. Digitalis toxicity may be the cause of first-degree AV block in AMI
C. Of patients with AMI and second-degree AV block, the majority have Mobitz type I or Wenckebach second-degree AV block
D. Mobitz type II second-degree AV block in AMI is almost always found with anterior infarction
E. In patients with anterior infarction who develop third-degree AV block, the conduction disturbance usually occurs without prior intraventricular conduction abnormalities

361. True statements about the natural history of untreated ventricular septal defect (VSD) include all of the following EXCEPT:

A. The natural history of VSD may differ depending on the size of the defect and the magnitude of the pulmonary vascular resistance
B. Regardless of size, the presence of a VSD confers an increased risk for endocarditis
C. Progressive pulmonary vascular disease with reversal of shunting (Eisenmenger complex) usually occurs during the 5th decade of life in those patients with VSD who will develop this complication
D. Infundibular pulmonic stenosis may develop gradually in occasional adult patients with isolated VSD
E. Women with VSDs that lead to ratios of pulmonary to systemic flow <2:1 generally tolerate pregnancy well

362. A 21-year-old intravenous drug abuser came to the hospital with fever and malaise of 3 weeks' duration. His chest x-ray showed right-sided pneumonia and bilateral pleural effusions. The initial examination was remarkable for inspiratory wheezes and dullness at the right base. There were prominent *c-v* waves in his jugular venous pulse and a hyperdynamic precordium was noted. A grade 3/6 systolic murmur was audible most prominently along the left sternal border. Five of six blood cultures were positive for *Pseudomonas aeruginosa* and he was started on tobramycin and piperacillin. However, after 3 weeks he had persistent fever to 100°F and 1+ pedal edema, and blood cultures were again positive for *Pseudomonas*. Appropriate therapy at this time would be:

A. an additional 4 weeks of treatment with higher doses of tobramycin and piperacillin
B. antibiotics changed to tobramycin and ceftazidime and given for an additional 4 weeks
C. tricuspid valvulectomy with replacement by a prosthetic valve and antibiotic treatment for 4 weeks
D. tricuspid valvulectomy with replacement by a Hancock porcine prosthesis and antibiotics for 4 weeks
E. tricuspid valvulectomy with replacement by a St. Jude mechanical prosthesis and continued antibiotics for 4 weeks

363. A 57-year-old white woman comes to the office complaining of dyspnea. She has no history of chest pain, denies smoking, and has never been hypertensive. She has a complicated medical history, including a long history of arthritis and adult-onset diabetes mellitus now requiring insulin. Her only current medication is NPH insulin. On examination she is a well-tanned woman with heart rate 90/min, respirations 16/min, blood pressure 140/85. Lungs: inspiratory crackles at the bases. Heart: elevated jugular venous pressure at 10 cm; normal carotid upstrokes and volume; normal cardiac impulse; S_1 and S_2 normal, loud S_3; holosystolic murmurs at left sternal border and apex, the former increasing with inspiration and the latter with handgrip. The liver is firm and palpable 2 cm below the right costal margin. There is 2+ pitting edema of both legs. ECG is unremarkable. An elevated transferrin saturation is found. The most likely cause for dyspnea is:

A. hemochromatosis
B. sarcoidosis
C. amyloidosis
D. Fabry's disease
E. ischemic cardiomyopathy

364. True statements about the diagnosis and treatment of right ventricular infarction (RVI) include all of the following EXCEPT:

A. Marked hypertension in response to small doses of nitroglycerin in patients with inferior infarction suggests RVI
B. The presence of unexplained systemic hypoxemia in RVI raises the possibility of a patent foramen ovale
C. Hemodynamic parameters in RVI often resemble those in patients with pericardial disease
D. Loss of atrial transport in RVI is primarily managed by increased fluid replacement in order to maintain appropriate right-sided filling pressures
E. ST-segment elevation in lead V_4R is a sensitive and specific sign of RVI

365. Each of the following statements about tetralogy of Fallot is correct EXCEPT:

A. Classic tetralogy of Fallot is composed of a large ventricular septal defect (VSD), infundibular and/or valvular pulmonic stenosis, right ventricular hypertrophy, and overriding aorta
B. In some cases, the VSD communicates with the right ventricle in an area just distal to the outflow tract obstruction
C. Survival of patients with tetralogy of Fallot into adult life usually reflects mild to at most moderate obstruction of right ventricular outflow

D. Pseudotruncus arteriosus is a variant of tetralogy of Fallot in which complete ventricular outflow tract obstruction occurs

E. Congestive heart failure is unusual in patients with tetralogy of Fallot

---

366. True statements about atheromatous emboli include all of the following EXCEPT:

A. The most common cause of atheromatous emboli is surgical manipulation of an atherosclerotic aorta

B. Cardiac catheterization may lead to embolism of atheromatous material

C. Hepatitis is an important complication of atheromatous embolism

D. Cholesterol emboli may be visible on direct inspection of the retinal arteries

E. Livido reticularis is one manifestation of atheromatous emboli

---

367. True statements about acute myocardial infarction (AMI) include all of the following EXCEPT:

A. Approximately one-fourth of all deaths in the United States are due to AMI

B. The majority of deaths caused by AMI occur during hours 2 to 4 after the beginning of the event

C. A decline by 25 per cent or more in the incidence of AMI has occurred in recent years in the United States

D. Most deaths among patients hospitalized with AMI are attributable to left ventricular failure and shock

E. Careful monitoring of cardiac rhythm and treatment of primary arrhythmias have reduced the incidence of in-hospital death from AMI

---

368. All of the following characteristics of chest pain would be unusual for coronary artery ischemia-induced angina EXCEPT:

A. pain that begins gradually and reaches maximum intensity over a period of minutes

B. pain aggravated or precipitated by one deep breath

C. pain relieved within seconds of lying horizontally

D. pain localized to an area the size of the tip of a finger

E. pain relieved within a few seconds by one or two sips of water

---

369. True statements about women, estrogen, and the risk for coronary artery disease (CAD) include all of the following EXCEPT:

A. The atherosclerotic process does not appear to be fundamentally different between men and women

B. In older women, triglyceride concentrations are an independent risk factor for CAD

C. Estrogen therapy in the postmenopausal woman has been shown to decrease the severity of angiographically demonstrable CAD

D. Oral contraceptives are associated with an increased risk of acute MI in some studies

E. The Nurse's Health Study suggested that oral contraceptive therapy leads to an increased risk of cardiovascular disease

---

370. True statements about supravalvular aortic stenosis (AS) include all of the following EXCEPT:

A. The clinical picture of supravalvular obstruction is indistinguishable from that of other forms of AS

B. Williams' syndrome is a distinctive clinical picture produced by coexistence of supravalvular AS and a multiple-system disorder

C. Accentuation of the aortic valve closure sound is a feature characteristic of supravalvular AS

D. A continuous murmur may be heard on physical examination of some patients with known or suspected supravalvular AS

E. Echocardiography is the most valuable technique for localization of the site of obstruction in supravalvular AS

---

371. A 65-year-old woman with an aortic valve replacement has a 2-week history of malaise and fever. After developing severe right flank pain, she seeks medical attention. On examination, she has a temperature of 100°F, heart rate 100/min, and respirations 16/min. Her lungs are clear. The cardiac examination is remarkable for a grade 3/6 systolic ejection murmur and a soft diastolic blowing murmur. Laboratory results include Hgb 10 gm/dl, WBC 14,000/mm³ with 80 per cent neutrophils, 5 per cent bands, and 15 per cent lymphocytes; urinalysis reveals 3+ heme; microscopic examination reveals 15 rbc/high-power field. The most likely diagnosis is:

A. focal glomerulonephritis

B. renal infarction

C. diffuse glomerulonephritis

D. cortical necrosis

E. renal abscess

372. All of the following statements with regard to *primary* endocardial fibroelastosis (EFE) are correct EXCEPT:

A. The condition is often familial
B. The mitral and aortic valve leaflets are usually thickened and distorted
C. The murmur of mitral stenosis is the most common murmur heard
D. Symptoms of primary EFE usually develop between 2 and 12 months of age
E. Echocardiographic features include a reduced ejection fraction and increased LA and LV dimensions

373. True statements regarding the use of nicotinic acid (niacin) in the treatment of dyslipidemias include all of the following EXCEPT:

A. Pharmacological doses of niacin are used in the treatment of dyslipidemias
B. Niacin is useful in each of the hyperlipidemia phenotypes except type I
C. Niacin may decrease HDL levels by 20 to 40 per cent
D. Flushing due to niacin is prostaglandin-mediated
E. Niacin has been shown in a clinical trial to decrease total mortality

374. A 26-year-old construction worker comes to the emergency room on Monday morning, January 2, in atrial fibrillation. He states that for the last few months he has had occasional episodes of palpitation, almost always on Mondays. His vital signs include heart rate 140/min, respirations 16/min, and blood pressure 160/95. His physical examination is unremarkable except for a soft systolic murmur, and while being observed in the hospital, he spontaneously reverts to normal sinus rhythm. The most likely precipitating drug or condition is:

A. caffeine
B. "uppers"
C. alcohol
D. hypertension
E. mitral valve prolapse

375. True statements about the diagnosis of pulmonary embolism include all of the following EXCEPT:

A. Clinical symptoms and signs often are not helpful in discriminating between patients with evidence of pulmonary embolism on a pulmonary arteriogram and those without such evidence
B. Dyspnea and pleuritic chest pain are common symptoms in pulmonary embolism

C. A majority of patients with pulmonary embolism have a normal respiratory rate
D. The differential diagnosis in suspected pulmonary embolism includes asthma
E. The differential diagnosis in outpatients with suspected pulmonary embolism includes rib fracture

376. A 48-year-old man is seen in the office because of episodic palpitations. His other symptoms include paroxysmal nocturnal dyspnea, nocturnal enuresis, and mild angina. His wife adds that he snores loudly. There is a history of several recent auto accidents. On examination, his blood pressure is elevated at 190/100 and he is mildly overweight. Laboratory examination reveals a hematocrit of 58 mm Hg. The most likely cardiac finding would be:

A. mitral valve stenosis
B. aortic valve stenosis
C. right ventricular hypertrophy
D. pulmonary valve stenosis
E. atrial septal defect

377. True statements about the coronary and pathological anatomy of acute myocardial infarction (AMI) include all of the following EXCEPT:

A. One-third to two-thirds of patients who die from AMI have critical obstruction of a single coronary artery at necropsy
B. In series of patients studied at necropsy, a small number of patients with MI are found to have normal coronary vessels
C. Angiography is relatively safe even during the acute phase of MI
D. During the early hours of transmural MI, 90 per cent of infarct-related vessels are totally occluded
E. Spontaneous thrombolysis may decrease the incidence of totally occluded vessels found in the period following MI

378. True statements about pulmonic stenosis (PS) with intact ventricular septum include all of the following EXCEPT:

A. Valvular PS is the most common form of isolated right ventricular obstruction
B. The most common symptoms of PS during infancy are acidemia and hypoxemia
C. Normal heart size and primarily left ventricular forces on electrocardiography are characteristic of PS with intact ventricular septum
D. Percutaneous transluminal balloon valvuloplasty is the initial procedure of choice in patients with typical valvular PS and moderate to severe degrees of obstruction

    E. The severity of obstruction due to PS is often suggested by findings on physical examination

379. True statements about Q-wave versus non-Q-wave myocardial infarction (MI) include all of the following EXCEPT:

    A. Patients with non-Q-wave MI have a natural history different from that of patients with a Q-wave MI

    B. In-hospital mortality is greater in patients with Q-wave infarcts than in patients with non-Q-wave infarcts

    C. Three years after the MI, the overall long term mortality in Q-wave and non-Q-wave MI patients is similar

    D. Diltiazem may be useful in patients who have sustained a recent non-Q-wave infarction

    E. The majority of patients with non-Q-wave infarction have total occlusion of the infarct-related vessel

380. All of the following are members of the fastidious, slow-growing group of HACEK organisms which may cause endocarditis EXCEPT:

    A. *Haemophilus*
    B. *Actinobacillus*
    C. *Cardiobacterium*
    D. *Escherichia coli*
    E. *Kingella*

381. A 1-year-old child presents with evidence of pericarditis. Three weeks earlier he had a fever that lasted for 10 days despite penicillin therapy. Associated findings at that time included congestion of the ocular conjunctivae and erythema of the palms and feet; a nonerupting rash; and dry, erythematous, and fissured lips. One week ago there was membranous desquamation of the fingertips. Present findings include ECG evidence of pericarditis and echocardiographic documentation of decreased LV function. The most likely diagnosis is:

    A. acute rubella myocarditis
    B. Coxsackie B myocarditis
    C. *Haemophilus influenzae* myocarditis
    D. Kawasaki disease
    E. Stevens-Johnson syndrome

382. True statements about the physical examination in acute myocardial infarction (AMI) include all of the following EXCEPT:

    A. The majority of patients with uncomplicated AMI have mild systolic hypertension

    B. The majority of patients with AMI have tachycardia

    C. The majority of patients with AMI develop a mild fever

    D. The majority of patients with AMI demonstrate a muffled S_1

    E. S_4 is audible in the majority of patients with AMI

383. A 28-year-old man presented with syncope. During his evaluation, a harsh systolic murmur was noted and a complete echocardiographic examination was obtained. A panel from the M-mode portion of the study is displayed *below*. True statements regarding this case include all of the following EXCEPT:

    A. Left ventricular hypertrophy is present

    B. The patient's syncope may be due to arrhythmia

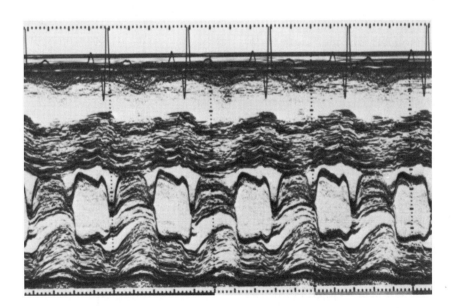

C. The E-to-F slope is markedly attenuated
D. The electrocardiogram is likely to be abnormal in this patient
E. Narrowing of the left ventricular outflow tract is present

---

384. True statements with regard to the HMG-CoA reductase inhibitors include all of the following EXCEPT:

A. These agents competitively inhibit 3-hydroxy-3-methylglutaryl coenzyme A reductase
B. Their primary mechanism of action is to decrease cholesterol synthesis
C. About 2 per cent of patients taking these agents will have a sustained rise in serum transaminase levels to three times the upper limit of normal
D. These agents usually cause a significant decrease in hepatic LDL receptors
E. Their main indication is to treat elevated LDL cholesterol

---

385. Increases in the following parameters directly increase cardiac $M\dot{V}O_2$ EXCEPT:

A. external mechanical work
B. left ventricular systolic pressure
C. left ventricular wall tension
D. left ventricular end-diastolic volume
E. none of the above

---

386. True statements about peripheral pulmonary artery stenoses include all of the following EXCEPT:

A. Pulmonary artery stenoses may occur anywhere from the main pulmonary trunk to the smallest peripheral arterial branches
B. Most often peripheral pulmonary artery stenoses are isolated findings, but occasionally they may be seen in conjunction with other cardiovascular defects
C. Intrauterine rubella infection is an important cause of pulmonary artery stenoses
D. Most children with peripheral pulmonary artery stenoses are asymptomatic
E. Percutaneous transcatheter balloon angioplasty may be used in the treatment of this disorder

---

387. A 59-year-old business executive complains of chest pain that is midsternal and that radiates primarily retrosternally. It is an aching, burning pain, occurring most frequently at night, occasionally awakening the patient shortly after he has fallen asleep. His internist prescribed nitroglycerin, which he has taken infrequently. However, it does relieve his pain, usually within 10 to 30 minutes. The previous day during a luncheon meeting, he had a severe episode while presenting a new financial plan; the pain seemed to lessen when he sat down and finished lunch. The most likely explanation for his chest pain is:

A. Prinzmetal's angina
B. esophageal reflux spasm
C. "fixed-threshold" angina
D. "variable-threshold" angina
E. biliary colic

---

388. Features common to type II hyperlipoproteinemia include all of the following EXCEPT:

A. increased low-density lipoprotein (LDL) levels
B. xanthomas of the extensor tendons
C. corneal arcus
D. premature atherosclerosis
E. recurrent pancreatitis

---

389. A 70-year-old man with multiple myeloma presented with new biventricular heart failure. An apical four-chamber view from a transthoracic echocardiographic study is displayed *at the top of the following page*. All of the following statements about this case are true EXCEPT:

A. Biventricular hypertrophy and enlarged atria are present
B. While not obvious on the present echocardiogram, a granular, sparkling texture of the thickened cardiac walls is seen in some instances with this disorder
C. In multiple myeloma, cardiac involvement of this type is uncommon
D. The most common clinical presentation of this disorder is restrictive cardiomyopathy
E. In some cases of this cardiac disorder, patients present with orthostatic hypotension

---

390. True statements about congestive heart failure in neonates and infants include all of the following EXCEPT:

A. Scalp edema, ascites, pericardial effusion, and decreased fetal movements are all findings in fetal heart failure
B. In the preterm infant, the most common cause of cardiac decompensation is a persistently patent ductus arteriosus
C. Tachycardia and pulmonary rales are uncommon manifestations of heart failure in the infant

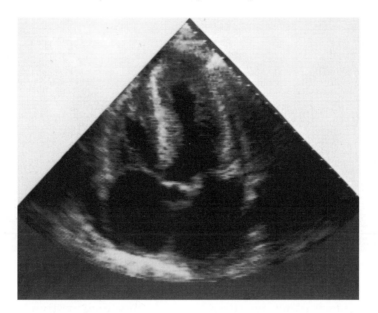

D. Pleural and pericardial effusions are rare in infants with cardiac decompensation

E. Hepatomegaly is a common finding in infants with heart failure

---

391. A 29-year-old woman presented with an atypical chest pain syndrome. During evaluation, a systolic murmur was heard at the apex, and an echocardiographic study was obtained. The panel *below* displays a portion of the M-mode echocardiogram from this study. True statements about this case include all of the following EXCEPT:

A. Systolic anterior motion of the mitral valve is evident

B. The C-D segment displays a typical finding in this study

C. M-mode echocardiography may be less sensitive in detecting this disorder than two-dimensional echocardiography

D. The presence of thickened valvular leaflets increases the risk for endocarditis in patients with this disorder

E. Color-flow Doppler may be useful in the echocardiographic examination of this disorder

---

392. A 75-year-old woman presented to her physician with severe fatigue and intermittent cyanosis. Initial evaluation revealed that cyanosis had been present for approximately 1 year and occurred chiefly during mild to moderate exertion. Transthoracic echocardiography yielded images that were suboptimal; there-

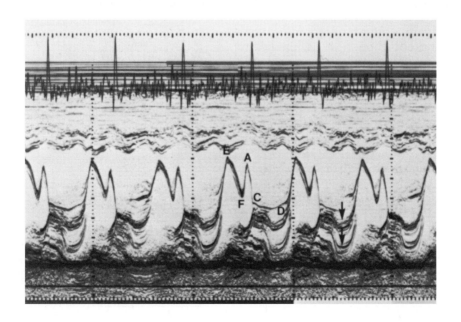

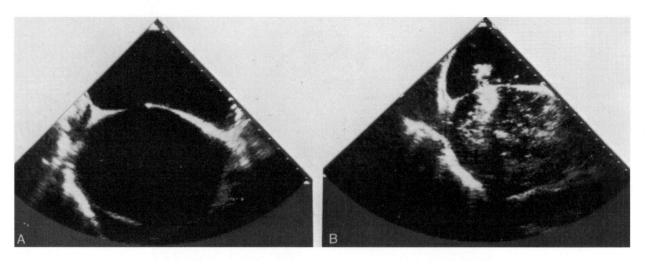

fore, transesophageal echocardiography was performed. Panel *A* shown *above* reveals a basal image from transesophageal echocardiogram, and Panel *B* shows an image obtained following injection of saline into an antecubital vein. True statements about this patient and the echocardiographic images displayed include all of the following EXCEPT:

A. The saline contrast image demonstrates right-to-left interatrial flow
B. The images verify a secundum-type atrial septal defect
C. An anomalous pulmonary vein is present
D. In transthoracic echocardiography, the subcostal position is most useful in studying the lesion displayed
E. When left atrial pressures exceed right atrial pressures in this condition, echocardardiography with saline contrast may demonstrate a negative contrast effect within the right atrium

---

393. A 29-year-old man is referred by his family practitioner for evaluation of a heart murmur first heard during childhood. He is entirely asymptomatic. Part of his evaluation included a full echocardiographic study. An M-mode echocardiogram from that study is displayed *at the right*. True statements about this case include all of the following EXCEPT:

A. A vegetation is probably present on the anterior leaflet of the mitral valve
B. The aortic valve in this disorder may be bicuspid
C. Infective endocarditis may lead to the lesion present in this case
D. This disorder is occasionally associated with ankylosing spondylitis
E. The M-mode echocardiographic findings may be present even in mild forms of this disease

394. A 62-year-old black man comes to the hospital in congestive heart failure. His symptoms include a 2-month history of progressive dyspnea and orthopnea and worsening pedal edema. The week prior to admission he had paroxysmal nocturnal dyspnea almost every night. He denies chest pain, fevers, or chills. His past history is remarkable for mild hypertension currently untreated with medication. He developed anemia 2 years ago, when a diagnosis of multiple myeloma was made. He has been stable since then on chlorambucil (Leukeran) 10 mg daily, and requiring transfusion of 1 unit of blood monthly.

On examination the heart rate was 100/min, respirations 22/min, and blood pressure 100/60. The chest showed inspiratory crackles halfway up the lung fields. His jugular venous pulse was 10 cm above the clavicle. The cardiac impulse was displaced laterally. S_1

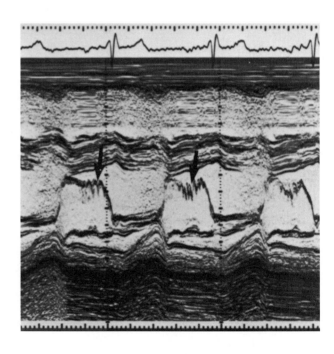

and S$_2$ were normal; a loud S$_3$ was present. A grade 2/6 holosystolic murmur radiated to the axilla. There was mild hepatosplenomegaly and 2+ pedal edema. Chest x-ray showed cardiomegaly, bilateral pleural effusions, and pulmonary vascular redistribution. ECG was normal except for low voltage. The most likely cause for his congestive heart failure is:

A. sarcoid heart disease
B. cardiac amyloidosis
C. Leukeran cardiotoxicity
D. alcoholic cardiomyopathy
E. hemochromatosis

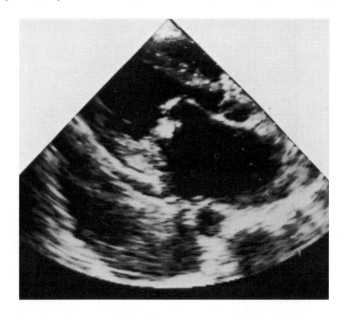

395. A 34-year-old woman presents with dyspnea and is found to be in atrial fibrillation. Following conversion to normal sinus rhythm, a full echocardiographic study is obtained. The figure *below* displays a continuous-wave Doppler recording through the mitral valve. True statements about this case include all of the following EXCEPT:

A. Doppler echocardiography is useful in quantifying the severity of mitral stenosis (MS)
B. The peak velocity of transmitral flow is usually decreased in MS
C. Mitral orifice size is better determined by two-dimensional echocardiography than by M-mode echocardiography
D. A reduced E-F slope is not pathognomonic of MS
E. In early diastole, the posterior leaflet of the mitral valve commonly moves in an anterior direction in patients with MS

396. A 42-year-old woman presents to the emergency room in pulmonary edema. Following stabilization, a complete workup is initiated. No cardiac murmurs are appreciated; the patient is referred for a full echocardiographic study. A parasternal long-axis view from the two-dimensional echocardiographic study is displayed *above*. True statements about this case include all of the following EXCEPT:

A. A left pleural effusion is present
B. Calcification is present on the mitral valve leaflet
C. The severity is directly correlated with the likelihood of developing infective endocarditis

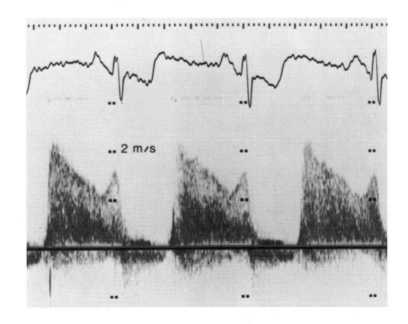

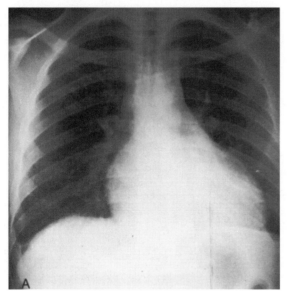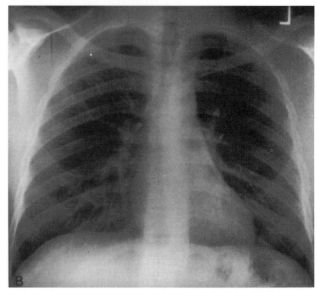

From Jay, M.: Plain Film in Heart Disease. Boston, Blackwell Scientific Publishing, 1992.

D. Approximately 15 per cent of patients with this disorder describe anginal chest pain

E. The disorder illustrated may occasionally lead to hoarseness

---

397. A 34-year-old man with known acquired immunodeficiency syndrome (AIDS) presented with the recent onset of fever and dyspnea. Physical examination revealed fever, sinus tachycardia, jugular venous distention, a pericardial friction rub, and hepatomegaly. During laboratory evaluation, the chest x-ray displayed in panel *A above* was obtained. A diagnosis was confirmed by obtaining both pericardial fluid and a pericardial biopsy specimen. The pericardial fluid was noted to have a high level of adenosine deaminase. The chest x-ray in panel *B above*, was obtained 3 weeks after the initiation of appropriate therapy. True statements about this case include all of the following EXCEPT:

A. In industrialized nations, the incidence of this disorder has steadily decreased except in immunosuppressed populations

B. Clinical detection of this disorder usually occurs either in the effusive stage or following the development of constrictive pericarditis

C. The acute onset of a characteristic severe pericardial pain is common in this disorder

D. This disorder is most likely to be diagnosed if both pericardial fluid and a pericardial biopsy specimen are obtained

E. The use of corticosteroids in addition to appropriate chemotherapy for this disorder may hasten clinical improvement

---

398. True statements regarding management of acute myocardial infarction (AMI) include all of the following EXCEPT:

A. Not all patients should receive reperfusion therapy

B. Unless contraindicated, all patients should receive aspirin

C. Thrombolytic therapy was first shown to decrease mortality in the GISSI trial

D. Thrombolytic therapy may lead to greater functional improvement for anterior infarcts than for inferior infarcts

E. An accelerated t-PA regimen is more cost effective in younger age groups

DIRECTIONS: Each question below contains suggested answers. For EACH of the alternatives, you are to respond either TRUE (T) or FALSE (F). In a given item, ALL, SOME, OR NONE OF THE ALTERNATIVES MAY BE CORRECT.

399. Acute myocardial infarction (AMI) may occasionally result from nonatherosclerotic causes. Examples of nonatherosclerotic causes of AMI include which of the following?

   A. Endocarditis
   B. Kawasaki disease
   C. Systemic lupus erythematosis
   D. Amyloidosis
   E. Cocaine abuse

400. True statements about regression of atherosclerosis include which of the following?

   A. Regression has been demonstrated in both animal and human studies
   B. When regression occurs, atherosclerotic lesions shrink in size, contain less lipid, and have a decreased collagen content
   C. Coronary angiographic studies in patients treated with aggressive lipid-lowering regimens demonstrate clear-cut regression
   D. Omega-3 fatty acids, a major component of fish oils, is the agent of choice to promote regression in patients following coronary artery bypass surgery
   E. Lovastatin has not yet been shown to promote atherosclerotic regression in patients with coronary artery disease

401. Noninvasive studies may be useful in the evaluation of patients with tetralogy of Fallot. True statements about such studies include which of the following?

   A. The electrocardiogram in tetralogy of Fallot is characterized by right ventricular hypertrophy
   B. The boot-shaped heart (coeur en sabot) is characteristic of the chest x-ray in infants and children
   C. The chest x-ray in tetralogy of Fallot is less typical in adults
   D. The abnormal relationship between the aortic annulus and the interventricular septum is rarely visible on M-mode echocardiography
   E. Magnetic resonance imaging may be helpful in assessment of tetralogy of Fallot

402. True statements with respect to the diagnosis of Prinzmetal's or variant angina include:

   A. Usually there is elevation of ST segments with pain

   B. Exercise testing of patients with variant angina is most likely to yield ST-segment elevation at low work thresholds
   C. Approximately two-thirds of patients have severe coronary artery stenosis at the site of the spasm
   D. Patients with normal coronary arteries and Prinzmetal's angina have a higher incidence of right coronary artery spasm and a more benign course
   E. Ergonovine testing with intravenous administration of 1 to 10 mg is sensitive and specific for provoking coronary artery spasm

403. With reference to the ostium primum atrial septal defect (ASD), true statements include which of the following?

   A. Ostium primum ASDs often displace and disfigure both the anterior and posterior leaflets of the mitral valve
   B. The clinical features of ostium primum ASDs are quite similar to those of the ostium secundum variety
   C. Chest roentgenography usually reveals both RA and RV enlargement
   D. The presence of an ostium primum ASD along with a ventricular septal defect in the posterobasal portion of the ventricular septum comprises the entity known as complete atrioventricular canal defect
   E. Streaming of contrast material through the ostium primum ASD into the right heart during left ventriculography creates the characteristic "gooseneck" deformity

404. True statements regarding cholesterol-lowering agents and atherosclerotic heart disease include:

   A. Regression of atherosclerosis by such agents has been demonstrated in both animal and human studies
   B. Primary prevention trials have shown a decrease in CAD mortality with HMG-CoA reductase inhibitors only
   C. Secondary prevention trials have demonstrated a decrease in atherosclerotic progression and reduction in CAD and total mortality
   D. The West of Scotland study showed a clear decrease in all-cause mortality
   E. The Scandinavian Simvastatin Survival Study included patients with CAD

405. Which of the following are true statements about the HMG-CoA reductase inhibitors?

    A. HMG-CoA reductase inhibitor therapy is most appropriate for the treatment of patients with both elevated VLDL cholesterol and decreased HDL cholesterol
    B. On average, lovastatin increases HDL cholesterol by 15 to 20 per cent
    C. The combination of an HMG-CoA reductase inhibitor and a bile-acid binding resin is especially effective in treating marked elevations of LDL
    D. Liver function test abnormalities occasionally occur with HMG-CoA reductase inhibitor therapy
    E. The HMG-CoA reductase inhibitors are efficiently cleared during first-pass circulation through the liver

406. True statements about the clinical manifestations of aortic dissection include:

    A. Men are more frequently affected than women
    B. Severe pain is the most common presenting symptom
    C. Patients with aortic dissection usually present with hypotension
    D. Aortic regurgitation is seen in the majority of patients with distal aortic dissection
    E. Pulse deficits are more common in proximal than in distal aortic dissection

407. Surgical *repair* of the mitral valve (e.g., annuloplasty and/or suture repair of the valve with repair of the chordae tendineae as necessary) might be prudent and is likely to be successful in the following patients:

    A. A 33-year-old man with Marfan syndrome and myxomatous degeneration
    B. A 62-year-old man with severe MR due to annular dilatation following MI
    C. A 40-year-old woman with MR due to a ruptured chordae tendineae with active infective endocarditis
    D. A 70-year-old woman with rheumatic heart disease, combined MS and MR with calcified mitral valve, and deformed leaflets
    E. A 23-year-old man with a congenitally cleft mitral valve

408. True statements regarding dietary therapy of dyslipidemias include which of the following?

    A. Dietary therapy has been demonstrated in angiographic studies to halt the rate of progression of atherosclerosis

    B. The appearance of new coronary lesions in patients following coronary artery bypass surgery has been shown to be influenced by dietary therapy
    C. In a Step I AHA diet, the recommended daily intake of total fat is <30 per cent of calories
    D. During pregnancy, third-trimester elevations in triglycerides and cholesterol are best approached with a Step I AHA diet
    E. Soluble fiber leads to an independent decrease in serum cholesterol of 10 to 15 per cent

409. With reference to management of ventricular septal defect (VSD), true statements include:

    A. In the absence of evidence of pulmonary hypertension, elective hemodynamic evaluation of VSD should occur between the ages of 3 and 6 years
    B. Surgical treatment for children with normal pulmonary arterial pressures and shunts >1.2:1.0 should be carried out before they begin school
    C. Right bundle branch block is the most significant surgically induced conduction system abnormality in the repair of VSD
    D. The presence of right bundle branch block with left anterior hemiblock and transient complete heart block in the postoperative period is an indication for permanent pacemaker therapy
    E. In patients who have repair of VSD, a normal resting pulmonary arterial pressure makes the presence of normal pulmonary pressures during exercise likely

410. True statements regarding PTCA as an adjunct to thrombolysis in the treatment of acute MI include:

    A. Routine empirical use of PTCA is associated with increased mortality
    B. Data from the RESCUE trial indicate a reduction in short-term mortality in the PTCA group
    C. Emergency PTCA in most studies is associated with an increased risk of abrupt closure of the infarct-related artery
    D. The success rate of rescue PTCA is <70 per cent
    E. Patients with a negative ETT following thrombolysis benefit more from PTCA than from medical therapy

411. A 62-year-old woman returns to the office for evaluation of mitral valve disease. Fifteen years earlier she had undergone a closed mi-

tral commissurotomy with excellent results. Five years ago she developed atrial fibrillation that persisted despite several attempts at cardioversion. Three years ago she was placed on warfarin because she suffered a small stroke. Her symptoms now include progressive dyspnea on exertion, rapid heart beat, and left-sided chest pain on exertion. Her clinical examination is consistent with moderate to severe mitral stenosis (MS). An echocardiogram reveals normal LV function, a markedly dilated left atrium, a heavily calcified poorly mobile aortic valve, and some mitral regurgitation. The other valves appear normal. You would advise the following:

A. cardiac catheterization
B. open commissurotomy and mitral valve repair
C. balloon mitral valvuloplasty
D. mitral valve replacement with a mechanical prosthetic valve
E. no further treatment

412. With regard to the management of tetralogy of Fallot, true statements include:

A. Early definitive repair is indicated
B. The size of the pulmonary arteries is the single most important determinant in assessing candidacy for primary repair of tetralogy of Fallot
C. If early corrective operation is not possible, a palliative procedure that leads to increased pulmonary blood flow is usually recommended
D. Postoperative increase in pulmonary vecnous return may lead to mild to moderate RV decompensation
E. Bleeding problems are a common complication in the postoperative period following repair of tetralogy of Fallot

413. Correct statements concerning the M-mode echocardiogram displayed *at right* include:

A. The mitral valve leaflets are thickened
B. The *a* wave is exaggerated
C. During diastole leaflet separation is decreased
D. The mitral valve area is probably normal
E. During diastole the posterior mitral valve leaflet moves posteriorly

414. Which of the following are true statements regarding the relationships between alcohol and coronary artery disease?

A. Alcohol use may be associated with increased blood pressure

B. An inverse correlation appears to exist between moderate alcohol use and cardiac events
C. Heavy drinkers tend to have a decreased prevalence of acute MI, although other serious morbidity exists in this group
D. CAD is inversely correlated with alcoholic intake in some angiographical studies
E. Moderate alcohol consumption tends to lower the LDL level

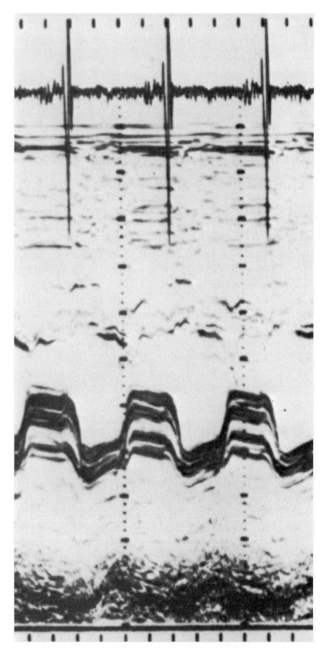

From Bloomfield, P., O'Boyle, J.E., and Parisi, A.F.: Non-invasive Investigations for the Diagnosis of Mitral Valve Disease. *In* Ionescu, M.I., and Cohn, L.H. (eds.): Mitral Valve Disease: Diagnosis and Treatment. London, Butterworths, 1985, p. 58.

415. Left ventricular aneurysm may develop as a consequence of acute myocardial infarction (AMI). True statements about left ventricular aneurysm include:

  A. Left ventricular aneurysm complicating AMI is usually due to total occlusion of the left anterior descending artery
  B. Aneurysms usually range in size from 1 to 8 cm in diameter
  C. Inferoposterior aneurysms are slightly more common than apical aneurysms
  D. When mortality in patients with left ventricular aneurysm is compared with that in patients without aneurysm but with similar ejection fractions, no substantial difference is evident
  E. Persistent ST-segment elevation in an electrocardiographic area of infarction indicates a large infarct but does not necessarily indicate an aneurysm

416. True statements about the pathophysiology of constrictive pericarditis include:

  A. Constriction leads to equalization of diastolic pressures in all four cardiac chambers
  B. Diastolic filling is unimpeded in early diastole in constrictive pericarditis
  C. Most ventricular filling occurs within the initial portion of diastole in constrictive pericarditis
  D. In general, the x descent is steeper than the y descent in constrictive pericarditis
  E. In constrictive pericarditis, the greatest acceleration of venous blood flow returning to the heart occurs during systole

417. Which of the following statements regarding risk stratification following myocardial infarction (MI) are true?

  A. Left ventricular function is the single most important factor in determining both short-term and long-term survival
  B. The presence of diabetes mellitus leads to an increased risk following MI
  C. If corrected for infarct size, the postinfarction risk for anterior wall MI and inferior MI is similar
  D. Silent postinfarction ischemia detected by ambulatory monitoring may have a prognosis similar to that of symptomatic ischemia following MI
  E. Women have a better prognosis than men following MI

418. Features typical of patients with familial myxoma include:

  A. transmission in an autosomal recessive fashion
  B. presence of multiple myxomas
  C. earlier age of initial presentation than for patients with sporadic myxoma
  D. increased incidence of pigmented nevi and lentigines
  E. increased incidence of myxomas outside the left atrium

419. Postinfarction angina may complicate acute myocardial infarction (AMI). True statements about postinfarction angina include:

  A. Both short- and long-term mortality are higher in patients with postinfarction angina
  B. Most patients who develop spontaneous angina in the early days following AMI should undergo cardiac catheterization
  C. No absolute increase in mortality is noted in patients who have true infarct extension
  D. Infarct extension occurs in <1 per cent of patients with AMI during the first 10 days after infarction

420. True statements about the management of constrictive pericarditis include:

  A. The therapy of choice for constrictive pericarditis is resection of the pericardial tissue from the anterior and inferior surfaces of the RV
  B. The operative mortality for pericardiectomy is approximately 10 to 15 per cent
  C. Most patients develop a low-output syndrome immediately following pericardiectomy for constrictive pericarditis
  D. Symptomatic improvement is reported in approximately 90 per cent of survivors of pericardiectomy
  E. In general, pericardiectomy should be performed early in the course of constrictive pericarditis in symptomatic patients

421. Myocarditis is not uncommon in association with the following viruses:

  A. Coxsackie
  B. Mumps
  C. Variola and vaccinia
  D. Echovirus
  E. Influenza

422. Perfusion lung scanning is a key diagnostic test used in screening for pulmonary embolism. True statements about perfusion lung scanning in the diagnosis of pulmonary embolism include:

A. A completely normal perfusion lung scan essentially rules out all but the smallest pulmonary emboli

B. The four designations *low*, *moderate*, *high*, and *indeterminate probability* for pulmonary embolism on perfusion lung scanning have been standardized by the American Society of Radiology

C. In general, patients with perfusion defects that are segmental or greater in size and with normal ventilation on scintigraphy in the same areas as the perfusion defects have an increased likelihood of pulmonary embolism

D. The presence of a chest x-ray abnormality in the area of a perfusion defect leads to the designation "indeterminate scan"

E. Subsegmental and nonsegmental perfusion defects that match ventilation defects may be present in patients with normal pulmonary angiography

423. Characteristics of abrupt closure following PTCA include:

A. Closure occurs in >15 per cent of cases

B. Risk factors for closure include age, gender, diabetes mellitus, and hemodialysis

C. The sole treatment objective in cases of abrupt closure is to establish adequate perfusion as a bridge to bypass surgery

D. Closure is often due to coronary vasospasm

E. Management strategies for abrupt closure include both perfusion catheters and stents

424. True statements with regard to the presentation of the patient with the valve shown *below* include:

A. The abnormality was most likely congenital

B. A systolic ejection murmur would be likely

C. Endocarditis frequently leads to this lesion

D. Diabetes mellitus and hypercholesterolemia are risk factors for development of this lesion

E. A loud diastolic blowing murmur would be likely

425. Which of the following statements regarding reperfusion injury following coronary artery occlusion are true?

A. Reperfusion injury adds substantially to the area of myocardium that is dying

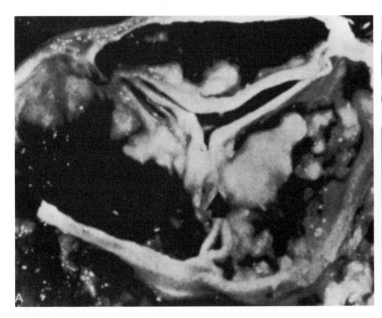

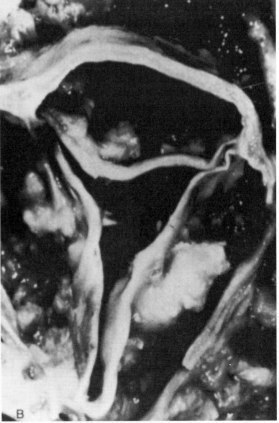

From Salem, D.N., and Isner, J.M.: Percutaneous aortic valvuloplasty. Chest *92*:326, 1987.

B. Reperfusion due to thrombolytic therapy may allow infarct extension caused by hemorrhage

C. Reasonable clinical evidence exists for the use of agents to scavenge oxygen-derived free radicals and prevent reperfusion injury

D. Reperfusion often leads to alterations in cardiac rhythm

E. Premature ventricular contractions are excellent clinical markers of reperfusion after thrombolytic therapy

426. While few absolute contraindications to physical activity exist for healthy people, there are cardiovascular contraindications to an exercise program. Absolute contraindications to such a program include:

A. resting blood pressure >200/110 mm Hg
B. unpaced third-degree heart block
C. diabetes
D. cardiomyopathy
E. ischemia

427. Appropriate steps in the *initial* management of acute pericarditis include:

A. bed rest
B. hospitalization
C. corticosteroid therapy
D. low-dose oral anticoagulants
E. antibiotics

428. Clinical features typical of mitral stenosis (MS) include:

A. greater incidence in women than in men
B. a loud first heart sound (S_1)
C. presence of a third heart sound (S_3)
D. hyperdynamic, enlarged LV
E. presence of a presystolic murmur

429. True statements about pericardiocentesis include:

A. Hydration prior to pericardiocentesis may prove useful

B. A major risk of percutaneous pericardiocentesis is laceration of the heart, coronary arteries, or lung

C. The size of the effusion is not well correlated with the probability of successfully obtaining pericardial fluid

D. Cardiac tamponade associated with malignant pericardial effusion can often be managed by pericardiocentesis

E. Pericardiocentesis is especially useful in situations in which a loculated effusion is present

430. True statements about the typical evolution of the ECG in acute pericarditis include:

A. In general, the serial appearance of four stages of abnormalities of the ST segments and T waves characterizes the electrocardiographic evolution of acute pericarditis

B. Stage I changes, or ST-segment elevation, are not often of great diagnostic value

C. The ST-segment elevation in stage I of acute pericarditis is usually most prominent in inferior leads

D. In acute pericarditis, the ST segment usually returns to baseline before the appearance of T-wave inversion

E. Stage IV electrocardiographic change is the reversion of T-wave changes to normal which may occur weeks or months following the acute episode of chest pain

431. True statements with regard to the clinical history of aortic stenosis (AS) include:

A. Average survival from the onset of syncope is approximately 3 years

B. Average survival from the onset of congestive heart failure is approximately 2 years

C. Average survival from the onset of angina pectoris is approximately 1 year

D. Sudden death in patients with AS usually occurs in previously symptomatic individuals

E. Development of atrial fibrillation is usually well tolerated in patients with moderately severe AS

432. Correct statements regarding comparisons between PTCA and CABG in ischemic heart disease include:

A. Mortality and nonfatal myocardial infarction rates in multivessel disease are similar after both PTCA and CABG

B. Relief of anginal symptoms is greater after surgery than PTCA

C. The BARI trial demonstrated a significant difference in mortality in favor of CABG among nondiabetic patients

D. The rate of subsequent revascularization as well as recurrence of angina is greater after PTCA than CABG

E. Patients who are treated with PTCA have lower initial in-hospital costs and less overall long-term expenditures

433. Asymmetrical or disproportionate septal hypertrophy may sometimes be documented by echocardiography in the following patients or conditions:

A. 6-month-old infant
B. pulmonic stenosis
C. beriberi
D. hyperthyroidism
E. following an anterior myocardial infarction

434. True statements with regard to penetrating chest wounds include:

A. Posttraumatic pericarditis is a common complication
B. Injuries to the atria are associated with a higher survival than are injuries to the ventricles
C. Rupture of the interventricular septum is often a late complication
D. The right coronary artery is the most commonly lacerated coronary artery

435. Which of the following are true statements about the management of ventricular premature beats (VPBs) in the setting of acute MI (AMI)?

A. Lidocaine is the only antiarrhythmic drug which has been shown conclusively to reduce mortality when used to treat VPBs in AMI
B. Early premature contractions (R-on-T phenomenon) in the setting of AMI are best treated with prophylactic lidocaine
C. Myocardial tissue appears to be more sensitive to procainamide in patients with AMI
D. Frequent or repetitive VPBs following AMI are an independent risk factor for sudden death
E. The CAST study results demonstrated that the drugs propafenone and ethmozine lead to an increase in sudden cardiac death in the post-AMI setting

436. Correct statements with regard to the mechanisms of action of nitrates in ischemic heart disease include:

A. Nitrates directly relax vascular smooth muscle
B. The vasodilator effects of nitrates predominate in the arterial circulation
C. Coronary arteries containing significant atherosclerotic plaque (>70 per cent stenosis) often dilate in response to nitrates
D. Nitrates increase myocardial contractility directly

E. An intact endothelium is required for nitrate-induced vasodilation

437. Patients at high risk for infective endocarditis should receive prophylactic antibiotics. Included in this group are patients with:

A. Isolated ostium secundum ASD
B. Post–coronary artery bypass
C. Hypertrophic obstructive cardiomyopathy
D. Repair of an ostium secundum ASD (without a patch) 1 year previously
E. Ventriculoatrial shunt for hydrocephalus

438. True statements about coronary arteriography and morphology in unstable angina include which of the following?

A. The left anterior descending (LAD) coronary artery is the vessel most commonly affected in patients with unstable angina
B. Patients with new onset of unstable angina have a lower incidence of three-vessel disease than those with prior angina
C. Coronary stenoses with scalloped or overhanging edges are more common in chronic stable angina than in unstable angina
D. Coronary thrombus is not commonly present in patients with rest angina
E. Plaque fissuring may be an antecedent of acute coronary syndromes such as unstable angina

439. Unusual clinical findings in a patient with hypertrophic obstructive cardiomyopathy include:

A. A prominent a wave in the jugular pulse
B. A slowing of the carotid upstroke
C. The murmur of aortic regurgitation
D. The murmur of mitral regurgitation
E. An S_3

440. Correct statements with regard to the oxygen-derived free radical system in myocardial ischemia include:

A. The superoxide anion is denoted as $\cdot O_2^-$
B. The superoxide anion can give rise to either hydrogen peroxide (H_2O_2) or the hydroxyl radical ($\cdot OH$)
C. Superoxide dismutase enzymes produce superoxide from hydrogen peroxide
D. Xanthine oxidase in the presence of xanthine may produce oxygen radicals
E. Free radicals are normally involved in cellular reactions such as oxidative phosphorylation

441. True statements concerning comparisons between PTCA and medical therapy in coronary artery disease (CAD) include:

A. PTCA confers a survival benefit in patients with single-vessel disease
B. In the Duke database, patients with multivessel disease who underwent PTCA had a better outcome and survival than those treated with medical therapy
C. The prognosis of patients with left ventricular dysfunction and CAD treated with PTCA is similar to those treated with CABG
D. In patients with single-vessel disease of the proximal LAD artery, PTCA and medical treatment lead to similar rates of MI and cardiac-related death
E. PTCA is superior to medical therapy in the relief of angina and improvement in exercise tolerance

442. Which of the following statements regarding surgery for coronary artery disease and perioperative complications are true?

A. Perioperative MI is seen in between 2 and 5 per cent of elective procedures
B. Intellectual dysfunction in the early hours after coronary artery surgery suggests the likelihood of perioperative stroke
C. Up to one-third of patients exhibit transient hypertension following coronary artery surgery
D. Patients with new fascicular conduction disturbances after coronary artery surgery have an increase in perioperative morbidity and mortality
E. Obesity is associated with an increased perioperative mortality in coronary artery surgery

443. Correct statements with regard to pathophysiological events associated with myocardial reperfusion following prolonged ischemia include:

A. Severely ischemic myocytes may demonstrate accelerated necrosis
B. Infarcts are more likely to be hemorrhagic with reperfusion
C. The reintroduction of oxygen causes marked damage to the sarcolemma and may lead to Ca^{++} overload in ischemic myocytes
D. The "no-reflow" phenomenon refers to the fact that mildly ischemic myocardium maintains sufficient vascular tone to prevent reperfusion

444. Which of the following are true statements regarding operative mortality in coronary artery bypass graft (CABG) surgery?

A. Impaired ventricular function continues to be a contraindication for CABG surgery
B. Patients of small stature have an increased operative mortality
C. Multiinstitutional data suggest that hospital death rates after CABG surgery are higher in community hospitals than in university hospitals
D. Internal mammary artery (MA) graft recipients have a reduction in long-term mortality but not in in-hospital mortality
E. The intraaortic balloon pump leads to a reduction in perioperative mortality for patients with poor left ventricular function

445. The Doppler echocardiogram illustrated *at the top of the following page* was obtained during evaluation of the mitral valve. Correct statements include:

A. Mitral stenosis is present
B. Early diastolic flow is abnormal at 2.5 m/sec
C. Mitral regurgitation is present
D. The "atrial kick" is absent
E. Panel *B* displays flow across a normal mitral valve

446. True statements about the demonstration of vegetations in endocarditis by echocardiography include:

A. Patients with one or more vegetations that are seen on echocardiography are at a higher risk for developing complications than those patients with no vegetations
B. Fungal endocarditis is more likely than bacterial endocarditis to reveal vegetations
C. *Streptococcus viridans* endocarditis rarely has demonstrable vegetations
D. A persistent vegetation usually indicates treatment failure

447. Associations of Ebstein's anomaly of the tricuspid valve include:

A. pulmonic stenosis
B. paroxysmal supraventricular tachycardia
C. Wolff-Parkinson-White syndrome
D. delay in tricuspid valve closure relative to mitral closure on M-mode echocardiography

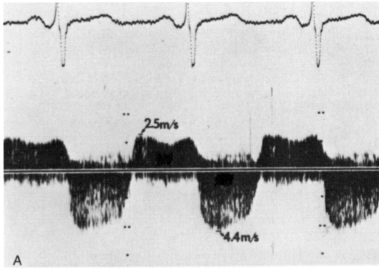

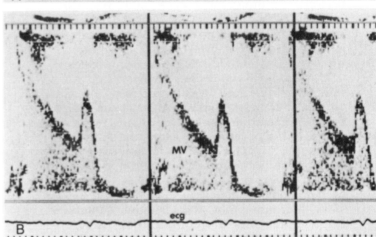

From Nishimura, R.A., Miller, F.A., Callahan, M.J., Benassi, R.C., Seward, J.B., and Tajik, A.J.: Doppler Echocardiography: Theory, Instrumentation, Technique, and Application. Mayo Clin. Proc. *60*:326, 1985.

448. True statements concerning restenosis following PTCA of native coronary arteries include:

   A. Restenosis occurs in >50 per cent of angioplastied vessels
   B. Restenosis is defined as stenosis involving >30 per cent of the vessel diameter
   C. Restenosis is due to neointimal thickening and hyperplasia, in part as a result of migration of smooth muscle cells
   D. The elastic properties of the vessel undergoing PTCA do not contribute to restenosis
   E. Male gender is associated with a high risk of restenosis

449. A 48-year-old man has a 2-week history of postprandial indigestion and nausea. On the evening of admission, after an argument with his wife, he developed abdominal pain in addition to his usual symptoms and sought medical attention. In the emergency room he had an unremarkable physical examination but his

ECG showed 2-mm ST-segment elevation in leads II, III, and aV_f. While preparations were being made for transfer to the CCU he stated that his pain suddenly disappeared; but within the next 30 sec his heart rate decreased to 30/min and his systolic pressure fell to 68 mm Hg. Likely explanation(s) include:

A. the Anrep effect
B. the Bezold-Jarisch reflex
C. rupture of an abdominal viscus
D. reperfusion of a thrombosed coronary artery

450. A 42-year-old man presents with Löffler's endocarditis. Typical findings include:

A. eosinophilia
B. ejection fraction ≤30 per cent
C. right ventricular pressure tracing showing a "square root" sign
D. asthma and nasal polyposis

451. True statements concerning cyanosis and cyanotic heart disease include:

   A. Cyanosis is due to levels of reduced hemoglobin in excess of 2 gm/dl
   B. Peripheral cyanosis is due to increased oxygen extraction from normally saturated arterial blood
   C. Cyanosis is not affected by physical exertion
   D. Differential cyanosis usually results from the presence of aortic coarctation and left-to-right shunting
   E. In cyanotic heart disease, cyanosis is sometimes improved by the squatting posture

452. A 55-year-old woman seeks medical attention because of progressive exertional dyspnea and rapid heart action. At age 12 she had rheumatic fever and has had a heart murmur since then. She has been in atrial fibrillation for 2 years with good rate control on digoxin 0.25 mg qid. Her vital signs are heart rate 80/min, blood pressure 130/80, and respirations 16/min. She has inspiratory rales at the lung bases. Her cardiac impulse is displaced laterally and is prominent. There are a loud S_1, single S_2, an opening snap, a holodiastolic rumbling murmur at the apex, and a soft diastolic blowing murmur along the left sternal border. Isometric handgrip augments the diastolic murmur while administration of amyl nitrite diminishes the murmur. She has 1+ peripheral edema. Her ECG is illustrated *at right*. The most likely diagnosis(es) is (are):

   A. tricuspid stenosis
   B. aortic regurgitation
   C. mitral regurgitation
   D. mitral stenosis

453. Characteristics of the opening snap (OS) in mitral stenosis (MS) include:

   A. The A_2-OS interval varies directly with left atrial pressure
   B. A short A_2-OS interval (<0.08 sec) is a reliable indicator of significant MS
   C. Sudden standing narrows the A_2-OS interval
   D. During exercise the A_2-OS interval narrows

454. Descriptions of the hemodynamic measurements characteristically obtained at cardiac catheterization in patients with cardiac tamponade include:

   A. prominent *y* descent
   B. an elevated right ventricular diastolic pressure

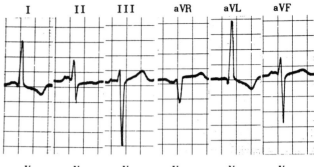

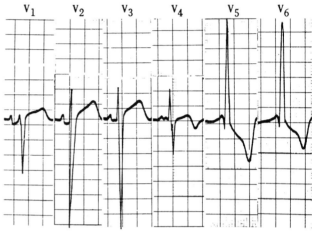

From Massie, E., and Walsh, T.J.: Clinical Vectorcardiography and Electrocardiography. Chicago, Year Book Medical Publishers, 1960, p. 136.

   C. an intrapericardial—right atrial pressure difference of 2 to 5 mm Hg
   D. the absence of a dip-and-plateau configuration in the right ventricular pressure tracing

455. Correct statements with regard to Chagas' disease include:

   A. The causative organism is *Brucella cruzi*
   B. The classic echocardiographic findings are those of a dilated cardiomyopathy with an apical aneurysm
   C. The most common ECG abnormality in chronic Chagas' disease is left bundle branch block
   D. The disease is transmitted to humans by the reduviid bug

456. Mechanisms that have been identified for cardiac dysfunction associated with excessive alcohol consumption include:

   A. direct toxic effect of alcohol and/or its metabolites
   B. beriberi heart disease

C. toxic effects due to additives in the beverage (e.g., cobalt)

D. hyperkalemia-induced contractile dysfunction

---

457. Correct statements about the rhythm displayed *below* in the setting of acute myocardial infarction (AMI) include:

A. This rhythm is present in between 10 and 15 per cent of patients with AMI

B. This rhythm is a consequence of left atrial ischemia in most cases

C. This rhythm in association with hemodynamic compromise should be treated by electrical cardioversion

D. This rhythm is the least common of atrial arrhythmias associated with AMI

---

458. Patent ductus arteriosus (PDA) in premature infants is characterized by:

A. significant deterioration in approximately one-third of infants

B. a normal cardiac silhouette on chest radiography

C. pharmacological responsiveness to indomethacin that leads to constriction and frequently to closure of the PDA

D. an absence of clinical findings on the cardiovascular examination

E. noninvasive evidence of shunting before physical findings are apparent

---

459. True statements regarding coronary bypass grafts include:

A. Approximately 10 per cent of saphenous venous grafts become occluded during the early perioperative period

B. Early graft closure is often due to thrombosis

C. In emergency bypass surgery, it is still often possible to use internal mammary artery conduits

D. Approximately 40 to 60 per cent of saphenous vein grafts are occluded at 10 years following bypass surgery

E. Patients receiving internal mammary artery conduits have a decreased risk of late death and myocardial infarctions

---

460. Correct statements regarding hemodynamic findings in patients with hypertrophic obstructive cardiomyopathy include:

A. Systolic function is usually impaired to a greater extent than diastolic function

B. The majority of ventricular emptying is more rapid than usual

C. Left ventricular end-diastolic pressure is usually normal

D. Ejection fraction is usually normal

E. The gradient may vary on a daily basis

---

461. Dynamic maneuvers to produce changes in the timing and intensity of the systolic click and murmur in the mitral valve prolapse (MVP) syndrome are helpful diagnostically. Correct statements include:

A. Sudden standing causes the click and murmur to occur earlier in systole

B. Propranolol causes the click and murmur to increase in intensity and to occur earlier

C. Handgrip causes a delay in onset of the click and murmur

D. During the straining phase of the Valsalva maneuver the click and murmur occur later in systole

---

462. True statements concerning tetralogy of Fallot include:

A. Tetralogy of Fallot accounts for 2 to 3 per cent of all forms of congenital heart disease

B. It is the most common cause of cardiac cyanosis after 1 year of age

C. Tetralogy of Fallot can be associated with anomalous coronary circulation

D. The degree of right-to-left shunting in tetralogy of Fallot depends to a large extent on the severity of the pulmonary obstruction

E. Overriding of the aorta in this anomaly is due to dextroposition of the aorta

---

463. In patients with combined aortic regurgitation (AR) and aortic stenosis (AS), cardiac output used in the Gorlin formula to calculate valve area should be the:

A. Fick output

B. dye indicator output

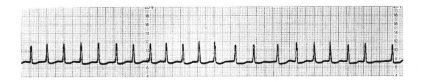

C. pulmonary artery saturation output

D. angiographic LV output

---

464. Characteristics of aortic injuries due to blunt trauma include:

    A. evidence of other thoracic trauma
    B. an abnormal chest x-ray
    C. an absence of specific symptoms
    D. survival for the majority of patients who reach the hospital alive
    E. excellent detection by CT scanning with contrast

---

465. Persistent patent ductus arteriosus is characterized by:

    A. exercise intolerance
    B. wide arterial pulse pressure
    C. normal sinus rhythm
    D. diagnostic M-mode echocardiogram
    E. differential cyanosis until pulmonary pressures rise

---

466. True statements regarding hypertension in infants and children include:

    A. Secondary causes of hypertension are more common than essential hypertension
    B. Blood pressure cuff sizes should be appropriate, since a cuff that is too small will produce spuriously low readings
    C. The most common cause of secondary hypertension is renal damage
    D. There is no familial tendency for susceptibility to hypertension
    E. Hypertension occurs in <0.5 per cent of infants and children

---

467. Myocardial contusion treatment normally includes:

    A. Bed rest, gradual ambulation over 7 to 10 days
    B. Analgesia with nonsteroidal antiinflammatory agents for chest pain

---

C. Cardiac monitoring for 3 to 5 days
D. Anticoagulation to prevent systemic embolization
E. Cardiac catheterization

---

468. Appropriate steps in the management of patients with acute aortic dissection include:

    A. combined sodium nitroprusside and beta blocker therapy
    B. administration of a loop diuretic
    C. surgical repair for cases of proximal dissection
    D. surgical repair for cases of distal dissection
    E. avoidance of narcotics for pain relief

---

469. The following may be considered primary hypercoagulable states:

    A. antithrombin III deficiency
    B. presence of lupus anticoagulant
    C. protein C deficiency
    D. oral contraceptive use

---

470. Correct statements about the arrhythmia illustrated *below* when seen in the setting of acute myocardial infarction (AMI), include:

    A. This rhythm may be seen in up to 20 per cent of patients with AMI
    B. This rhythm confers a small but significant increase in morbidity and mortality
    C. This rhythm commonly occurs due to slowing of the sinus rhythm
    D. This rhythm is initiated almost exclusively by the occurrence of a premature beat

---

471. The following events will increase the gradient and systolic murmur of hypertrophic obstructive cardiomyopathy:

    A. sudden standing from a squatting position
    B. a spontaneous premature contraction
    C. administration of amyl nitrite
    D. the Müller maneuver

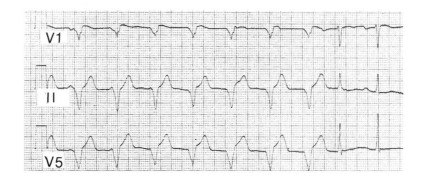

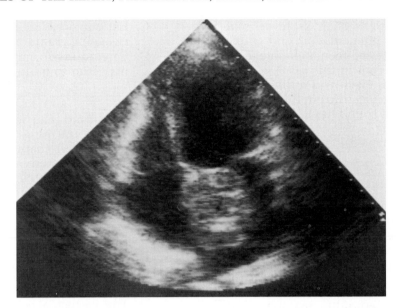

472. A 52-year-old man suffered a large anterior myocardial infarction (MI) (CPK maximum, 4000 given intravenously) 2 months ago. Since then he has had symptoms of persistent mild congestive heart failure despite taking 80 mg furosemide qid. His ECG shows ST-segment elevations in V_2–V_4. An enlarged cardiac silhouette is present on chest x-ray. Correct statements with regard to diagnosis and management include:

A. Anticoagulation for 4 to 6 months is prudent
B. Biplane left ventriculography is more likely to define accurately his problem than two-dimensional echocardiography
C. He is likely to have multivessel coronary artery disease
D. Surgical intervention should be planned within the next 1 to 2 weeks

473. A 55-year-old businessman presents to the office complaining of increasing fatigue and shortness of breath. He has also noticed that he is more comfortable sleeping on three pillows. He denies any change in his usual habits and also denies chest pain or pleuritic pain. His only medications are hydrochlorthiazide and a beta blocker for hypertension of 10 years' duration. His past medical history is remarkable for an appendectomy. He smokes $1/2$ to 1 pack of cigarettes per day. He drinks whiskey socially and admits to one or two martinis at lunch. There is no family history of heart disease.

On examination the heart rate is 104/min, respirations 20/min, blood pressure 150/90. There are grade II hypertensive changes in the fundi. His lungs reveal bibasilar rales over the lower third of the lung fields; the carotid up-strokes are normal. The apical impulse is lat-

erally displaced and sustained. S_1 and S_2 are normal with an increased A_2. There is a loud S_4 and a moderately loud S_3. There is a grade 2/6 holosystolic murmur that radiates to the axilla. The remainder of the examination is normal except for a trace of pedal edema. The chest x-ray and ECG show left ventricular hypertrophy. The most likely cause(s) for this man's congestive heart failure is (are):

A. hypertension
B. alcohol
C. coronary atherosclerosis
D. idiopathic hypertrophic subaortic stenosis

474. True statements with regard to blood flow in the subendocardium as compared with the subepicardium include:

A. Systolic flow is less in the subendocardium
B. Total subendocardial flow under normal conditions is equal to or greater than subepicardial flow
C. An elevation of ventricular end-diastolic pressure will reduce subendocardial flow to a greater extent than subepicardial flow
D. The reserve for vasodilatation in the subendocardium is greater than in the subepicardium

475. A 50-year-old woman presented following a recent transient neurological event. During her evaluation, she underwent a transthoracic echocardiogram. An apical four chamber view from the study is displayed *above*. Which of the following statements about this case are true?

A. The echocardiographic appearance makes thrombus the most likely diagnosis for the lesion displayed

B. Systemic symptoms such as fever, malaise, Raynaud's phenomenon, and an elevated erythrocyte sedimentation rate (ESR) might all be present in this case
C. The neurological event was unlikely to be related to the echocardiographic findings
D. A soft first heart sound might be expected in this patient
E. The lesion displayed is most likely to be malignant

476. Which of the following statements regarding aortic balloon valvuloplasty are true?

A. A retrograde (aorta-to-left ventricle) approach is preferred for aortic balloon valvuloplasty
B. The procedural mortality for aortic valvuloplasty is approximately 5 per cent
C. In general, the need for repeat aortic valvuloplasty is low (<10 per cent)
D. Orifice improvement after aortic valvuloplasty is usually more marked than that seen after mitral valvuloplasty
E. Vascular injury at the access site occurs in 5 to 10 per cent of aortic valvuloplasty procedures

477. Tissue plasminogen activator (t-PA) may play a role in the thrombolytic treatment of acute pulmonary embolism. True statements about t-PA in this setting include:

A. t-PA causes more fibrin-specific thrombolysis and less hemorrhage than either urokinase or streptokinase in animal models
B. The majority of patients who receive t-PA demonstrate significant clot lysis within 6 hours
C. In clinical trials to date, there is approximately a 5 per cent incidence of major bleeding with t-PA
D. For large or massive pulmonary embolism, t-PA is the current therapy of choice

478. True statements regarding sarcoid heart disease include:

A. Less than 10 per cent of patients with pulmonary sarcoidosis have clinical manifestations of sarcoid heart disease
B. Conduction disturbances are the most frequent clinical indication of sarcoid heart disease

C. Endomyocardial biopsy may reveal noncaseating granulomas and fibrosis
D. Sarcoid involvement of the cardiac valves may lead to mitral and/or aortic stenosis

479. A 49-year-old man with metastatic adenocarcinoma of the lung presents with anasarca. An apical four-chamber view from an echocardiographic study is displayed *on the following page*. Which of the following statements regarding this case are true?

A. Diastolic collapse of the free wall of the right atrium is present
B. Diastolic collapse of the right ventricle is evident
C. Malignant disease is the most common cause of cardiac tamponade
D. The absence of echocardiographic evidence of a pericardial effusion would virtually exclude the diagnosis of cardiac tamponade in this case
E. The presence of right ventricular hypertrophy may obscure right ventricular diastolic collapse in the presence of tamponade physiology

480. True statements regarding primary tumors of the heart include:

A. Benign tumors are more common than malignant tumors
B. The most common malignant cardiac tumors are angiosarcomas and rhabdomyosarcomas
C. The presence of a hemorrhagic pericardial effusion is consistent with a malignant tumor
D. Malignant tumors are more likely to occur on the left side of the interatrial septum

481. True statements about chylomicrons include:

A. They are composed mainly of triglycerides
B. Chylomicrons are frequently present in fasting plasma
C. Chylomicronemia per se is not thought to contribute to premature coronary artery disease
D. Chylomicrons are cleared from the blood in the liver by action of the enzyme acyl cholesterol acyl transferase (ACAT)

482. The following is (are) commonly associated with viral pericarditis:

A. Coxsackie virus group B
B. peak incidence in the spring and fall

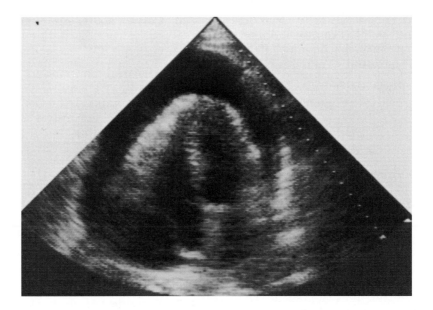

C. frequent prodromal syndrome
D. short-term recurrence rate of between 15 and 40 per cent
E. frequent relapses

483. Correct statements with respect to low-density lipoproteins (LDLs) include:

A. LDLs are the major cholesterol-carrying components of plasma
B. The major lipid components of LDL are triglyceride and esterified cholesterol
C. LDL is mainly formed from VLDL metabolism
D. Apo A-I is the dominant protein present in LDL

484. A 66-year-old woman with chronic stable angina returns to her home in New York from a Florida vacation. After carrying her suitcases up two flights of stairs, she develops her usual anginal pain. She cannot locate her nitroglycerin pills in her purse, so she uses some pills on the window sill in her kitchen. Despite taking three tablets, she obtains no relief. Finally, she locates her other nitroglycerin and obtains relief in 5 minutes. Her other medications include propranolol 40 mg qid and isosorbide dinitrate 40 mg qid. The most likely explanation(s) for the failure of the initial three pills to relieve her angina is (are):

A. poor absorption due to dry mouth
B. development of an anxiety state

C. loss of potency
D. nitrate tolerance

485. Features of constrictive pericarditis on physical examination include:

A. pulsus paradoxus
B. systolic retraction of the apical impulse
C. midsystolic pericardial knock
D. hepatomegaly

486. Passive collapse of a stenotic coronary artery when myocardial flow increases is due to the following hemodynamic principles:

A. As flow increases, there is an exponential rise in the pressure gradient across the stenosis
B. As flow increases, turbulence causes a rise in intraluminal pressure
C. A rise in the transstenotic pressure gradient causes a fall in intraluminal pressure
D. As flow increases intromyocardial pressure rises, which causes increased extrinsic compression of blood vessels

487. Criteria that necessitate prophylaxis for deep venous thrombosis (DVT) and pulmonary embolism in general surgical patients include:

A. obesity
B. age ≥40 years
C. a surgical procedure >1 hour in duration
D. known cancer

488. The following drugs are typically used for treatment of chronic stable (exercise-induced) angina. Drugs that cause detrimental effects in patients with Prinzmetal's angina include:

    A. Ca^{++} channel antagonists
    B. aspirin
    C. nitrates
    D. beta blockers

489. True statements with regard to acquired aortic stenosis (AS) due to rheumatic disease as compared with degenerative (senile) calcific disease include:

    A. AS secondary to rheumatic disease is more likely to have associated aortic regurgitation (AR)
    B. Commissural fusion is the hallmark of the rheumatic aortic valve
    C. There is an increased incidence of degenerative AS in patients with hypercholesterolemia or diabetes mellitus
    D. In degenerative AS, calcific deposits at the tips of the valve leaflets narrow the opening to blood flow

490. Correct statements with regard to the severity of obstruction in pure mitral stenosis (MS) include:

    A. Atrial contraction increases the presystolic transmitral valvular gradient by approximately 30 per cent
    B. When the mitral valve area is ≤2.0 cm^2, little additional flow can be achieved regardless of the transvalvular pressure gradient
    C. At any given valve area the transvalvular pressure gradient is a function of the square of the transvalvular flow rate
    D. At any given valve area the transvalvular pressure gradient is directly proportional to the transvalvular flow rate

491. Secondary causes of type IV hyperlipoproteinemia (primary increased VLDL) include:

    A. diabetes mellitus
    B. hypothyroidism
    C. nephrotic syndrome
    D. neurofibromatosis

DIRECTIONS: The group of questions below consists of lettered headings followed by a set of numbered items. For each numbered item select the ONE lettered heading with which it is MOST closely associated. Each lettered heading may be used ONCE, MORE THAN ONCE, OR NOT AT ALL.

For each statement, match the appropriate substance.

    A. Elevate(s) HDL cholesterol
    B. Elevate(s) LDL cholesterol
    C. Have (has) no significant effect on lipoproteins
    D. Lower(s) cholesterol
    E. Lower(s) VLDL cholesterol

492. Thiazide diuretics

493. Propranolol

494. Estrogens

495. Calcium channel antagonists

For each congenital cardiac abnormality listed, match the appropriate descriptive phrase.

    A. Persistent truncus arteriosus
    B. Coronary arteriovenous fistula
    C. Anomalous pulmonary origin of the coronary artery
    D. Ruptured aortic sinus aneurysm
    E. Aortic arch obstruction

496. This defect is always accompanied by ventricular septal defect (VSD)

497. Myocardial infarction is the most common clinical presentation

498. This malformation usually involves the right coronary artery

499. This anomaly is frequently characterized by a history of chest pain of recent onset

Match the following cell types potentially involved in atherogenesis listed below with the appropriate descriptive phrase.

    A. Endothelial cell
    B. Smooth muscle cells
    C. Macrophage
    D. Platelet

500. Demonstrate(s) proliferation in the intima in atherosclerosis

501. Is (are) the principal cell(s) of the fatty streak

502. Secrete(s) prostacyclin

503. Is (are) capable of little or no protein synthesis

For each disease, match the appropriate statement.

    A. Viral myocarditis
    B. Diphtheritic cardiomyopathy
    C. Trypanosomal myocarditis
    D. None of the above

504. Cardiac symptomatology may occur after a symptom-free interval of many years

505. The majority of children who develop this condition recover with few or no sequelae

506. Papillary muscle involvement may lead to a characteristic murmur of mitral regurgitation

507. The typical electrocardiographic presentation includes left ventricular hypertrophy and inverted T waves in the left precordial leads

508. Electrocardiographic changes range from ST-segment and T-wave changes to arrhythmias and conduction disturbances

---

For each aortic outflow tract disease, match the appropriate finding.

    A. Acquired nonrheumatic aortic stenosis
    B. Hypertrophic obstructive cardiomyopathy
    C. Congenital subvalvular stenosis
    D. Congenital supravalvular stenosis
    E. Congenital valvular stenosis

509. Normal carotid pulse on the right but slow rise on the left

510. Mitral regurgitation is frequently present

511. Aortic ejection sound is commonly present

512. Murmur of mitral regurgitation due to Gallavardin phenomenon is suggested

---

For each statement, match the appropriate lesion.

    A. Osler nodes
    B. Janeway lesions
    C. Roth spots
    D. Subungual hemorrhages
    E. Bracht-Wächter bodies

513. Small (1 to 4 mm diameter), irregular, erythematous nontender macules present on the thenar and hypothenar eminences of the hands

514. Small, raised red (or purple) tender lesions present in the pulp spaces of the terminal phalanges of the fingers

515. Collections of lymphocytes in the nerve layer of the retina

516. Collections of lymphocytes and mononuclear cells in the myocardium

---

For each drug, match the appropriate statement.

    A. Nicotinic acid
    B. Neomycin sulfate
    C. Cholestyramine
    D. Probucol
    E. Gemfibrozil

517. May decrease prothrombin time in patients taking warfarin

518. May increase prothrombin time in patients taking warfarin

519. Most likely to cause impaired glucose tolerance and hyperuricemia

520. Most likely to lower HDL

For each drug(s) listed, match the effect on concomitant use of beta-blocking agents.

    A. Cimetidine
    B. Aluminum hydroxide gel
    C. Barbiturates
    D. Lidocaine
    E. Calcium carbonate antacids

521. Enhance(s) metabolism of beta blockers and reduce(s) plasma level(s)

522. Reduce(s) hepatic metabolism of beta blockers and increase(s) plasma levels

523. Reduce(s) gastrointestinal absorption of beta blockers and reduce(s) plasma levels

For each prosthetic device, match the appropriate statement.

    A. Starr Edwards valve
    B. Carpentier-Edwards valve
    C. St. Jude valve
    D. Hancock valve
    E. Lillehei-Kaster valve

524. Pivoting-disc valve that has relatively high incidence of thrombosis in small sizes or in aortic position

525. Lowest profile mechanical valve

526. Least thrombogenic mechanical prosthesis for the mitral position

527. The tissue valve with the better hemodynamic profile

For each, match the most appropriate statement.

    A. Constrictive pericarditis
    B. Restrictive cardiomyopathy
    C. Both
    D. Neither

528. Atrial fibrillation, diffuse low QRS voltage

529. RV systolic pressure >60 mm Hg

530. Normal motion of the crista supraventricularis present on angiography

531. 80 per cent of LV filling occurs in the first half of diastole

    A. Behçet's syndrome
    B. Systemic sclerosis
    C. Ankylosing spondylitis
    D. Reiter's syndrome
    E. Giant cell arteritis

532. Granuloma formation in the coronary arteries

533. Uveitis and urethritis

534. Myocardial fibrosis and contraction band necrosis

535. Histologically similar to syphilitic aortitis

536. Occlusion of the subclavian artery and aneurysms of the common carotid artery

---

    A. Myxoma
    B. Sarcoma
    C. Rhabdomyoma
    D. Lipoma
    E. Papillary fibroelastoma

537. Right atrial involvement is most common

538. May be accompanied by multiple blue nevi

539. Most common cardiac valve tumor

540. Often seen in the intraatrial septum

541. May be seen in patients with tuberous sclerosis

DIRECTIONS: The group of questions below consists of four lettered headings followed by a set of numbered items. For each numbered item select

A if the item is associated with (A) *only*
B if the item is associated with (B) *only*
C if the item is associated with *both* (A) and (B)
D if the item is associated with *neither* (A) nor (B)

Each lettered heading may be used ONCE, MORE THAN ONCE, OR NOT AT ALL.

A. Supravalvular aortic stenosis
B. Discrete subaortic stenosis
C. Both
D. Neither

542. Commonly associated with mental retardation

543. Associated with idiopathic infantile hypercalcemia

544. Commonly accompanied by tricuspid stenosis

545. Mild degrees of aortic regurgitation are commonly observed

546. Dilatation of the ascending aorta is common

A. Heparin
B. Alpha-methyldopa
C. Procainamide
D. Nitroglycerin

547. Erythematous rash, anemia

548. Coombs'-positive hemolysis

549. Chocolate-colored blood, normal P_{O_2}

550. Thrombocytopenia with thromboemboli

A. Heparin
B. Thrombolytic therapy
C. Both
D. Neither

551. May be effective up to 2 weeks after the onset of symptoms of pulmonary embolism

552. Dissolution of recently formed thrombus is a major action

553. In general, should be used along with an antiplatelet agent

554. May cause aldosterone depression

555. Inhibits erythrocyte aggregation and leukocyte plugging

A. Type II glycogen storage disease
B. Mucocutaneous lymph node syndrome (Kawasaki disease)
C. Both
D. Neither

556. Inherited as an autosomal dominant disorder

557. Congestive heart failure may be an important complication

558. Intravenous gamma globulin may be a useful therapy

559. The etiology of the disorder remains unknown

560. The electrocardiogram may demonstrate a short P-R interval

---

A. Fatty streak
B. Fibrous plaque
C. Both
D. Neither

561. Earliest lesion of atherosclerosis

562. Lipid-filled smooth muscle cells are present

563. Is composed primarily of macrophages

564. Is commonly found within the length of the renal arteries

565. Is grossly white in appearance

A. Tricuspid stenosis
B. Pulmonic stenosis
C. Both
D. Neither

566. Usually rheumatic in origin

567. May be associated with carcinoid heart disease

568. Most adults are asymptomatic

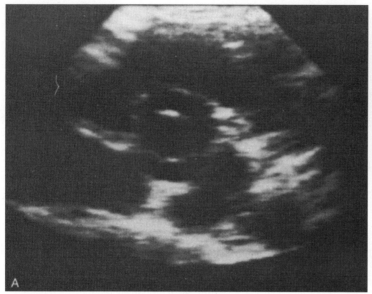
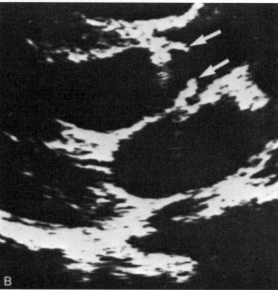

From Stewart, W.J., King, M.E., Gillam, L.D., et al.: Prevalence of aortic valve prolapse with bicuspid aortic valve and its relation to aortic regurgitation: A cross-sectional echocardiographic study. Am. J. Cardiol. *54*:1277, 1984.

From Stewart, W.J.: The diagnosis of clinically suspected left ventricular outflow tract obstruction. *In* Miller, D.D., Burns, R.J., Gill, J.B., and Ruddy, T.D. (eds.): Clinical Cardiac Imaging. New York, McGraw-Hill, 1988, p. 466.

569. Ascites is common on physical examination

570. Balloon valvuloplasty is the treatment of choice

    A. Emphysema
    B. Chronic bronchitis
    C. Both
    D. Neither

571. Cardiomegaly on chest x-ray

572. Pulmonary hypertension at rest

573. Markedly decreased oxygen-diffusion capacity

574. Repeated episodes of right heart failure

    A. ⎱
    B. ⎰ *See illustration above*
    C. Both
    D. Neither

575. The most common congenital cardiac anomaly

576. Patients having dental procedures require antibiotic prophylaxis

577. Often associated with ankylosing spondylitis

578. May be associated with aortic valve prolapse

579. May be associated with angina

    A. Acute ventricular septal rupture in the presence of acute myocardial infarction (AMI)
    B. Acute mitral regurgitation in the presence of AMI
    C. Both
    D. Neither

580. A murmur due to this lesion may decrease in intensity as arterial pressure falls

581. Pulmonary artery wedge pressure tracings may demonstrate large *v* waves

582. A characteristic diastolic murmur is usually present

583. Occurs primarily with large infarctions

    A. Chronic constrictive pericarditis
    B. Cardiac amyloidosis
    C. Both
    D. Neither

584. Right ventricular pressure tracing showing a deep and rapid early decline at the onset of diastole, with a rapid rise to a plateau in early diastole ("square root" sign)

585. Left ventricular end-diastolic pressure (LVEDP) 10 mm Hg greater than right ventricular end-diastolic pressure (RVEDP)

586. Peak RV systolic pressure = 35 mm Hg, RVEDP = 18 mm Hg

587. Pulmonary artery systolic pressure = 60 mm Hg, RVEDP = 15 mm Hg

---

A. Takayasu's arteritis
B. Giant cell arteritis
C. Both
D. Neither

588. Occurrence is predominantly in women

589. Onset is typically during teenage years

590. Jaw muscle claudication suggests the diagnosis

591. Fever is almost always present

592. Steroid therapy is a cornerstone of management

A. Mitral regurgitation (not due to prolapse)
B. Aortic stenosis
C. Both
D. Neither

593. Systolic murmur decreases in intensity during the strain of the Valsalva maneuver

594. Systolic murmur increases in intensity with handgrip

595. Systolic murmur becomes softer after administration of amyl nitrite

596. Systolic murmur intensity varies significantly from beat-to-beat in atrial fibrillation

---

A. Complete transposition of the great arteries
B. Total anomalous pulmonary venous connection
C. Both
D. Neither

597. An interatrial communication is frequently present

598. A majority of patients have symptoms during the first year of life

599. Cardiac murmurs are not a prominent clinical feature

600. The electrocardiogram most commonly shows right atrial enlargement and right ventricular hypertrophy

601. Balloon atrial septostomy may provide dramatic palliation

---

A. Amoxicillin 3.0 gm orally 1 hour before procedure; then 1.5 gm 6 hours after initial dose
B. Erythromycin ethlysuccinate 800 mg, or erythromycin stearate 1.0 gm orally 2 hours before procedure; then half the dose 6 hours after initial dose
C. Ampicillin 2 gm IV (or IM) and gentamicin 1.5 mg/kg IV (or IM) 30 minutes before procedure followed by amoxicillin 1.5 gm orally 6 hours after initial dose
D. No antibiotic prophylaxis required

602. Extraction of a tooth in a penicillin-allergic patient with a mechanical aortic valve

603. Cystoscopy in a patient with hypertrophic obstructive cardiomyopathy

604. Laminectomy in a patient with an implanted defibrillator

605. Tonsillectomy in a child with a ventricular septal defect

---

A. Myocardial infarction
B. Endocardial fibrosis
C. Capillary leak syndrome
D. Congestive heart failure

606. Interleukin-2

607. 5-Fluorouracil

608. Ifosfamide

609. Busulfan

A. Patent ductus arteriosus
B. Complete atrioventricular canal defect
C. Both
D. Neither

610. A common AV orifice is frequently present

611. An association with rubella infection during the first trimester is noted

612. Heart failure in early infancy is common

613. A "gooseneck" deformity is seen during left ventricular angiography.

614. A blowing, high-pitched decrescendo diastolic murmur is common at the left sternal border

---

A. Atenolol
B. Propranolol

C. Both
D. Neither

615. Relatively lipid-soluble

616. Accumulates in renal failure

617. Has intrinsic sympathomimetic activity

618. Relatively selective for beta$_2$-adrenoceptors

Part III
Diseases of the Heart, Pericardium, Aorta, and Pulmonary Vascular Bed

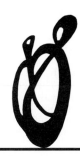

CHAPTERS 29 THROUGH 47

ANSWERS

286-A *(Braunwald, pp. 896–898)*

Atrial septal defect is one of the more common acyanotic congenital heart diseases, which is commonly not diagnosed until late in childhood or adulthood. Although ASD is commonly asymptomatic, children, especially those with larger shunts, tend to be physically somewhat underdeveloped, and may experience exertional dyspnea and easy fatigability. They may also present with frequent respiratory tract infections. Atrial arrhythmias and pulmonary hypertension as presenting complaints are uncommon. Physical examination usually reveals the diagnostic wide fixed splitting of the second heart sound. The first heart sound is normal, with some patients having an accentuated tricuspid valve component. It is never widely split on the basis of ASD alone. The electrocardiogram may be helpful in determining the type of ASD. Secundum ASD patients exhibit right axis deviation on ECG, while those with primum ASD characteristically exhibit left axis deviation. Patients with sinus venosus ASD exhibit left axis deviation of the P wave axis (not the QRS axis), and P-R prolongation can be seen with all types of ASD. Operative repair is advised for all patients with pulmonary-systemic flow ratios ≥1.5:1.0.[1,2] Repair is ideally carried out in those 2 to 4 years old.

REFERENCES

1. Konstantinides, S., and Geibel, A., Olschewski, M., et al.: A comparison of surgical and medical therapy for atrial septal defect in adults. N. Engl. J. Med. *333*:469–473, 1995.
2. Gatzoulis, M.A., Redington, A.N., Somerville, J., and Shore, D.F.: Should atrial septal defects in adults be closed? Ann. Thorac. Surg. *61*:657–659, 1996.

287-C *(Braunwald, pp. 1039–1041)*

The Doppler recording displayed demonstrates a velocity of 4 m/sec, which is consistent with a peak instantaneous systolic gradient across the aortic valve of 64 mm Hg. The patient in question thus presents with symptomatic aortic stenosis (AS). Angina pectoris, syncope, and heart failure are the cardial symptoms of AS.[1] The onset of symptoms in patients with AS is an ominous sign: Survival curves show that the time of death following symptom occurrence is approximately 5 years for patients with angina, 3 years for those with syncope, and 2 years for patients with heart failure.[2] Dyspnea is the most frequent presenting complaint in AS, and angina is present as well in approximately two-thirds of patients with critical AS. Angina may occur in the absence of significant coronary artery obstruction in up to half of patients presenting with the symptom, owing to both increased oxygen demands by the hypertrophied left ventricle and decreased oxygen delivery from excessive compression of the smaller coronary vessels.[3] Symptoms of congestive heart failure are due to varying degrees of pulmonary venous hypertension and usually occur late in the course of AS.

Syncope in AS is most commonly due to systemic vasodilatation in the setting of a fixed cardiac output. Syncope may also rise because of atrial arrhythmias, such as atrial fibrillation with loss of the "atrial kick," and ventricular rhythm disorders, such as transient ventricular fibrillation. Extension of the valvular calcification into the adjacent conduction system may also occasionally lead to transient atrioventricular block and syncope in AS. Gastrointestinal bleeding is associated with calcified AS and may be due to either angiodysplasia or idiopathic causes. Interestingly, this association may resolve following aortic valve replacement.[4]

REFERENCES

1. Kennedy, K.D., Nishimura, R., Holmes, D.R., et al.: Natural history of moderate aortic stenosis. J. Am. Coll. Cardiol. *17*:313, 1991.
2. Ross, J., Jr., and Braunwald, E.: The influence of corrective operations on the natural history of aortic stenosis. Circulation *37*(Suppl. V):61, 1968.
3. Marcus, M.L., Dot, D.B., Hiratzka, L.F., et al.: Decreased coronary reserve. A mechanism for angina pectoris in patients with aortic stenosis and normal coronary arteries. N. Engl. J. Med. *307*:1362, 1982.
4. Love, J.W.: The syndrome of calcific aortic stenosis and gastrointestinal bleeding. Resolution following aortic valve replacement. J. Thorac. Cardiovasc. Surg. *87*:779, 1982.

288-D   *(Braunwald, pp. 1295–1297)*

This patient presents a difficult problem. He has a history that is consistent with exercise-induced chest pain but has had two negative standard exercise tolerance tests (ETTs). However, the relatively low sensitivity of exercise testing (~73 per cent sensitivity for all coronary artery disease) and the fact that this patient appears to have variable threshold angina as indicated by the relationship of the pain to cold weather makes the standard ETT an unsatisfactory test to rule out coronary artery disease. In fact, the standard ETT is particularly insensitive for patients with single-vessel disease. In a study by Goldschlager et al., patients with single-vessel disease had a significantly lower incidence of downsloping ST segments or ST depression of 2 mm than that noted for patients with two- or three-vessel disease.[1]

Thus in this patient, in whom your clinical suspicion for coronary artery disease is relatively high, a further workup is mandatory. Of the other tests available, a stress thallium-201 scintigram would be the one most likely to yield a positive result.[2] Echocardiography might reveal other causes for chest pain, such as mitral valve prolapse, but again would not rule out significant coronary artery disease. Changing medications to nifedipine might be a successful therapeutic intervention but should be done along with further diagnostic workup. Coronary arteriography might eventually be indicated if the stress thallium study showed a large perfusion defect or if the patient was not helped by medical treatment.

Another option would be to perform an exercise radionuclide ventriculogram. This test has also been shown to have a high sensitivity and specificity for coronary artery disease, with measurement of both ejection fraction and regional wall motion aiding in the diagnosis.[3] The greater sensitivity of the two radionuclide techniques compared with the standard ETT is probably related to the fact that abnormalities of perfusion and of left ventricular contraction occur at a lower ischemic threshold than does exercise-induced ST-segment depression. In patients with normal resting ventricular wall motion, exercise echocardiography offers another sensitive, highly specific test to detect coronary artery disease.[4]

REFERENCES

1. Goldschlager, N., Selzer, A., and Cohn, K.: Treadmill stress tests and indicators of presence and severity of coronary artery disease. Ann. Intern. Med. *85*:277, 1976.
2. Port, S.C., Oshima, M., Ray, G., et al.: Assessment of single-vessel coronary artery disease: Results of exercise electrocardiography, thallium-201 myocardial perfusion imaging, and radionuclide angiography. J. Am. Cardiol. *6*:75, 1985.
3. Gibbons, R.J., Fyke, F.E., Clements, I.P., et al.: Noninvasive identification of severe coronary disease using exercise radionuclide angiography. J. Am. Coll. Cardiol. *11*:28, 1988.
4. Ryan, T., Vasey, C.G., Presti, C.F., et al.: Exercise echocardiography: Detection of coronary artery disease in patients with normal left ventricular wall motion at rest. J. Am. Coll. Cardiol. *11*:993, 1988.

289-D   *(Braunwald, p. 1133)*

The Scandinavian Simvastatin Survival Study (4S) was a randomized, double-blind, placebo-controlled study of 4444 patients with angina pectoris or previous myocardial infarction, and serum cholesterol 5.5 to 8.0 mmol/liter (210 to 310 mg/dl), that sought to determine the effect of simvastatin therapy on overall mortality.[1] Men and women were enrolled and the study population was followed for a median follow-up period of 5.4 years. Mean change in serum total cholesterol, LDL cholesterol, HDL cholesterol, and triglycerides were −25, −35, +8, and −10 per cent, respectively. The primary endpoint of the study, total mortality, was reduced by 30 per cent (from 11.5 per cent to 8.2 per cent, p = 0.0003). There was also a significant reduction in all coronary mortality (relative risk, 0.58), and in all cardiovascular mortality (relative risk, 0.65). The risk of having any coronary event (fatal and nonfatal) was also significantly reduced (relative risk, 0.73). Risk reduction was observed in those older than 60 years and, importantly, was similar in each quartile of baseline serum total cholesterol, LDL cholesterol, and HDL cholesterol.[2]

REFERENCES

1. Scandinavian Simvastatin Survival Study Group: Randomized trial of cholesterol lowering in 4444 patients with coronary heart disease: The Scandinavian Simvastatin Survival Study (4S). Lancet *344*:1383, 1994.
2. Scandinavian Simvastatin Survival Study Group: Baseline serum cholesterol and treatment effect in the Scandinavian Simvastatin Survival Study (4S). Lancet *345*:1274, 1995.

290-D   *(Braunwald, pp. 32–49)*

This patient probably has subacute infective endocarditis. The exact incubation period of subacute endocarditis is difficult to define. Starkebaum et al.[1] suggested that the time from transient bacteremia to the development of symptoms was about a week, with symptoms appearing in 2 weeks in 84 per cent of the patients. In many cases the onset of subacute infective endocarditis is characterized by the general manifestations of infection without any signs or symptoms specific to diseases of the heart or any other organ. This patient's complaints of malaise, myalgias, chills, and fever are nonspecific. The classic findings, such as subungual (splinter) hemorrhages, Osler nodes, Janeway lesions, and Roth spots, were much more prominent in the preantibiotic era than in the current era because of the previous longer course of active disease. Nevertheless, the presence of microscopic hematuria is consistent with glomerulonephritis or renal infarction, which are common in subacute endocarditis, occurring in 80 and 50 per cent of patients, respectively.[2]

Although it is possible that the patient's murmur may be a consequence of acute endocarditis, it is more likely that the patient has had longstanding mitral valve prolapse. This is further suggested by his complaints of palpitations and chest pain; these could be due either to the endocarditis or to underlying mitral valve prolapse. Because of the uncertainty in diagnosis of mitral valve prolapse, it is difficult to determine precisely the contributing risk of mitral valve prolapse to endocarditis. In a case-controlled study of patients with valvular endocarditis, Clemens et al.[3] found that 13 of 51 (25 per cent) patients had mitral valve prolapse, while only 11 of 153 (7 per cent) of patients hospitalized for other causes had mitral valve prolapse. This indicates a three- to fourfold higher risk of endocarditis in such patients. Others have found a much lower relative risk,[4] suggesting that although the risk of bacterial endocarditis is greater in patients with mitral valve prolapse than in the patients without this lesion, the absolute risk remains low. As a generalization, it is probable that patients who have only a mitral valve click without significant mitral regurgitation are at minimal risk. On the other hand, patients with large myxomatous valves with significant mitral regurgitation probably are at significantly increased risk and should receive prophylactic therapy for dental manipulations and other procedures that could cause bacteremia.

REFERENCES

1. Starkebaum, M., Durack, D., and Beeson, P.: The "incubation period" of subacute bacterial endocarditis. Yale J. Biol. Med. 50:59 1977.
2. Feinstein, E.I.: Renal complications of bacterial endocarditis. Am. J. Nephrol. 5:457, 1985.
3. Clemens, J.D., Horwitz, R.J., Jaffee, C.C., et al.: A controlled evaluation of the risk of bacterial endocarditis in persons with mitral valve prolapse. N. Engl. J. Med. 30:776, 1982.
4. Retchin, S.M., Fletcher, R.H., and Waugh, R.A.: Endocarditis and mitral valve prolapse: What is "risk?" Int. J. Cardiol. 5:653, 1984.

291-A *(Braunwald, pp. 1110–1111, 1114–1116; Figs. 34–7 and 34–12)*

Macrophages are derived from circulating monocytes and are the major predecessor to the lipid-laden cell that forms the basis for the fatty streak, the "foam" cell. Macrophages are capable of secreting chemotactic agents as well as at least six different growth factors.[1] Therefore, the macrophage is a central cell in the proliferative response of connective tissue that accompanies chronic inflammation. While the mechanism is not well understood, hypercholesterolemia seems to increase the adhesion of monocytes to the endothelium.[2] As these cells become localized to the subendothelium, they become macrophages and take up modified or oxidized LDL via the scavenger receptors on their surface to become foam cells.[3] These cells are well situated to elaborate oxidative metabolites that might injure the overlying endothelium, as well as growth factors that might stimulate smooth muscle cell proliferation. These two potential effects of the macrophages account for the central role of the cell in the response-to-injury hypothesis (see Braunwald, Fig. 34–7, p. 1110). "Contractile state" and "synthetic state" describe two different forms recognized for smooth muscle cells, not macrophages.

REFERENCES

1. Ross, R., Raines, E.W., and Bowen-Pope, D.F.: The biology of platelet-derived growth factor. Cell 46:155, 1986.
2. Ross, R.: The pathogenesis of atherosclerosis—an update. N. Engl. J. Med. 314:496, 1986.
3. Parthasarathy, S., Quinn, M.T., Schwenke, D.C., et al.: Oxidative modification of beta—very low density lipoprotein. Potential role in monocyte recruitment and foam cell formation. Arteriosclerosis 9:398, 1989.

292-C *(Braunwald, pp. 1198–1199)*

The clinical history remains an important part of the diagnosis of acute myocardial infarction. While a prodrome may be elicited in between 20 and 60 per cent of these patients, it may not be disturbing enough to cause them to seek immediate medical attention. In fact, only about 20 per cent of all patients with prodromal symptoms will seek medical help in the first 24 hours.[1] Approximately one-third of such patients will have had symptoms for 1 to 4 weeks before hospitalization, and in many cases these symptoms are of unstable angina, occurring at rest or with less activity than usual.

Morphine is usually capable of relieving the pain of AMI, although a dull pressure or ache may persist following analgesic treatment. Interestingly, the longer a patient suspected of having ischemic chest pain requires administration of analgesic therapy after hospital admission, the more likely that the diagnosis of AMI will be confirmed.[2] A variety of studies, including those in patients receiving thrombolytic therapy, have supported the notion that the ischemic zone of viable myocardium surrounding the necrotic central area of infarction gives rise to the pain sensation. This has important clinical ramifications for the care of patients in the periinfarction setting.

The majority of patients with transmural myocardial infarction and chest discomfort have nausea and vomiting,[3] which is thought to be due to activation of vagal reflexes. Attempts to quantify the number of infarctions that occur in a "silent" fashion through population studies have suggested that between 20 and 60 per cent of nonfatal infarctions are unrecognized by the patient and are discovered at the time of routine ECG.[4] However, further analysis reveals that approximately half of these patients will indeed have some recollection of an event characterized by symptoms compatible with AMI and that the infarction was not truly silent. Unrecognized or silent infarction occurs more commonly in patients without prior angina pectoris and in those with a history of hypertension or diabetes, although the association with diabetes is still controversial.

REFERENCES

1. Harper, R.W., Kennedy, G., DeSanctis, R.W., and Hutter, A.M., Jr.: The incidence and pattern of angina prior to acute myocardial infarction: A study of 577 cases. Am. Heart J. *97*:178, 1979.
2. Baker, P.: Suspected myocardial infarction: Early diagnostic value of analgesic requirements. Br. Med. J. *290*:27, 1985.
3. Ingram, D.A., Fulton, R.A., Portal, R.W., and Aber, C.P.: Vomiting as a diagnostic aid in acute ischemic cardiac pain. Br. Med. J. *281*:636, 1980.
4. Margolis, J.R., Kannel, W.B., Feinleib, M., et al.: Clinical features of unrecognized myocardial infarction: Silent and symptomatic. Eighteen-year follow-up: The Framingham Study. Am. J. Cardiol. *32*:1, 1973.

293-E   *(Braunwald, pp. 1221–1222; 1375–1376)*

Primary PTCA for AMI has several important differences and potential advantages when compared with pharmacological thrombolysis.[1] The safety and success rate in establishing reperfusion (>90 per cent) is clearly superior to that of thrombolytic agents and there is less likelihood of developing complications such as reocclusion, reinfarction, and stroke with primary PTCA. This, however, did not translate into large differences between patients randomized to primary PTCA versus thrombolytic agents in several small randomized trials.[2–4] The Primary Angioplasty in Myocardial Infarction (PAMI) trial was the largest such trial and randomized 395 patients to PTCA or t-PA using standard dosing of t-PA (*not* the accelerated t-PA regimen of the GUSTO trial). PAMI demonstrated a lower incidence of death or reinfarction by hospital discharge and a 6-month follow-up among those treated with PTCA compared with thrombolysis.[4] Primary PTCA may be especially of value in patients with acute myocardial infarction presenting in cardiogenic shock. This group showed minimal benefit from thrombolysis with

better outcomes using primary angioplasty in several small series.[5–7] In addition, in experienced centers, primary angioplasty may be associated with better outcome, significantly shorter hospital stay, and less follow-up costs compared with thrombolysis.[8]

REFERENCES

1. Lieu, T.A., Gurley, R.J., Lundstrom, R.J., and Parmley, W.W.: Primary angioplasty and thrombolysis for acute myocardial infarction: An evidence summary. J. Am. Coll. Cardiol. *27*:737–750, 1996.
2. Gibbons, R.J., Holmes, D.R., Reeder, G.S., et al.: Immediate angioplasty compared with the administration of a thrombolytic agent followed by conservative treatment for myocardial infarction. The Mayo Coronary Care Unit and Catheterization Laboratory Groups. N. Engl. J. Med. *328*:685–691, 1993.
3. Zijlstra, F., de Boer, M.J., Hoorntje, J.C., et al: A comparison of immediate coronary angioplasty with intravenous streptokinase in acute myocardial infarction. N. Engl. J. Med. *328*:680–684, 1993.
4. Grines, C.L., Browne, K.F., Marco, J., et al.: A comparison of immediate angioplasty with thrombolytic therapy for acute myocardial infarction. The Primary Angioplasty in Myocardial Infarction Study Group. N. Engl. J. Med. *328*:673–679, 1993.
5. Eltchaninoff, H., Simpfendorfer, C., Franco, I., et al.: Early and 1-year survival rates in acute myocardial infarction complicated by cardiogenic shock: A retrospective study comparing coronary angioplasty with medical treatment. Am. Heart J. *130*:459–464, 1995.
6. Bengtson, J.R., Kaplan, A.J., Pieper, K.S., et al.: Prognosis in cardiogenic shock after acute myocardial infarction in the interventional era. J. Am. Coll. Cardiol. *20*:1482–1489, 1992.
7. Hibbard, M.D., Holmes, D.R., Jr., Bailey, K.R., et al.: Percutaneous transluminal coronary angioplasty in patients with cardiogenic shock. J. Am. Coll. Cardiol. *19*:639–646, 1992.
8. Goldman, L.: Cost and quality of life: Thrombolysis and primary angioplasty. J. Am. Coll. Cardiol. *25*(Suppl. 7):38S–41S, 1995.

294-C   *(Braunwald, p. 1505)*

Effusive-constrictive pericarditis, which may represent an intermediate stage in the development of chronic constrictive pericarditis, is defined as the simultaneous presence of a tense pericardial effusion and of visceral pericardial restriction. This pathophysiology leads to the hemodynamic hallmark of the condition, which is continued elevation of right atrial pressure following aspiration of the pericardial fluid and the resultant return of intrapericardial pressures to zero. The etiologies for this entity are the same as those for chronic constrictive pericarditis. The most common include idiopathic or presumed viral pericarditis, as well as tuberculosis, neoplastic infiltration of the pericardium, and mediastinal irradiation. The physical findings seen most commonly in effusive-constrictive pericarditis include pulsus parodoxus, abnormal or diminished pulse pressure, and jugular venous distention with a predominant *x* descent. They therefore more closely resemble the physical findings of cardiac tamponade than they do those of chronic constrictive pericarditis.

The chest x-ray in this condition usually shows cardiac enlargement, and the ECG may reveal diffuse low QRS voltage and/or ST- or T-wave abnormalities. Echocardiography may demonstrate both the pericardial effusion and a thickened pericardium.[1] The diagnosis of effusive-constrictive pericarditis is ultimately made at cardiac catheterization, with careful hemodynamic monitoring of intrapericardial and right atrial pressures before and after pericardiocentesis. Although restoration or intrapericardial pressure to zero following pericardiocentesis may allow some improvement in hemodynamics, pressures do not return entirely to normal. Wave forms may convert to a patient more consistent with constrictive pericarditis following pericardiocentesis, with a prominent *y* descent in the left atrial pressure tracing as well as a dip-and-plateau pattern in the right ventricular pressure tracing. As might be expected from the pathophysiology, pericardiocentesis provides only partial and transient relief, and definitive therapy for this condition consists of total parietal and visceral pericardiectomy.

REFERENCE

1. Martin, R.P., Bowden, R., Filly, K., and Popp, R.L.: Intrapericardial abnormalities in patients with pericardial effusion. Circulation *61*:568, 1980.

295-A   *(Braunwald, p. 1176)*

Myocardial stunning is defined as the prolonged myocardial dysfunction that follows a brief episode of severe ischemia, with gradual return of contractile activity. Myocardial hibernation, on the other hand, is the term applied to myocardial dysfunction resulting from chronic hypoperfusion. Myocardial stunning affects both systolic and diastolic functions, and may occur in the globally as well as the regionally ischemic myocardium. Clinically stunning is most frequently seen in patients recovering from ischemic arrest during cardiopulmonary bypass. It is also seen in ischemic regions adjacent to infarcted zones and in territories that are severely ischemic in patients with unstable angina. The sequence of biochemical events and reactions causing this transient myocardial dysfunction to follow ischemic results is not clear. Proposed mechanisms include transient calcium overload, excitation contraction uncoupling, and generation of oxygen free radicals.[1-3]

REFERENCES

1. Schipke, J.D., Korbmacher, B., Dorszewski, A., et al.: Hemodynamic and energetic properties of stunned myocardium in rabbit hearts. Heart *75*:55–61, 1996.
2. Sun, J.Z., Tang, X.L., Park, S.W., et al.: Evidence for an essential role of reactive oxygen species in the genesis of late preconditioning against myocardial stunning in conscious pigs. J. Clin. Invest. *97*:562–576, 1996.
3. Hess, M.L., and Kukreja, R.C.: Free radicals, calcium homeostasis, heat shock proteins, and myocardial stunning. Ann. Thorac. Surg. *60*:760–766, 1995.

296-A   *(Braunwald, pp. 1148–1149)*

Patients with lipid disorders are often taking other medications that may affect the underlying metabolism of lipoproteins. Common antihypertensive agents, such as noncardioselective beta blockers and diuretics, both tend to alter lipid profiles. Some of the thiazide diuretics may lead to elevations in total cholesterol. Similarly, noncardioselective beta blockers tend to increase VLDL levels, an effect that is thought to be due to the inhibition of adrenergic lipoprotein lipase stimulation. It should be remembered, however, that both nonselective and cardioselective beta blockers have been shown to decrease cardiac mortality in clinical studies and that lipid alterations do not mandate discontinuation of these drugs in many patients. The alpha-adrenoceptor beta blocking agent prazosin does not adversely affect the lipoprotein profile and may actually increase HDL levels. Calcium blockers, centrally acting alpha$_2$ agonists, and angiotensin-converting enzyme inhibitors all tend to have a neutral effect on blood lipids. Estrogen replacement therapy tends to raise HDL levels as well as VLDL and triglyceride levels, while reducing LDL. While the effects of estrogen therapy on cardiac risk remain controversial, recent evidence suggests that estrogen use may reduce the incidence of cardiovascular mortality and coronary heart disease.[1]

REFERENCE

1. Stampfer, M.J., et al.: Postmenopausal estrogen therapy and cardiovascular disease. Ten-year follow-up from the Nurses' Health Study. N. Engl. J. Med. *325*:756, 1991.

297-C   *(Braunwald, pp. 893)*

In general, the electrocardiogram is less helpful in the diagnosis of congenital heart disease in premature and newborn infants than it is in older children or adults. Right ventricular hypertrophy is a *normal* finding in the neonate, and the range of normal voltages is wide in this age group. Initial septal depolarization may be assessed from the ECG even in the neonate. While septal Q waves may not be clearly seen in the lateral precordial leads in the first 72 hours of life, a *leftward, posteriorly directed septal vector* giving rise to Q waves in the right precordial leads is abnormal and may suggest the presence of marked right ventricular hypertrophy, single ventricle, or inversion of the ventricles.

T-wave inversions may be a normal finding in the neonatal ECG, and by the age of 72 hours T waves should be inverted in right precordial leads and upright in the lateral precordium. The persistence of upright T waves in right precordial leads is a sign of significant, abnormal right ventricular hypertrophy. Flattening or inversion of lateral T waves may suggest subendocardial ischemia or obstruction to left ventricular outflow. In addition, these findings may be seen in electrolyte disturbance, acidosis, and hypoxemia.

The electrocardiographic findings of myocardial infarction in an infant suggest the diagnosis of anomalous origin of a coronary artery. Finally, heart block or supraventricular tachycardia as well as other arrhythmias may be detected by the ECG. Thus, while the ECG is not as useful in neonates and infants as it is in older age groups, it is capable of offering significant clues to the presence of underlying cardiovascular disease.

298-D (Braunwald, pp. 1368–1370)

Abrupt vessel closure is one of the most serious complications of coronary angioplasty and is defined as the sudden occlusion of the target or adjacent segment of a coronary vessel during or after percutaneous revascularization. It occurs in about 4 to 8 per cent of interventions and carries a mortality of up to 8 per cent, with up to 6 per cent risk of periprocedural myocardial infarction. Most cases occur before the patient leaves the catheterization laboratory, but up to 25 per cent occur shortly afterwards. The mechanism of closure is a consequence of the expected intimal dissection caused by balloon inflation. Deep and extensive disruption of the medial layer may lead to an occlusive flap and/or intramural hematoma that will initiate thrombus formation. In this instance, exposure of the underlying subendothelium results in activation of platelets and thrombosis, both of which are aided by blood stasis. The initial management usually consists of repeat balloon dilatation with long inflations. Stents have been used with very good results. Thrombolytic agents may be of value in select cases of abrupt closure with extensive thrombosis.

299-C (Braunwald, pp. 1320–1321)

Venous graft occlusion occurs in between 8 and 12 per cent of patients before they ever leave the hospital, and by 1 year between 12 and 20 per cent of vein grafts have become occluded.[1] Graft occlusion within the first year usually involves thrombosis, with or without marked intimal hyperplasia of the underlying vessel. Following the first year, atherosclerotic changes begin to accumulate in saphenous grafts. The histological evolution of atherosclerosis in venous bypass grafts is indistinguishable from that seen in arterial vessels.[2] The annual occlusion rate for vessels following the first year is on the order of 2 per cent,[1] though in grafts that are between 6 and 11 years old, an annual attrition rate of 4 per cent is noted.[3] Therefore, an overall occlusion rate for each distal anastomosis is noted of between 25 and 30 per cent at 5 to 7 years, and 40 to 50 per cent at 10 years. Disease progression continues in nongrafted arteries and occurs at a rate of 18 to 38 per cent over the first decade.[4] Interestingly, the risk of disease progression in the native circulation is three to six times higher in those vessels to which a graft is placed, as compared with ungrafted native arteries.[4] In general, this progression in the native vessel usually occurs proximal to the site of graft insertion. These data are the basis for the recommendation that arteries with minimal disease not receive a bypass graft.

REFERENCES

1. Grondin, C.M., Campeau, L., Thornton, J.C., et al.: Coronary artery bypass grafting with saphenous vein. Circulation 79(Suppl. I):24, 1989.
2. Lie, J.T., Lawrie, G.M., and Morris, G.C.: Aortocoronary bypass saphenous vein graft atherosclerosis. J. Am. Cardiol. 40:906, 1977.
3. Campeau, L., Enjalbert, M., Lesperance, J., et al.: Atherosclerosis and late closure of aortocoronary saphenous vein grafts: Sequential angiographic studies at 2 weeks, 1 year, 5 to 7 years, and 10 to 12 years after surgery. Circulation 68(Suppl. II):1, 1983.
4. Kroncke, G.M., Kosolcharoen, P., Clayman, J.A., et al.: Five year changes in coronary arteries of medical and surgical patients of the Veterans Administration randomized study of bypass surgery. Circulation 78(Suppl. I):144, 1988.

300-D (Braunwald, pp. 901–904; Fig. 29–16)

Ventricular septal defect is among the most prevalent of congenital cardiac malformations and is the most frequently diagnosed congenital heart disease beyond the neonatal period. Most commonly, the defect occurs in the region of the membranous septum and is thus referred to as a perimembranous defect. Other types of VSD include muscular defects (which tend to be multiple), subpulmonary defects, and subaortic defects. Spontaneous closure is more likely to occur in the membranous type of VSD, which is infrequently associated with other defects. VSD closure occurs on the basis of adherence of the septal leaflet of the tricuspid valve to the defect, hypertrophy of the septal muscle, or ingrowth of fibrous tissue, not by continuous growth of the septum. Spontaneous closure occurs by the age 3 years in 45 per cent of patients and can occur as late as 8 or 10 years of age.[1] Diagnosis is usually suspected on clinical grounds and echocardiography greatly facilitates the diagnosis, localization, and quantitation of VSD. In children with single defects, surgical repair is preferable over pulmonary artery banding. Operative management is not indicated for patients with normal pulmonary artery pressures and small VSD. Complete heart block (CHB) is the most significant conduction system abnormality complicating surgery, but occurs immediately after surgery in <1 per cent of patients.[2] Late-onset CHB occasionally is a problem complicating VSD repair, especially in patients with postoperative evidence of fascicular or bundle branch block on ECG.

REFERENCES

1. Weldman, W.H., Blount, S.G., Jr., DuShane, J.W., et al.: Clinical course in ventricular septal defect: Natural history study. Circulation 56:I-56, 1977.

2. Houyel, L., Vaksmann, G., Fournier, A., and Davignon, A.: Department of Pediatric Cardiology, Sainte-Justine Hospital, Montreal, Quebec, Canada. Ventricular arrhythmias after correction of ventricular septal defects: Importance of surgical approach. J. Am. Coll. Cardiol. 16:1224–1228, 1998.

301-A (Braunwald, pp. 911–914)

In most cases, coarctation of the aorta consists of an eccentric narrowing of the thoracic aortic lumen just *distal* to the origin of the subclavian artery, which is frequently dilated.[1] Less commonly the coarctation may be proximal to or involve the origin of the left subclavian artery itself. Coarctation is frequently associated with other congenital cardiac malformations, the most common of which are bicuspid aortic valve, patent ductus arteriosus, ventricular septal defect, and mitral valve abnormalities.[2] Adult patients with coarctation of the aorta are usually asymptomatic, and suspicion is the key to the diagnosis of the condition. In adults with this condition, the most common complaints are headaches, leg fatigue, and intermittent claudication. Patients may also come to medical attention because of symptoms associated with left ventricular failure, infective endarteritis, or aortic rupture or dissection. Endocarditis may occur on an associated bicuspid valve as another presentation of this disorder.

While patients with coarctation usually appear normal, this is the most common anomaly associated with Turner syndrome and coarctation should be specifically sought in patients with this syndrome. In most cases, simultaneous palpation of pulses in the upper and lower extremities reveals diminished and delayed femoral pulses when compared with radial pulses. In questionable cases, exercise may exacerbate the difference and accentuate these physical findings. A suprasternal thrill is often present in coarctation of the aorta. In addition, auscultation usually demonstrates the ejection murmur that may be caused by the coarctation itself or by an associated bicuspid aortic valve. The presence of an ejection click should further raise the possibility of this aortic valve abnormality.

REFERENCES

1. Maron, B.J.: Aortic isthmic coarctations. *In* Roberts, W.C. (ed.): Adult Congenital Heart Disease. Philadelphia, F.A. Davis, 1987, pp. 443–454.
2. Serfas, D., and Borow, K.M.: Coarctation of the aorta. Anatomy, pathophysiology, and natural history. J. Cardiovasc. Med. 8:575, 1983.

302-A (Braunwald, pp. 1466–1467)

The two-dimensional echocardiogram illustrated demonstrates a tumor in the right atrium attached to the intraatrial septum (IAS). Since the tumor appears to be pedunculated, it is much more likely that it is a myxoma rather than a rhabdomyoma or a lymphosarcoma, both of which tend to be adherent to the wall. Myxomas are the most common type of primary cardiac tumor, comprising 30 to 50 per cent of total tumors in most pathological series. Approximately 85 per cent of myxomas occur in the left atrium; the number in the right atrium is only about 15 per cent. In more than 90 per cent of cases myxomas are solitary. The most common site of attachment for myxomas is in the area of the fossa ovalis. Rhabdomyosarcomas are tumors of smooth muscle, which usually diffusely infiltrate the myocardium. Lymphosarcomas are quite rare in contrast to metastatic systemic lymphoma, which involves the heart in 25 per cent of cases. Lymphosarcomas can mimic hypertrophic cardiomyopathy due to the extensive myocardial infiltration. A pericardial cyst would be relatively easy to discern based on the echocardiographic appearance of a liquid-filled space.

303-C (Braunwald, p. 1146; Table 35–2)

Genetic disorders of triglyceride metabolism have been defined that lead to each of three HLP phenotypes: type III, type IV, and type V. Type III HLP, also called familial dysbetalipoproteinemia or broad-beta-lipoproteinemia, is a rare disorder due to an abnormality in the apoprotein E isoform that is present. Patients usually demonstrate roughly equal elevations of cholesterol and triglycerides, and lipoprotein electrophoresis reveals an increase both in VLDL and in a pre-beta band adjacent to VLDL (hence the name broad-beta-lipoproteinemia). A characteristic lesion on the palms of the hands (xanthoma striatum palmare) is associated with the disorder.

Two different genetic disorders have been described that lead to the phenotype for type IV hyperlipoproteinemia. Primary or familial endogenous hypertriglyceridemia is an autosomal dominant disease that occurs in approximately 1 per cent of the general population. Triglyceride levels are usually in the 200 to 500 mg/dl range, and are in part due to an oversynthesis of hepatic triglyceride and VLDL. Familial combined hyperlipidemia (FCH) is a second genetic disorder which may yield a type IV pattern. While a predisposition to coronary disease is documented for FCH patients, the association between primary (familial) endogenous hypertriglyceridemia and CAD is less clear.[1]

The type V HLP phenotype is uncommon and occurs less frequently in women. The disorder usually is first recognized in adults and may be precipitated by chronic alcohol ingestion or exogenous estrogen therapy.[2] A type V pattern is also seen on occasion in patients with genetic forms of hypertriglyceridemia. Because the type V phenotype is frequently associated with diabetes and other risk factors for premature atherosclerosis, it is not entirely clear whether the underlying lipid disorder itself predisposes to CAD.[3]

REFERENCES

1. Sniderman, A.D., Wolfson, C., Teng, B., et al.: Association of hyperapobetalipoproteinemia with endogenous hypertriglyceridemia and atherosclerosis. Ann. Intern. Med. 97: 833, 1982.
2. Fallet, R.W., and Glueck, C.J.: Familial and acquired type V hyperlipoproteinemia. Atherosclerosis 23:41, 1976.
3. Zilversmit, D.B.: Atherogenesis: A postprandial phenomenon. Circulation 60:473, 1979.

304-E   (Braunwald, p. 1337; Fig. 38–24)

Although most patients with unstable angina have severe obstructive coronary disease, substantial evidence exists to support the role of platelet aggregation and subsequent formation of coronary thrombi in the precipitation of ischemic symptoms. In addition, several randomized clinical trials have established the value of aspirin therapy in reducing mortality, recurrent unstable angina, and myocardial infarction.[1-3] In these trials, use of aspirin was associated with 50 per cent reduction in mortality and in the incidence of subsequent myocardial infarction. A recent landmark trial by Theroux established the value of heparin therapy in relation to aspirin therapy.[2,4] In this trial, 479 patients with unstable angina were randomized soon after their admission to the hospital to receive either 325 mg of aspirin twice a day, heparin at 1000 units/hour intravenously, both drugs, or placebo. The incidence of myocardial infarction was decreased by aspirin and to a greater extent by heparin (with and without aspirin). Heparin use (with or without aspirin) was associated with significant reduction in the incidence of refractory angina compared to placebo or aspirin alone (p = 0.002). However, more recent data have shown that the use of heparin alone in this group of patients is associated with increased risk of rebound symptoms following the discontinuation of heparin therapy.[5] This is believed to be secondary to an increase in thrombin activity after cessation of heparin. More gradual "weaning" of heparin infusion and coadministration of aspirin reduce this risk.

To minimize the side effects associated with aspirin intake, several small randomized trials have examined the effect of smaller doses of aspirin on outcome in patients with unstable angina. Doses as low as 75 mg/day showed comparable benefits to higher doses, with lesser side effects.[3] However, based on doses given in large randomized clinical trials, current recommendations are 160 to 325 mg/day. In patients who are intolerant of aspirin, ticlopidine is a very good alternative. Although its side-effect profile is different and may include neutropenia, a randomized controlled trial recently using 250 mg twice a day of ticlopidine reported a 47 per cent reduction in cardiovascular death and a 46 per cent reduction in nonfatal infarction at 6 months.

REFERENCES

1. Cairns, J.A., Gent, M., Singer, J., et al.: Aspirin, sulfinpyrazone, or both in unstable angina. Results of a Canadian multicenter trial. N. Engl. J. Med. 313:1369–1375, 1985.
2. Theroux, P., Ouimet, H., McCans, J., et al.: Aspirin, heparin, or both to treat acute unstable angina. N. Engl. J. Med. 319: 1105–1111, 1988.
3. Wallentin, L.C.: Aspirin (75 mg/day) after an episode of unstable coronary artery disease: Long-term effects on the risk for myocardial infarction, occurrence of severe angina and the need for revascularization. Research Group on Instability in Coronary Artery Disease in Southeast Sweden. J. Am. Coll. Cardiol. 18:1587–1593, 1991.
4. Theroux, P., Waters, D., Qiu, S., et al.: Aspirin versus heparin to prevent myocardial infarction during the acute phase of unstable angina. Circulation 88(5 Pt 1):2045–2048, 1993.
5. Theroux, P., Waters, D., Lam, J., et al.: Reactivation of unstable angina after the discontinuation of heparin. N. Engl. J. Med. 327:141–145, 1992.
6. Balsano, F., Rizzon, P., Violi, F., et al.: Antiplatelet treatment with ticlopidine in unstable angina. A controlled multicenter clinical trial. The Studio della Ticlopidina nell'Angina Instabile Group. Circulation 82:17–26, 1990.

305-D   (Braunwald, pp. 1192–1193)

Autopsy studies over the last 4 decades have revealed that true atrial infarction occurs in between 7 and 17 per cent of autopsy-proven cases of MI.[1] Atrial infarction is often seen in conjunction with left ventricular infarction and more commonly involves the right atrium. This may be due to the presence of well-oxygenated blood in the left atrium, which may nourish the thin atrial wall despite the presence of obstructive coronary disease involving the coronary arterial system perfusing the left atrium. Atrial infarction may lead to rupture of the atrial wall and is more frequently noted in the atrial appendages than in the lateral or posterior aspects of the atrium itself. Because right atrial infarction is usually associated with obstructive disease of the sinus node artery, it is frequently accompanied by atrial arrhythmias.

REFERENCE

1. Gardin, J.M., and Singer, D.H.: Atrial infarction: Importance, diagnosis and localization. Arch. Intern. Med. 141:1345, 1981.

306-C   (Braunwald, pp. 1079–1080; Table 33–3)

Prosthetic valve endocarditis (PVE) may occur "early," within the first 60 days following placement of the valve, or "late," in subsequent months or years. While this distinction is somewhat arbitrary, differences in both the clinical features and microbial patterns have been documented in these two groups. Cases of early prosthetic valve endocarditis usually are due to contamination in the immediate operative or perioperative setting. Staphylococcus epidermidis is the most common organism isolated in this group, occurring in 25 to 30 per cent of cases. Staphylococcus aureus is seen in 20 to 25 per cent of this group as well. The risk for developing prosthetic valve endocarditis peaks in the first several weeks following the operation and then declines to a relatively low rate, with an incidence of 0.2 to 0.5 per cent per patient year.

In late cases, as in the question, the source of infection is often difficult to identify but is presumed to be seeding of the valve by a transient bacteremia. The bacteriology in late PVE is thus similar to that of native valvular endocarditis (see Braunwald, Table 33–3, p. 1079). The most common organism isolated in this setting is *Streptococcus viridans*. In the first year following surgery, the incidence of methicillin-resistant organisms is greater than 80 per cent. However, in the subsequent months and years, methicillin resistance is only on the order of 20 to 30 per cent.[1] The transesophageal echocardiographic image displayed demonstrates that the mitral valve prosthesis is well-seated in the appropriate position without any evidence of valvular dehiscence or dysfunction. The prominent vegetations seen on the atrial side of the valve are well delineated by the technique and provide an excellent example of the increased sensitivity of this form of echocardiography as compared with transthoracic studies.[2]

REFERENCES

1. Calderwood, S.B., Swinski, L.A., Waternaux, C.M., et al.: Risk factors for the development of prosthetic valve endocarditis. Circulation *72*:31, 1985.
2. Mugge, A., Daniel, W.G., Frank, G., et al.: Reassessment of prognostic implications of vegetation size determined by the transthoracic and the transesophageal approach. J. Am. Coll. Cardiol. *14*:631, 1989.

307-B   *(Braunwald, pp. 1016–1017; 1044–1045)*

In 1982, pediatric cardiologists began to use balloon dilatation catheters with inflated diameters of 1 to 2 cm to produce commissural splitting of stenotic pulmonary valves and were able to achieve reductions of pulmonic valve gradients to approximately one-third of their baseline value. In addition, this technique proved to have a very high success rate and has now essentially replaced open surgical repair for valvular pulmonic stenosis. Theoretical concerns existed regarding the efficacy of balloon valvuloplasty in the treatment of adult acquired rheumatic and/or calcific stenosis of either the mitral or aortic valves. In 1985, despite these concerns, successful balloon valvuloplasty using a transseptal approach was first reported in young adult patients with rheumatic mitral stenosis. This technique is now being used successfully in a variety of centers and is capable of achieving physiologically adequate enlargement of the mitral orifice. Mitral valvuloplasty is especially useful in patients without mitral valvular calcification or thickening.[1] Moderate or severe mitral regurgitation occurs rarely following balloon valvuloplasty, provided that patients are preselected for the absence of left atrial thrombus. One minor complication without significant hemodynamic consequence is that approximately one-third of patients show some evidence of a persistent, small left-to-right shunt at the site of atrial septal puncture from transseptal left heart catheterization.

Aortic valvuloplasty using a retrograde approach has also proven to be of use in some patients, especially those at high risk for surgical aortic valve replacement. However, the magnitude of orifice improvement during aortic valvuloplasty appears to be suboptimal, and less than that achieved by the mitral procedure. In addition, a high percentage of patients have poor results at 24 months, with either death or recurrence of critical aortic stenosis.[2]

REFERENCES

1. Kirklin, J.W.: Percutaneous balloon versus surgical closed commissurotomy for mitral stenosis. Circulation *83*:1450, 1991.
2. Bashore, T.M., Davidson, C.J., and the Mansfield Scientific Aortic Valvuloplasty Registry Investigators: Follow-up recatheterization after balloon aortic valvuloplasty. J. Am. Coll. Cardiol. *17*:1188, 1991.

308-E   *(Braunwald, pp. 1467–1469)*

Myxomas are by far the most common type of cardiac tumors, comprising 50 per cent of the total in most series.[1] They can be either sporadic or familial. Less than 10 per cent are of the latter type, which is transmitted as an autosomal dominant disease, usually occurs in younger patients, tends to occur in more than one location, and is more likely to lead to recurrence. Sporadic myxoma is the more common type, is more common in females, and is usually a single tumor rising in the left atrium. Sporadic myxomas are the most common cardiac source of tumor emboli due to their friability and intracavitary location. Although the majority of myxomas are benign, certain features should raise suspicion of malignant behavior. These features include the presence of local invasion or distant metastasis; evidence of rapid growth; hemorrhagic pericardial effusion; precordial pain; location of the tumor on the right side of the heart, on the free wall, or in the ventricals, as well as an intramural location; and extension into the pulmonary veins.[2] These features, like features suggestive of the familial variety, predict an increased recurrence rate following surgical removal. Recurrence rate for the majority of patients with sporadic myxoma is in the range of 1 to 5 per cent.[3]

REFERENCES

1. Reynen, K.: Cardiac myxomas. N. Engl. J. Med. *333*:1610–1617, 1995.
2. Salcedo, E.E., Cohen, G.I., White, R.D., and Davison, M.B.: Cardiac tumors: Diagnosis and treatment. Curr. Probl. Cardiol. *17*:73, 1992.
3. Waller, D.A., Ettles, D.F., Saunders, N.R., and Williams, G.: Recurrent cardiac myxomas: The surgical implications of two distinct groups of patients. Thorac. Cardiovasc. Surg. *37*:226, 1989.

309-D   *(Braunwald, p. 1674)*

The patient described has the classic clinical signs and findings of *type II glycogen storage disease*. This disease is a consequence of the deficiency of alpha-1,4-glucosidase (acid maltase), a lysosomal enzyme that hydrolyzes glycogen into glucose. The condition commonly presents in the neonatal period. Characteristic symptoms include failure to thrive, progressive hypotonia, lethargy, and a weak cry. Of all the glycogen storage diseases, type II (or Pompe's disease) is the most likely to cause cardiac symptoms. The ECG shows extremely tall, broad QRS complexes with a short P-R interval (commonly <0.09 sec). A short P-R interval may be the result of enhanced AV conduction due to myocardial glycogen deposition. Chest x-ray frequently shows cardiomegaly with pulmonary vascular redistribution. Diagnosis is confirmed by demonstrating the enzymatic deficiency in lymphocytes, skeletal muscle, or liver.[1]

Cardiac glycogenosis may be confused with other entities that cause cardiac failure, particularly in association with cardiomegaly in the early months of life. *Endocardial fibroelastosis*, a disease of unknown etiology, differs from Pompe's disease in lacking the short P-R interval and the fact that symptoms are limited to the cardiac system, while in Pompe's disease skeletal muscle hypotonia is prominent. Furthermore, in endocardial fibroelastosis, mitral regurgitation and abnormalities of the cardiac valves, especially mitral and aortic, are frequent. *Coarctation of the aorta*, another common cause of congestive heart failure in infants, can readily be distinguished by the presence of pulse and blood pressure discrepancies between the upper and lower extremities. *Myocarditis*, another cause of congestive heart failure in children, is usually of abrupt onset and is not associated with hypotonia. *Anomalous pulmonary origin of the left coronary artery* can cause cardiomegaly but usually has a distinctive ECG pattern of anterolateral MI.

Shone syndrome is a developmental complex that consists of four obstructive anomalies: (1) a supravalvular ring of the left atrium; (2) a parachute mitral valve; (3) subaortic stenosis; and (4) coarctation of the aorta. It frequently presents with mitral stenosis, since flow from the left atrium must pass through the intrachordal spaces of the mitral valve causing functional mitral stenosis. Pulmonary venous hypertension is a common finding in this illness because of left ventricular inflow and outflow obstruction. However, Shone syndrome frequently presents in early childhood rather than infancy and lacks the skeletal muscle changes of Pompe's disease.

Friedreich's ataxia is a hereditary autosomal recessive disease that affects the individual during late childhood and presents with progressive ataxia. The limbs, in addition to being ataxic, generally show considerable weakness. About 50 per cent of patients with Friedreich's ataxia have cardiac involvement, which typically presents as a hypertrophic cardiomyopathy associated with arrythmias. Coronary arteries may either be normal or show extensive intimal proliferation leading to ob-

struction while atherosclerosis and thrombosis are generally not present.

REFERENCE

1. Caddell, J.L.: Metabolic and nutritional diseases. *In* Adams, F.H., and Emmanouilides, G.C. (eds.): Moss' Heart Disease in Infants, Children and Adolescents. 3rd ed. Baltimore, Williams & Wilkins, 1983, pp. 596–626.

310-D   *(Braunwald, pp. 1140–1141)*

Nicotinic acid is a B vitamin with lipid-lowering effects that occur when given at pharmacological (high) doses. Nicotinic acid's role as a coenzyme in carbohydrate metabolism is not related to its lipid-lowering effects. Its primary action is to reduce VLDL, which causes a subsequent reduction in IDL and LDL levels. In addition, nicotinic acid decreases the release of free fatty acids from adipocytes (which are used by the liver for triglycerides synthesis), thus reducing triglycerides levels.[1] In therapeutic doses (1.5 to 6 gm/day), nicotinic acid reduces LDL cholesterol by 10 to 25 per cent and triglycerides by 20 to 50 per cent. It also increases HDL cholesterol by 15 to 35 per cent. The increase in HDL cholesterol is caused by decreased catabolism of HDL and apo A-I.[2] Nicotinic acid also reduces circulating levels of Lp(a).[3] Despite these marked effects on lipid profile, its widespread use has been limited because of the frequency of side effects. The most common side effect is the development of flushing, which can be reduced by preadministration of aspirin or other prostaglandin inhibitors. Hepatotoxicity is a serious and potentially life-threatening complication that has been reported more often with sustained-release preparations. Mild elevations in liver enzymes, however, are not life threatening and do not necessitate termination of therapy.

REFERENCES

1. Lavie, C.J., and Milani, R.V.: Nicotinic acid. *In* Messerli, F.H. (ed.): Cardiovascular Drug Therapy. 2nd ed. Philadelphia, W.B. Saunders Co., 1996.
2. Shepherd, J., Packard, C., Patch, J.R., et al.: Effects of nicotinic acid therapy on plasma high density lipoprotein subfraction distribution and composition and on lipoprotein A metabolism. J. Clin. Invest. *63*:858, 1979.
3. Carlson, L.A., Hamsten, A., and Asplund, A.: Pronounced lowering of serum levels of lipoprotein LP(a) in hyperlipidemic subjects treated with nicotinic acid. J. Intern. Med. *226*:271, 1989.

311-D   *(Braunwald, pp. 1174–1176)*

Collaterals are vascular channels that interconnect ordinary arteries. Preexisting collaterals are thin-walled channels that are closed in the normal human heart due to the lack of pressure differential. However, with acute coronary occlusion, distal pressure decreases, and the pressure gradient (and possibly other stimuli) causes these preexisting collaterals to open instantly. With continued obstruction, maturation of these collaterals then takes place. This occurs in three stages and over a period of up to 6 months. In the first two stages the luminal diameter of these collaterals increased nearly tenfold. In the mature stage a collateral may reach 1 mm in diameter, and it becomes a three-layer structure, similar to a normal coronary artery. In addition these collaterals have the capacity to respond to different agents (e.g., they dilate in response to beta-agonists and nitrates and constrict in response to vasopressin and serotonin).

The value of collaterals is seen in patients with large collaterals following coronary occlusion, where their presence with sufficient density can mitigate the severity of myocardial ischemia and necrosis. The presence of angiographically visible collaterals is associated with reduced fibrosis and better contractile function in the area of the myocardium which they supply.[1] Patients may even show absence of myocardial dysfunction in the territory of a large occluded coronary artery. For this reason, there has been much interest in finding agents or methods to enhance collateral function or increase their density. Exercise effects on coronary collaterals has been studied extensively in animals and in clinical trials using serial angiography.[2,3] The results from these studies indicate that exercise has no effect on the size or function of collateral vessels: an increase in collaterals was seen only with progression of underlying coronary stenoses, but not with exercise programs. Preliminary studies have suggested that heparin may improve collateral blood flow following myocardial infarction, and when combined with exercise.[4]

REFERENCES

1. Schwarz, F., Flameng, W., Ensslen, R., et al.: Effect of collaterals on left ventricular function at rest and during stress. Am. Heart J. *95*:570, 1978.
2. Franklin, B.A.: Exercise training and coronary collateral circulation. Med. Sci. Sports Exerc. *23*:648–653, 1991.
3. Ferguson, R.J., Petitclerc, R., Choquette, G., et al.: Effect of physical training on treadmill exercise capacity, collateral circulation and progression of coronary disease. Am. J. Cardiol. *34*:764, 1974.
4. Fujita, M., Sasayama, S., Asanoi, H., et al.: Improvement of treadmill capacity and collateral circulation as a result of exercise with heparin pretreatment in patients with effort angina. Circulation *77*:1022, 1988.

312-C *(Braunwald, pp. 1486–1492)*

The accumulation of pericardial fluid to the point of cardiac compression is termed cardiac tamponade and is characterized by an increase in intracardiac pressures, progressive limitation of diastolic filling of the ventricles, and an ultimate reduction in stroke volume. Normal intrapericardial pressures are several mm Hg lower than right and left ventricular diastolic pressures and are very close to intrapleural pressures. As fluid is accumulated in the pericardial space, intrapericardial pressure rises to the level of the RA and RV dia-

stolic pressures, and cardiac tamponade occurs. At this point, the transpericardial pressure distending the cardiac chambers declines to zero. While the rise of RA and intrapericardial pressures may be less dramatic in the presence of hypovolemia, cardiac tamponade can occur during this state and may be masked because the pressures in these two spaces equalize at a lower absolute value. As intrapericardial fluid continues to accumulate, pericardial and RV diastolic pressures rise together toward the level of LV diastolic pressure. Subsequently, all three pressures equalize and, as they continue to rise, lead to a marked decrease in transmural distending pressures, with a decrease in the diastolic volumes of the ventricles and a fall in stroke volume.[1] Cardiac output in this setting may initially be maintained by a reflex tachycardia. However, as the accumulation of pericardial fluid continues, compensatory mechanisms are no longer able to maintain systemic blood pressure and cardiac output begins to decline, with an accompanying impairment of the perfusion of vital organs.

In the most extreme examples of cardiac tamponade, transmural diastolic ventricular pressures may actually be negative. This implies that ventricular filling in this situation occurs by diastolic suction. Both the cardiac depressor branches of the vagus nerve and sinoatrial node ischemia are believed to contribute to the sinus bradycardia that may occur during severe cardiac tamponade.[2] Hemodynamic deterioration during tamponade has been noted to be markedly influenced by the presence of atrial compression during diastole and subsequent impairment of cardiac filling. Echocardiographic studies have demonstrated that right atrial and ventricular diastolic collapse are often present in patients with tamponade, while left atrial and/or left ventricular diastolic collapse are more variable findings.[3]

REFERENCES

1. Spodick, D.H.: The normal and diseased pericardium: Current concepts of pericardial physiology, diagnosis, and treatment. J. Am. Coll. Cardiol. *1*:240, 1983.
2. Kostreva, D.R., Castaner, A., Pedersen, D.H., and Kampine, J.P.: Nonvagally mediated bradycardia during cardiac tamponade or severe hemorrhage. Cardiology *68*:65, 1981.
3. Singh, S., Wann, L.S., Schuchard, G.H., et al.: Right ventricular and right atrial collapse in patients with cardiac tamponade—a combined echocardiographic and hemodynamic study. Circulation *70*:966, 1984.

313-C *(Braunwald, pp. 1126–1127)*

The apoprotein components of lipoproteins have several functions, including structural support, receptor recognition, and in some cases, enzymatic activity. Apo A-I is the major protein in HDL and in at least one study has been inversely correlated with arteriographic evidence of coronary disease.[1] The apo A-I protein also activates the enzyme lecithin:cholesterol acyltransferase (LCAT). LCAT allows the HDL particle to convert cholesterol obtained from peripheral tissues to cholesteryl ester, an important step in the so-called "reverse" cholesterol transport pathway. The two forms of apoprotein B, apo B-48 and apo B-100, arise from a single gene that displays a unique editing mechanism which allows for synthesis of both proteins.[2] Apo B-100 is the primary apoprotein of LDL, allowing recognition of the particle by the LDL receptor on cell surfaces. Apoprotein E may be found in VLDL particles as well as in chylomicrons, in IDL particles, and, to a small extent, in HDL as well. Most patients with type III hyperlipoproteinemia are homozygous for a particular apoprotein E phenotype (E_{2-2}). This disorder is characterized by premature atherosclerosis and is notable for the presence of hypercholesterolemia and hypertriglyceridemia due to an increase in IDL and/or VLDL particle populations.

REFERENCES

1. Kottke, B.A., Zinsmeister, A.R., Holmes, D.R., Jr., et al.: Apolipoproteins and coronary artery disease. Mayo Clin. Proc. *61*:313, 1986.
2. Higuchi, K., Hospattankar, I.V., Law, S.W., et al.: Human (apolipoprotein B) mRNA: Identification of two distinct apo B-100 mRNA containing a premature w-frame translational stop codon in both liver and intestine. Proc. Natl. Acad. Sci. U.S.A. *85*:1772, 1988.

314-B   (Braunwald, pp. 1054–1055)

This 67-year-old woman presents with the classic physical findings and symptoms of tricuspid regurgitation (TR). By history, the course of her illness is relatively rapid and includes systemic symptoms such as fatigue, weight loss, and peculiar episodes of rapid heartbeat, flushing, and diarrhea. The most likely diagnosis is the carcinoid syndrome. Carcinoid is a slowly growing tumor that leads to focal or diffuse deposits of fibrous tissue in the endocardium of the valvular cusps and cardiac chambers. The white fibrous carcinoid plaques are most extensive on the right side of the heart, usually because the tumor begins in the portal circulation and drains through the inferior vena cava into the right side of the heart. The plaques are deposited on the ventricular surfaces of the tricuspid valve and cause the cusps to adhere to the underlying right ventricle, producing TR.[1] Carcinoid syndrome is suggested by the coexistence of TR, flushing, and diarrhea due to the release of vasoactive amines (predominantly 5'-hydroxytryptamine) by the tumor cells.

The causes of isolated TR may be divided into those involving an anatomically abnormal valve and those involving an anatomically normal valve. The latter, in which functional TR is present due to dilatation of the RV and tricuspid annulus, is actually more common. The most common cause of functional TR is RV hypertension, especially as a result of mitral valve disease, RV infarction, congenital heart disease, primary pulmonary hyperten-

sion, or cor pulmonale. This woman had no evidence for chronic elevations in her pulmonary pressures, nor did she have an RV lift. RV infarction may also cause TR in the absence of pulmonary hypertension, secondary to RV dilatation.

A variety of disease processes may affect the tricuspid valve directly leading to regurgitation. Among these are: (1) Ebstein's anomaly, in which there is abnormal attachment and elongation of the tricuspid valve with ventricularization of the atrium; (2) common atrioventricular canal, in which the tricuspid valve is involved in the formation of an aneurysm of the ventricular septum; (3) rheumatic fever, which usually causes both regurgitation and stenosis as well as coexisting mitral valve disease; (4) infarction, rupture, or ischemia of the papillary muscles of the RV in coronary disease; (5) infective endocarditis; and (6) Marfan syndrome. Less common causes of TR include cardiac tumors (particularly right atrial myxomas), endomyocardial fibrosis, methysergide-induced valvular disease, and systemic lupus erythematosus.

REFERENCE

1. Callahan, J.A., Wroblewski, E.M., Reeder, G.S., et al.: Echocardiographic features of carcinoid heart disease. Am. J. Cardiol. *50*:762, 1982.

315-A   (Braunwald, pp. 1241–1242)

Left ventricular free wall rupture is one of the most dramatic and rapidly fatal complications of acute myocardial infarction. It is likely that it is responsible for a significant proportion of sudden death that occurs a few days after an infarct. The incidence of free wall rupture is estimated to be around 10 per cent in hospitalized patients, and a recent autopsy series found the incidence as high as 30 per cent among autopsied cases.[1] The early use of thrombolytic agents appears to reduce the incidence of this complication, although delayed use may actually increase the risk despite improving overall survival.[2] Free wall rupture is more common in the elderly and possibly in women, and is seen more often in hypertensive patients. It frequently involves the anterior or lateral left ventricular walls more than the inferior wall. Typical rupture patients are recovering from a first large myocardial infarction when hemopericardium and cardiac tamponade occur and cause rapid death. This complication can occur between days 1 and 21 of the infarct but most commonly occurs 1 to 4 days following the infarction. The tear usually occurs near or involves the junction between the infarcted myocardium and normal muscle.

REFERENCES

1. Reddy, S.G., and Roberts, W.C.: Frequency of rupture of the left ventricular free wall or ventricular septum among necropsy cases of fatal acute myocardial infarction since introduction of coronary care units. Am. J. Cardiol. *63*:906, 1989.

2. Honan, M.B., Harrell, F.E., Reimer, K.A., et al.: Cardiac rupture, mortality and the timing of thrombolytic therapy: A meta-analysis. J. Am. Coll. Cardiol. *16*:359, 1990.

316-B   *(Braunwald, pp. 1078–1079)*

The vast majority of intravenous drug abusers with right-sided endocarditis are noted to have either pneumonia or multiple septic emboli on chest x-ray. Recent echocardiographic studies also document mild degrees of tricuspid and pulmonic regurgitation in such patients without a history of prior endocarditis or frank vegetations.[1] However, the murmur of tricuspid regurgitation is frequently absent, and when the pulmonic valve is involved by endocarditis, murmurs may be overlooked or ascribed to a function or flow murmur.[2] The patient in the example shown has a large tricuspid valve vegetation, the most common site of endocardial involvement based on clinical studies.[3] However, in autopsy studies, an increased incidence of left-sided valvular involvement is noted, reflecting the increased mortality of infectious endocarditis in addicts when the mitral and/or aortic valves are involved. *Staphylococcus aureus* is isolated from approximately 60 per cent of cases of endocarditis in drug addicts, because the skin serves as the most common source of microorganisms in this setting.[4] Streptococci and enterococci account for nearly 20 per cent of lesions, while gram-negative bacilli and fungi account for approximately 10 and 5 per cent, respectively. *Staphylococcus aureus* is the organism most commonly isolated in this setting, and in 70 to 80 per cent of cases documented *S. aureus* endocarditis, only tricuspid valvular involvement is present.

REFERENCES

1. Eichacker, P.Q., Miller, K., Robbins, M., et al.: Echocardiographic evaluation of heart valves in IV drug abusers without a previous history of endocarditis. Clin. Res. *32*:670a, 1984.
2. Burns, J.M.A., Hogg, K.J., Hillis, W.S., and Dunn, F.G.: Endocarditis in intravenous drug abusers with staphylococcal septicemia. Br. Heart J. *61*:356, 1980.
3. Baddour, L.M.: Twelve-year review of recurrent native valve infective endocarditis: A disease of the modern antibiotic era. Rev. Infect. Dis. *10*:1163, 1988.
4. Levine, D.P., Crane, L.R., and Zervos, J.J.: Bacteremia in narcotic addicts at the Detroit Medical Center. II. Infectious endocarditis: A prospective comparative study. Rev. Infect. Dis. *8*:374, 1986.

317-B   *(Braunwald, pp. 1535–1537)*

The most common cause of blunt cardiac trauma is motor vehicle accidents. Direct cardiac compression usually results from impact with the steering wheel. Indirect compression occurs with impact to the abdominal wall. Other causes of blunt cardiac trauma include direct blows to the chest and following cardiac resuscitation. Fracture of the sternum or ribs does not necessarily accompany blunt cardiac trauma, but its presence should alert the clinician to the high likelihood and potential seriousness of underlying cardiac damage. In addition, lack of early manifestations by no means excludes the presence of cardiac injury. Manifestations of trauma are typically not seen for days or even weeks following the injury.

Blunt cardiac trauma can result in injury to one or more of the cardiac structures. The pericardium, myocardium, endocardial structures (including cardiac valves, chordae and papillary muscles), the coronary arteries, and the major vessels (aorta and the pulmonary artery) can be involved. Evidence of traumatic pericarditis may be seen in patients without evidence of pericardial tears or lacerations. Important complications of pericardial involvement include tamponade, cardiac herniation through a tear, and constrictive pericarditis.

Myocardial involvement can be in the form of contusion or laceration. Myocardial contusion often goes unrecognized because of a lack of symptoms. The most common symptom is precordial pain resembling myocardial infarction. ECG is most helpful in recognizing contusion of the left ventricle, and may demonstrate nonspecific ST-segment and T-wave changes or changes consistent with pericarditis. Because CK may be elevated by trauma to noncardiac structures, CK values are of limited use in the diagnosis of myocardial contusion. In addition, because skeletal muscle contains a small amount of CK-MB, the value of this isoenzyme is especially limited in cases of skeletal muscle trauma with large elevations in total CK activity. When myocardial rupture occurs it is due to either direct myocardial laceration or infarction leading to thinning and rupture. Most commonly, rupture from trauma involves the right ventricle and usually results in the rapid development of cardiac tamponade and death.

318-C   *(Braunwald, pp. 1438–1439)*

Cardiac involvement in HIV can be due to direct involvement by HIV, by other infecting organisms, due to malignant involvement by Kaposi's sarcoma, or due to immune and drug-induced cardiomyopathy. Cardiac involvement occurs in up to 50 per cent of cases, although symptoms develop in only 10 per cent.[1-3] In symptomatic patients, the most common presentation is with symptoms of heart failure due to LV dysfunction. Other findings suggestive of cardiac involvement in these patients include pericardial effusions (which are rarely associated with tamponade), arrythmias, endocarditis, and nonspecific ECG changes. The etiology of cardiomyopathy (the co-called HIV cardiomyopathy) in these patients is unclear. Myocarditis is frequently seen in these patients and is likely to be multifactorial. Recently, HIV was isolated from cardiac myocytes, suggesting that the virus itself may be cardiotoxic.[4] Treatment of HIV patients follows the same approach used for treating patients with other causes of heart failure. Therapy can offer some degree of symptomatic relief, but overall prognosis is poor.

REFERENCES

1. De Castro, S., d'Amati, G., Gallo, P., et al.: Frequency of development of acute global left ventricular dysfunction in human immunodeficiency virus infection. J. Am. Coll. Cardiol. 24:1018–1024, 1994.
2. Reilly, J.M., Cunnion, R.E., Anderson, D.W., et al.: Frequency of myocarditis, left ventricular dysfunction and ventricular tachycardia in the acquired immune deficiency syndrome. Am. J. Cardiol. 62:789–793, 1988.
3. Cohen, I.S., Anderson, D.W., Virmani, R., et al.: Congestive cardiomyopathy in association with the acquired immunodeficiency syndrome. N. Engl. J. Med. 315:628–630, 1986.
4. Calabrese, L.H., Proffitt, M.R., Yen-Lieberman, B., et al.: Congestive cardiomyopathy and illness related to the acquired immunodeficiency syndrome (AIDS) associated with isolation of retrovirus from myocardium. Ann. Intern. Med. 107:619–692, 1987.

319-D   (Braunwald, pp. 1144–1146)

A number of secondary causes of hypertriglyceridemia have been identified. These include diabetes mellitus, chronic renal failure, cigarette use, alcohol use, obesity, and some drugs, such as the noncardioselective beta blockers. Triglyceride elevation is an independent cardiac risk factor for women, and it is likely that other patient populations with elevated triglycerides and increased risk for cardiovascular disease will be identified in the coming years. In further analysis of CLAS trial, triglyceride levels predicted atherosclerotic disease. Current guidelines in the United States for triglyceridemia are based on the NIH-sponsored Consensus Conference of 1984.[2] Levels under 250 mg/dl are considered normal, those between 250 and 500 are borderline, and levels above 500 mg/dl are classified as "high risk." The risks of hypertriglyceridemia include pancreatitis that may be severe, and thus recommendations for patients with fasting triglyceride levels of ≥500 mg/dl include aggressive treatment first with diet and then pharmacological agents. The European Atherosclerosis Society is more aggressive and suggests treating any fasting triglyceride level over 200 mg/dl.

REFERENCES

1. Blankenhorn, D.H., Alaupovic, P., Wickham, E., et al.: Prediction of angiographic change in native human coronary arteries and aortocoronary bypass grafts. Lipid and nonlipid factors. Circulation 81:470, 1990.
2. Consensus Conference. Treatment of hypertriglyceridemia. JAMA 251:1196, 1984.

320-B   (Braunwald, pp. 896–898)

There are a variety of clinical findings in ASD that may provide evidence of the underlying condition. On physical examination, common findings include a prominent RV impulse, palpable pulmonary artery pulsations, accentuation of the tricuspid valve closure sound leading to splitting of the first heart sound, and a midsystolic pulmonary ejection murmur due to increased flow across the pulmonic valve. If the shunt is large, a mid-diastolic rumbling murmur may be audible at the lower left sternal border. This murmur results from increased blood flow across the tricuspid valve.

The ECG may be particularly helpful in the diagnostic evaluation of a patient with suspected ASD. The ECG in patients with an ostium secundum ASD usually shows right-axis deviation and an rSR′ or rsR′ pattern in the right precordial leads with a normal QRS duration. The presence of left-axis deviation of the P wave in the frontal plane in association with the aforementioned constellation suggests the presence of a sinus venosus defect. Left-axis deviation and superior orientation of the QRS complex in the frontal plane suggest the presence of either an ostium primum defect or, less commonly, a secundum atrial defect in association with mitral valve prolapse. Prolongation of the P-R interval may be seen with all types of ASDs. It is believed to result both from the increased size of the atrium in this condition and the increased distance for intranodal conduction produced by the defect itself.[1]

Chest x-ray may reveal enlargement of the RA and RV, pulmonary arterial dilatation, and increased pulmonary vascular markings. Echocardiographic evaluation of ASD may reveal pulmonary arterial and RV dilatation as well as anterior systolic (paradoxical) supraventricular septal motion, especially if significant RV volume overload is present.[2] The defect itself may be visualized by two-dimensional echocardiography, particularly utilizing a subcostal view of the interatrial septum. In many institutions, two-dimensional echocardiography along with Doppler flow analysis has become the primary confirmatory test for ASD.[3] Cardiac catheterization may be employed in clinical situations in which the diagnosis is in question or if insignificant pulmonary hypertension is suspected. In children with ASD, pressures on the right side of the heart are usually normal, even in the presence of a large left-to-right shunt. Pulmonary hypertension and resultant right ventricular failure are serious complications of ASD and most commonly begin in the third or fourth decade of life.

REFERENCES

1. Clark, E.B., and Kugler, J.D.: Preoperative secundum atrial septal defect with coexisting sinus node and atrioventricular node dysfunction. Circulation 65:976, 1982.
2. DiSessa, T.G., and Friedman, W.F.: Echocardiographic evaluation of cardiac performance. In Friedman, W.F., and Higgins, C.B. (eds.): Pediatric Cardiac Imaging. Philadelphia, W.B. Saunders Company, 1984, p. 219.
3. Freed, M.D., Nadas, A.S., Norwood, W.I., and Castaneda, A.R.: Is routine preoperative cardiac catheterization necessary before repair of secundum and sinus venosus atrial septal defects? J. Am. Coll. Cardiol. 4:333, 1984.

321-B *(Braunwald, pp. 1420–1421)*

The auscultatory hallmark of hypertrophic cardiomyopathy (HCM) associated with an outflow tract gradient in the presence of a harsh crescendo-decrescendo murmur. The murmur is labile in intensity and duration (dynamic) and responds differently than fixed obstruction (e.g., aortic valve stenosis) to a variety of maneuvers that alter left ventricular (LV) filling, afterload, and contractility. In general, any maneuver that decreases left ventricular filling, decreases afterload or increases contractility, will increase the gradient and the murmur. With the Valsalva maneuver, for example, there is decreased LV filling and reduction in afterload. This increases the gradient and the intensity of the murmur. Similarly, with the administration of amyl nitrate (decreased afterload and increased contractility) and with tachycardia (increased contractility), there is an increase in outflow tract obstruction, and subsequent increase in the gradient and the murmur. With the Mueller maneuver (inspiration against closed glottis, increasing both preload and afterload), administration of phenylephrine (increased afterload), or beta blockers (decreased contractility and increased preload), there is a decrease in outflow tract obstruction, and subsequent decrease in the gradient and the murmur.

322-E *(Braunwald, pp. 1146–1147)*

In several retrospective studies Lp(a) has been shown to be an independent risk factor for coronary artery disease. The Lp(a) molecule includes a part that is identical to LDL, which is linked to apo(a), a protein that has close structural homology to plasminogen. This latter structural feature is thought to play a role in the increased incidence of coronary thrombosis in patients with increased Lp(a) levels. The primary determinant of Lp(a) level is genetic, and more than 90 per cent of the variation in Lp(a) levels is attributable to variations in the apo(a) gene.[1,2] Given the increased risk of coronary events associated with increased levels of Lp(a), it is logical to think that reducing Lp(a) levels would be associated with reduction in coronary risk. This hypothesis, however, has not yet been proven, in part because Lp(a) measurement has only recently become widely available, and also because levels are not affected by most lipid-lowering agents. Nicotinic acid, estrogen, and bezafibrate can lower Lp(a) levels, but the impact of these therapies on coronary events has not been determined yet.

REFERENCES

1. Scanu, A.M.: Identification of mutations in human apolipoprotein(a) kringle 4-37 from the study of the DNA of peripheral blood lymphocytes: Relevance to the role of lipoprotein(a) in atherothrombosis. Am. J. Cardiol. *75:* 588–618, 1995.
2. Trommsdorff, M., Kochl, S., Lingenhel, A., et al.: A penta-nucleotide repeat polymorphism in the 5′ control region

of the apolipoprotein(a) gene is associated with lipoprotein(a) plasma concentrations in Caucasians. J. Clin. Invest. *96:*150–157, 1995.

323-B *(Braunwald, pp. 1240–1241)*

Patients with right ventricular infarction (RVI) may have a hemodynamic profile resembling that of patients with pericardial disease. For example, elevations in right atrial and ventricular filling pressures, as well as a rapid right atrial x descent and an early diastolic dip-and-plateau ("square root sign"), may be present. In addition, Kussmaul's sign may occur in patients with RVI and is highly predictive for right ventricular involvement in the setting of inferior wall infarction.[1] Patients who are admitted with inferior wall infarction should have an ECG with the precordial leads placed on the right chest in a mirror-image pattern to the usual placement on the left chest. Most patients with right ventricular infarction have ST-segment elevation of 1 mm or more in lead V_4R.[2] Echocardiography may confirm the absence of pericardial fluid and the presence of abnormal right ventricular wall motion, as well as right ventricular dilatation and depression of right ventricular function. RVI must be distinguished from other causes of hypotension with acute myocardial infarction, including pericardial tamponade as already mentioned, constrictive pericarditis, and pulmonary embolus.

Treatment is aimed at increasing right atrial, right ventricular, and thus left-sided filling pressures by increasing total intravascular volume through the administration of intravenous saline. A marked hypotensive response to small doses of nitroglycerin may be a clinical clue to the presence of RVI.[3] Because atrial transport may be very important in patients with RVI, patients who become pacemaker dependent may benefit from atrioventricular sequential pacing, which has been shown to improve hemodynamics in this condition.[3]

REFERENCES

1. Baigrie, R.S., Haq, A., Morgan, C.D., et al.: The spectrum of right ventricular involvement in inferior wall myocardial infarction: A clinical hemodynamic and noninvasive study. J. Am. Coll. Cardiol. *1:*1396, 1983.
2. Croft, C.H., Nicod, P., Corbett, J.R., et al.: Detection of acute right ventricular infarction by right precordial electrocardiography. Am. J. Cardiol. *50:*421, 1982.
3. Haffajee, C.I., Love, J., Gore, J.M., and Alpert, J.S.: Reversibility of shock by atrial or atrioventricular sequential pacing in right ventricular infarction. Am. J. Cardiol. *49:*1025, 1982.

324-B *(Braunwald, pp. 1317–1319)*

Presently, most surgeons believe that IMA grafts should be placed during bypass grafting procedures whenever technically feasible. Loop and colleagues first published the data on improved 10-year survival in patients receiving an IMA graft.[1] Subsequent studies[2] have confirmed the findings of these investigators, and further studies of the longevity of these grafts have proved that the patency rate for IMA grafts at 10 to 12 years exceeds 90 per cent.[3] In recent years, surgeons have also begun to use multiple IMA grafting procedures. Such procedures are technically more demanding, but do not appear to be associated with an increase in either operative morbidity or mortality[4] (see Braunwald, Fig. 38–12, p. 1318). An interesting recent report suggests that endothelium-dependent relaxation of an IMA graft is more pronounced than in a comparable vein graft, suggesting that flow-dependent autoregulation may be enhanced in such grafts.[5]

REFERENCES

1. Loop, F.D., Lytle, B.W., Cosgrove, D.M., et al.: Influence of the internal mammary artery graft on 10-year survival and other cardiac events. N. Engl. J. Med. 314:1, 1986.
2. Cameron, A., Davis, K.B., Green, G.E., et al.: Clinical implications of internal mammary bypass grafts: The Coronary Artery Surgery Study experience. Circulation 77:815, 1988.
3. Loop, F.D., Lytle, B.W., Cosgrove, D.M., et al.: New arteries for old. Circulation 79(Suppl. I):40, 1989.
4. Morris, J.J., Smith, R., Glower, D.D., et al.: Clinical evaluation of single versus multiple mammary artery bypass. Circulation 82(Suppl. IV):214, 1990.
5. Luscher, T.F., Diederich, D., Siebenmann, R., et al.: Difference between endothelium-dependent relaxation in arterial and in venous coronary bypass grafts. N. Engl. J. Med. 319:462, 1986.

325-C   (Braunwald, pp. 1547–1550)

Complete repair is recommended for any patients with AAA ≥6 cm in diameter by placement of a synthetic prosthesis and resection of aneurysmal segments of the aorta. The management of asymptomatic aneurysms <6 cm in diameter remains controversial and depends on the clinical status of the individual patient. In poor-risk patients with aneurysms between 4 and 6 cm, close follow-up and frequent ultrasound examination are warranted. In persons who are otherwise clinically stable and in good health, elective resection of aneurysms between 4 and 6 cm in diameter may be appropriate.[1]

Prior to careful hemodynamic monitoring, "declamping shock" was a difficult problem, characterized by marked hypotension following release of the aortic crossclamp after surgery. This problem has been virtually eliminated in modern surgical care. Improvements in cardiac protection have also been realized by the use of vasodilator therapy to diminish changes in afterload caused by clamping and unclamping of the aorta.[2] Similar advances in renal and pulmonary management have relegated complications affecting these organ systems to a much less frequent status. Because patients who do not survive repair of AAA suffer MI 50 per cent of the time,[3] routine coronary angiography and selective coronary bypass surgery prior to aneurysm resection may be appropriate in this population.

The operative risk in the lowest-risk patients from AAA repair is approximately 2 to 5 per cent. If the aneurysm is unstable and has been expanding, mortality is 5 to 15 per cent; in the event of frank rupture, mortality is approximately 50 per cent. Only 5 to 10 per cent of patients survive for 5 years with unrepaired aneurysms >6 cm, compared with more than 50 per cent of those who undergo successful resection and compared with 80 per cent for an age-matched "normal" population.

REFERENCES

1. Gleidman, M.L., Ayers, W.B., and Vestal, B.L.: Aneurysms of the abdominal aorta and its branches. A study of untreated patients. Ann. Surg. 217:1537, 1982.
2. Shenaq, S.A., Chelly, J.E., Karlberg, H., et al.: Use of nitroprusside during surgery for thoracoabdominal aortic aneurysm. Circulation 70(Suppl. I):7, 1984.
3. Hertzer, N.R.: Fatal myocardial infarction following abdominal aortic aneurysm resection. Three hundred forty-three patients followed 6–11 years postoperatively. Ann. Surg. 192:671, 1980.
4. Hertzer, N.R., Bevin, E.G., Young, J.R., et al.: Coronary artery disease in peripheral vascular patients. Ann. Surg. 199: 223, 1984.

326-E   (Braunwald, pp. 1025–1026; Table 32–4)

Several clinical features are helpful in distinguishing acute from chronic MR.[1] In acute MR the ECG is usually normal, while in chronic MR abnormalities such as P mitrale, atrial fibrillation, and left ventricular hypertrophy are frequently present. The heart size is usually normal in acute MR; cardiomegaly and left atrial enlargement are prominent in chronic MR. An apical thrill is commonly present in chronic MR and frequently absent in acute MR. There are also several differences in the systolic murmurs of acute and chronic MR. In chronic MR the primary location of the murmur is usually at the apex, and in acute MR it is usually at the base of the heart. While the murmur frequently radiates to the axilla in chronic MR, it can radiate to the neck, spine, and top of the head in acute MR depending on the location of the jet. Furthermore, in patients with acute MR who have a normal-sized left atrium, the left atrial pressure rises abruptly, frequently leading to pulmonary edema and elevated JVP. Because the v wave is markedly elevated in acute MR, the pressure gradient between the left ventricle and atrium declines at the end of systole. The murmur may not be holosystolic but instead may be decrescendo, ending well before A_2. It is also usually lower pitched and softer than the murmur of chronic MR.

REFERENCE

1. Blumenthal, P., et al.: Noninvasive investigations with a diagnosis of mitral valve disease. In Ionescu, M.I., and Cohn, L.H. (eds.): Mitral Valve Disease: Diagnosis and Treatment. London, Butterworth's, 1985.

327-B *(Braunwald, pp. 1489–1490)*

Several forms of cardiac tamponade are evident clinically and can be distinguished by their distinct features. In patients in whom pericardial fluid collects rapidly, such as those who suffer intrapericardial hemorrhage from a penetrating heart wound or aortic dissection, the appearance of Beck's triad may be noted. This includes a profound decrease in systemic arterial pressure, concomitant elevation of systemic venous pressure, and a small, quiet heart, as first described by Beck in 1935.[1] Patients who develop tamponade rapidly may show evidence of decreased cerebral perfusion—as well as an absent or difficult-to-perceive pulsus paradoxus because of the profound hypotension that usually accompanies this scenario.

In patients in whom cardiac tamponade develops at a more gradual rate, dyspnea is often the major complaint. Such patients may appear acutely ill, although not morbidly so, if the tamponade has developed in a chronic manner. Systemic symptoms such as weight loss and profound weakness may also be present. The most common physical findings in tamponade include jugular venous distention, tachypnea, tachycardia, pulsus paradoxus, and hepatomegaly. The presence of pulsus paradoxus is extremely helpful in suggesting the diagnosis of cardiac tamponade. The differential diagnosis of a patient with the triad of pulsus paradoxus, systemic venous distention, and clear lungs includes obstructive pulmonary disease, constrictive pericarditis, restrictive cardiomyopathy, and massive pulmonary embolism.

Low-pressure cardiac tamponade may be seen in patients who are normotensive and in whom the physical examination is normal except for a moderate elevation of jugular venous pressure. This entity has been reported in tuberculous and neoplastic pericarditis and may be associated with severe dehydration.[2] It represents the earliest stages of developing cardiac tamponade in which intrapericardial pressures and right atrial pressures are equalized at a relatively low absolute pressure reading. With rehydration, the clinical picture of tamponade becomes more pronounced.

REFERENCES

1. Beck, C.S.: Two cardiac compression triads. JAMA *104*:714, 1935.
2. Labib, S.B., Udelson, J.E., and Pandian, N.G.: Echocardiography in low pressure cardiac tamponade. Am. J. Cardiol. *63*:1156, 1989.

328-A *(Braunwald, pp. 1511–1512)*

Two types of pericarditis can follow acute myocardial infarction: early and delayed. Early acute fibrinous pericarditis is frequently seen following acute myocardial infarction, usually within the first few days. Its incidence varies depending on the size of the infarct, which seems to be the primary determinant of its development. The use of thrombolytic therapy caused a 50 per cent reduction in the incidence of this complication, and observations from the GISSI trial suggest that the earlier the thrombolytic agent is given, the lower is the incidence of pericarditis.[1] In addition, pericarditis is less common following non-Q-wave infarction. The use of heparin has not been associated with increased risk of pericarditis or tamponade. Clinical evidence of pericarditis can be found as early as 12 hours after the infarction, and the earliest sign may be a pericardial friction rub. In about 70 per cent of patients, the rub may be accompanied by pleuritic chest pain. Appearance of symptoms and signs of pericarditis more than 10 days following an infarction suggests the onset of Dressler syndrome. Typical diagnostic ECG changes of pericarditis are uncommon in post-MI pericarditis or Dressler syndrome. Rather, two types of atypical T-wave changes that have been described carry a high sensitivity (>95 per cent) and moderate specificity (~75 per cent) for the diagnosis of post-MI pericarditis.[2,3] They consist of either T waves that remain persistently positive 48 hours or more after infarction, or premature reversal of initially inverted T waves to positive deflections. Other causes of such T-wave changes include CPR, reinfarction, and very small infarcts.

REFERENCES

1. Correale, E., Maggioni, A.P., Romano, S., et al.: Comparison of frequency, diagnostic and prognostic significance of pericardial involvement in acute mycardial infarction treated with and without thrombolytics. Gruppo Italiano per lo Studio della Sopravvivenza nell'Infarto Miocardico (GISSI). Am. J. Cardiol. *71*:1377–1381, 1993.
2. Oliva, P.B., Hammill, S.C., and Talano, J.V.: T wave changes consistent with epicardial involvement in acute myocardial infarction. Observations in patients with a postinfarction pericardial effusion without clinically recognized postinfarction pericarditis. J. Am. Coll. Cardiol. *24*:1073–1077, 1994.
3. Oliva, P.B., Hammill, S.C., and Talano, J.V.: Effect of definition on incidence of postinfarction pericarditis. It is time to redefine postinfarction pericarditis? Circulation *90*:1537–1541, 1994.

329-D *(Braunwald, pp. 1564–1567)*

Acute aortic dissection is a medical and surgical emergency. Without treatment, mortality is very high, especially in the first few hours. Mortality in untreated cases can exceed 25 per cent in the first 24 hours and 50 per cent in the first week following the onset. Immediate medical management should focus on reduction of blood pressure, reduction of arterial dP/dt (which reflects the force of ejection of the left ventricle), fluid resuscitation if necessary, and preparation of the patient for operative intervention if indicated. Beta blockers are the agents of choice for lowering blood pressure and nitroprusside can be added for further blood pressure control. Labetalol is a very good initial therapy because it combines blood-pressure-lowering effects (alpha and beta blockade) with reduction in dP/dt (beta blockade). In general, proximal acute dissection involving the ascending aorta is best managed by surgery. This is because any progression of proximal dissection can compromise flow to one of the major vessels, including the coronaries, cause rupture into the pericardium resulting in rapid tamponade and death, or lead to severe aortic valve regurgitation. Uncomplicated distal dissections, however, can be managed with medical therapy or surgery; both approaches have shown similar impact on outcome.

A small percentage of patients present with chronic dissections. By surviving the acute stage, these patients represent a selected subset of lower risk patients who can be managed conservatively with medical therapy regardless of the location of the dissection, unless the dissection is complicated by aneurysm, rupture, vascular compromise, or aortic regurgitation. When aortic regurgitation complicates acute dissection, decompression of the false lumen may be all that is required to correct the geometry of the aortic valve and allow resuspension of the leaflets.[1,2] This technique has had favorable results with low incidence of recurrent aortic regurgitation in long-term follow-up. Because of this and the risk associated with valve replacement, an attempt should be made to preserve the native aortic valve if possible in cases of dissection complicated by regurgitation.

REFERENCES

1. von Segesser, L.K., Lorenzetti, E., Lachat, M., et al.: Aortic valve preservation in acute type A dissection: Is it sound? J. Thorac. Cardiovasc. Surg. 111:381–390, 1996.
2. Mazzucotelli, J.P., Deleuze, P.H., Baufreton, C., et al.: Preservation of the aortic valve in acute aortic dissection: Long-term echocardiographic assessment and clinical outcome. Ann. Thorac. Surg. 55:1513–1517, 1993.

330-C   (Braunwald, pp. 1516–1517)

Pericardial injury and pericarditis may occur early during the course of radiation therapy. However, it is more common months or even years later. This is especially true when cases of delayed constrictive pericarditis are included. The risk of radiation pericarditis depends on multiple factors including the radiation dose, duration, volume of the heart included in the radiation field, use of ^{60}Co source, and anterior weighting of the radiation dose.[1,2] When the whole pericardium is included in the radiation field, the risk of pericarditis is about 20 per cent, while the use of subcarinal block, which protects the heart from the radiation field, decreases the risk by about 2.5 per cent. In its early stages, there is usually a small pericardial effusion that may resolve spontaneously or may organize and progress to a fibrous stage causing constrictive pericarditis. The acute form of radiation injury is seldom evident clinically. The delayed

form, however, can present with symptoms of acute pericarditis or present as an asymptomatic pericardial effusion. Up to 20 per cent of these patients will progress to chronic pericarditis that will require pericardiectomy. Surgical pericardiectomy is required for treatment of patients with large recurrent pericardial effusion or severe effusive-constrictive pericarditis. Operative mortality in these patients is high (21 per cent) when compared with pericardiectomy in patients with idiopathic constrictive pericarditis (~5 per cent).

REFERENCES

1. Benoff, L.J., and Schweitzer, P.: Radiation therapy-induced cardiac injury. Am. Heart J. 129:1193–1196, 1995.
2. Arsenian, M.A.: Cardiovascular sequelae of therapeutic thoracic radiation. Prog. Cardiovasc. Dis. 33:299–311, 1991.

331-A   (Braunwald, pp. 1414–1416)

The echocardiogram shown is from a patient with hypertrophic cardiomyopathy (HCM) and illustrates marked systolic anterior motion of the mitral valve with prolonged near contact between the anterior leaflet and the ventricular septum at the arrow. The ventricular septum is somewhat thickened while the mitral valve leaflets appear normal—without calcification, abnormal fluttering, or failure to appose in systole. Although a characteristic feature of HCM is disproportionate septal hypertrophy, generalized LV hypertrophy may also be present. Another feature in many patients with HCM is a narrowed LV outflow tract, which is formed by the inner ventricular septum anteriorly and the anterior leaflet of the mitral valve posteriorly. When HCM is associated with obstruction to LV outflow, as in the patient whose echocardiogram is illustrated, there is abnormal systolic anterior motion of the anterior leaflet and occasionally the posterior leaflet of the mitral valve. There is a close relationship between the degree of this abnormal motion and the size of the outflow gradient.

Three explanations have been offered for systolic anterior motion: (1) the mitral valve is pulled against the septum by contraction of the papillary muscles because of the abnormal location and orientation of these muscles due to the hypertrophy; (2) the mitral valve is pushed against the septum because of its abnormal position in the LV outflow tract; and (3) the mitral valve is drawn toward the septum because of the lower pressure that occurs distal to the obstruction as blood is ejected at high velocity through a narrowed outflow tract (Venturi effect). It should be noted that systolic anterior motion may occasionally be found in other conditions, including hypercontractile states, transposition of the great arteries, and infiltration of the septum.

Other common echocardiographic findings in HCM include a small LV cavity, reduced septal thickening during systole, reduced rate of closure of the mitral valve in mid-diastole, mitral valve prolapse, good systolic function, and a large *a* wave during atrial contraction.

332-C (Braunwald, pp. 1218–1219)

The three currently approved thrombolytic agents for intravenous use in patients with acute MI are streptokinase, t-PA, and APSAC. Streptokinase has been the most widely used of these agents, in part because of its long-standing availability, low cost, and proven efficacy in reducing mortality.[1] APSAC is an agent that may be administered rapidly (usually by intravenous injection as a bolus) and that provides a sustained fibrinolytic effect. However, early hopes that APSAC would be more clot-selective than streptokinase have not been realized.[2] The ease of administration of this compound, however, provides a distinct advantage over the other two agents, which must be administered by continuous intravenous infusion. t-PA is a component of the endogenous fibrinolytic system and is produced for therapeutic use by recombinant DNA techniques. The agent is given in a total dose of 100 mg, with 60 mg given in the first hour, followed by 20 mg per hour over the next 2 hours. Six to 10 mg of the initial 60-mg dose is given as a bolus in the currently recommended protocol.

A great deal of controversy surrounds the relative merits of t-PA with respect to streptokinase. In general, trials have suggested that the patency rate of the infarct-related artery is higher with t-PA, and in the trials that have employed early angiography, this has consistently been the case.[3,4] Larger mortality trials comparing the two agents have not shown a significant difference in overall mortality rates.[5] These trials have been criticized because of a failure to employ intravenous heparin early during therapy with t-PA as has been the case in most other trials. At the present time, cardiologists remain divided about which of these two agents is the drug of first choice in the setting of acute MI, although in the United States the majority at present probably favor rt-PA.

REFERENCES

1. Yusuf, S., Collins, R., Peto, R., et al.: Intravenous and intracoronary fibrinolytic therapy in acute myocardial infarction. Overview of results on mortality, reinfarction and side effects from 33 randomized control trials. Eur. Heart J. *6*:556, 1985.
2. Lavie, C.J., Gersh, B.J., and Chesebro, J.H.: Reperfusion in acute myocardial infarction. Mayo Clin. Proc. *65*:549, 1990.
3. Collen, D.: Coronary thrombolysis: Streptokinase or recombinant tissue-type plasminogen activator? Ann. Intern. Med. *112*:529, 1990.
4. Chesebro, J.H., Knatterud, G., Roberts, R., et al.: Thrombolysis in myocardial infarction (TIMI) trial, phase I: A comparison between intravenous tissue plasminogen activator and intravenous streptokinase. Circulation *76*:142, 1987.
5. The International Study Group: In-hospital mortality and clinical course of 20,891 patients with suspected acute myocardial infarction randomized between alteplase and streptokinase with or without heparin. Lancet *2*:71, 1990.

333-D (Braunwald, pp. 914–918)

Congenital valvular AS is a relatively common congenital anomaly. It has been estimated to occur in 3 to 6 per cent of patients with congenital cardiovascular defects and is seen much more frequently in males than in females, with a sex ratio of approximately 4:1. Up to 20 per cent of individuals with congenital valvular AS have associated cardiovascular anomalies, of which patient ductus arteriosus and coarctation of the aorta are most frequent. The majority of children with congenital AS develop and grow in a normal manner and are asymptomatic. The diagnosis is therefore usually suspected when a murmur is detected on routine physical examination. When symptoms do occur the most common include fatigability, exertional dyspnea, syncope, and angina pectoris. In general, the presence of symptoms suggests critical stenosis.

Findings on physical examination for children with congenital valvular AS are similar to those in adults. In general, the presence of a fourth heart sound is associated with severe obstruction.

In patients <10 years of age, the electrocardiogram provides a more reliable guide to the severity of congenital AS than it does in older patients.[1] The presence of LVH with "strain" generally indicates that severe obstruction is present (see Braunwald, Fig. 29–32, p. 916). Other findings in the younger age group that are associated with severe obstruction include a T-wave axis <-40 degrees, a widening of the angle between the mean QRS and T forces in the frontal plane >100 degrees, an S wave in V_1 >16 mm, and an R wave in V_5 >20 mm.

Echocardiography is useful in diagnosing the presence and severity of congenital AS. The most accurate noninvasive approach to quantification of the severity of obstruction is a combination of continuous-wave Doppler flow analysis and two-dimensional echocardiography.[2]

Cardiac catheterization in infants and young children with valvular AS is most important for establishing the site and severity, rather than the presence, of the lesion, since the malformation is often readily detected by physical examination and noninvasive studies. Catheterization is indicated in children with a clinical diagnosis of AS and the possibility of severe obstruction. The appearance of symptoms that are consistent with AS or that may be related to such a lesion should prompt cardiac catheterization. Management of the child with congenital AS includes antibiotic prophylaxis to prevent infective endocarditis regardless of the severity of aortic valvular obstruction. Participation in competitive sports is usually restricted in patients with milder degrees of obstruction, and strict avoidance of more strenuous physical activity is advisable if severe AS is present. Aortic valvulotomy appears to be a safe, effective treatment for congenital valvular AS.[3]

REFERENCES

1. Braunwald, E., Goldblatt, A., Aygen, M.M., et al.: Congenital aortic stenosis. I. Clinical and hemodynamic findings in 100 patients. Circulation 27:426, 1963.
2. Robinson, P.J., Wyse, R.K.H., Deanfield, J.E., et al.: Continuous wave Doppler velocimetry as an adjunct to cross-sectional echocardiography in the diagnosis of critical left heart obstruction in neonates. Br. Heart J. 52:552, 1984.
3. DeBoer, B.A., Robbins, R.C., Maron, B.J., et al.: Late results in aortic valvotomy for congenital valvular aortic stenosis. Ann. Thorac. Surg. 50:69, 1990.

334-D   (Braunwald, pp. 1334–1335)

Holter monitoring commonly demonstrates silent ischemia in patients with unstable angina. Recent data suggest that the vast majority (>85 to 90 per cent) of the ischemic episodes in this condition are silent, and that the presence of such episodes predicts unfavorable outcomes, both during hospitalization and over the subsequent months.[1,2] Silent ischemic changes on Holter monitoring are correlated with reductions in both myocardial perfusion and ventricular function.[3] The control of anginal symptoms in patients with unstable angina does not guarantee that silent ischemic episodes have also been eradicated.[1] Therefore, patients with unstable angina may benefit from predischarge Holter monitorings, and persistent silent ischemia may merit early angiography and revascularization,[2] since such patients are at high risk for adverse clinical events in the months following their hospitalization.[4]

REFERENCES

1. Nademanee, K., Intrachot, V., Josephson, M.A., et al.: Prognostic significance of silent myocardial ischemia in patients with unstable angina. J. Am. Coll. Cardiol. 10:1, 1987.
2. Gottlieb, S.O., Weisfeldt, M.L., Ouyang, P., et al.: Silent ischemia predicts infarction and death during 2 years follow-up of unstable angina. J. Am. Coll. Cardiol. 10:756, 1987.
3. Cohn, P.F., Brown, A.J., Jr., Wynne, J., et al.: Global and regional left ventricular ejection fraction abnormalities during exercise in patients with silent myocardial ischemia. J. Am. Coll. Cardiol. 1:931, 1983.
4. Gottlieb, S.O., Weisfeldt, M.L., Ouyang, P., et al.: Silent ischemia as a marker for early unfavorable outcomes in patients with unstable angina. N. Engl. J. Med. 314:1214, 1986.

335-E   (Braunwald, pp. 877–879)

While the true incidence of congenital cardiovascular malformation is difficult to determine accurately, it has been estimated that approximately 0.8 per cent of live births are complicated by some such disorder. The most common malformation seen is the ventricular septal defect, which is followed in frequency of occurrence by atrial septal defect and patent ductus arteriosus. These data do not take into account the congenital, nonstenotic bicuspid aortic valve or mitral valve prolapse, both of which may be quite prevalent. While the major-

ity of children with congenital heart disease are male, specific defects may show a definite sex predilection. Thus patent ductus arteriosus and atrial septal defects are more common in females, whereas valvular aortic stenosis, congenital aneurysms of the sinus of Valsalva, coarctation of the aorta, tetralogy of Fallot, and transposition of the great arteries are seen more frequently in males. Extracardiac anomalies occur in approximately 25 per cent of infants born with significant cardiac disease and often are multiple.

Approximately one-third of infants with both cardiac and extracardiac anomalies have some established syndrome. For example, maternal rubella during pregnancy may lead to the *rubella syndrome*, which consists of cataracts, deafness, microcephaly, and some combination of patent ductus arteriosus, pulmonic valvular and/or arterial stenosis, and atrial septal defect. Chronic maternal alcohol abuse may lead to the *fetal alcohol syndrome*. This consists of microcephaly, micrognathia, microphthalmia, prenatal growth retardation, developmental delay, and cardiac defects such as ventricular septal defect, which occur in approximately 45 per cent of the affected infants. Maternal systemic lupus erythematosus during pregnancy has been linked to congenital complete heart block but not to any specific anatomical abnormality.

336-E   (Braunwald, pp. 1080–1082, 1089–1093)

The majority of cases of endocarditis are caused by one of the streptococcal organisms, most commonly *S. viridans*, which cause 30 to 65 per cent of native valve endocarditis (NVE). However, other species of streptococci are occasionally responsible for more fulminant episodes of endocarditis. *S. pneumoniae*, for example, accounts for only 1 to 3 per cent of NVE, frequently involves a previously normal aortic valve, and is commonly associated with concurrent pneumonia or meningitis. Mortality rates from *S. pneumoniae* range from 30 to 50 per cent. Enterococci, which were once considered to be group D streptococci, are responsible for 5 to 15 per cent of cases of NVE. They are more frequently encountered in elderly males with underlying urinary tract pathology, and can involve normal or abnormal valves, presenting as either acute or subacute endocarditis. These organisms are resistant to semisynthetic penicillinase-resistant penicillins and cephalosporins.

Treatment with bactericidal activity can be achieved only by combining a cell wall–active agent (e.g., penicillin, ampicillin, or vancomycin) and an appropriate aminoglycoside, intravenously, for at least 4 to 6 weeks. Strains that are highly resistant to penicillin and ampicillin must be treated with vancomycin *plus* gentamicin intravenously for 4 to 6 weeks. Such intense antimicrobial therapy is not necessary, however, in cases of uncomplicated *S. viridans* or *S. bovis* endocarditis, which can be treated with a single agent for 4 weeks or with penicillin plus gentamicin for 2 weeks.[1,2] Finally, NVE due to group B streptococci (*S. agalactiae*), which have been associated with colonic villous adenoma and other neoplasms (as is *S. bovis*), can cause large vegetations and a highly morbid NVE characterized by frequent systemic emboli due to the organisms' failure to produce fibrinolysin.[3,4]

REFERENCES

1. Bansal, R.C.: Infective endocarditis. Med. Clin. North Am. *79*:1205–1240, 1995.
2. Bisno, A.L., Dismukes, W.E., Durack, D.T., et al.: Antimicrobial treatment of infective endocarditis due to viridans streptococci, enterococci, and staphylococci. JAMA *261*: 1471–1477, 1989.
3. Pringle, S.D., McCartney, A.C., Marshall, D.A., and Cobbe, S.M.: Infective endocarditis caused by *Streptococcus agalactiae*. Int. J. Cardiol. *24*:179–183, 1989.
4. Scully, B.E., Spriggs, D., and Neu, H.C.: *Streptococcus agalactiae* (group B) endocarditis—a description of twelve cases and review of the literature. Infection *15*:169, 1987.

337-C *(Braunwald, pp. 1018–1019)*

The progressive development of mitral regurgitation in this 60-year-old patient following an inferior myocardial infarction (MI) is most consistent with infarction of the posterior papillary muscle. Since papillary muscles are perfused via a terminal portion of the coronary vascular bed, they are particularly vulnerable to ischemia. The posterior papillary muscle, supplied usually by only the posterior descending branch of the right coronary artery, is more susceptible to ischemia and infarction than the anterolateral papillary muscle, which has a dual blood supply from the diagonal branches of the left anterior descending artery and the marginal branches from the left circumflex artery. Although necrosis of a papillary muscle is a frequent complication of MI, particularly of inferior infarction,[1] frank rupture of a papillary muscle is far less common. Total rupture of a papillary muscle is usually fatal because of the extremely severe and rapid MR that it produces. MR may also occur significantly later in the course of MI, in which case it is usually due to left ventricular dilatation. In this case, dyskinesis of the left ventricle results in an abnormal spatial relationship between the papillary muscles and the chordae tendineae, resulting in MR.

Ruptures of the chordae tendineae are also important causes of MR, although such ruptures bear no special relationship to MI. Common causes of chordal rupture include congenitally abnormal chordae, spontaneous idiopathic rupture, infective endocarditis, trauma, rheumatic fever, and myxomatous degeneration.[2] In idiopathic rupture an increase in mechanical strain of undetermined cause is believed to cause rupture. The posterior chordae rupture spontaneously more frequently than do the anterior chordae.

REFERENCES

1. Balu, V., Hershowitz, S., Masud, A.R.Z., et al.: Mitral regurgitation in coronary artery disease. Chest *81*:550, 1982.
2. Hickey, A.J., Wilcken, D.E.L., Wright, J.S., and Warren, B.A.: Primary (spontaneous) chordal rupture: Relation to myxomatous valve disease and mitral valve prolapse. J. Am. Coll. Cardiol. *5*:1341, 1985.

338-C *(Braunwald, pp. 1547–1550)*

The normal abdominal aorta has a diameter of approximately 2 cm; clinically significant aneurysms measure 4 cm or more. The majority of such aneurysms are asymptomatic and are found either on routine physical examination or during radiographic evaluation for other reasons. A variety of noninvasive methods exist for the diagnosis and accurate sizing of abdominal aortic aneurysms. Among these, physical examination is the *least* accurate. As of this writing, abdominal ultrasound is both the simplest and most accurate method to detect and size abdominal aortic aneurysms. Experience with computed tomography (CT) scanning and digital subtraction angiography is still being evaluated. Abdominal aortic angiography may be less accurate in predicting size in some instances because the aneurysm's full width may be masked by the presence of nonopacified thrombus. Aortography is currently used in patients with diagnostic dilemmas, patients with associated renal or vascular disease, or patients who are being prepared for surgical repair of AAA.

Natural history studies of AAA have revealed a critical relationship between aneurysm size and subsequent rupture. Thus, half of all aneurysms >6 cm in diameter will rupture within a year of diagnosis, while smaller aneurysms rupture far less frequently (i.e., about 15 to 20 per cent within the first year). Aneurysms appear to expand at an approximate rate of 0.2 to 0.5 cm per year.[1,2]

REFERENCES

1. Delin, A., Ohlsén, H., and Swedenborg, J.: Growth rate of abdominal aortic aneurysms as measured by computed tomography. Br. J. Surg. *72*:530, 1985.
2. Nevitt, M.P., Ballard, D.J., and Hallett, J.W., Jr.: Prognosis of abdominal aortic aneurysms: A population-based study. N. Engl. J. Med. *321*:1009, 1989.

339-B *(Braunwald, pp. 1088–1089)*

The patient described had subacute bacterial endocarditis, with an aortic valve vegetation that is well seen in the illustration. The aortic valve vegetation actually prolapses into the left ventricular outflow tract in the image displayed. The diagnosis of aortic regurgitation itself, as with all valvular regurgitation, is best made echocardiographically by applying Doppler techniques.[1] Valvular vegetations are not well visualized by standard transthoracic echocardiography until the vegetations reach sizes >3 to 4 mm in diameter.[2] When the vegetation leads to valvular destruction or if the vegetation is pedunculated, both M-mode and two-dimensional echocardiography may display the abnormality. However, for smaller vegetations, transesophageal echocardiography is emerging as the diagnostic modality of choice.[3] Echocardiography is also quite useful in identifying the complications of infective endocarditis. These complications may include valvular regurgitation (new onset), premature closure of the mitral valve due to elevated left ventricular diastolic pressures, or the development of an aortic abscess.[4]

REFERENCES

1. Grayburn, P.A., Smith, M.D., Handshoe, R., et al.: Detection of aortic insufficiency by standard echocardiography, pulsed Doppler echocardiography, and auscultation. Ann. Intern. Med. *104*:599, 1986.
2. Dillion, J.C., Feigenbaum, H., Konecke, L.L., et al.: Echocardiographic manifestations of valvular vegetations. Am. Heart J. *86*:698, 1973.
3. Klodas, E., Edwards, W.D., and Khandheria, B.K.: Use of transesophageal echocardiography for improving detection of valvular vegetations in subacute bacterial endocarditis. J. Am. Soc. Echocardiogr. *2*:386, 1989.
3. Saner, H.E., Asinger, R.W., Homans, D.C., et al.: Two-dimensional echocardiographic identification of complicated aortic root endocarditis. Implications for surgery. J. Am. Coll. Cardiol. *10*:859, 1987.

340-E   (Braunwald, pp. 1061–1066)

Tilting-disc valves are generally characterized by being less bulky and having a lower profile than other types of mechanical cardiac valves. The St. Jude valve is currently the most widely used valve. It has semicircular discs and a very favorable hemodynamic profile, with a lower transvalvular gradient at any outer valve diameter or cardiac output than other valve types.[1,2] For this reason, and because of an excellent durability record, the St. Jude valve is especially useful in children. In addition, thrombogenicity of this valve in the mitral position may be less than that of other tilting-disc valves. However, perivalvular regurgitation appears to be more common with this and other mechanical valves than with biprosthetic valves.

The risk of thromboembolism and valve thrombosis involving prosthetic cardiac valves appear to be greatest with mechanical valves in the first postoperative year and is most common in the tricuspid position, followed by the mitral and then aortic locations. It is therefore recommended that patients with mechanical prosthetic valves, regardless of design or position, receive long-term therapeutic anticoagulation with warfarin. The target INR should be between 2.5 and 3.5.[3] It is also recommended that valve replacement in the tricuspid position be carried out using bioprosthetic valves to lower the risk of thromboembolism and valve thrombosis.[4–6] With bioprosthetic valves, despite a lower risk of thromboembolism, it is highly desirable to anticoagulate patients for the first 3 months, while endothelialization of the sewing ring takes

place. Anticoagulation beyond the first 3 months is recommended for bioprosthetic valves in the mitral position when heart failure, history of thromboembolism, or atrial fibrillation are present.[3]

The major drawback to bioprosthetic valves is their limited durability. Tears, degeneration, perforation, and calcifications, are seen earlier than with mechanical valves, and by 10 years after surgery, failure rate averages 30 per cent, and reach 60 per cent by 15 years. Structural bioprosthetic valve failure is more common in the mitral position, and in younger patients. The time after surgery at which these valves fail is inversely related to the age at which they were implanted. Degeneration is particularly rapid when bioprosthetic valves are implanted in patients <35 to 40 years of age, and is extremely rare when they are implanted in those older than 70 years.

REFERENCES

1. Khan, S, Chaux, A., Matloff, J., et al.: The St. Jude Medical valve. Experience with 1,000 cases. J. Thorac. Cardiovasc. Surg. *108*:1010–1019, 1994.
2. Nakano, K., Koyanagi, H., Hashimoto, A., et al.: Twelve years' experience with the St. Jude Medical valve prosthesis. Ann. Thorac. Surg. *57*:697–702, 1994.
3. Cannegieter, S.C., Rosendaal, F.R., Wintzen, A.R., et al.: Optimal oral anticoagulant therapy in patients with mechanical heart valves. N. Engl. J. Med. *333*:11–17, 1995.
4. Scully, H.E., and Armstrong, C.S.: Tricuspid valve replacement. Fifteen years of experience with mechanical prostheses and bioprostheses. J. Thorac. Cardiovasc. Surg. *109*: 1035–1041, 1995.
5. Nakano, K., Eishi, K., Kosakai, Y., et al.: Ten-year experience with the Carpentier-Edwards pericardial xenograft in the tricuspid position. J. Thorac. Cardiovasc. Surg. *111*:605–612, 1996.
6. Van Nooten, G.J., Caes, F., Taeymans, Y., et al.: Tricuspid valve replacement: Postoperative and long-term results. J. Thorac Cardiovasc. Surg. *110*:672–679, 1995.

341-A   (Braunwald, pp. 1255–1256)

Echocardiographic studies document some degree of pericardial effusion in 17 to 25 per cent of patients with AMI.[1] Effusions are seen more commonly in patients with larger infarcts, when congestive heart failure is present, and in the setting of an anterior MI. Pericarditis due to AMI generally occurs between days 2 and 4 after the infarction. The diagnosis is often based on the presence of a pericardial friction rub, which may be present in approximately 7 per cent of AMI patients.[2] Electrocardiographic changes or obvious symptoms of pericarditis are less common than the presence of the rub itself. The Dressler or postmyocardial infarction syndrome typically occurs between 2 and 10 weeks following infarction, although some overlap between this syndrome and typical post-MI pericarditis does exist. The Dressler syndrome has been observed much less commonly recently, owing in part to both the decrease in chronic anticoagulation in the setting of AMI and an increase in the use of antiinflammatory drugs. Treatment of the syndrome typically involves high-dose salicylates.

Other nonsteroidal antiinflammatory agents are relatively contraindicated due to their association with impaired infarct healing and, potentially, ventricular rupture.

REFERENCES

1. Pierard, L.A., Albert, A., Henrard, L., et al.: Incidence and significance of pericardial effusion in acute myocardial infarction as determined by two-dimensional echocardiography. J. Am. Coll. Cardiol. 8:517, 1986.
2. Krainin, F.M., Flessas, A.P., and Spodick, D.H.: Infarction-associated pericarditis. Rarity of diagnostic electrocardiogram. N. Engl. J. Med. 311:1211, 1984.

342-A (Braunwald, pp. 1010–1011)

The diastolic murmur of MS is a low-pitched rumbling murmur best heard at the apex. This murmur is caused by the increased velocity of blood flow across a narrowed orifice with resulting turbulence. The most useful feature of the murmur with regard to the assessment of the severity of stenosis is the duration of the murmur. In patients with MS the murmur persists as long as the gradient across the mitral valve exceeds approximately 3 mm Hg. Furthermore, persistence of the murmur throughout diastole usually corresponds to a mean transvalvular gradient exceeding 10 mm Hg. The intensity of the murmur is much less closely related to the severity of the stenosis and is determined by factors such as the configuration of the patient's chest, the presence of sinus rhythm, and the compliance of the mitral valve leaflets.

The murmur usually commences shortly after the opening snap and in mild MS quickly fades away to be followed by a presystolic murmur. The diastolic murmur of MS can be distinguished from that of tricuspid stenosis because in MS the murmur is reduced during inspiration, augmented during expiration, and reduced during the strain of the Valsalva maneuver, all of which tend to decrease inflow into the left atrium. The opposite findings occur in tricuspid stenosis.

Several other conditions can mimic the rumbling diastolic murmur of MS including the Austin-Flint murmur heard in aortic regurgitation, due to fluttering of the mitral valve in diastole. In a dilated ventricle or in a hypertrophied ventricle with a restrictive cardiomyopathy, a diastolic murmur due to abnormal diastolic filling may also be present. As mentioned previously, tricuspid stenosis closely mimics the murmur of MS but may be distinguished by several maneuvers. Finally, a left atrial myxoma may impede flow across a normal mitral valve, causing both a diastolic murmur and mitral regurgitation.

343-B (Braunwald, pp. 1343–1344)

Syndrome X, the combination of an angina-like chest pain syndrome and normal coronary arteriography, usually has an excellent prognosis.[1] This syndrome is more frequently seen in women and is characterized by chest pain that has *atypical* features in the majority of patients. One study demonstrated that two-thirds of patients with chest pain and normal coronary arteries had predominantly psychiatric disorders.[2] However, other studies have shown that some patients of this type have inadequate coronary vasodilator reserve.[3] The cardiovascular physical examination in such patients is usually normal. The resting ECG usually contains only nonspecific abnormalities, and most patients have a normal exercise test, although approximately 20 per cent will have a positive exercise test. Studies of esophageal motility may be useful in patients with chest pain and normal arteriography; documented esophageal reflux in the setting of chest pain is often successfully treated.[4] Most data suggest that patients of this type have an excellent prognosis for long-term survival. However, a subset of patients that have chest pain, normal arteriography, and left bundle branch block have significant decreases in left ventricular function over subsequent years.[5] This may represent a group of patients with occult cardiomyopathy at the time of presentation.

REFERENCES

1. Papanicolaou, M.N., Cliff, R.M., Hlatky, M.A., et al.: Prognostic implications of angiographically normal and insignificantly narrowed coronary arteries. Am. J. Cardiol. 58: 1181, 1986.
2. Bass, C., and Wade, C.: Chest pain with normal coronary arteries. A comparative study of psychiatric and social morbidity. Psychol. Med. 14:51, 1984.
3. Cannon, R.O., III, Schenke, W.H., Quyyumi, A., et al.: Comparison of exercise testing with studies of coronary flow reserve in patients with microvascular angina. Circulation 83(Suppl. III):77, 1991.
4. DeMeester, T.R., O'Sullivan, G.C., Bermudez, G., et al.: Esophageal function in patients with angina-type chest pain and normal coronary angiograms. Ann. Surg. 196: 488, 1982.
5. Opherk, D., Schuler, G., Wetterauer, K., et al.: Four year follow-up study in patients with angina pectoris and normal coronary arteriograms ("syndrome X"). Circulation 80:1610, 1989.

344-A (Braunwald, pp. 1049–1050)

Hill's sign refers to a marked difference between popliteal and brachial systolic cuff pressures seen in AR. This difference in chronic severe AR exceeds 60 mm Hg and is due to the marked increase in stroke volume in cases of chronic AR, causing larger "standing waves," which explains its rare occurrence in patients with acute AR. This sign may be absent in patients with concomitant AS or heart failure. The AR murmur is a high-frequency diastolic murmur that begins immediately after A_2. The severity of regurgitation correlates better with the duration rather than severity of the murmur, and in cases of severe AR, a holodiastolic murmur with a "rough" quality may be heard. However, with the development of heart failure, equilibration of aortic and LV diastolic pressures abolishes the late diastolic component and the murmur becomes shorter. When the murmur is musical ("cooing dove" murmur), it usually signifies eversion or perforation of a cusp, and when it is louder on the right side, it usually signifies the presence of a dilated ascending aorta, which may be the underlying cause of the valvular insufficiency. In general, maneuvers that decrease afterload decrease the diastolic regurgitant murmur as well as any Austin Flint murmur (which results from the rapid antegrade flow across a mitral orifice that is narrowed by the rapidly rising LV diastolic pressure and partial closure of the anterior mitral leaflet). Examples of maneuvers that decrease afterload include inhalation of amyl nitrite and the Valsalva maneuver. Conversely, AR murmurs are augmented by isometric exercise and vasopressors.

345-B (Braunwald, pp. 1508–1510)

Bacterial (purulent) pericarditis tends to occur via one of several mechanisms, including contiguous spread from a postoperative infection, an infection related to infective endocarditis, a subdiaphragmatic infection, or hematogenous spread during bacteremia. Of note, direct pulmonary extension from bacterial pneumonia or empyema now accounts for only about 20 per cent of cases of bacterial pericarditis.[1] Several factors may predispose to the development of purulent pericarditis, including a preexisting pericardial effusion from uremic pericarditis as well as the immunosuppressed state such as that seen in burns, following immunosuppressive therapy, or with hematological malignancies or the acquired immunodeficiency syndrome. Bacterial pericarditis is usually an acute fulminant illness of short duration that is characterized by high spiking fevers, shaking chills, night sweats, and dyspnea. Typical symptoms of pericarditis may be absent and the process may thus appear for the first time as new jugular venous distention and pulsus paradoxus with the development of cardiac tamponade.

In the patients described by Rubin and Moellering,[1] cardiac tamponade developed acutely in 38 per cent of patients with previously unsuspected bacterial pericarditis. Thus, the key to the diagnosis is a high index of suspicion. However, despite the lower incidence of purulent pericarditis in the antibiotic era, overall survival continues to be very poor, with a mortality of approximately 30 per cent in most series. This poor prognosis is in large part due to the lack of recognition of the entity clinically prior to death. Early complete surgical drainage and appropriate parenteral antibiotic therapy are important parts of the treatment of this devastating disorder. High concentrations of antibiotics may be achieved in pericardial fluid with parenteral therapy; therefore, installation of antibiotics directly into this space is not warranted. Surgical drainage of the percardium is essential in almost all patients with this condition.[2]

REFERENCES

1. Rubin, R.H., and Moellering, R.C., Jr.,: Clinical, microbiologic and therapeutic aspects of purulent pericarditis. Am. J. Med. 59:68, 1975.
2. Morgan, R.J., Stephenson, L.W., Woolf, P.K., et al.: Surgical treatment of purulent pericarditis in children. J. Thorac. Cardiovasc. Surg. 85:527, 1983.

346-A (Braunwald, pp. 1424–1425)

This 16-year-old youth has an examination consistent with hypertrophic cardiomyopathy. Recommendations of the American College of Cardiology[1] are that competitive sports not be allowed if any of the following clinical features are present: (1) marked ventricular hypertrophy, (2) evidence of significant outflow gradient by echocardiography or catheterization, (3) important superventricular or ventricular arrhythmias, and (4) history of sudden death in relatives with hypertrophic cardiomyopathy. It is recommended that low-intensity competitive sports be allowed if none of these conditions are present. This boy has evidence of left ventricular hypertrophy on ECG and chest x-ray, a possible significant outflow gradient by examination, and a history of sudden death in a cousin. Thus, competitive sports would be prohibited. Further workup should obviously be carried out, including echocardiography, and perhaps cardiac catheterization, and ambulatory ECG monitoring should be performed to assess the extent of ventricular arrhythmias.

REFERENCE

1. Maron, B.J., et al.: Task Force III: Hypertrophic cardiomyopathy, other myopericardial diseases and mitral valve prolapse. J. Am. Coll. Cardiol. 6:1215, 1985.

347-C (Braunwald, pp. 1202–1203)

Serum creatine kinase is the most commonly used serum marker for the diagnosis of acute myocardial infarction. CK levels increase within 4 to 6 hours after the onset of symptoms. They normally peak around 24 hours and decline back to normal within 2 to 3 days, except in cases of early reperfusion (spontaneously or following chemical or mechanical reperfusion). In such cases, serum CK peaks earlier, and is no longer useful in the estimation of infarct size. Although elevation of CK activity is a sensitive marker of acute myocardial infarction, false-positive results may be obtained when CK is released from other organs or when its clearance is reduced. Analysis of the MB isoenzyme of CK is considered a more specific marker for cardiac muscle injury. However, other tissues contain small amounts of CK-MB, which can cause elevation of its activity with inflammation or following trauma or surgery. These tissues include the tongue, intestine, uterus, prostate, and the diaphragm. Normal human skeletal muscle also contains a small amount (1 to 3 per cent) of CK-MB.[1]

A subset of patients presenting with chest discomfort or other symptoms suggestive of myocardial ischemia may have elevated levels of CK-MB activity with normal total CK activity. These patients generally have a prognosis that is worse than that for patients with suspected acute myocardial infarction without increased total CK or CK-MB.[2] Recently, CK-MM and CK-MB isoforms were identified. Some of these isoforms appear to be released into the circulation within 2 hours on the onset of symptoms, and measurement of their level may provide a rapid and specific test to evaluate patients suspected of acute myocardial infarction.[3,4]

REFERENCES

1. Tsung, J.S., and Tsung, S.S.: Creatine kinase isoenzymes in extracts of various human skeletal muscle. Clin. Chem. *32*: 1568–1570, 1986.
2. Califf, R.M., and Ohman, E.M.: The diagnosis of acute myocardial infarction. Chest *101*:106S–115S, 1992.
3. Abendschein, D.R.: Rapid diagnosis of myocardial infarction and reperfusion by assay of plasma isoforms of creatine kinase isoenzymes. Clin. Biochem. *23*:399–407, 1990.
4. Guest, T.M., and Jaffe, A.S.: Rapid diagnosis of acute myocardial infarction. Cardiol. Clin. *13*:283–294, 1995.

348-D   (Braunwald, pp. 896–898)

ASD may be overlooked and only uncommonly results in disability in children or adolescents.[1] The anatomical sites of intraatrial defects include the sinus venosus or high ASD, the ostium secundum ASD, and the ostium primum ASD. The sinus venosus defect is usually associated with anomalous connections of the pulmonary veins from the right lung to the junction of the superior vena cava or right atrium.[2] The ostium secundum type of ASD should be distinguished from a patent foramen ovale that may occur in up to 25 per cent of adults; a widely patent foramen ovale may be considered an acquired form of ASD. Ten to 20 per cent of patients with ostium secundum ASD also have prolapse of the mitral valve.[3]

Patients with ASD are usually asymptomatic in early life. Children with ASD occasionally experience exertional dyspnea and easy fatigability, but in generally symptoms are not prominent. Children with ASD tend to be somewhat underdeveloped physically and prone to respiratory infections. However, the symptoms and signs of ASD in the adult, such as atrial arrhythmias, pulmonary vascular obstruction, and heart failure, are very uncommon in the pediatric age group. In children, the diagnosis of ASD is most often entertained after detection of a heart murmur on routine physical examination.

REFERENCES

1. Hunt, C.E., and Lucas, R.V., Jr.: Symptomatic atrial septal defect in infancy. Circulation *42*:1042, 1973.
2. Davea, J.E., Cheitlin, M.D., and Bedynek, J.L.: Venosus atrial septal defect. Am. Heart J. *85*:177, 1973.
3. Leachman, R.D., Cokkinos, D.V., and Cooley, D.A.: Association of ostium secundum atrial septal defects with mitral valve prolapse. Am. J. Cardiol. *38*:167, 1976.

349-E   (Braunwald, pp. 1378–1382)

The use of stents in the treatment of coronary stenoses has revolutionized the field of interventional cardiology.[1] Stents are currently approved for the treatment of abrupt or threatened closure (Gianturco-Roubin stent), and for the prevention of restenosis (Palmaz-Schatz stent) in de novo atherosclerotic lesions. Both stents are made of stainless steel and are highly thrombogenic. Combined with incomplete deployment, this led to a high incidence of stent thrombosis in earlier clinical trials. Anticoagulation with warfarin decreased the incidence of subacute thrombosis to about 5 per cent. More recently, the use of aspirin and ticlopidine following optimal stent deployment with high inflation pressures has led to a further reduction in the incidence of this complication to about 1 to 2 per cent.[2] The risk of stent thrombosis continues to be high, however, in smaller vessels, in the presence of a thrombus, and with the use of multiple stents. The mechanism by which stents reduce the incidence of restenosis is related to the significant improvement in acute angiographic gain (minimal luminal diameter) relative to balloon angioplasty alone. This occurs despite significantly higher late loss in luminal diameter over the subsequent 6 months. However, there is no reduction in intimal hyperplasia with stents.[3]

REFERENCES

1. Eeckhout, E., Kappenberger, L., and Goy, J.L.: Stents for intracoronary placement: Current status and future directions. J. Am. Coll. Cardiol. *27*:757–765, 1996.
2. Schomig, A., Neumann, F.J., Kastrati, A., et al.: A randomized comparison of antiplatelet and anticoagulant therapy after the placement of coronary-artery stents. N. Engl. J. Med. *334*:1084–1089, 1996.
3. Carter, A.J., Laird, J.R., Kufs, W.M., et al.: Coronary stenting with a novel stainless steel balloon-expandable stent: Determinants of neointimal formation and changes in arterial geometry after placement in an atherosclerotic model. J. Am. Coll. Cardiol. *27*:1270–1277, 1996.

350-C   (Braunwald, pp. 1038–1039)

The LV responds to the sudden production of severe obstruction to outflow by dilatation and reduction of stroke volume. However, in most adults with AS, the obstruction develops slowly over a long period of time, resulting in significant compensatory measures. Fundamentally, LV output is maintained by development of LV hypertrophy. This enables the heart to sustain a large pressure gradient across the aortic valve without reduction in cardiac output, LV dilatation, or development of symptoms. This is due in large part to coexisting hypertrophy of the LA with an increased role for atrial contraction in maintaining appropriate LV filling. This is frequently manifested by the development of large *a* waves in the LA pressure pulse with elevated LV end-diastolic pressure. The latter is also increased by the reduction of diastolic compliance of the LV due to ventricular hypertrophy. However, it is only the patient with LV failure in whom dilatation and an increase in LV end-diastolic volume occur.

351-C (*Braunwald, pp. 1079–1080; see also Question 359*)

Infection superimposed on prosthetic valves poses difficult management problems. In general, treatment should involve two drugs with a bactericidal effect on the organism that has been isolated. If the patient appears responsive, antibiotics should be continued for 6 to 8 weeks. Late streptococcal endocarditis involving a bioprosthesis is the infection most amenable to intensive antibiotic therapy. Early prosthetic valve endocarditis (<60 days following operation) is rarely responsive to medical therapy. The mortality with early prosthetic valve endocarditis is very high, approximately 40 per cent.

There are several *absolute* indications for operation[1]: the presence of congestive heart failure, ongoing sepsis, fungal etiology, valvular obstruction, unstable prosthesis, and recent-onset heart block. *Relative* indications for operation include mild congestive failure, nonstreptococcal etiology, early prosthetic valve endocarditis, embolism, perivalvular leak, vegetations on echocardiography, relapse, and culture-negative endocarditis without clinical response to empiric antibiotic therapy. It should be noted that early failure of therapy necessitates surgical treatment and that the mortality with medical therapy alone in patients with heart failure approaches 100 per cent.

At operation, all infected material and tissue and potential sources of emboli should be excised and major hemodynamic abnormalities corrected. In totalling the results in major series, overall mortality of patients with prosthetic valve endocarditis managed with antibiotics was 61 per cent, whereas mortality of those treated surgically (generally a sicker group of patients) was 39 per cent.[1]

REFERENCE

1. Cowgill, L.D., Addonizio, V.P., Hopeman, A.R., and Harken, A.H.: Prosthetic valve endocarditis. Curr. Probl. Cardiol. *11*:617, 1986.

352-C (*Braunwald, pp. 1340–1343*)

Prinzmetal's or variant angina patients typically suffer from angina at rest, with ECG evidence of ST-segment elevation during pain (see Braunwald, Fig. 38–26, p. 1341). The management of this syndrome may be difficult, but relies upon the use of agents that are capable of exerting a direct vasodilatory effect on spastic coronary arteries. Sublingual, intravenous, and long-acting nitrate preparations have all been proved useful in treating and preventing Prinzmetal's anginal attacks.[1] Similarly, calcium channel antagonists have been found to be quite effective in the treatment of this syndrome, with similar efficacy noted for nifedipine, diltiazem, and verapamil.[2] Prazosin has also been found to be of use in patients with Prinzmetal's angina.[3] In contrast, beta blockers may be without effect or may actually exacerbate symptoms in patients with Prinzmetal's angina. Aspirin also may increase the severity of ischemic events in Prinzmetal's patients, perhaps because aspirin therapy inhibits production of the endogenous vasodilator prostaglandin I_2 (prostacyclin).[4] Patients with coronary artery spasm due to variant angina and no underlying obstructive disease are not candidates for revascularization. However, patients with variant angina in the setting of discrete, noncalcified, proximal lesions obstructing a single major coronary artery may actually benefit from PTCA.[5] In the rare patient with Prinzmetal's angina who requires coronary artery bypass surgery, verapamil in the priming solution may help prevent perioperative coronary vasospasm.[6] Interestingly, internal mammary artery grafts do not appear to have the vasospastic properties of the native coronary arteries in patients with this syndrome.[7]

REFERENCES

1. Ginsburg, R., Lamb, I.H., Schroeder, J.S., et al.: Randomized double blind comparison of nifedipine and isosorbide dinitrate therapy in variant angina pectoris due to coronary artery spasm. Am. Heart J. *103*:44, 1982.
2. Beller, G.: Calcium antagonists in the treatment of Prinzmetal's angina and unstable angina pectoris. Circulation *80*(Suppl. IV):78, 1989.
3. Tzivoni, D., Keren, A., Benhorin, J., et al.: Prazosin therapy for refractory variant angina. Am. Heart J. *105*:262, 1983.
4. Miwa, K., Kambara, H., and Kawai, C.: Effect of aspirin in large doses on attacks of variant angina. Am. Heart J. *105*:351, 1983.
5. Corcos, T., David, P.R., Bourassa, M.G., et al.: Percutaneous transluminal coronary angioplasty for the treatment of variant angina. J. Am. Coll. Cardiol. *5*:1046, 1985.
6. Katsumoto, K., and Niibori, T.: Prevention of coronary spasms during aorto-coronary (A-C) bypass surgery for variant angina and effort angina with ST segment elevation. J. Cardiovasc. Surg. *29*:343, 1988.
7. Kitamura, S., Morita, R., Kawachi, K., et al.: Different responses of coronary artery and internal mammary artery bypass grafts to ergonovine and nitroglycerin in variant angina. Ann. Thorac. Surg. *47*:756, 1989.

353-C (*Braunwald, pp. 1308–1311; Table 38–9*)

Although the calcium antagonists differ significantly in structure, they have relatively similar effects on myocardial function. They appear to be beneficial in controlling angina and improving exercise tolerance in patients with chronic stable angina due to coronary atherosclerosis as well as in patients with Prinzmetal's variant angina. Many calcium antagonists are becoming available in the United States. Nifedipine, verapamil, and diltiazem—the three first-generation agents—are all effective in causing relaxation of vascular smooth muscle in both the systemic and coronary arterial beds. The number of second-generation calcium antagonists is rapidly expanding, and some appear to have unique features that may be clinically relevant.[1] *Nicardipine*, for example, is water-soluble but not light-sensitive and may therefore prove to be a useful intravenous form of calcium antagonist. *Amlodipine* has a plasma half-life of 36 hours, which may make it especially beneficial for treatment of hypertension and/or stable angina. Several differences are seen in the side effects of calcium antagonists. With respect to hypotension, flushing, and headache, nifedipine causes moderate and sometimes severe effects due to its potent vasodilator properties, considerably more than diltiazem and verapamil at normal doses. Because nifedipine causes the greatest reduction in systemic vascular resistance, it tends to cause less left ventricular dysfunction than either diltiazem or verapamil. However, at high doses, all of these agents may be associated with a fall in cardiac output.

The calcium antagonists, unlike the beta blockers, are less likely to affect the heart rate and conduction system. However, verapamil has significant inhibitory effects on AV conduction, and in patients with AV conduction disease may cause P-R interval prolongation. Verapamil also decreases the heart rate in patients with sick sinus syndrome. Diltiazem is less likely to do this than verapamil, and nifedipine often raises heart rate. Although all the calcium channel antagonists also reduce gastrointestinal motility, verapamil is significantly more likely to cause gastrointestinal symptoms such as nausea and constipation. Finally, none of the calcium channel antagonists cause bronchoconstriction, which is a significant advantage over the beta blockers.

REFERENCE

1. Opie, L.H.: Calcium channel antagonists. Part V. Second generation agents. Cardiovasc. Drugs Ther. 2:191, 1988.

354-C   *(Braunwald, pp. 1376–1378)*

Coronary atherectomy involves the removal of atheromatous material from diseased coronary arteries. It is done with one of three devices. Directional and extraction atherectomy use a spinning blade to cut the stenosis, while rotational atherectomy abrades the plaque. The directional atherectomy (DCA) catheter was the first device to win U.S. Food and Drug Administration (FDA) approval for clinical use. Data from an observational registry shows an overall procedural success rate of about 85 to 90 per cent for DCA.[1] Results may be further improved by the use of adjunctive balloon angioplasty. Several randomized controlled trials compared the effect of DCA on subsequent restenosis with PTCA. Despite significantly better angiographic results, DCA was associated with

only marginally smaller restenosis rates.[1-3] More importantly, there was an increased risk of acute procedural ischemic complications (including death or myocardial infarction) in patients randomized to DCA, and a similar trend also was seen at the 6-month time point. In the CAVEAT-1 cohort, there was also higher mortality in the DCA group (2.2 per cent versus 0.6 per cent, p = 0.035).[1,4,5]

Rotational atherectomy is performed with a device that uses a rapidly spinning burr with an abrasive tip to grind and abrade the atheromatous plaque. It produces particles that are 10 μm in diameter, and generally pass downstream without adverse effects. The Rotablator is designed to operate on the principal of differential cutting, where rigid material such as calcified plaque constituents are preferentially abraded and the elastic components of the arterial wall are spared. For this reason, this technique has been particularly advocated for heavily calcified or nondilatable lesions.[6,7]

REFERENCES

1. Holmes, D.R., Jr., Topol, E.J., Adelman, A.G., et al.: Randomized trials of directional coronary atherectomy: Implications for clinical practice and future investigation. J. Am. Coll. Cardiol. 24:431–439, 1994.
2. Landau, C., Lange, R.A., and Hillis, L.D.: Percutaneous transluminal coronary angioplasty. N. Engl. J. Med. 330: 981–993, 1994.
3. Baim, D.S., and Kuntz, R.E.: Directional coronary atherectomy: How much lumen enlargement is optimal? Am. J. Cardiol. 72:65E–70E, 1993.
4. Carrozza, J.P., Jr., and Baim, D.S.: Complications of directional coronary atherectomy: Incidence, causes, and management. Am. J. Cardiol. 72:47E–54E, 1993.
5. Elliott, J.M., Berdan, L.G., Holmes, D.R., et al.: One-year follow-up in the Coronary Angioplasty Versus Excisional Atherectomy Trial (CAVEAT I). Circulation 91:2158–2166, 1995.
6. MacIsaac, A.I., Bass, T.A., Buchbinder, M., et al.: High speed rotational atherectomy: Outcome in calcified and noncalcified coronary artery lesions. J. Am. Coll. Cardiol. 26: 731–736, 1995.
7. Guerin, Y., Spaulding, C., Desnos, M., et al.: Rotational atherectomy with adjunctive balloon angioplasty versus conventional percutaneous transluminal coronary angioplasty in type B2 lesions: Results of a randomized study. Am. Heart J. 131:879–883, 1996.

355-E   *(Braunwald, pp. 1507–1508)*

While tuberculous pericarditis is now an uncommon cause of pericarditis in industrialized nations, the disease continues to be an important problem among the disadvantaged and in immunosuppressed patients. Tuberculous pericarditis usually develops by retrograde spread from peritracheal, peribronchial, or mediastinal lymph nodes, or by early hematogenous spread from the primary tuberculous infection. The process is usually chronic. Symptoms may be systemic and nonspecific, and clinical detection of tuberculous pericarditis usually does not occur until the effusive or late constrictive pericarditic stages are reached. The typical pericardial chest pain of acute viral or idiopathic pericarditis is uncommon in tuberculous pericarditis.[1] In addition, typical signs or symptoms of cavitary pulmonary tuberculosis are usually absent.

Typical examination in patients with tuberculous pericarditis usually reveals evidence of chronic cardiac compression, which may mimic heart failure. For example, in one series,[2] 88 per cent of patients had jugular venous distention, 95 per cent had hepatomegaly, and 73 per cent had ascites, whereas a pericardial friction rub was heard in only 18 per cent. While the chest x-ray usually shows an enlarged cardiac silhouette and pleural effusions may be present, the apices and hila of the lung are usually normal. Definitive diagnosis of tuberculous pericarditis is usually difficult because of the low yield of the bacillus in the pericardial fluid, failure of the bacillus to grow on an appropriate medium, and/or the need to observe cultures for a minimum of 8 weeks. The probability of a definitive diagnosis is greatest if both pericardial fluid and a pericardial biopsy are obtained in the effusive stage of the disease.[3]

Initial therapy of tuberculous pericarditis includes hospitalization with bed rest and a three-drug chemotherapy regimen ordinarily consisting of isoniazid, rifampin, and streptomycin or ethambutol. The use of corticosteroids in order to reduce pericardial inflammation has not been shown to reduce the risk of developing constrictive pericarditis and therefore should be reserved for critically ill patients with recurrent large effusions who do not respond to the initial antituberculosis drugs alone.[4]

REFERENCES

1. Hageman, J.T., D'Esopo, N.D., and Glenn, W.W.L.: Tuberculosis of the pericardium: A long-term analysis of forty-four cases. N. Engl. J. Med. 270:327, 1964.
2. Strang, J.I.G.: Tuberculosis pericarditis in Transkei. Clin. Cardiol. 5:667, 1984.
3. Barr, J.F.: The use of pericardial biopsy in establishing etiologic diagnosis in acute pericarditis. Arch. Intern. Med. 96:693, 1955.
4. Rooney, J.J., Crocco, J.A., and Lyons, H.A.: Tuberculosis pericarditis. Ann. Intern. Med. 72:73, 1970.

356-B   (Braunwald, pp. 1440–1441)

This 32-year-old woman presents with transient high-grade AV block and syncope. Her history is most consistent with the development of Lyme disease. This disease is caused by a tick-borne spirochete (Borrelia burgdorferi), which is distributed throughout the northeast, midwest, and western United States, with many cases found in northeastern resorts such as Nantucket. The disease usually is seen during the summer, beginning with a characteristic skin rash (erythema chronicum migrans), and followed in weeks to months by neurological, synovial, and cardiac involvement.

About 10 per cent of patients with Lyme disease develop evidence of cardiac involvement, with the most common manifestation being variable degrees of AV block. Syncope due to severe AV block occurs occasionally.[1] There may also be transient left ventricular dysfunction, and a positive gallium scan may indicate cardiac involvement. It appears that treatment as soon as possible with tetracycline or erythromycin may improve the prognosis.

Development of rheumatic fever would be unusual without any antecedent febrile episodes or sore throat. Although systemic lupus erythematosus may cause AV block, it would be unusual for this patient to have a normal physical examination and negative antinuclear antibody. Trichinella spiralis infection, which causes the clinical syndrome trichinosis, may occur following ingestion of this helminth in contaminated meat. It rarely causes cardiac disease. In severe cases of trichinosis, there may be congestive heart failure; associated electrocardiographic abnormalities include T-wave abnormalities, prolongation of the QRS complex, diminished QRS voltage, and first-degree AV block. Hemochromatosis, which is related to iron overload, may cause arthritis and joint symptoms, but usually presents with findings of a restrictive or dilated cardiomyopathy and would be unlikely to occur in an otherwise healthy woman.

REFERENCE

1. McAlister, H.F., Klementowicz, P.T., Andrews, C., et al.: Lyme carditis: An important cause of reversible heart block. Ann. Intern. Med. 110:339, 1989.

357-E   (Braunwald, pp. 1385–1386)

Since the successful application of balloon mitral valvuloplasty in young adults with rheumatic mitral stenosis in 1985,[1] the technique has evolved rapidly and has been applied widely. The technique uses a transseptal approach, in which a small balloon catheter is passed across the mitral valve into the apex of the left ventricle (which is an adequate position for most mitral valvuloplasty procedures and is easier to obtain than the descending aorta placement that was originally used for this procedure). Overall mortality for the procedure is presently between 1 and 2 per cent, and cardiac perforation occurs in approximately 1 per cent of patients. One-fifth of patients have a small residual atrial septal defect due to the transseptal approach, although about half of these shunts resolve spontaneously by the time of the follow-up catheterization.[2] Four echocardiographic features predict unfavorable early and late hemodynamic results for balloon mitral valvuloplasty. These include (1) poor leaflet mobility, (2) subvalvular thickening, (3) valvular thickening, and (4) valvular calcification. Patients with little or no evidence of any of these four features have an initial success rate >90 per cent and a rate of significant restenosis at 1 year of approximately 4 per cent. A physiologically adequate increase in mitral valve area (from 0.9 to 2.0 cm^2) is achieved with most successful dilatations.

REFERENCES

1. Lock, J.E., Khalilullah, M., Shrivastava, S., et al.: Percutaneous catheter commissurotomy in rheumatic mitral stenosis. N. Engl. J. Med. 313:1515, 1985.
2. Casale, P., Block, P.C., O'Shea, J.P., and Palacios, I.F.: Atrial septal defect after percutaneous mitral balloon valvuloplasty: Immediate results and follow-up. J. Am. Coll. Cardiol. 15:1300, 1990.
3. Block, P.C., and Palacios, I.F.: Aortic and mitral balloon valvuloplasty: The United States experience. In Topol, E.J. (ed.): Textbook of Interventional Cardiology. Philadelphia, W.B. Saunders Company, 1990.

358-A *(Braunwald, pp. 1536–1538)*

Myocardial contusion is a common occurrence with chest injuries. It has been documented in several series in 7 to 17 per cent of cases of chest trauma. It usually produces no significant symptoms and often goes unrecognized. The most common symptom of myocardial contusion is precordial pain resembling that of myocardial infarction, but pain from musculoskeletal chest trauma can confuse the clinical picture. The ECG is helpful in recognizing contusion, with nonspecific ST-T wave abnormalities or ST-T wave changes of pericarditis being quite common. Although transmural injury with pathological Q waves does occur, it is considerably rarer and is usually masked during the initial presentation by findings of pericarditis. Cardiac muscle enzymes, specifically the CPK-MB band, are very useful, with increases in CPK-MB reported in 17 per cent of patients with chest trauma coming to the Henry Ford Hospital.[1]

Other diagnostic tests include radionuclide imaging; technetium-labeled pyrophosphate shows a positive uptake at sites of myocardial contusion. Two-dimensional echocardiography is useful for documenting regional wall motion abnormalities. ECG monitoring frequently reveals a variety of arrhythmias, including most commonly atrial arrhythmias, atrial fibrillation, and atrioventricular and intraventricular conduction defects, as well as sinus node dysfunction and sinus bradycardia.

The development of congestive heart failure is unusual in uncomplicated cases of myocardial contusion and should raise the issue of an associated pathological event. The most common pathological events associated with congestive heart failure in this setting are ruptures of the right or left ventricle or the ventricular septum. These are somewhat rare events and are more common in cases of severe chest wall trauma, especially with motor vehicle accidents.

On the basis of a series of 546 autopsy cases of nonpenetrating injury to the heart, the incidence of rupture of the ventricular septum was estimated to be about 5 per cent, with a similar number of patients experiencing rupture of the atrial septum.[2] In these patients, diagnostic catheterization and two-dimensional echocardiography should be performed quickly, with survival often possible following emergency surgery.

REFERENCES

1. Torres-Mirabal, P., Gruenberg, J.C., Brown, R.S., and Obeid, F.N.: Spectrum of myocardial contusion. Am. Surg. 48:383, 1982.
2. Parmley, L.F., Manion, W.C., and Mattingly, T.W.: Nonpenetrating traumatic injury of the heart. Circulation 18:371, 1958.

359-A *(Braunwald, pp. 1079–1080; 1092)*

Prosthetic valve endocarditis (PVE) has now increased to account for 10 to 20 per cent of all cases of infective endocarditis in developed countries. The risk is not uniform over time, and the greatest risk appears to be during the first 6 weeks after valve surgery, but remains high for the first 6 months. After 1 year of valve implantation, there remains a persistent risk of about 0.2 to 0.35 per cent per year. This decrease in risk seems to coincide with a change in the microbiology of the organisms responsible for PVE. Most infections occurring before 1 year, and certainly before 60 days, following surgery are likely to represent nosocomial infections. The predominant organism in this period is coagulase-negative staphylococci (*Staphylococcus epidermidis*).[1,2] Other organisms that are seen include *S. aureus*, gram-negative bacteria, diphtheroides, and fungi. PVE with onset more than 1 year after surgery is most commonly caused by streptococci, while coagulase-negative staphylococci constitute <20 per cent of infections in this period. Mechanical valves have a higher risk of PVE in the first few months after surgery, while bioprosthetic valves have higher risk of PVE beyond 12 months. The reason for this difference is unclear.

Cases of staphylococcal PVE are optimally treated with triple antibiotic regimens. The recommended combination includes rifampin and gentamicin plus nafcillin or oxacillin (for methicillin-susceptible staphylococci) or plus vancomycin (for methicillin-resistant staphylococci). Treatment is continued intravenously for at least 6 weeks.[3,4]

REFERENCES

1. Cowgill, L.D., Addonizio, V.P., Hopeman, A.R., and Harken, A.H.: A practical approach to prosthetic valve endocarditis. Ann. Thorac. Surg. 43:450–457, 1987.
2. Lytle, B.W., Priest, B.P., Taylor, P.C., et al.: Surgical treatment of prosthetic valve endocarditis. J. Thorac. Cardiovasc. Surg. 111:198–207, 1996.
3. Bayer, A.S., Nelson, R.J., and Slama, T.G.: Current concepts in prevention of prosthetic valve endocarditis. Chest 97:1203–1207, 1990.
4. Bisno, A.L., Dismukes, W.E., Durack, D.T., et al.: Antimicrobial treatment of infective endocarditis due to viridans streptococci, enterococci, and staphylococci. JAMA 261:1471–1477, 1989.

360-E *(Braunwald, pp. 1250–1252)*

A variety of atrioventricular conduction disturbances occur in AMI. First-degree AV block occurs in between 4 and 14 per cent of patients with AMI admitted to coronary care units. In almost all patients with first-degree AV block, the disturbance is intranodal (above the bundle of His) and generally does not require specific treatment. Digitalis intoxication may also lead to this conduction disturbance, and may require stopping of the medication. First-degree AV block may also be a manifestation of increased vagal tone and thus may be associated with sinus bradycardia and hypotension which is responsive to atropine in select circumstances.

While second-degree AV block occurs in between 4 and 10 per cent of patients with AMI admitted to coronary care units, about 90 per cent of patients with second-degree AV block have Mobitz type I (Wenckebach block). Mobitz type II second-degree AV block is a rare conduction defect in this setting and appears in a distinctly different clinical setting from that in which Mobitz type I occurs. Mobitz type I second-degree AV block occurs most commonly in patients with inferior myocardial infarction, is usually transient, and rarely progresses to complete AV block. It usually resolves within 72 hours following infarction and does not require specific therapy. In contrast, Mobitz type II block usually occurs below the bundle of His, is associated with a widened QRS complex, and almost always occurs in the setting of anterior infarction. In this situation, Mobitz type II second-degree AV block usually reflects trifascicular block and impaired conduction distal to the bundle of His and therefore frequently progresses to complete heart block. This AV conduction disturbance is generally treated with a temporary demand pacemaker.

Complete AV block (third-degree AV block) may occur in either anterior or inferior infarction. This disturbance occurs in between 5 and 8 per cent of patients with AMI and has a different prognosis based on the location of the inciting infarction. In inferior infarction, complete heart block usually evolves from first-degree and type I second-degree AV block, usually has a stable escape rhythm, and is usually transient, with resolution within a week after infarction.[1] The mortality in this setting is approximately 15 per cent. In contrast, patients with anterior infarction develop third-degree AV block more suddenly, although it is usually preceded by Mobitz type II second-degree AV block. In general, patients in this setting have unstable escape rhythms, wide QRS complexes, and a mortality in the range of 70 to 80 per cent.[2]

REFERENCES

1. Strasberg, B., Pinchas, A., Arditti, A., et al.: Left and right ventricular function in inferior acute myocardial infarction and significance of advanced atrioventricular block. Am. J. Cardiol. 54:985, 1984.
2. Hindman, M.C., Wagner, G.S., JaRo, M., et al.: The clinical significance of bundle branch block complicating acute myocardial infarction. 2. Indications for temporary and permanent pacemaker insertion. Circulation 58:689, 1978.

361-C   (Braunwald, pp. 901–904)

The size of the VSD and the degree to which pulmonary vascular resistance is altered by increased pulmonic flow from the VSD leads to differing clinical presentations in adults with this lesion. In general, patients with small defects are asymptomatic and are not at risk for the development of pulmonary vascular obstructive disease. However, all patients with VSD are at increased risk for the development of infective endocarditis, which may occur in up to 4 per cent of patients with VSD.[1] This complication usually occurs by the third or fourth decade of life. The infection is usually located at the right ventricle at the site where shunted blood impacts against the ventricular wall.

VSDs in the presence of normal pulmonary artery pressures and pulmonary-systemic flow ratios <1.5:1 in asymptomatic persons in general do not require surgical closure. Women with VSDs that lead to pulmonary-systemic flow ratios <2:1 and only modest pulmonary hypertension generally tolerate pregnancy very well. In women with larger left-to-right shunts, however, left ventricular failure may occur during pregnancy. In those who have Eisenmenger complex, pregnancy is extremely poorly tolerated. The development of Eisenmenger complex due to progressive pulmonary vascular disease is one of the most dreaded complications noted in patients with VSD.[2] This usually occurs sometime between the end of the second or during the third decade of life[3] and may be complicated by hemoptysis, chest pain resembling angina, cerebral abscess, paradoxical emboli, and sudden death. Although patients with a VSD and shunt reversal may survive for 5 to 10 years, prognosis is very poor in general and death usually occurs by the fourth decade of life.

REFERENCES

1. Corone, P., Doyon, F., Gaudeau, S., et al.: Natural history of ventricular septal defect: A study involving 790 cases. Circulation 55:908, 1977.
2. Friedman, W.F., and Heiferman, M.F.: Clinical problems of postoperative pulmonary vascular disease. Am. J. Cardiol. 50:631, 1982.
3. Graham, T.P., Jr.: The Eisenmenger syndrome. In Roberts, W.C. (ed.): Adult Congenital Heart Disease. Philadelphia, F.A. Davis, 1987, pp. 567–582.

362-E   (Braunwald, pp. 1078–1079)

This patient presents with findings typical of right-sided endocarditis, which almost invariably involves the tricuspid valve. Typical features include the subacute course lasting between 2 weeks and several months, presence of pneumonia and pleural effusions of the chest x-ray, and evidence on examination of tricuspid regurgitation, including c-v waves in the jugular venous pulse and a murmur of tricuspid regurgitation. Right-sided endocarditis usually involves infection from the use of contaminated needles and syringes. S. aureus is isolated in 60 per cent of cases; the vast majority of patients with right-sided endocarditis will demonstrate findings consistent with pneumonia or septic emboli. There is an associated incidence of left-sided endocarditis in these patients as well, which must be sought carefully during the initial workup, since mortality appears to be greater in such instances.[1]

This particular patient had a *Pseudomonas* infection with valvular destruction and significant tricuspid regurgitation. He was treated with appropriate antibiotic therapy but after 3 weeks had persistent evidence of both bacteremia and systemic infection. The chance of curing infection of the tricuspid valve caused by *Pseudomonas* and other gram-negative bacteria or fungi may be improved by surgically removing the infected valve. It has been noted that young patients tolerate tricuspid valvulectomy without valve replacement quite well, provided that there is no associated pulmonary hypertension.[2] In intravenous drug addicts with right-sided endocarditis there is a high incidence of recurrence of intravenous drug abuse and endocarditis, underscoring the potential risk of placing a prosthetic valve. Thus, unless the patient is in refractory congestive heart failure due to left-sided as well as right-sided endocarditis, and unless the patient has pulmonary hypertension, recommended treatment consists of valvulectomy without prosthetic valve placement, followed by an additional 4 to 6 weeks of appropriate antibiotic therapy.

REFERENCES

1. Dressler, F.A., and Roberts, W.C.: Infective endocarditis in opiate addicts: Analysis of 80 cases studied at necropsy. Am. J. Cardiol. *63*:1240, 1989.
2. Yee, E.S., and Khonsari, S.: Right-sided infective endocarditis: Valvuloplasty, valvectomy or replacement. J. Cardiovasc. Surg. *30*:744, 1989.

363-A   *(Braunwald, pp. 1430; 1790–1792)*

This 57-year-old woman has a history and physical examination suggesting myocardial dysfunction. It appears that her dysfunction is more right-sided than left-sided, with significant pitting edema, elevated jugular venous pressure, and a slightly enlarged liver. Furthermore, there is evidence for AV valvular regurgitation with both tricuspid and mitral valve regurgitant murmurs audible. Several factors in the history and physical examination suggest a diagnosis of hemochromatosis. Specifically, the association of arthritis and diabetes is common in hemochromatosis because of disposition of iron in the pancreas and in synovial tissue. An enlarged liver is also frequently present. Furthermore, her tanned skin may well represent the bronzing that commonly occurs in this disease. Her cardiac examination is consistent with a restrictive cardiomyopathy manifested by AV regurgitation and mild congestive failure.

Hemochromatosis may occur as a familial or idiopathic disorder, or in association with a defect in hemoglobin synthesis resulting in ineffective erythropoiesis, in chronic liver disease, and with excessive oral intake of iron over many years. The severity of myocardial dysfunction is proportional to the amount of iron present in the myocardium. Extensive deposits of myocardial iron are invariably associated with cardiac dysfunction, usually chronic congestive heart failure. The clinical manifestations vary but usually involve signs of congestive heart failure and right-sided failure. The diagnosis is aided by finding elevated plasma iron levels, normal or low total iron-binding capacity, and markedly elevated transferrin saturation. Cardiac failure is usually progressive and refractory to therapy, although repeated use of the iron-chelating agent desferroxamine may be beneficial, especially in patients presenting earlier in the course of the disease.[1]

Sarcoidosis may cause similar findings, but would be unlikely in a white woman of this age. The lack of pulmonary involvement would also be atypical.

Amyloidosis is another possibility, but significant cardiac amyloidosis is usually associated with immunocyte dyscrasias such as multiple myeloma; it would be unusual in association with rheumatoid arthritis.

A diagnosis of Fabry's disease is possible but less likely. This is an inherited disease of glycosphingolipid metabolism caused by a deficiency of the enzyme ceramide trihexosidase. It is characterized by intracellular accumulation of a neutral glycolipid and prominent involvement of the skin and kidneys. Symptomatic cardiovascular involvement is most common in males rather than females, who are usually asymptomatic carriers. Common findings are systemic hypertension, renovascular hypertension, mitral valve prolapse, and congestive heart failure.

Ischemic cardiomyopathy is possible, especially in the setting of adult-onset diabetes, but the presence of a normal electrocardiogram makes this unlikely.

REFERENCE

1. Cutler, D.J., Isner, J.M., Bracey, A.W., et al.: Hemochromatosis heart disease: An unemphasized cause of potentially reversible restrictive cardiomyopathy. Am. J. Med. *69*:923, 1980.

364-D   *(Braunwald, pp. 1240–1241; Table 37–10)*

RVI frequently accompanies inferior left ventricular infarction and may be recognized by a characteristic clinical and hemodynamic pattern. Hypotension or a marked hypotensive response to low-dose nitroglycerin in patients with inferior infarction suggests a diagnosis of RVI.[1] The hemodynamic picture in RVI is similar to that in pericardial disease, and may include an elevated right ventricular filling pressure, a steep right atrial *y* descent, and a square root sign in the RV pressure tracing. Kussmaul's sign may also be present in RVI. The presence of unexplained systemic hypoxemia in the setting of unidentified RVI suggests the possibility of right-to-left shunting through a patent foramen ovale.[2]

The right-sided placement of the precordial ECG leads may be quite helpful in establishing the diagnosis of RVI. ST-segment elevation in lead V_4R is relatively specific and sensitive for the diagnosis of RVI, as is the presence of ST elevation of 0.1 mV or more in any of the right-sided leads V_4R through V_6R.[3] Because left-sided filling pressures are dependent upon a compromised right-sided transport of blood, loss of atrial transport in patients with RVI may lead to a marked reduction in stroke volume and systemic arterial hypotension. In such instances, the use of atrial or atrioventricular sequential pacing must be considered.[4]

REFERENCES

1. Ferguson, J.J., Diver, D.J., Boldt, M., and Pasternak, R.C.: Significance of nitroglycerin-induced hypotension with acute myocardial infarction. Am. J. Cardiol. *64*:311, 1989.
2. Bansal, R.C., Marsa, R.J., Holland, D., et al.: Severe hypoxemia due to shunting through a patent foramen ovale: A correctable complication of right ventricular infarction. J. Am. Coll. Cardiol. *5*:188, 1985.
3. Robalino, B.D., Whitlow, P.L., Underwood, D.A., and Salcedo, E.E.: Electrocardiographic manifestations of right ventricular infarction. Am. Heart J. *118*:138, 1989.
4. Matangi, M.F.: Temporary physiologic pacing in inferior wall acute myocardial infarction with right ventricular damage. Am. J. Cardiol. *59*:1207, 1987.

365-B   *(Braunwald, pp. 929–932)*

Classic tetralogy of Fallot is marked by a large VSD in association with infundibular and/or valvular pulmonic stenosis, right ventricular hypertrophy, and an overriding aorta. In all cases, the VSD is located *proximal* to the level of the right ventricular outflow tract obstruction and is therefore associated with elevated right ventricular systolic pressure and right-to-left shunting. This is in contrast to the situation in patients who have a double-chambered right ventricle and a membranous VSD, in whom the septal defect communicates with the low-pressure distal portion of the right ventricle and leads to simple VSD physiology rather than the right-to-left shunting and cyanosis that marks tetralogy of Fallot.

Symptoms and clinical findings of tetralogy of Fallot depend on the severity of right ventricular outflow tract obstruction. In mild right ventricular outflow tract obstruction, a left-to-right shunt is predominant and the patient may remain acyanotic. The condition in patients with right ventricular obstruction severe enough to cause cyanosis usually is recognized during infancy or early childhood; the patients may then undergo palliative or total surgical repair. Patients with uncor-

rected tetralogy of Fallot who survive into adult life usually have at most moderate obstruction to right ventricular outflow in association with relatively well-preserved pulmonary blood flow. At the other end of the spectrum, if obstruction to right ventricular outflow is complete, a large obligatory right-to-left shunt will be present, and the lungs are then perfused through collaterals that arise from systemic vessels. In these patients there is severe cyanosis, absence of a systolic heart murmur, and presence of a continuous murmur that originates from bronchial collaterals. This variant of tetralogy of Fallot is termed *pseudotruncus arteriosus*.

Because the large VSD allows for decompression of the right ventricle in tetralogy of Fallot, the right ventricular systolic pressure does not exceed that in the aorta, even in the presence of severe obstruction to right ventricular outflow. Congestive heart failure is unusual in patients with tetralogy of Fallot. Instead, a decrease in cardiac reserve in adults with tetralogy of Fallot is more typical. Exertional dyspnea and poor exercise tolerance are present in about one-third of tetralogy of Fallot patients without operation who survive into the third decade of life.[1]

REFERENCE

1. Higgins, C.B., and Mulder, D.G.: Tetralogy of Fallot in the adult. Am. J. Med. *29*:837, 1972.

366-C   *(Braunwald, pp. 1570–1571)*

Showers of microemboli that arise from atherosclerotic plaques in the aortic or major arterial trunks lead to clinical and pathological changes as the particulate material lodges in small arterial branches. Atheromatous embolism, also known as cholesterol embolism, occurs most commonly following surgery involving manipulation of an atherosclerotic aorta, such as major abdominal vascular procedures, especially resection of abdominal aortic aneurysms. Showers of atherosclerotic emboli may also be provoked by cardiac catheterization, cardiopulmonary bypass, and intraarterial cannulations of any type, and may occasionally occur spontaneously as well. Some studies have suggested a casual relationship between cholesterol embolism and long-term anticoagulant therapy with drugs of the warfarin sodium type. Clinical findings in this disorder may include bilateral lower extremity pain, livido reticularis, and a host of purpuric and ecchymotic lesions in the lower extremities. In addition, abdominal pain may occur.

Two important recognized complications of cholesterol emboli following abdominal aortic surgery are pancreatitis and renal failure due to diffuse microinfarction of the organ in question. The resulting renal failure may be severe and irreversible. Hepatitis is not part of the clinical syndrome. Because showers of cholesterol emboli may be widely scattered, cerebral involvement may occur, and in some instances, visualization of cholesterol particles in the retinal arteries is possible.[1] Unfortunately, there is no specific therapy for cholesterol emboli; specific treatment of the resulting complications of the disorder is the cornerstone of management. The use of anticoagulants to prevent further episodes of embolization remains controversial and does not appear to be of any great value.

REFERENCE

1. Coppello, J.R., Lessell, S., Greco, T.P., and Eisenberg, M.S.: Diffuse disseminated atheroembolism. Arch. Ophthalmol. *102*:255, 1984.

367-B (Braunwald, pp. 1184–1185)

Statistics compiled by the American Heart Association reveal that approximately one-fourth of all deaths in the United States are due to AMI, and that nearly 1.5 million patients suffer this disorder annually. The majority of deaths associated with AMI occur *within the first hour* of the event and are attributable to ventricular fibrillation or other arrhythmias. Over 500,000 patients with confirmed AMI are hospitalized yearly in the United States, and another group of patients at least as large in number as this are admitted because of suspected AMI. The mortality rate during hospitalization and during the first year following infarction is approximately 12 per cent. Although a decline in the death rate from coronary artery disease has been noted in recent years, the precise explanation for this occurrence is not yet entirely clear. A fall in mortality due to a decrease in the incidence of AMI by 25 per cent has been noted, and a similar fall in the fatality rate associated with each case of myocardial infarction has also been documented.[1] At least some of the latter reduction in mortality is due to the interventions that have been developed over the last several decades for in-hospital care of the patient with AMI, including the development of coronary care units and newer methods of treatment of AMI.

Careful monitoring of cardiac rhythm and prompt treatment of primary arrhythmias in coronary care units have led to a reduction in the incidence of in-hospital deaths from AMI due to arrhythmias. Most deaths in hospitalized patients with AMI presently are caused by left ventricular failure and shock and occur within the first 3 to 4 days following the onset of infarction.[2]

Before the widespread use of coronary care units, treatment of AMI was primarily directed toward allowing healing of the infarct. Subsequently, major emphasis was placed on prevention and aggressive treatment of arrhythmias. Currently, attempts to limit infarct size by restoring perfusion of ischemic tissue, particularly using thrombolytic therapy, have become very important.

REFERENCES

1. Pell, S., and Fayerweather, W.E.: Trends in the incidence of myocardial infarction and in associated mortality and morbidity in a large employed population. 1957–1983. N. Engl. J. Med. *312*:1005, 1985.
2. Ong, L., Green, S., Reiser, P., and Morrison, J.: Early prediction of mortality in patients with acute myocardial infarction: A prospective study of clinical and radionuclide risk factors. Am. J. Cardiol. *57*:33, 1986.

368-A (Braunwald, pp. 1291–1292)

The differential diagnosis of chest pain is difficult because the discomfort of angina due to coronary artery disease is nonuniform, and other disease entities can mimic it. Constant[1] has suggested that physicians should ask specific questions to differentiate nonanginal chest pain from angina. Several characteristics that would tend to rule out ischemic chest pain are listed in Question 368; others include a pain lasting less than 5 sec. or more than 20 or 30 minutes, pain precipitated by a single movement of the trunk or arm, and pain associated with tenderness of the chest wall.

Differentiating the discomfort of noncardiac disorders from angina pectoris is possible when the quality of the pain, its duration, precipitating factors, and associated symptoms are taken into consideration (see Braunwald, Table 1–3, p. 5). In general, typical angina usually begins gradually and reaches maximum intensity over a period of minutes before dissipating. The discomfort is usually not sharp but rather is a dull, continuous ache or a squeezing pain. It is usually precipitated by exertion or anxiety and relieved by rest. Associated symptoms frequently include shortness of breath, diaphoresis, and anxiety. Posture can affect the pain of myocardial ischemia; it is often intensified by assuming the horizontal position and relieved by assuming the vertical position.

REFERENCE

1. Constant, J.: The clinical diagnosis of nonanginal chest pain: The differentiation of angina from nonanginal chest pain by history. Clin. Cardiol. *6*:11, 1983.

369-E (Braunwald, p. 1153, Refer to pp. 1704–1711)

While CAD is relatively uncommon in women prior to menopause, the rates of CAD for men and women begin to converge following the onset of menopause. The primary pathological process of atherosclerosis does not appear to be different between the sexes. Thus, much of the attention regarding the premenopausal differences between men and women in cardiovascular disease rates has been focused upon circulating levels of steroid hormones (testosterone in men and estrogen in women). Androgens are associated with a disease in the HDL fraction. The triglyceride concentration, which varies inversely with the HDL level, has also been shown to be an independent risk factor for coronary disease in older women studied in the Framingham cohort.[1] Following menopause, a gradual decline in serum HDL is noted, and a gradual increase in both total and LDL cholesterol levels occurs. These changes appear to be diminished or halted by hormone-replacement therapy with estrogens.

Case-control studies have shown significant benefit in delaying coronary disease in angiographic studies of women receiving estrogen therapy after menopause.[2] Oral contraceptives, which contain both estrogen and progesterone, have a more complex effect. The risk of acute MI has been clearly demonstrated to increase in the setting of oral contraceptive therapy.[3] However, the Nurse's Health Study evaluated the risk for cardiovascular disease in a prospective fashion in 120,000 women taking oral contraceptives over an 8-year period, and found no increase in cardiovascular risk.[4] Several recent studies have highlighted the role of physician bias in treating coronary disease in the female population.[5,6] These studies demonstrated that women receive a less aggressive therapeutic approach than men with the equivalent clinical level of disease, though the reasons for this bias are complex and only partially understood.[7]

REFERENCES

1. Kannel, W.B.: Metabolic risk factors for coronary heart disease in women: Perspective from the Framingham Study. Am. Heart J. *114*:413, 1987.
2. Sullivan, J.M., Vander-Zwag, R., Lemp, G.F., et al.: Postmenopausal estrogen use and coronary atherosclerosis. Ann. Intern. Med. *108*:358, 1988.
3. Mann, J.L., Vessey, M.P., Thorogood, M., and Doll, R.: Myocardial infarction in young women with special reference to oral contraceptive practice. Br. Med. J. (Clin. Res.) *2*: 241, 1975.
4. Stampfer, M.J., Willett, W.C., Colditz, G.A., et al.: A prospective study of past use of oral contraceptive agents and risk of cardiovascular disease. N. Engl. J. Med. *319*:1313, 1988.
5. Ayanian, J.Z., and Epstein, A.M.: Differences in the use of procedures between women and men hospitalized for coronary heart disease. N. Engl. J. Med. *325*:221, 1991.
6. Steingart, R.M., Packer, M., Hamm, P., et al.: Sex differences in the management of coronary artery disease. N. Engl. J. Med. *325*:226, 1991.
7. Healy, B.: The Yentl syndrome. N. Engl. J. Med. *325*:274, 1991.

370-A   (Braunwald, pp. 919–921)

Supravalvular AS is a congenital narrowing of the ascending aorta that may be either diffuse or localized, and originates at the superior margin of the sinuses of Valsalva above the level of the coronary arteries. The clinical picture of supravalvular obstruction usually differs in many ways from that observed in other forms of AS. The lesion may be associated with idiopathic infantile hypercalcemia or may be one finding in the "Williams syndrome." This condition is marked also by a peculiar elfin facies (see Braunwald, Fig. 29–36, p. 920), mental retardation, auditory hyperacusis, narrowing of peripheral systemic and pulmonary arteries, and abnormalities of dental development. The occurrence of the distinctive elfin facies appearance—even in infancy—should alert the physician to the possibility of a multisystem disease and underlying supravalvular AS.

In general, the major physical findings resemble those observed in patients with valvular AS. Accentuation of the aortic valve closure sound due to elevated pressure in the aorta proximal to the stenosis, and the occurrence of a late systolic continuous murmur that results from coexisting narrowing of peripheral pulmonary arteries, may help distinguish this anomaly from valvular AS. Occasionally, a disparity in upper extremity pulses may be noted, with a higher systolic pressure in the right arm than that in the left. This is caused by streaming of blood from the supravalvular lesion preferentially to the right arm circulation.

Electrocardiography generally reveals LV hypertrophy when obstruction is severe, and chest x-ray rarely reveals poststenotic dilatation of the ascending aorta, in contrast to valvular and discrete subvalvular AS. Electrocardiography is the single most valuable technique for localization of the site of obstruction in supravalvular AS. Doppler examination and subsequent retrograde aortic catheterization may determine further the degree of hemodynamic abnormality present. The success of operative repair of this condition depends upon the extent of the abnormality; it is most successful when the obstruction is discrete and there is relatively little accompanying hypoplasia.

371-B   (Braunwald, pp. 1084–1086)

The kidneys are frequently involved in endocarditis by a variety of pathological processes. The patient described has subacute endocarditis most likely involving her prosthetic aortic valve. The mild anemia and leukocytosis are consistent with this finding. Urinalysis shows the presence of hematuria. A common lesion in the kidney caused by endocarditis is renal infarction, which occurs in two-thirds of untreated cases. This is consistent with her history of severe right flank pain and the urinary findings. Another common lesion is a focal glomerulonephritis. This complication occurs in up to 50 per cent of untreated cases and 15 per cent of treated ones. It may be also associated with renal failure and the nephrotic syndrome. A diffuse glomerulonephritis occurs in 30 to 60 per cent of untreated cases and in 10 per cent of treated cases.

Renal cortical necrosis is not a primary lesion associated with infective endocarditis but in severe cases will accompany disseminated intravascular coagulation. Renal abscesses may occur with a long course of endocarditis and are most common in association with highly invasive organisms such as *Staphylococcus aureus*. It should be noted that antimicrobial therapy may also be associated with such renal lesions as interstitial nephritis, toxic nephropathy, and acute tubular necrosis.[1]

REFERENCE

1. Feinstein, E.I., Eknoyan, G., and Lister, B.J.: Renal complications of bacterial endocarditis. Am. J. Nephrol. *5*:457, 1985.

372-C *(Braunwald, pp. 991–992)*

In infants and children the important nonobstructive causes of cardiomyopathy are congestive cardiomyopathy, which include the familial and nonfamilial forms of endocardial fibroelastosis (EFE).[1] This classification does not include patients whose myocardial dysfunction is caused by infection, cardiac anomaly, or conditions of increased preload or afterload. Congestive cardiomyopathy in the pediatric age group usually is a disease of infants, with most cases becoming manifested before the age of 1 year.

Pathologically, both primary and secondary forms of EFE have been recognized. In the secondary variety *focal* areas of opaque fibroelastic thickening of the mural endocardium or cardiac valves are observed in association with other types of cardiac malformations. Primary EFE usually involves the entire left ventricle and mitral and aortic valves and is not associated with significant cardiac defects. Primary EFE often occurs in a familial form, although the mode of inheritance has not been defined. Although several pathological mechanisms have been proposed, the most likely one appears to be inadequate subendocardial blood flow. Typically, the LA and LV are dilated with microthrombi found adherent to the endocardium. The aortic and mitral valve leaflets are thickened and distorted, with a murmur of mitral regurgitation audible in approximately 40 per cent of infants. Papillary muscles and chordae tendineae are also part of the fibroelastic process and are shortened and distorted, contributing to the mitral regurgitation.

Clinical features reflect left ventricular dysfunction and congestive heart failure. Infants frequently present with fatigue (during feeding), failure to thrive, cyanosis, wheezing, and cough. Chest x-ray reveals marked generalized cardiomegaly, frequently with pulmonary congestion. Typical ECG findings include left ventricular hypertrophy with inverted T waves in the left precordial leads. Echocardiographic features include a dilated LA and LV, reduced LV ejection fraction, and abnormal mitral valve motion. Differential diagnosis includes anomalous pulmonary origin of the left coronary artery, myocarditis, and glycogen storage diseases. Optimal management includes early and prolonged treatment with digitalis. Results of mitral valve replacement have been disappointing.

REFERENCE

1. Tripp, M.E.: Congestive cardiomyopathy of childhood. *In* Barness, L.A. (ed.): Advances in Pediatrics. Chicago, Year Book Medical Publishers, 1984, pp. 179–203.

373-C *(Braunwald, pp. 1140–1141)*

Niacin is given at maximum doses of 3 to 6 gm/day, which far exceeds the amount of this B vitamin necessary to achieve a nutrient effect. Niacin acts in part by reducing hepatic VLDL synthesis and thus LDL production.[1] The drug affects each lipoprotein class in a beneficial way: LDL and VLDL are decreased, while HDL levels are *increased* by 20 to 40 per cent. The common side effects of niacin include flushing and pruritus, both of which are thought to be mediated by prostaglandin release. They may therefore be inhibited by aspirin prophylaxis given 1 to 2 hours preceding the dose of niacin. The drug also impairs glucose tolerance and raises uric acid levels, making patients with diabetes or gout poor candidates for niacin. In the niacin arm of the Coronary Drug Project study, both coronary and total mortality were seen to decrease significantly following termination of the trial.[2] Until recently, this was the only trial to demonstrate a decrease in total mortality with therapy of hypercholesterolemia. However, the Scandanavian Simvastatin Survival Study showed recently that treatment of hypercholesterolemic patients with stable CAD with the HMG-CoA reductase inhibitor simvastatin also can reduce overall mortality.[3]

REFERENCES

1. Grundy, S.M., Mok, H.Y., Zech, L., and Berman, M.: Influence of nicotine acid on metabolism of cholesterol and triglycerides in man. J. Lipid Res. *22*:24, 1981.
2. Canner, P.L., Berge, K.G., Wenger, N.K., et al.: Fifteen year mortality in the Coronary Drug Project patients. Long term benefit with niacin. J. Am. Coll. Cardiol. *8*:1245, 1986.
3. Randomized trial of cholesterol lowering in 4,444 patients with coronary heart disease: The Scandinavian Simvastatin Survival Study (4S). Lancet *344*:1383, 1994.

374-C *(Braunwald, pp. 1412–1413)*

This 26-year-old man presents with atrial fibrillation (AF) after New Year's Eve. Furthermore, most of his episodes of atrial fibrillation have occurred on Mondays. These facts should prompt consideration of the "holiday heart syndrome," which is the occurrence with palpitations, chest discomfort, and syncope following a binge of alcohol consumption. Thus, it is not unreasonable to suspect that this young man had been partying over the New Year's Eve holiday and because of this has developed AF from the holiday heart syndrome.[1]

The most common arrhythmia associated with this syndrome is AF, followed by atrial flutter and frequent ventricular premature contractions. Alcohol consumption may predispose nonalcoholics to atrial fibrillation or flutter. It is suspected that hypokalemia may play a role in the genesis of some of these arrhythmias. The atrial fibrillation usually occurs several hours following the last drink and may be related to the onset of some early withdrawal symptoms, especially sympathetic hyperactivity. The treatment is conservative, with primary focus on decreasing alcohol consumption. In patients with more severe alcoholic disease, AV conduction disturbances (most commonly first-degree heart block), bundle branch block, and left ventricular hypertrophy may be observed. In patients with documented cardiomyopathy and the holiday heart syndrome, the prognosis is poor, with sudden death and ventricular tachyarrhythmia common.

REFERENCE

1. Greenspan, A.J., and Schaal, S.F.: The "holiday heart": Electrophysiologic studies of alcohol effects in alcoholics. Ann. Intern. Med. *98*:135, 1983.

375-C   *(Braunwald, pp. 1585–1587; Tables 46–4, 46–5 and 46–7)*

The clinical presentation of pulmonary embolism may be subtle or may be easily confused with a variety of diagnoses and therefore requires a high index of suspicion. In the Urokinase-Streptokinase Pulmonary Embolism trial (UPET), the most common symptoms reported were dyspnea and pleuritic chest pain, and the most common physical sign was tachypnea, with more than 92 per cent of patients having a respiratory rate >16 breaths/min.[1]

The use of symptoms and signs alone to identify patients with this condition may be difficult; in one study, symptoms and signs were not often helpful in discriminating between patients with true pulmonary embolism and those with no evidence of it on pulmonary arteriography.[2] Therefore, in patients in whom this diagnosis is suspected clinically the diagnosis must be pursued by obtaining radionuclide scans or by angiography. The differential diagnosis of pulmonary embolism depends in part on the patient population being examined. In an outpatient population, costochondritis, rib fracture, the early stages of pneumonia, and pleurodynia may all enter into the differential diagnosis. In addition, pneumonia, congestive heart failure, myocardial infarction, asthma, chronic obstructive pulmonary disease, and pneumothorax may all enter into the differential diagnosis of pulmonary embolism in outpatients or inpatients.

REFERENCES

1. Bell, W.R., Simon, T.I., and DeMets, D.L.: The clinical features of submassive and massive pulmonary emboli. Am. J. Med. *62*:355, 1977.
2. Stein, P.D., Willis, P.W., III, and DeMets, D.L.: History and physical examination in acute pulmonary embolism in patients without preexisting cardiac or pulmonary disease. Am. J. Cardiol. *47*:218, 1981.

376-C   *(Braunwald, pp. 1614–1615)*

This man has the classic findings of the sleep apnea syndrome.[1] These patients frequently present with daytime sleepiness, nighttime snoring with apnea, nocturnal awakenings, difficulties in their jobs, and frequent automobile accidents due to falling asleep at the wheel. Physically, these patients can be distinguished from pickwickian patients, who are invariably very obese. Specific symptoms include paroxysmal nocturnal dyspnea,

morning headaches, cardiac arrhythmias (more frequently at night), which are predominantly ventricular arrhythmias, truncal obesity, pulmonary hypertension, nocturnal enuresis, peripheral edema, hypertension, and an elevated hematocrit on laboratory examination.

Although the precise cause of the sleep apnea syndrome is unclear, three types of patterns have been recorded: central apnea, obstructive apnea, and mixed apnea. In central apnea, there appears to be a decrease in central nervous system sympathetic outflow to the respiratory effort. On the other hand, in obstructive apnea, it seems that the upper airway becomes transiently obstructed, causing airflow to stop despite continuing efforts of the respiratory muscles. These patients experience apneic periods, which can occur between 40 and 100 times per hour. During prolonged periods of apnea, the pO_2 can reach values of 20 to 25 mm Hg with saturations below 50 per cent. Sustained hypoxemia of this type leads to arrhythmias, including sinus bradycardia, sinus arrest, long asystoles, frequent atrial premature beats, and ventricular arrhythmias. Acute elevations of pulmonary capillary wedge pressure during these episodes result in development of pulmonary hypertension and right ventricular hypertrophy.

Treatment can be difficult; however, in general it involves relief of obstruction in patients with obstructive apneas and administration of drugs such as progesterone and tricyclic antidepressants to patients with central apnea.

REFERENCE

1. Burrek, B.: The hypersomnia-sleep apnea syndrome: Its recognition in clinical cardiology. Am. Heart J. *107*:543, 1984.

377-A   *(Braunwald, pp. 1185–1190)*

In general, patients with AMI who come to autopsy have more than one coronary artery severely narrowed, and between one- and two-thirds of such patients will have a critical obstruction of all three coronary arteries. The remainder are equally divided between those having single-vessel disease and those having two-vessel disease.[1] Most transmural infarctions occur distal to the occlusion of a coronary artery, although total occlusion of a coronary artery is not always associated with MI, largely because of the presence of collateral blood flow. In most series of patients with AMI studied at autopsy or by coronary arteriography, a small number are found to have normal coronary vessels.[2] Possible explanations in these patients include an embolus that has lysed or migrated or a prolonged episode of severe coronary arterial spasm that may have led to myocardial necrosis.

While in the past coronary arteriography was avoided in the acute setting of MI because of potential complications, experience over the last decade has shown that angiography is safe even during the acute phase of MI.[3] Studies in the early hours of AMI have revealed an approximate 90 per cent incidence of total occlusion of infarct-related vessels.[4] Recanalization secondary to spontaneous thrombolysis contributes to a diminished prevalence of total occlusion in vessels studied in the postinfarction period. The incidence of coronary thrombosis in subendocardial infarction is less well established; however, evidence that thrombosis plays a major role in patients with unstable ischemic syndromes[4] suggests that a similar pathophysiology may exist in the majority of cases of nontransmural AMI.

REFERENCES

1. Buja, L.M., and Willerson, J.T.: Clinicopathologic correlates of acute ischemic heart disease syndromes. Am. J. Cardiol. *47*:343, 1981.
2. Betriu, A., Castaner, A., Sanz, G.A., et al.: Angiographic finding 1 month after myocardial infarction: A prospective study of 259 survivors. Circulation *65*:1099, 1982.
3. deFeyter, P.J., van den Brand, M., Serruys, P.W., and Wijns, W.: Early angiography after myocardial infarction: What have we learned? Am. Heart J. *109*:194, 1985.
4. DeWood, M.A., Spores, J., Notske, R., et al.: Prevalence of total coronary occlusion during the early hours of transmural myocardial infarction. N. Engl. J. Med. *303*:897, 1980.

378-C *(Braunwald, pp. 924–926)*

Valvular PS results from the fusion of the pulmonic valve cusps during mid to late intrauterine development and is the most common form of isolated RV obstructive heart disease. The severity of the pulmonic obstruction and the degree to which the RV and its outflow tract have developed determine the clinical presentation and course in the newborn with PS. Severe PS is characterized by cyanosis due to right-to-left shunting through the foramen ovale, by cardiomegaly, and by diminished pulmonary blood flow. Thus, hypoxemia and metabolic acidemia are principal clinical disturbances noted in the symptomatic neonate.

Clinical distinction between tetralogy of Fallot or tricuspid or pulmonary atresia and PS is usually possible in infants, since those with tetralogy generally do not have x-ray evidence of cardiomegaly while those with PS do. Also, infants with tricuspid or pulmonary atresia generally show primarily LV hypertrophy by electrocardiography in contrast to RV hypertrophy observed with critical PS in the neonate. The severity of obstruction is often suggested by the physical findings. Thus, prominent *a* waves in the jugular venous pulse, an S_4, and presystolic pulsations of the liver reflect vigorous atrial contraction and suggest the presence of severe PS. A systolic ejection sound is often heard following the first heart sound at the upper left sternal border. The ejection sound typically is louder during expiration and when it is inaudible or occurs less than 0.08 sec from the onset of the Q wave, severe obstruction is suggested. The electro-

cardiogram is usually normal in mild PS, whereas moderate and severe PS is associated with right axis deviation and RV hypertrophy.

The severity of obstruction is the most important clinical determinant of subsequent course in PS. In the presence of a normal cardiac output, moderate stenosis is considered to be present if the peak systolic transvalvular pressure gradient is between 50 and 80 mm Hg or the peak systolic RV pressure is between 75 and 100 mm Hg. Reliable localization of the site of obstruction and an assessment of its severity may be obtained by combined continuous-wave Doppler and two-dimensional echocardiography.

Cardiac catheterization and angiocardiography may localize the site of obstruction, evaluate its severity, and document the coexistence of other cardiac abnormalities. Patients with mild and moderate PS in general have a favorable course. Approximately three-fourths of such patients reveal unchanged pressure gradients over 4- to 8-year intervals. Percutaneous transluminal balloon valvuloplasty is the initial procedure of choice in patients with valvular PS and moderate to severe degrees of obstruction. In addition, surgical relief can be accomplished at an extremely low risk if necessary.

379-E *(Braunwald, pp. 1258–1261)*

Clinical data suggest that the patient with a non-Q-wave infarction will have a natural history following the event that is different from that observed in patients with Q-wave MI. Patients with non-Q-wave MI have smaller infarcts initially and have a lower mortality in the early (in-hospital) phase following the MI.[1] In addition, patients who have sustained non-Q-wave MI have a lower incidence of heart failure, more frequent angina (which is presumed related to the residual myocardium at risk), and a relatively infrequent incidence of total occlusion of the infarct-related vessel. However, the 12-month period following a non-Q-wave infarct is marked by instability or recurrent events more frequently than in patients who have sustained Q-wave infarction. Sixty per cent of patients with a non-Q-wave MI have a critical obstruction in two or more major coronary arteries, and many will develop an acute Q-wave infarct in the following year.[1] In one series, nearly half of the patients with non-Q-wave MI had unstable angina that emerged during the subsequent 11 months.[2] It thus appears that non-Q-wave infarction is a relatively unstable condition that may be associated with a lower initial mortality, but carries a higher risk of subsequent events. The early and late risk patterns for the two different types of MI tend to cancel each other out and lead to an overall long-term mortality that is quite similar for both Q-wave and non-Q-wave MI.[3] In a large multicenter study the use of diltiazem in a patient with a non-Q-wave infarction led to a 50 per cent reduction in the cumulative incidence of postinfarction angina or recurrent MI.[4] Patients with clear evidence of ischemia in the periinfarction or postinfarction period must be approached aggressively, and should have coronary arteriography and revascularization if appropriate.

REFERENCES

1. O'Brien, T.X., and Ross, J.: Non-Q-wave myocardial infarction. Incidence, pathophysiology, and clinical course compared with Q wave infarction. Clin. Cardiol. *12*(Suppl. III): 3, 1989.
2. Madigan, N.P., Rutherford, B.D., and Frye, R.L.: The clinical course, early prognosis and coronary anatomy of subendocardial infarction. Am. J. Med. *60*:634, 1976.
3. Nicod, P., Gilpin, E., Dittrich, H., et al.: Short- and long-term clinical outcome after Q-wave and non-Q-wave myocardial infarction in a large patient population. Circulation *79*:528, 1989.
4. Gibson, R.S., Boden, W.E., Theroux, P., et al.: Diltiazem and reinfarction in patient with non-Q-wave infarction. N. Engl. J. Med. *315*:423, 1986.

380-D   *(Braunwald, pp. 1082–1083; 1092)*

The HACEK group of organisms refers to a number of gram-negative bacilli that are among the less common causes of endocarditis. The E in HACEK stands for *Eikenella*, not *E. coli*. All of these organisms share a sensitivity to ampicillin, although treatment frequently includes an aminoglycoside as well (see Table 33–12, p. 1093). The most common of these organisms to cause endocarditis is *Haemophilus influenzae*.

381-D   *(Braunwald, pp. 994–997)*

The child described in the case presentation has several of the classic findings of the mucocutaneous lymph node syndrome of infancy, *Kawasaki disease*. The syndrome generally presents as a febrile illness in children that occurs before the age of 10 years and usually before the age of 2. Classically these children have fever and ocular and oral manifestations followed in several days by a rash and indurative edema of the hands and feet with palmar and plantar erythema. Finally, after about 2 weeks, cutaneous desquamation occurs.

Diagnostic criteria for Kawasaki disease include (1) a fever lasting 5 days or more that is unresponsive to antibiotics; (2) bilateral congestion of the conjunctivae; (3) indurative edema of the palms and feet, followed by membranous desquamation of the fingertips; (4) changes in the lips and mouth including dry erythematous and fissured lips with a strawberry tongue and injected oral pharynx; and (5) a polymorphous exanthem of the trunk without crusts or vesicles. Diagnosis is accepted when the first criterion and at least three of the remainder are present.

Multiple organ system involvement has been noted, including arthritis, cerebral spinal fluid pleocytosis, pulmonary infiltrates, and hydrops of the gallbladder. Adenopathy, diarrhea, leukocyto-

sis, thrombocytosis, sterile pyuria and proteinuria, and abnormal liver functions are also frequently present. Pathologically, the disease starts as an acute perivasculitis of the small arteries at which time pericarditis, interstitial myocarditis, and endocardial inflammation are seen. It then progresses to a panvasculitis involving the major coronary arteries resulting in aneurysm and thrombus formation, potentially leading to coronary artery thrombosis and myocardial infarction. The syndrome has an associated mortality of 1 to 3 per cent secondary to complications from coronary artery involvement, myocarditis, or pericarditis, with the majority of deaths occurring in the fourth week. Cardiac involvement includes ECG evidence of myocarditis and pericarditis, echocardiographic evidence of poor LV function, cardiomegaly, and pericardial effusion.

High-dose salicylate therapy appears to be useful by preventing platelet thrombus formation and decreasing the development of occluded coronary arteries. Empiric treatment with high-dose intravenous gamma globulin and salicylates has resulted in decreased formation of coronary artery aneurysms.[1] Prognosis is variable; approximately half of the children with coronary aneurysms diagnosed early after the acute phase of the disease subsides have normal-appearing vessels by angiography 1 or 2 years later.[2]

Rubella myocarditis occurs in utero and can cause varying degrees of myocardial damage. Invariably, cardiovascular manifestations of the rubella syndrome, other than myocarditis, dominate the clinical picture.

Coxsackie B infection usually occurs as part of an epidemic myocarditis. The illness is characterized by fever, tachycardia, and symptoms of encephalitis or hepatitis. The characteristic rash and desquamation common to Kawasaki disease are not present. *Haemophilus influenzae* can cause a purulent pericarditis following upper respiratory infection and croup but is not known to cause myocarditis. *Stevens-Johnson syndrome* is a desquamating skin illness involving mucous membranes associated with an autoimmune response to a variety of agents but does not commonly include cardiac manifestations.

REFERENCES

1. Newburger, J.W., Takahasi, M., Burns, J.C., et al.: The treatment of Kawasaki syndrome with intravenous gamma globulin. N. Engl. J. Med. *315*:341, 1986.
2. Anderson, T., Meyer, R.A., and Kaplan, S.: Long-term evaluation of cardiac size and function in patients with Kawasaki disease. J. Am. Coll. Cardiol. *1*:714, 1983.

382-A   *(Braunwald, pp. 1199–1201)*

In uncomplicated AMI, subtle changes in the vital signs reflect the underlying pathological process. Most patients with uncomplicated AMI are *normotensive*, although a small group of patients have a mild decrease in systolic blood pressure and an elevation in diastolic pressure due to the reduction in stroke volume that accompanies the usual tachycardia. While the heart rate may vary from marked bradycardia to a variety of tachycardias, the most common underlying rhythm in AMI is a mild sinus tachycardia, with a return to a more normal rate following treatment of pain and anxiety. Almost all patients with AMI have ventricular premature beats. Most patients with AMI develop some elevation in temperature, which begins between 4 and 48 hours after the onset of the MI and is probably a nonspecific response to tissue necrosis. Rectal temperatures of 100 and 101°F are usual, and the fever usually abates by the 4th or 5th day following the infarction. The presence of higher fever should prompt the clinician to search for other potential causes of temperature elevation. In uncomplicated AMI, the respiratory rate is often slightly elevated soon after the development of the infarct because of both anxiety and pain. However, it usually returns to normal upon appropriate treatment. In patients with LV failure, however, the respiratory rate correlates with the severity of underlying congestive heart failure. Many patients with pulmonary edema have respiratory rates exceeding 40/min.

Despite the severity of infarction present, the underlying cardiac examination is often surprisingly unremarkable. The most common finding on palpation is the presence of a presystolic pulsation that is consistent with vigorous atrial contraction in the setting of reduced left ventricular compliance (a palpable S_4). The heart sounds, especially the first heart sound, are frequently muffled.[1] The heart sounds return to normal intensity during recovery. The presence of left ventricular dysfunction or left bundle branch block may lead to paradoxical splitting of the second heart sound. Patients with postinfarction angina may also develop transient paradoxical splitting of the second heart sound due to prolongation of left ventricular ejection during anginal or ischemic episodes. An S_4 is almost always present in patients with sinus rhythm with AMI and reflects atrial contraction against a left ventrice with reduced compliance mentioned above. The presence of an S_3 in AMI is usually a reflection of extensive left ventricular dysfunction and heralds a higher risk of death than that in patients without such a sound.[2] Soft systolic murmurs are also commonly present in patients with AMI and generally reflect mild mitral regurgitation due to papillary muscle dysfunction or left ventricular dilatation.

REFERENCES

1. Stein, P.D., Sabbah, H.N., and Barr, I.: Intensity of heart sounds in the evaluation of patients following myocardial infarction. Chest *75*:679, 1979.
2. Riley, C.P., Russell, R.O., Jr., and Rackley, C.E.: Left ventricular gallop sound and acute myocardial infarction. Am. Heart J. *86*:598, 1973.

383-C *(Braunwald, pp. 1134, 1421–1422)*

The M-mode echocardiogram displayed demonstrates a markedly hypertrophied left ventricle with an asymmetric increase in the dimension of the septum. In addition, the anterior leaflet of the mitral valve is seen to move in an anterior direction during systole, so-called "systolic anterior motion" of the valve (SAM). These findings are characteristic of hypertrophic cardiomyopathy (HCM). Most patients with HCM are asymptomatic or only mildly symptomatic, though with large outflow tract gradients, symptoms may intervene. The most common symptom is dyspnea, which is present in close to 90 per cent of symptomatic patients with HCM and is felt to be due to the elevated left ventricular diastolic pressures that occur in this disorder as a consequence of diastolic dysfunction.[1] Angina, fatigue, presyncope, and syncope are also commonly observed. Syncope may result from inadequate cardiac output during exertion or increases in heart rate, or it may be due to cardiac arrythmias. This symptom is most commonly observed in younger patients with both small left ventricular dimensions and evidence of ventricular tachycardia on ambulatory Holter monitoring.[2]

The hallmark of HCM on physical examination is the presence of a systolic murmur associated with the outflow tract gradient. The murmur is crescendo-decrescendo in configuration and often harsh. It is best differentiated from the murmur of valvular aortic stenosis by the brisk initial phase of the carotid pulse, and by changes in the murmur following specific maneuvers (see Braunwald, Table 41–10, p. 1420). In patients with HCM who are symptomatic, the electrocardiogram is usually abnormal. The most common abnormalities are nonspecific ST and T wave changes, as well as left ventricular hypertrophy, which is often characterized by QRS complexes that are tallest in the mid precordial leads.[3] Abnormal Q waves are also relatively common in HCM and may be found in 20 to 50 per cent of patients. Echocardiography in HCM demonstrates left ventricular hypertrophy, with a good deal of variability in the degree and pattern of the hypertrophic muscle. The presence of a markedly thickened septum, as in the example displayed, provides strong evidence for the diagnosis. In addition, when a pressure gradient exists across the left ventricular outflow tract in HCM, the anterior leaflet of the mitral valve moves forward abnormally during systole.[4] The degree of SAM is closely correlated to the magnitude of the outflow gradient, though it is unclear whether SAM itself produces this gradient. A decreased E-to-F slope is an M-mode echocardiographic finding characteristic of mitral stenosis, not HCM.

REFERENCES

1. Spirito, P., Chiarella, F., Carratino, L., et al.: Clinical course and prognosis of hypertrophic cardiomyopathy in an outpatient population. N. Engl. J. Med. *320*:749, 1989.

2. Nienebar, C.A., Hiller, S., Spielman, R.P., et al.: Syncope in hypertrophic cardiomyopathy: Multivariate analysis of prognostic determinants. J. Am. Coll. Cardiol. *15*:948, 1990.
3. Maron, B.J., Wolfson, J.K., Ciro, E., and Spirito, P.: Relation of electrocardiographic abnormalities and patterns of left ventricular hypertrophy identical by two-dimensional echocardiography in patients with hypertrophic cardiomyopathy. Am. J. Cardiol. *51*:189, 1983.
4. Madeira, H.C.: The mitral valve in hypertrophic cardiomyopathy—an echocardiographic approach. Postgrad. Med. J. *62*:563, 1986.

384-D   *(Braunwald, p. 1141)*

The HMG-CoA reductase inhibitors are a class of drugs useful for the treatment of hyperlipoproteinemia. These agents are competitive inhibitors of the enzyme 3-hydroxy-3-methylglutaryl coenzyme A reductase, the rate-limiting enzyme in cholesterol biosynthesis. By inhibiting this enzyme they reduce cholesterol synthesis and cause a secondary *increase* in the level of hepatic LDL receptors.

Lovastatin, the first of these drugs to gain approval, appears to be quite well tolerated with few side effects, except for infrequent but sustained rises in serum transaminase levels. Therefore, it is recommended that liver function tests be performed every 2 to 3 months during the first year of therapy. These drugs may also cause myositis, and rarely, a frank rhabdomyolysis syndrome, especially in patients also receiving immunosuppressive regimens with cyclosporine A. Because of the ability of HMG-CoA reductase inhibitors to increase the number of LDL receptors, they reduce LDL cholesterol very significantly, even in patients who are heterozygotes for familial hypercholesterolemia. They act in an additive manner when used with bile acid sequestrants. These drugs are significantly less effective in patients who are homozygotes for familial hypercholesterolemia, probably because patients with this syndrome have essentially no LDL receptors. However, for unclear reasons, some patients with this disorder do respond somewhat to these drugs. Currently, four HMG-CoA reductase inhibitors are available: simvastatin, lovastatin, pravastatin and flurastatin. A fifth, atorvastatin, will be released in 1997.

385-E   *(Braunwald, pp. 1161–1163)*

Myocardial oxygen consumption ($M\dot{V}O_2$) provides an accurate measure of total cardiac metabolism. Over the years, it has been observed that the energy needs of the myocardium cannot be calculated simply from the external work as a product of the developed pressure and stroke volume. In addition, it has been shown that the ratio of the work performed to the oxygen consumed, i.e., the myocardial efficiency, varies widely depending on hemodynamic conditions. Simplistically, the $M\dot{V}O_2$ is determined by the tension time index (which is defined by the area under the LV pressure curve) and the velocity of myocardial contraction. Thus the developed wall tension or stress is an important determinant of $M\dot{V}O_2$. Wall stress can be calculated by LaPlace's law and is related directly to the radius of the heart and the intraventricular pressure but *inversely* related to ventricular wall thickness. Thus, it is an established clinical finding that with increased pressure and volume, there is compensatory wall thickening, which decreases wall stress.[1,2]

The other major determinant of $M\dot{V}O_2$ is contractility, which is related to the extent of inotropic stimuli and neural influences. Heart rate itself increases contractility and therefore also increases $M\dot{V}O_2$. The maintenance of the active contractile state, which requires continued excitation-contraction coupling, may increase $M\dot{V}O_2$. Finally, $M\dot{V}O_2$ is influenced by the substrate utilized (free fatty acids versus glucose or lactic acid),[3] although this effect is important only in ischemic and failing myocardium. In ischemia there is decreased oxidation of fatty acids with increased utilization of anaerobic substrates resulting in decreased $M\dot{V}O_2$.

REFERENCES

1. Teplick, R., Haas, G.S., Trautman, E., et al.: Time dependence of the oxygen cost of force development during systole in the canine left ventricle. Circ. Res. *59*:27, 1986.
2. Suga, H., Yamada, Y., Goto, Y., and Igarashi, Y: Oxygen consumption and pressure volume area of abnormal contractions in canine heart. Am. J. Physiol. *26*:H154, 1984.
3. Vik-Mo, H., and Mjos, O.E.: Influence of free fatty acids on myocardial oxygen consumption and ischemic injury. Am. J. Cardiol. *48*:361, 1981.

386-B   *(Braunwald, p. 924)*

Stenoses of the pulmonary artery may be single or multiple and may occur from the main pulmonary artery trunk to the smaller peripheral arterial branches. In general, pulmonary artery stenosis is associated with other cardiovascular defects including ventricular septal defect, tetralogy of Fallot, supravalvular aortic stenosis, and pulmonic valvular stenosis. Perhaps the most important cause of significant pulmonary artery stenoses in the newborn is intrauterine rubella infection.[1] Associated cardiovascular malformations in this syndrome include patent ductus arteriosus, pulmonic valve stenosis, and atrial septal defect. Systemic findings may include cataracts, microphthalmia, thrombocytopenia, hepatitis, deafness, and blood dyscrasias.

The clinical features vary, but most infants and children remain asymptomatic. A continuous murmur may be present due to the pulmonary artery stenosis, especially if the lesion is in a main branch pulmonary artery or if an associated anomaly leads to increased pulmonary blood flow. Electrocardiography often demonstrates right ventricular hypertrophy when obstruction is severe.

In the rubella syndrome, left axis deviation with counterclockwise orientation of the QRS complex in the frontal plane is commonly seen. The diagnosis of peripheral pulmonary arterial stenosis may be confirmed by detecting pressure gradients within the pulmonary arterial system at cardiac catheterization. Mild to moderate unilateral or bilateral stenoses do not require surgical relief, and multiple stenoses may not be amenable to correction. Intraoperative or percutaneous balloon angioplasty has been used successfully to treat this disorder.[2]

REFERENCES

1. Venables, A.W.: The syndrome of pulmonary stenosis complicating maternal rubella. Br. Heart J. *27*:49, 1965.
2. Kan, J.S., Marvin, W.J., Jr., Bass, J.L., et al.: Balloon angioplasty-branch pulmonary artery stenosis: Results from the valvuloplasty and angioplasty of congenital anomalies registry. Am. J. Cardiol. *65*:798, 1990.

387-B   *(Braunwald, pp. 1291–1292)*

This man has classic findings of chest pain caused by esophageal reflux and spasm. Differentiation of esophageal disorders from ischemic heart disease can be difficult, since the pains are located in similar areas and are frequently associated with emotional stress. However, while ischemic pain may produce substernal burning, certain features, including substernal burning, are more suggestive of esophageal than anginal pain. They include a prolonged, continuous ache, a discomfort that is primarily retrosternal and that does not radiate into the arms, a pain not associated with exercise, and a pain that disturbs sleep. Classically, esophageal disease associated with regurgitation causes "water brash," a taste in the mouth consistent with regurgitation of gastric contents. Frequently, patients with esophageal spasm experience relief with nitroglycerin. Unlike angina, however, esophageal pain is often relieved by milk, antacids, or food.[1]

Esophageal spasm may be documented by performing the Bernstein test, which consists of alternate infusions of dilute acid and normal saline into the esophagus via a nasogastric catheter. In patients with gastroesophageal acid reflux, acid infusion will reproduce the pain within 2 to 4 minutes. It should be noted that ECG changes can occur with gastric reflux and also that coexisting coronary artery disease may be exacerbated by gastroesophageal disorders.

Biliary colic also may be confused with angina pectoris. It is usually caused by a rapid rise in biliary pressure due to obstruction of the cystic or bile ducts. Thus the pain is usually abrupt in onset, steady in nature, and lasts from minutes to hours. It should be suspected when a history of dyspepsia, flatulence, fatty food intolerance, and indigestion is present.

REFERENCE

1. Constant, J.: The clinical diagnosis of nonanginal chest pain: The differentiation of angina from nonanginal chest pain by history. Clin. Cardiol. *6*:11, 1983.

388-E   *(Braunwald, pp. 1142–1144)*

Type II hyperlipoproteinemia is an elevation of total plasma cholesterol, predominantly LDL cholesterol. There are two types: in type IIa fasting triglycerides and VLDL are normal while in type IIb they are elevated. The most common cause of an isolated elevation of cholesterol and LDL is polygenic hypercholesterolemia, which may account for the condition in as many as 85 per cent of patients shown to have elevated cholesterol levels. Type IIa hyperlipoproteinemia may be due to familial hypercholesterolemia (FH), which is an autosomal dominant disease having a frequency of 1 in 500 for the heterozygote and 1 in one million for the homozygote. Finally, familial combined hyperlipidemia may also present as a type II phenotype.

These patients have protean manifestations clinically. Tendinous xanthomas appearing on the extensor tendons such as the achilles and forearm tendons suggest underlying FH. These patients may have corneal arcus and xanthomas in other areas. Premature development of atherosclerosis is common. However, recurrent pancreatitis is not associated with the type II phenotype. It is seen in type I hyperlipoproteinemia and familial hypertriglyceridemia in which chylomicronemia leads to abdominal pain and pancreatitis.

389-C   *(Braunwald, pp. 1427–1429)*

The apical four-chamber view illustrated demonstrates biventricular hypertrophy, enlarged atria, and a small pericardial effusion, all of which are typical findings of cardiac amyloidosis. In multiple myeloma, amyloid heart disease is a common finding and proves to be a frequent cause of death.[1] Clinically apparent cardiac amyloidosis occurs in one-third to one-half of patients with multiple myeloma, and the most common presentation is that of restrictive cardiomyopathy. In such cases, right-sided findings predominate on the physical examination. Another common presentation of cardiac amyloidosis is congestive heart failure due to systolic dysfunction. In approximately 10 per cent of cases, orthostatic hypotension occurs and is presumed to be a result of amyloid infiltration of the autonomic nervous system or of the blood vessels themselves. A fourth, rare presentation of cardiac amyloidosis is an abnormality of cardiac impulse formation and conduction. Such patients may demonstrate arrythmia and conduction disturbances, and when these are apparent, sudden death that is presumed to be due to arrythmia is relatively common.[2]

The example displayed demonstrates several classic echocardiographic findings of amyloidosis. These findings may also be accompanied by a distinctive granular, sparkling appearance of the thickened cardiac walls in some patients, which is presumed to be due to amyloid deposition in myocardial tissue.[3] The presence of low voltage of the electrocardiogram and thickened left ventricular walls helps distinguish cardiac amyloidosis from pericardial disease or left ventricular hypertrophy and is thought to be characteristic of myocardial infiltration with amyloid fibrils.[4]

REFERENCES

1. Falk, R.H.: Cardiac amyloidosis. *In* Zipes, D.P., and Rowland, D.J.(eds.): Progress in Cardiology. Philadelphia, Lea & Febiger, 1989, p. 143.
2. Smith, T.J., Kyle, R.A., and Lie, J.T.: Clinical significance of histopathologic patterns of cardiac amyloidosis. Mayo Clin. Proc. *59*:547, 1984.
3. Hongo, M., and Ikeda, S.I.: Echocardiographic assessment of the evolution of amyloid heart disease: A study with familial amyloid polyneuropathy. Circulation *73*:249, 1986.
4. Cueto-Garcia, L., Reeder, G.S., Kyle, R.H., et al.: Echocardiographic findings in systemic amyloidosis. Spectrum of cardiac involvement and relation to survival. J. Am. Coll. Cardiol. *6*:737, 1985.

390-C *(Braunwald, pp. 889–890)*

While the development of congestive heart failure is a common pathological consequence of congenital cardiac lesions, the manifestations of this syndrome in neonates are somewhat different from those observed in the adult population. The advent of fetal echocardiography has allowed the early identification of intrauterine cardiac failure, which is manifested by scalp edema, pericardial effusion, ascites, and decreased fetal movements.

In infants born prematurely, persistent patent ductus arteriosus is the most common cause of cardiac decompensation; other forms of structural heart disease are rare. In the full-term newborn the earliest important causes of heart failure are coarctation of the aorta, hypoplastic left heart, paroxysmal atrial tachycardia, cerebral or hepatic arteriovenous fistula, and myocarditis. While heart failure in newborn infants is most commonly the result of a structural defect, it may occur secondary to severe metabolic abnormalities, such as hypoxemia and acidemia. The signs of pulmonary and systemic venous congestion in infants are somewhat different from those of the older child or adult. Among the most common symptoms and signs of heart failure in the infant are feeding difficulties and failure to gain weight and grow, tachycardia, pulmonary rales and rhonchi, liver enlargement, and cardiomegaly. It is much less common to see peripheral edema and ascites, while gallop rhythms and pleural or pericardial effusions are distinctly rare in infants.

The distinction between left and right heart failure is much less obvious in the infant than it is in the older child or adult. This results from left-to-right shunting in the presence of left heart failure, which leads to concomitant right-sided dysfunction. When right ventricular filling pressure is elevated, it causes a greater apparent reduction in left ventricular compliance in neonates and infants than in adults.

391-A *(Braunwald, pp. 1029–1035)*

The M-mode echocardiogram displayed is taken from a young woman with typical late systolic prolapse of the mitral valve. Following atrial contraction (A), the anterior and posterior mitral leaflets coapt (C). However, coaptation does not persist until the start of diastole (D point) as is usually the case. Rather, a U- or hammock-shaped configuration in the C-D segment is present and arises from posterior movement of the mitral valve leaflets in midsystole.[1] Marked bowing of the mitral valve leaflets toward the posterior left atrial wall is noted (arrows), with midsystolic buckling of the leaflets clearly evident. Systolic *anterior* motion of the mitral valve occurs in midsystole in patients with hypertrophic obstructive cardiomyopathy. Two-dimensional echocardiography may detect mitral valve prolapse in some patients in whom M-mode echocardiography has not detected the disorder.[2] The presence of thickened or redundant mitral valve leaflets confers an increased risk of developing endocarditis or severe mitral regurgitation[3] (see Braunwald, Fig. 32–25, p. 1034). Moderate or severe mitral regurgitation occurs in approximately 10 per cent of patients with mitral valve prolapse, is most frequently found in men over the age of 50, and may require color flow Doppler in order to identify the location and severity of the regurgitant jet.[4] In approximately 20 per cent of patients with mitral valve prolapse, some prolapse of the tricuspid and/or aortic valves may be detected. Prolapse of these valves is quite uncommon, however, in the absence of mitral valve prolapse.

REFERENCES

1. Pollick, C., and Sutton, M.S.: Acquired mitral and tricuspid disease. *In* Sutton, M.S., and Oldershaw, P. (eds.): Textbook of Adult and Pediatric Echocardiography Doppler. Cambridge, Blackwell Scientific Publications, Inc., 1989, pp. 184–191.
2. Abbasi, A.S., DeCristofaro, D., Anabtawi, J., and Irwin, L.: Mitral valve prolapse. Comparative value of M-mode, two-dimensional and Doppler echocardiography. J. Am. Coll. Cardiol. *2*:1219, 1983.
3. Marks, A.R., Choong, C.Y., Sanfilippo, A.J., et al.: Identification of high-risk and low-risk subgroups of patients with mitral valve prolapse. N. Engl. J. Med. *320*:1031, 1989.
4. Panadis, I.P., McAllister, M., Ross, J., and Mintz, G.S.: Prevalence and severity of mitral regurgitation in the mitral valve prolapse syndrome. A Doppler echocardiographic study of 80 patients. J. Am. Coll. Cardiol. *7*:975, 1986.
5. Rodger, J.C., and Morley, P.: Abnormal aortic valve echoes in mitral prolapse. Echocardiographic features of floppy aortic valve. Br. Heart J. *47*:337, 1982.

392-C *(Braunwald, pp. 896–898)*

These images reveal a secundum type of atrial septal defect between the right and left atria. In general, transthoracic two-dimensional echocardiography, especially from the subcostal position, can allow direct examination of the interatrial septum. The technique may be quite helpful both in identification of an ASD and in differentiating the various types of ASD from one another. A primum ASD, which coexists with endocardial cushion defects and cleft mitral valve, may be readily identified by echocardiography. The sinus venosus type ASD may be difficult to identify with two-dimensional echocardiography,[1] and other ASDs may also prove difficult to image transthoracically. In such cases, transesophageal echocardiography may be of assistance. Both color flow Doppler and saline contrast echocardiography (panel *B*) may be used to evaluate the direction of flow across a shunt of this type. When flow is predominantly from left to right, left atrial blood (noncontrast) passes through the ASD and leads to a negative contract effect within the right atrium.[2] Conversely, when Eisenmenger syndrome has intervened, as in the case described, there is a right-to-left interatrial shunt and contrast is seen first within the left atrium and then the left ventricle following a saline injection.[3] Anomalous pulmonary venous return is more commonly associated with a sinus venosus defect, in which additional echoes may be found posterior to the left atrium or associated with the right atrium or the inferior or superior vena cavae. These images exemplify the usefulness of transesophageal echocardiography in patients in whom standard transthoracic imaging is difficult due to anatomical or pathological reasons.

REFERENCES

1. Nasser, F.N., Tajik, A.J., Stewart, J.B., and Hagler, D.J.: Diagnosis of sinus venosus atrial septal defect by two-dimensional echocardiography. Mayo Clin. Proc. 56:568, 1981.
2. Weyman, A.E., Wann, L.S., Caldwell, R.L., et al.: Negative contrast echocardiography: A new method for detecting left-to-right shunts. Circulation 59:498, 1979.
3. Van Hare, G.G., and Silverman, N.H.: Contrast two-dimensional echocardiography in congenital heart disease: techniques, indications and clinical utility. J. Am. Coll. Cardiol. 13:673, 1989.

393-A *(Braunwald, pp. 1045–1046, 1050–1051; Figs. 32–36 and 32–37)*

This M-mode study displays high-frequency fluttering of the anterior leaflet of the mitral valve in diastole. This finding is characteristic of both acute and chronic aortic regurgitation (AR). This sign is an echocardiographic correlate of the Austin Flint rumble, although unlike the ausculatory finding, it may occur even in cases of mild AR.[1] AR may arise from primary disease of the aortic valve itself, due to dilatation of the aortic root, or for both reasons. A steady increase in the percentage of patients with pure aortic root disease has been documented over the past several decades.[2] Common causes of valvular AR include rheumatic fever and infective endocarditis. Trauma may also lead to prolapse of the aortic cusp, as may a congenitally bicuspid valve. While isolated congenital AR is uncommon, when present it is often associated with such a bicuspid valve.[3] A variety of less common diseases are as-

sociated with aortic regurgitation, including connective tissue diseases such as Marfan syndrome, Ehlers-Danlos syndrome, and myxomatous proliferation of the aortic valve, as well as systemic lupus erythematosus, rheumatoid arthritis, and ankylosing spondylitis.[4] AR due to dilatation of the ascending aorta may arise from a variety of disorders, including systemic hypertension, cystic medionecrosis of the aorta (isolated or in association with Marfan syndrome), giant cell arteritis, ankylosing spondylitis, rheumatoid arthritis, and syphilis (see Braunwald, Table 32–8, p. 1049). Regardless of the underlying disorder that leads to AR, dilatation and hypertrophy of the left ventricle as well as dilatation of the mitral valve annulus (and even of the left atrium) are commonly observed.

REFERENCES

1. Louie, E.K., Mason, T.J., Shah, R., et al.: Determinants of anterior mitral leaflet fluttering in pure aortic regurgitation from pulsed Doppler study of the early diastolic interaction between the regurgitant jet and mitral inflow. Am. J. Cardiol. 61:1085, 1988.
2. Olson, L.J., Subramanian, R., and Edwards, W.D.: Surgical pathology of pure aortic insufficiency. A study of 225 cases. Mayo Clin. Proc. 59:835, 1984.
3. Darvill, F.R., Jr.: Aortic insufficiency of unusual etiology. JAMA 184:753, 1963.
4. DeMoulin, J.C., Lespagnard, J., Bertholet, M., and Soumagna, D.: Acute fulminant aortic regurgitation in ankylosing spondylitis. Am. Heart J. 105:859, 1983.

394-B *(Braunwald, pp. 1427–1429; see also Answer 389)*

This patient has a history of progressive congestive heart failure. His past medical history is remarkable for mild hypertension, a diagnosis of multiple myeloma, transfusion of 1 unit of blood monthly, and administration of Leukeran. The most likely diagnosis is cardiac amyloidosis, which is associated with immunocyte dyscrasias, most commonly multiple myeloma, as in this patient.

Amyloidosis of the heart may lead to several clinical syndromes.[1] The most common is congestive heart failure due to systolic dysfunction. Hemodynamic evidence of restriction of ventricular filling is not prominent in these patients. There is frequently cardiomegaly, and progression to death is rapid. A second presentation of cardiac amyloidosis is a restrictive cardiomyopathy with predominant right-sided findings producing a picture similar to constrictive pericarditis. Orthostatic hypotension is a third mode of presentation occurring in about 10 per cent of the cases; it is frequently aggravated by coexisting renal amyloidosis leading to hypovolemia. Finally, abnormalities of cardiac impulse formation and conduction resulting in arryhthmias and conduction disturbances is the least common mode of presentation.

The chest x-ray in this disorder usually shows cardiomegaly, and pleural effusions are common. The ECT is usually abnormal; the most characteristic feature is diminished voltage followed by axis shifts and various conduction disturbances.

Echocardiography most commonly reveals increased thickness of the walls of the ventricles, small ventricular chambers, dilated atria, and impaired left ventricular function. A classic finding, which is infrequently seen, is a granular sparkling texture observed on two-dimensional echocardiography, most typically in the interatrial septum. Treatment of this form of cardiomyopathy is limited, although various efforts are being made to prevent the development of the immune reaction leading to the appearance of amyloid.

REFERENCE

1. Falk, R.H.: Cardiac amyloidosis. *In* Zipes, D.P., and Rowlands, D.J. (eds.): Progress in Cardiology. Philadelphia, Lea & Febiger, 1989, p. 143.

395-B   *(Braunwald, p. 1012)*

A full echocardiographic study in a patient with MS often provides a wealth of information and allows development of a full therapeutic plan. Information is made available by M-mode, two-dimensional, and Doppler echocardiography in this disorder. The diagnosis is often quite straightforward by M-mode echocardiography (see for example, Braunwald, Fig. 3–45, p. 71), although the M-mode technique is not able to quantitate the severity of the valve lesion. Typical findings of MS on M-mode echocardiography include a reduced E-F slope, leaflet thickening, decreased leaflet separation in diastole, and anterior movement of the posterior mitral valve leaflet during early diastole. While the E-F slope is reduced in MS, this finding may also be present in other conditions in which left ventricular compliance and the velocity of left ventricular filling are reduced.

A more accurate determination of mitral orifice size is available with two-dimensional echocardiography (see Braunwald, Fig. 32–3, p. 1012).[1] Planimetry of the mitral orifice in the parasternal short-axis view often allows an accurate determination of the valve area. Two-dimensional echocardiography also is useful in detecting mitral annular calcification and in estimating pulmonary artery pressure. The latter determines (and is correlated with) the degree of tricuspid regurgitation present, as assessed by Doppler echocardiography. Doppler echocardiography is especially useful in quantifying the severity of MS.[2] Peak velocity of transmitral flow is *increased* in MS, and the rate of decline of this flow is reduced during early diastole. In the continuous-wave Doppler flow velocity signal illustrated, peak velocity exceeds 2 msec. The peak transmitral gradient in this patient is 18 mm Hg, consistent with severe mitral stenosis.[3] In addition, a direct correlation between the size of the mitral orifice and the time required for peak velocity to reach half its initial level in MS ($T_{1/2}$)

may be used to direct calculations of mitral valve area.

REFERENCES

1. Smith, M.D., Handshoe, R., Handshoe, S., et al.: Comparative accuracy of two-dimensional echocardiography and Doppler pressure half-time methods of assessing severity of mitral stenosis in patients with and without prior commisurotomy. Circulation 73:100, 1986.
2. Zoghbi, W.A., Farmer, K.L., Soto, J.G., et al.: Accurate noninvasive quantification of stenotic aortic valve area by Doppler echocardiography. Circulation 73:452, 1986.
3. Pollick, C., and Sutton, M.S.: Acquired mitral and tricuspid disease. *In* Sutton, M.S., and Oldershaw, P. (eds.): Textbook of Adult and Pediatric Echocardiography and Doppler. Cambridge, Blackwell Scientific Publications, Inc., 1989, pp. 175–181.

396-C   *(Braunwald, pp. 1010–1011)*

The long-axis view displays typical rheumatic deformity of the mitral valves with left atrial enlargement. The mitral leaflets are heavily calcified and their motion in diastole is severely constrained. Calcification is also seen extending into the perivalvular and subvalvular structures.[1] A left pleural effusion is also seen and is a direct consequence of the elevated pulmonary venous pressure in this patient. The full two-dimensional study likely demonstrates restricted mitral valve motion and doming of the valvular leaflets.[2] Pulmonary edema is usually observed in patients with critical obstruction to left atrial emptying and mitral valve areas of 1 cm^2 or less. Pulmonary edema in this setting is often precipitated by conditions that increase cardiac output or that lead to an increased heart rate and a reduction in the time available for transmitral flow. Examples of such precipitants include exertion, emotional stress, pregnancy, respiratory infection, fever, and sexual intercourse. Atrial fibrillation with a rapid ventricular response is another common precipitant of pulmonary edema in mitral stenosis. Approximately 15 per cent of patients with MS experience chest discomfort that is anginal in nature.[3] While this symptom may arise from right ventricular hypertension, concomitant atherosclerosis, or even coronary obstruction due to embolization of left atrial thrombus, in many cases the explanation for chest pain in MS remains obscure. Ineffective endocarditis in MS tends to be more common in patients with milder forms of the disease and tends to occur *less* frequently on thickened and calcified mitral valves. In some instances, direct compression of the left recurrent laryngeal nerve by a dilated left atrium may lead to hoarseness, a condition termed Ortner's syndrome.[4]

REFERENCES

1. Pollick, C., and Sutton, M.S.: Acquired mitral and tricuspid disease. *In* Sutton, M.S., and Oldershaw, P. (eds.): Textbook of Adult and Pediatric Echocardiography and Doppler. Cambridge, Blackwell Scientific Publications, Inc., 1989, pp. 169–191.

2. Glover, M.U., Warren, S.E., Vieweg, W.V.R., et al.: M-mode and two-dimensional echocardiographic correlation with findings at catheterization and surgery in patients with mitral stenosis. Am. Heart J. *105*:98, 1983.
3. Wood, P.: An appreciation of mitral stenosis. Br. Med. J. *1*: 1051 and 1113, 1954.
4. Sharma, N.G.K., Kapoor, C.P., Mahambre, L., and Borker, M.P.: Ortner's syndrome. J. Indian Med. Assoc. *60*:427, 1973.

397-C *(Braunwald, pp. 1507–1508; see also Answer 355)*

This case illustrates a patient with AIDS presenting with tuberculous pericarditis during the effusive stage of the illness. While the incidence of tuberculous pericarditis has decreased in industrialized nations over the past 3 decades, the disorder remains an important problem in immunosuppressed patients, including those with AIDS.[1,2] This disorder is also a major cause of pericarditis among developing populations, especially South and West African blacks, the black poor of the United States, and Asian and African immigrants. Tuberculous pericarditis usually presents in the effusive stage as in this case or late in its course, following the development of constrictive pericarditis. The disease usually develops slowly and is marked by nonspecific systemic findings including fever, night sweats, dyspnea, and fatigue.[3] The acute onset of severe pericardial pain, which is seen frequently in viral or idiopathic pericarditis, is *uncommon* in tuberculous pericarditis.[3] In addition, the disease may present as an acute illness of less than 2 weeks' duration.[4] Abnormalities on physical examination are common and may be especially helpful in making this diagnosis. Fever, sinus tachycardia, and pericardial friction rub, as well as jugular venous distention, and hepatomegaly, are all important findings suggestive of tuberculous pericarditis in the appropriate population. Ascites may be found commonly in this disorder,[3] but a pericardial friction rub is heard in only a minority of cases.

The chest roentgenogram illustrated displays many of the classic features of effusive tuberculous pericarditis. These include an enlarged cardiac silhouette, with accompanying mediastinal widening suggestive of a pericardial effusion, normal lung hila and apices, and a small pleural effusion, which is seen in approximately half of patients. Patients may also occasionally present with chronic constrictive pericarditis and symptoms and signs consistent with severe chronic systemic venous congestion. The diagnosis of tuberculous pericarditis requires a high index of suspicion and is best made by obtaining both pericardial fluid and a pericardial biopsy specimen during the early effusive stage.[5] The measurement of a high level of adenosine deaminase activity (>45 units/liter) is also supportive of the diagnosis.[5] Without antituberculous chemotherapy, the disease is rapidly fatal, with an early mortality >80 per cent. However,

while mortality following treatment with a three-drug regimen (oral isoniazid, oral ethambutol, and intramuscular streptomycin) is still significant, it is markedly reduced. In one trial, the addition of corticosteroids to the three-drug regimen described led to a lower mortality at 24 months (4 versus 11 per cent), a more rapid clinical improvement, and a decreased requirement for subsequent pericardiectomy.[6]

REFERENCES

1. Dalli, E., Quesada, A., Juan, G., et al.: Tuberculous pericarditis as the first manifestation of acquired immunodeficiency syndrome. Am. Heart J. *114*:905, 1987.
2. Kinney, E.L., Monsuez, J.J., Kitzis, M., and Vittecoq, D.: Treatment of AIDS-related heart disease. Angiology *40*: 970, 1989.
3. Strang, J.I.G.: Tuberculous pericarditis in Transkei. Clin. Cardiol. *5*:667, 1984.
4. Permanyer-Miralda, G., Sagrista-Sauleda, J., and Soler-Soler, J.: Primary acute pericardial disease: A prospective series of 231 consecutive patients. Am. J. Cardiol. *56*:623, 1985.
5. Sagrista-Sauleda, J., Permanyer-Miralda, G., and Soler-Soler, J.: Tuberculous pericarditis: Ten-year experience with a prospective protocol for diagnosis and treatment. J. Am. Coll. Cardiol. *11*:724, 1988.
6. Strang, J.I., Kakaza, H.H., Gibson, D.G., et al.: Controlled atrial of prednisolone as adjuvant in the treatment of tuberculous constrictive pericarditis in Transkei. Lancet *2*: 1418, 1987.

398-E *(Braunwald, pp. 1207–1212, 1215–1218)*

Myocardial infarction continues to be an important health issue in the United States. It is estimated that 1.5 million patients suffer annually from AMI infarction. Despite aggressive and improved management strategies over the past 10 years, up to one-third of MI patients still die in the periinfarction period. Treatment strategies for AMI have focused on ways to limit infarct size, early recognition of malignant arrythmias, and secondary prevention. Several factors have played an important role in decreasing mortality in AMI. The coronary care unit concept was introduced in the mid 1960's to focus on early recognition and management of cardiac arrythmias. Pulmonary flotation catheters next were introduced for detailed bedside hemodynamic monitoring and management of patients with heart failure and cardiogenic shock.

The coronary reperfusion era began with intracoronary thrombolytics and then proceeded to the more clinically feasible use of intravenous thrombolytics. Thrombolytic therapy's impact on infarct size and survival first was clearly demonstrated in the GISSI trial, in which 11,000 patients with AMI received intravenous streptokinase within 6 hours of onset of symptoms, which lead to a significant reduction in mortality in treated patients.[1] In a recent comprehensive review of nine large trials of thrombolytic therapy, the Fibrinolytic Therapy Trialists' (FTT) Collaborative Group found an average 18 per cent reduction in short-term mortality in

AMI in treated patients.[2] There was a greater reduction in these studies in mortality in patients with anterior ST-segment elevation (22 per cent) than those with inferior ST elevation (11 per cent). Greater improvement of left ventricular function was also seen in anterior infarcts when compared to inferior infarcts, even when normalized for infarct size.[2]

Of all the available thrombolytics, accelerated t-PA is the most effective in restoring early perfusion in the infarct-related artery (GUSTO).[3,4] Accelerated t-PA appears to be more cost effective in the *elderly* population, since this age group has in general a higher mortality with AMI. Nevertheless, not all patients benefit from reperfusion. For example, the LATE and EMERAS trials provide evidence that a reduction in mortality is still possible in patients receiving thrombolytics between 6 and 12 hours following the onset of AMI, but this effect appears to be lost by 12 hours after the MI has begun.[5,6]

REFERENCES

1. Gruppo Italiano per lo Studio Della Streptochinasi Nell'Infarct Miocardio (GISSI): Effectiveness of intravenous thrombolytic treatment in acute myocardial infarction. Lancet *1*:397, 1986.
2. Fibrinolytic Trialists' Collaboration: Indications for fibrinolytic therapy in suspected acute myocardial infarction: Collaborative overview of early mortality and major morbidity results from all randomized trials of more than 1,000 patients. Lancet *343*:311, 1995.
3. Simoons, M.L.: Another coronary reperfusion regimen. Lancet *346*:324, 1995.
4. Lee, K.L., Woodlief, L.H., Topol, E., et al.: Predictors of 30-day mortality in the era of reperfusion for acute myocardial infarction. Results from an international trial of 41,021 patients. Circulation *91*:659, 1995.
5. LATE (Late Assessment of Thrombolytic Efficacy) Study Group: Late assessment of thrombolytic efficacy (LATE) study with alteplase 6–24 hours after onset of acute myocardial infarction. Lancet *342*:759, 1993.
6. EMERAS (Estudio Multicentrico Estroptoquinasa Republicas de America del SUR) Collaborative Group: Randomized trial of late thrombolysis in acute myocardial infarction. Lancet *342*:767, 1993.
7. Stewart, R.E., and O'Neill, W.W.: Direct angioplasty for acute myocardial infarction. Curr. Opin. Cardiol. *10*:367, 1995.

399 A-T, B-T, C-T, D-T, E-T   *(Braunwald, p. 1193)*

While uncommon, there are a number of nonatherosclerotic causes of AMI. Embolic phenomena may involve the coronary arteries, such as those that result from endocarditis, either infective or marantic in nature. Such emboli most frequently lodge in the left anterior descending coronary artery. Inflammatory processes can also involve the coronary artery and may occasionally lead to AMI. Kawasaki disease, necrotizing arteritis, systemic lupus erythematosus, and syphilis can all lead to coronary occlusion by such a mechanism. MI may also result from the coronary arterial involvement in amyloidosis, Hurler syndrome, pseudoxanthoma elasticum, and homocystinuria. In these cases, coronary mural thickening due to the metabolic disease in question or simultaneous intimal proliferative disease leads to restriction of coronary blood flow. Cocaine abuse has been shown to precipitate AMI in patients with normal coronary arteries, those with a prior history of MI, and those with known coronary spasm. An extensive list of the further potential causes of MI without coronary atherosclerosis may be found in Braunwald, Table 37–1, p. 1193.

400 A-T, B-T, C-T, D-F, E-F   *(Braunwald, p. 1121)*

A number of studies, both in animals and in humans, have demonstrated that atherosclerotic lesions may be induced to regress. In monkeys that have developed early experimental atherosclerosis after being placed on a high-fat, high-cholesterol diet, regression may become evident within 1 month following resumption of a normal diet.[1] Animals with more advanced atherosclerotic lesions also demonstrate regression following the lowering of plasma cholesterol.[2] Interestingly, in these experiments lesions in the aorta and coronary arteries appeared to regress more fully than those at the carotid bifurcation.

One of the first clear-cut demonstrations of regression in a clinical population was made in the Cholesterol-Lowering Atherosclerosis Study (CLAS), in which patients with recent coronary artery bypass grafting were aggressively treated to lower plasma cholesterol levels.[3] Following 2 years of therapy, a high significant rate of regression was noted in the treatment group. This study was also striking for the rapidity with which the regression in atherosclerotic lesions took place. The Familial Atherosclerosis Treatment Study (FATS) also used angiography to demonstrate regression in coronary disease following aggressive lipid-lowering therapy with either lovastatin or combined niacin-binding resin therapy.[4] This study used quantitative angiography and, unlike the CLAS study, was performed on patients with known coronary disease, prior to bypass graft surgery.

Ingestion of omega-3 fatty acids, a major component of fish oils, leads to the production of thromboxane A_3, instead of thromboxane A_2. Unlike thromboxane A_2, thromboxane A_3 is not a potent platelet aggregatory agent, and thus fish oils have a net antiplatelet effect. However, to date, the use of fish oils to treat atherosclerotic disease remains controversial and the role of these agents in promoting regression of atherosclerosis remains unclear.

REFERENCES

1. Faggiotto, A., Ross, R., and Harker, L.: Studies of hypercholesterolemia in the nonhuman primate: I. Changes that lead to fatty streak formation. Arteriosclerosis *4*:323, 1984.
2. Clarkson, T.B., Bond, M.G., Bullock, B.C., et al.: A study of atherosclerotic regression in Macaca mulatta: V. Changes in abdominal aorta and carotid and coronary arteries from animals with atherosclerosis induced for 38 months and

then regressed for 24 or 48 months at plasma cholesterol concentrations of 300 or 200 mg/dl. Exp. Mol. Pathol. *41:* 96, 1984.

3. Blankenhorn, D.H., Nessim, S.A., Johnson, R.L., et al.: Beneficial effects of combined colestipol-niacin therapy on coronary atherosclerosis and coronary venous bypass grafts. JAMA *257:*3233, 1987. (Published erratum appears in JAMA *259:*2698, 1988.)

4. Brown, G., Albers, J.J., Fisher, L.D., et al.: Regression of coronary artery disease as a result of intensive lipid-lowering therapy in men with high levels of apolipoprotein. B. N. Engl. J. Med. *323:*1289, 1990.

401 A-T, B-T, C-T, D-F, E-T *(Braunwald, pp. 930–932)*

The electrocardiogram in tetralogy of Fallot is characterized by right axis deviation, as well as right ventricular hypertrophy. Older patients with uncorrected tetralogy of Fallot may develop atrial flutter or fibrillation as well. The classic boot-shaped heart that is seen in conjunction with decreased pulmonary blood flow in infants and children with tetralogy of Fallot is less typically seen in adults. A right-sided aortic arch may be apparent on x-ray examination in approximately 30 per cent of patients with tetralogy of Fallot. In adults, especially those who are acyanotic, pulmonary vascularity may be normal or even increased in up to half the patients.

M-mode echocardiography is usually capable of demonstrating the abnormal relationship between the aortic annulus and interventricular septum that exists in this disorder. Two-dimensional echocardiography may give further information regarding the extent and location of infundibular obstruction, the integrity of the pulmonary valve and artery, and the extent of right ventricular hypertrophy, as well as the location of the VSD. Doppler analysis may also be employed to assess blood flow across the VSD as well as to quantitate right ventricular outflow tract systolic gradients. More recently, magnetic resonance imaging has been used to diagnose and assess tetralogy of Fallot and the associated cardiac anomalies.

402 A-T, B-F, C-T, D-T, E-F *(Braunwald, pp. 1340–1343; Figs. 38–26 and 38–27)*

Prinzmetal's angina, or variant angina pectoris, is characterized by the development of chest pain and ischemic ECG changes in the absence of an increase in cardiac work or oxygen consumption. Thus, unlike in chronic stable angina (effort-induced), episodes of Prinzmetal's angina occur without increases in heart rate, arterial pressure, or myocardial contractility. Spasm of a proximal coronary artery with resultant transmural ischemia has been convincingly documented arteriographically. This is classically associated with elevation of ST segments. Exercise testing in patients with variant angina is of limited value because there is such a variable response of the patients to exercise. Studies have demonstrated approximately equal

numbers of patients who show ST-segment elevation, ST-segment depression, or no change in ST segments during exercise. This reflects the presence of underlying fixed coronary artery disease in some patients and the absence of significant disease in others.

Approximately two-thirds of patients with Prinzmetal's angina will demonstrate severe proximal coronary artery stenosis at coronary angiography. In these patients spasm usually occurs within 1 cm of the stenosis. The other one-third of patients have normal coronary arteries in the absence of ischemia.[1] Patients with normal coronary arteriograms are more likely to have purely nonexertional angina and ST-segment elevations. These patients frequently have an increased incidence of right coronary artery spasm. Patients with mild fixed coronary stenoses tend to experience a more benign course than do patients with associated severe obstructive lesions.[2]

A number of provocative tests for coronary spasm have been developed, among which the ergonovine test is one of the most sensitive and useful. *Ergonovine maleate*, an ergot alkaloid, stimulates both alpha-adrenergic and serotonin receptors and therefore exerts a direct constrictive effect on vascular smooth muscle. In patients with Prinzmetal's angina, the sensitivity to this particular vasoconstrictor is heightened. In general, patients with Prinzmetal's angina will develop a sudden and severe vasoconstriction in response to intravenous doses ranging from 0.05 to 0.40 mg. In normal subjects, doses of this magnitude will cause a uniform, mild vasoconstriction of all the coronary vessels, as opposed to a sudden, dramatic spasm of one coronary artery.[3] Finally, intracoronary acetylcholine has recently been demonstrated to induce coronary spasm in patients with variant angina with high specificity and sensitivity.[4]

REFERENCES

1. Matsuda, Y., Ozaki, M., Ogawa, H., et al.: Coronary arteriography and left ventriculography during spontaneous and exercise-induced ST-segment elevation in patients with variant angina. Am. Heart J. *106:*509, 1983.

2. Cipriano, P.R., Koch, F.H., Rosenthal, S.J., and Schroeder, J.S.: Clinical course of patients following the demonstration of coronary artery spasm by angiography. Am. Heart J. *101:*127, 1981.

3. Winniford, M.D., Johnson, S.M., Mauritson, D.R., and Hillis, L.D.: Ergonovine provocation to assess efficacy of long-term therapy with calcium antagonists in Prinzmetal's variant angina. Am. J. Cardiol. *51:*684, 1983.

4. Okumura, K., et al.: Sensitivity and specificity of intracoronary injection of acetylcholine for the induction of coronary spasm. J. Am. Coll. Cardiol. *12:*883, 1988.

403 A-F, B-T, C-T, D-T, E-F *(Braunwald, pp. 898–899)*

Atrioventricular (AV) septal defects include malformations characterized by varying degrees of incomplete development of the atrial septum, the inflow portion of the ventricular septum, and the atrioventricular valves (see Braunwald, Fig. 29–1, p. 879). These anomalies are also known as endocardial cushion defects or atrioventricular (AV) canal defects. AV septal defects may be encountered in association with other congenital abnormalities, including trisomy 21, Ellis–van Creveld syndrome, and asplenia or polysplenia syndromes.

Ostium primum ASDs occur immediately adjacent to the AV valves, either of which may be deformed or incompetent. Most commonly it is only the anterior or septal leaflet of the mitral valve that is displaced and cleft; more often than not the posterior leaflet of the mitral valve and the tricuspid valve are not involved. Ostium primum ASDs lead to large left-to-right intraatrial shunting and have clinical features that are quite similar to those seen in ostium secundum defects.

In addition to similar findings on physical examination, chest x-ray often reveals RA and RV prominence as well as increased pulmonary vascular markings. Left ventriculography performed at the time of cardiac catheterization may reveal the pathognomonic "gooseneck" deformity. This results from the altered relationship between the anterior components of the mitral valve and the right border of the left ventricular cavity as it leads to the aorta.

When a ventricular septal defect accompanies the ostium primum septal defect and a common AV orifice is therefore present, the malformation is known as a complete atrioventricular canal defect. Approximately 35 per cent of patients with common AV canal have accompanying cardiovascular abnormalities including tetralogy of Fallot, double-outlet right ventricle, transposition of the great arteries, total anomalous pulmonary venous connections, left ventricular outflow tract obstruction, pulmonic stenosis, and persistent left superior vena cava. In addition, common AV canal is seen quite commonly in patients with trisomy 21.

404 A-T, B-F, C-T, D-F, E-T   *(Braunwald, pp. 1127–1134)*

Hypercholesterolemia, particularly elevated levels of LDL, is associated with an increased risk for CAD. This association has been established in both observational and interventional epidemiological studies. The Multiple Risk Factor Intervention Trial (MRFIT) showed a positive correlation between total cholesterol level and CAD mortality.[1] Many clinical trials with cholesterol-lowering drugs have been undertaken to evaluate the efficacy of these agents in preventing CAD events in patients without obvious CAD (primary prevention). In one of the first such trials, the Lipid Research Clinics Coronary Primary Prevention Trial (LRC-CPPT), a 19 per cent reduction in nonfatal MI and CAD death was demonstrated in patients receiving cholestyramine.[2] These results give rise to the clinical rule of thumb that a 1 per cent decrease in total cholesterol reduces the incidence of CAD events by 2 to

3 per cent. The recent West of Scotland Coronary Primary Prevention Study randomized patients with LDL levels of approximately 150 mg/dl or more to receive the HMG-CoA reductase inhibitor pravastatin or placebo.[3] The pravastatin group had a 31 per cent reduction in death resulting from coronary disease after approximately 5 years.

Many secondary prevention trials have also been undertaken to examine the effects of lipid-lowering therapies in patients with known atherosclerotic disease. Secondary prevention trials also have demonstrated a decrease in CAD mortality with lipid-lowering therapy. The Cholesterol Lowering Atherosclerosis Study (CLAS) evaluated the effects of intensive combination drug therapy on atherosclerosis in native coronary vessels and bypass venous grafts.[4] Coronary angiograms were obtained at baseline and at 2-year follow-up. Regression was demonstrated at 15 per cent of the treated group compared to 6 per cent in the placebo group. Recently, the large Scandinavian Simvastatin Survival Study[5] showed a 30 per cent decrease in total mortality and a 42 per cent decrease in coronary mortality in patients with known CAD, the first such trial to show a clear effect on all-cause mortality during the period of the study. Importantly, this study made it clear there are no differences in death due to cancer, accidents, or other causes between patients treated with HMG-CoA reductase inhibitor and those on placebo.

REFERENCES

1. Stamler, J., Wentwork, D., and Neaton, J.D., for the MRFIT Research Group: Is relationship between serum cholesterol and risk of premature death from coronary heart disease continuous and graded? JAMA 256:2823, 1986.
2. Lipid Research Clinics Program: The Lipid Research Clinics Coronary Primary Prevention Trial results. I. Reduction in incidence of coronary heart disease. JAMA 251:351, 1984.
3. West of Scotland Coronary Primary Prevention Study. N. Engl. J. Med., Nov. 1995.
4. Blankenhorn, D.H., Nessim, S.A., and Johnson, R.L.: Beneficial effects of combined colestipolniacin therapy on coronary atherosclerosis and coronary bypass venous grafts. JAMA 257:3233, 1987.
5. Scandinavian Simvastatin Survival Study Group: Randomized trial of cholesterol lowering in 4,444 patients with coronary heart disease. Lancet 344:1383, 1994.

405 A-F, B-F, C-T, D-T, E-T   *(Braunwald, p. 1141; Table 35–8)*

The HMG-CoA reductase inhibitors are all effective in the treatment of patients with elevated levels of LDL cholesterol. Only a modest increase (5 to 10 per cent) in the HDL cholesterol has been noted in large clinical trials of these drugs. The effect of HMG-CoA reductase inhibitors on Lp(a) is currently controversial, and some studies have demonstrated that Lp(a) does not change or may even increase with HMG-CoA reductase inhibitor therapy.[1] Combinations of the HMG-CoA reductase inhibitors and bile-acid–binding resins are particularly effective in lowering LDL cholesterol and may lead to a net decrease in LDL of 50 to 60 per cent.

Serious side effects are uncommon with HMG-CoA reductase inhibitors. Liver function test abnormalities have been reported and on occasion (in fewer than 1 per cent of patients) require discontinuation of therapy. A myositis of frank rhabdomyolysis syndrome has been reported, especially in patients receiving concomitant immunosuppressive therapy. This is felt to be due to an increase in blood levels of lovastatin in the presence of cyclosporine therapy. Current data suggest that reductase inhibitors are effectively removed in first-pass clearance by the liver, which helps account for the relative safety and efficacy of these agents.

REFERENCE

1. Kostner, C.M., Gavish, D., Leopold, B., et al.: HMG-CoA reductase inhibitors lower LDL cholesterol without reducing Lp(a) levels. Circulation 80:1313, 1989.

406 A-T, B-T, C-F, D-F, E-T *(Braunwald, pp. 1556–1557)*

Aortic dissection affects twice as many men as women, and is seen most commonly in the sixth and seventh decades of life. Over 90 per cent of patients presenting with aortic dissection will complain of severe pain. The pain is usually sudden in onset, most severe at its inception, and may be unbearable; adjectives such as "tearing" and "ripping" are frequently used to describe the discomfort. The discomfort tends to migrate in association with dissection of the hematoma into the aortic wall. The diagnosis is often easily confirmed by physical examination. While patients may appear to be in shock, the blood pressure measured is often elevated, especially in patients with distal dissection. The characteristic physical findings associated with aortic dissection, such as pulse deficits and aortic regurgitation, are more commonly seen in proximal dissection. For example, approximately 50 per cent of patients with a proximal dissection will display some form of a pulse deficit, often involving decrease or loss of pulses associated with the brachiocephalic vessels. Similarly, aortic regurgitation is most commonly seen in association with proximal dissection and occurs in more than 50 per cent of patients with aortic dissection.[1]

A variety of clinical conditions in which chest pain consistent with aortic dissection may occur can be confused with this entity, especially if another manifestation such as aortic regurgitation or a neurological abnormality is associated with the chest discomfort. Included in the differential diagnosis are myocardial infarction, acute aortic regurgitation without dissection, thoracic nondissecting aneurysm, mediastinal tumors, musculoskeletal pain, and pericarditis. The most crucial study in the diagnosis of aortic dissection is aortic angiography, which almost always confirms the diagnosis and is well tolerated, even by critically ill patients.

REFERENCE

1. Hirst, A.E., and Gore, I.: The etiology and pathology of aortic regurgitation. In Doroghazi, R.M., and Slater, E.E. (eds.): Aortic Dissection. New York, McGraw-Hill Book Company, 1983, p. 13.

407 A-F, B-T, C-T, D-F, E-T *(Braunwald, pp. 1026–1029)*

Once the decision is made to operate on a patient with predominant mitral regurgitation (MR), several options are available. Excellent results have been obtained with reconstructive procedures that employ a rigid or semirigid prosthetic annulus such as the Carpentier ring. Direct suture repair of the valve and replacement, reimplantation, elongation, or shortening of the chordae tendineae as necessary to make the valve nonregurgitant are usually performed. The impetus to repair as opposed to replace the mitral valve is that many of the hazards of chronic anticoagulation and thromboembolism that accompany use of a mechanical prosthesis are largely eliminated. This procedure can be performed in a wide range of patients, including those with ruptured chordae tendineae, annular dilatation, and even active endocarditis.

However, there are two classes of patients who, in general, should not have a reconstructive procedure. First, patients whose MR originates from myxomatous degeneration (such as occurs in Marfan syndrome) frequently will have progression of underlying disease following reconstruction and will require valve replacement. Second, patients with severe calcification both of the annulus and of the valve, such as elderly persons, do not have enough pliable mitral valve tissue to make a nonregurgitant orifice; these patients are usually more effectively treated with valve replacement.[1]

REFERENCE

1. Kirklin, J.W.: Mitral valve repair for mitral incompetence. Mod. Concepts Cardiovasc. 56:7, 1987.

408 A-T, B-T, C-T, D-F, E-F *(Braunwald, pp. 1136–1138; Tables 35–4 and 35–5)*

In general, the initial therapeutic intervention in all patients with dyslipidemia should be dietary therapy. The Leiden Intervention Trial, a 2-year angiographic study of the effects of dietary therapy, demonstrated that the progression of coronary atherosclerosis could be significantly decreased by a vegetarian diet that contained increased polyunsaturated fat.[1] The CLAS study of patients following coronary artery bypass surgery also showed that dietary therapy could decrease the appearance of new coronary lesions, as assessed by angiography.[2] These and other studies led the National Cholesterol Education Program expert panel to recommend that progressive initiation of dietary therapy be implemented for any patient with an LDL cholesterol level of 160 mg/dl or higher. The Step I AHA diet, the initial therapy plan, includes a total fat intake of <30 per cent of total calories, with saturated fatty acids accounting for <10 per cent of total calories. Total cholesterol intake is limited to <200 mg/day in this plan. The more aggressive Step II AHA diet is reserved for patients who do not have the expected response to Step I diet. This second plan reduces saturated fatty acids to <7 per cent of total calories and total daily cholesterol intake to <200 mg. It is considered appropriate to replace dietary fat with complex carbohydrates, including vegetable fiber. A modest (4 to 5 per cent) independent effect of soluble fiber in serum cholesterol reduction is usual. During pregnancy, elevated levels of cholesterol and triglycerides often occur in the third trimester and are not of clinical significance. These elevations usually return to baseline within the first several months after delivery and need not be specifically treated with dietary therapy.

REFERENCES

1. Arntzenius, A.C., Kromhout, D., Barth, J.D., et al.: Diet, lipoproteins, and the progression of coronary atherosclerosis. The Leiden Intervention Trial. N. Engl. J. Med. 312: 805, 1985.
2. Blankenhorn, D.H., Johnson, R.L., Mack, W.J., et al.: The influence of diet on the appearance of new lesions in human coronary arteries. JAMA 263:1646, 1990.

409 A-T, B-F, C-F, D-F, E-F *(Braunwald, pp. 901–904)*

The management of VSD in infants and children begins with elective hemodynamic evaluation between the ages of 3 and 6 years provided that no evidence of pulmonary hypertension is noted. In children with pulmonary systemic flow ratios <1.5:1, surgical treatment is *not* recommended because the risk of infective endocarditis does not exceed the risk of operation.[1] In addition, although the operative repair of VSD has a low morbidity and mortality, postoperative heart block, infection, and other complications do occur occasionally. With larger shunts, elective operation is usually advised before the child enters school in order to minimize any subsequent differences in development between the patient and normal classmates.

The most significant surgically induced abnormality of the conduction system following repair of VSD is complete heart block, which occurs immediately postoperatively in <1 per cent of patients. Late-onset complete heart block may occur occasionally, especially in the 10 to 25 per cent of patients whose postoperative ECG findings show complete right bundle branch block with left anterior hemiblock.[2] The presence of the latter pattern defines two populations of patients, those with pe-

ripheral damage to the conduction system and those with damage to the bundle of His or its proximal branches.[3] Therefore, the presence of this ECG pattern and accompanying transient heart block in the early postoperative period suggests the need for electrophysiological studies in the postoperative period but may not require permanent pacemaker therapy.

Exercise studies in patients with repair of VSD may uncover late abnormalities in circulatory function despite normal or only moderately elevated pulmonary vascular resistance. An impaired cardiac output response to exercise as well as a markedly abnormal increase in pulmonary arteriovenous pressure gradient may be noted.[4] The precise etiology of these abnormalities remains undefined but may be related to abnormal LV function after closure of the defect and/or to persistent changes in the pulmonary arterioles or to abnormal pulmonary vascular reactivity.

REFERENCES

1. deLeval, M.: Ventricular septal defects. *In* Stark, J., and deLeval, M. (eds.): Surgery for Congenital Heart Defects. New York, Grune & Stratton, 1983, p. 271.
2. Godman, M.J., Roberts, N.K., and Izukawa, T.: Late postoperative conduction disturbances after repair of ventricular septal defect in tetralogy of Fallot. Circulation 49:214, 1974.
3. Okarama, E.O., Guller, B., Molony, J.D., and Weidman, W.H.: Etiology of right bundle branch block pattern after surgical closure of ventricular septal defects. Am. Heart J. 90:14, 1975.
4. Otterstad, J.E., Simonsen, S., and Erikssen, J.: Hemodynamic findings at rest and during mild supine exercise in adults with isolated uncomplicated ventricular septal defects. Circulation 71:650, 1985.

410 A-T, B-T, C-T, D-F, E-F *(Braunwald, pp. 1221–1223)*

It is now established that successful coronary reperfusion can be achieved with PTCA in acute MI in two principal settings: (1) when used as primary therapy (primary PTCA), or (2) as an adjunct to thrombolysis. The latter is used when thrombolysis fails to achieve coronary reperfusion, in which case PTCA may be performed as "rescue" therapy.

A variety of outcomes have been reported in the literature for rescue PTCA after failed thrombolysis.[1] Although the procedural success is generally high (>80 per cent), the average rate of reocclusion also is high (18 per cent), with an average mortality of around 10 per cent. Two randomized trials[2,3] have addressed the effects of rescue PTCA versus a more conservative approach following thrombolysis. One of these, the RESCUE[3] trial did report a reduction in mortality and heart failure at 30 days in the PTCA group.

There also have been numerous trials evaluating the effect of adjunctive or deferred PTCA following thrombolysis in relation to outcome and mortality. Several trials compared immediate, early (within several hours to a few days), or deferred PTCA (more than 4 days) versus no PTCA in patients who appear to have reperfused with thrombolysis. In a metaanalysis of clinical trials of more than 6000 patients, routine use of PTCA was associated with a trend toward increased mortality.[4] This analysis also showed higher rates of abrupt closure, reinfarction, and urgent coronary bypass surgery, but not benefit in ventricular recovery. In patients who do not demonstrate any provocable ischemia following thrombolysis, there are no data to support the use of empirical PTCA. The TIMI II trial, which addressed this issue directly, showed no clear benefit of the invasive strategy after thrombolysis over the conservative strategy for either mortality or reinfarction rates.[5] Similarly, the TOPS[6] trial also randomized patients with a negative ETT following thrombolysis to either medical therapy or PTCA. The PTCA group also did worse in this study, with a higher rate of abrupt closure and a lower rate of infarct-free survival at the 1-year follow-up visit.

REFERENCES

1. Belenkie, I., Traboulsi, M., et al.: Rescue angioplasty during myocardial infarctions has a beneficial effect on mortality. Can. J. Cardiol. 8:357, 1992.
2. Ellis, S.G., and Van de Werf, F.: Present status of rescue PTCA. Current polarization of opinion and randomized trials. J. Am. Coll. Cardiol. 19:681, 1992.
3. Ellis, S.G.: Randomized comparison of rescue PTCA with conservation management of patients with early failure of thrombolysis for acute anterior MI. Circulation 90:2280, 1994.
3. Michels, K.B., and Yusuf, S.: Does PTCA in acute MI affect mortality and reinfarction rates? A quantitative overview of the randomized trials. Circulation 91:476, 1995.
5. The TIMI Study Group: Comparison of invasive and conservative strategies after treatment with intravenous tPA in acute myocardial infarction: Results of the thrombolysis in myocardial infarction phase II trial. N. Engl. J. Med. 320:618, 1989.
6. Ellis, S.G., and Mooney, M.R.: Randomized trial of late PTCA versus conservative management for patients with residual stenosis after thrombolytic therapy of MI: Treatment of post thrombolysis stenoses (TOPS) study group. Circulation 86:1400, 1992.

411 A-T, B-F, C-F, D-T, E-F   *(Braunwald, pp. 1013–1017)*

This woman clearly has at least moderately severe MS, and her age and complaint of left-sided chest pain suggest that she may have coexistent coronary artery disease. In addition, her echocardiogram raises the possibility of coexistent aortic stenosis (AS). Therefore, it would be prudent to carry out cardiac catheterization and coronary arteriography to evaluate the coronary artery disease to rule out AS and to confirm the presence of significant MS. It would not be acceptable to defer further treatment in a patient who has symptoms of progressive dyspnea on exertion, arrhythmias, and chest pain. At cardiac catheterization it is likely that a mitral valve area <1.0 cm² will be found, in which case surgical treatment should be recommended.

Open commissurotomy and mitral valve repair would be a reasonable suggestion for first-time operation for MS in certain patients. At open commissurotomy, cardiac bypass is established, any thrombi in the left atrium are removed, and then the commissures are incised, the papillary muscles split, and the valves débrided of calcium. This procedure is useful for patients with mild calcific disease and also is helpful in patients with mild to moderate mitral regurgitation. However, this woman is not an ideal candidate for repair for two reasons. First, she has been in atrial fibrillation for many years and has a dilated atrium, which means anticoagulation cannot be avoided following repair. Second, the operation would be technically difficult because of extensive calcification. Therefore, it likely would be necessary, if she is to undergo open heart surgery, to carry out mitral valve replacement with a mechanical prosthesis.

Finally, although balloon mitral valvuloplasty is useful in some patients,[1] in this patient with significant calcification and potentially coexisting aortic and coronary disease, it would be less likely to be an option. In addition, the prior surgery may have significantly altered the intraatrial septum, making the balloon valvuloplasty attempt more dangerous, especially during the initial crossing of the foramen ovale. It would therefore be more appropriate to proceed with mitral valve replacement in this patient.

REFERENCE

1. Tuzcu, E.M., Block, P.C., and Palacios, I.F.: Comparison of early versus late experience with percutaneous mitral balloon valvuloplasty. J. Am. Coll. Cardiol. 17:1121, 1991.

412 A-T, B-T, C-T, D-F, E-T   *(Braunwald, pp. 970–971)*

In general, total correction of tetralogy of Fallot is advised for almost all patients, even in infancy.[1] The successful early correction appears to prevent the consequences of progressive infundibular obstruction and acquired pulmonary atresia, delayed growth and development, and the complications secondary to hypoxemia and polycythemia with bleeding tendencies that arise in this population. It is the size of the pulmonary arteries that is most important in determining candidacy for primary repair of tetralogy of Fallot, as opposed to the age or size of the infant or child. Marked hypoplasia of the pulmonary arteries is a relative contraindication for a total corrective operation and when present usually leads to a palliative procedure designed to increase pulmonary blood flow by establishing a systemic–pulmonary arterial anastomosis.[2] The total correction of the tetralogy then may be carried out later in childhood or adolescence at lower risk. Such palliative procedures relieve hypoxemia and polycythemia and their attendant complications.

The postoperative period after palliative or corrective surgery is marked by a variety of common complications. A sudden increase in pulmonary venous return may lead to mild to moderate *left* ventricular decompensation, while varying degrees of pulmonic valvular regurgitation may increase right ventricular cavity size.[3] In addition, bleeding problems may frequently be seen, especially in older polycythemic patients. Complete right bundle branch block or left anterior hemiblock is often observed postoperatively. The greatest cause of early and late mortality and poor surgical results is restriction in pulmonary arterial flow due to persistent problems with right-sided outflow tract obstruction. In general, surgical repair leads to relief of symptoms of hypoxemia and the severe exercise intolerance that mark the preoperative period.

REFERENCES

1. Kirklin, J.K., Pacifico, A.D., and Kirklin, J.W.: Tetralogy of Fallot: Principles of surgical managements. Mod. Probl. Paediatr. *22*:139, 1983.
2. Kirklin, J.W., Blackstone, E.H., Kirklin, J.K., et al.: Surgical results and protocols in the spectrum of tetralogy of Fallot. Ann. Surg. *198*:251, 1983.
3. Naito, Y., Fujita, T., Yagihara, T., et al.: Usefulness of left ventricular volume in assessing tetralogy of Fallot for total correction. Am. J. Cardiol. *56*:356, 1985.

413 A-T, B-F, C-T, D-F, E-F   *(Braunwald, p. 1012; see also Answer 395)*

The M-mode echocardiogram displayed comes from a patient with mitral stenosis (MS). The classic features of MS include thickening of the leaflets, decreased maximal leaflet separation in diastole, and absence of the *a* wave in the setting of normal LV function. Shown in this echocardiogram are redundant echoes consistent with a thickened calcified rheumatic valve. Decreased leaflet separation can be readily seen in diastole. Furthermore, there is minimal reopening during atrial contraction. In normal subjects the posterior leaflet of the mitral valve moves posteriorly during early diastole, while in the example shown here it can be seen that the posterior mitral leaflet moves anteriorly, as does the anterior leaflet. Thus, the anterior and posterior leaflets appear to be fused. The LV cavity size and systolic function measured by movement of the septum and the posterior LV wall appear normal, which is characteristic of MS. It should be noted that determination of mitral valve area is not possible by M-mode echocardiography. However, using two-dimensional echocardiography in the parasternal short-axis view the mitral valve orifice can be observed in cross-section and the innermost portion of the mitral valve orifice planimetered to obtain a measure of the area. Doppler echocardiography, however, is the most accurate noninvasive technique for estimating the transmitral valvular pressure gradient, and for estimating the valve area.

REFERENCE

1. Glover, M.U., Warren, S.E., Vieweg, W.V.R., et al.: M-mode and two-dimensional echocardiographic correlation with findings at catheterization and surgery in patients with mitral stenosis. Am. Heart J. *105*:98, 1983.

414 A-T, B-T, C-F, D-T, E-F   *(Braunwald, pp. 1153–1154)*

The interactions between alcohol and the cardiovascular system are complex and only partially understood. Excessive alcohol consumption is clearly associated with elevations in blood pressure[1] and with a primary dilated cardiomyopathy as well. However, a potential beneficial effect of mild to moderate alcohol intake on cardiovascular morbidity and mortality has been recognized by some studies. In four of the five major prospective studies on moderate alcohol intake and atherosclerosis, a clear inverse relationship between alcohol intake and the incidence of CAD was documented.[2] Other studies have found the same inverse relationship between CAD and the anatomical degree of atherosclerosis.[3] The reason for this potential cardioprotective effect of alcohol is unclear. Despite these associations, alcohol cannot be specifically recommended as a preventive measure because of the increase in overall morbidity and mortality that is associated with alcohol abuse. Alcoholism is clearly correlated with overt CAD, and heavy alcohol intake has been positively correlated with the prevalence of acute MI in several studies. Alcohol is known to raise HDL levels, although the specific subfraction (HDL_2, $HHDL_3$, or both) varies depending on the study.[4]

REFERENCES

1. Regan, T.J.: Alcohol and the cardiovascular system. JAMA *264*:377, 1990.
2. Hennekens, C.H.: Alcohol. *In* Kaplan, N.M., and Stamler, J. (eds.): Prevention of Coronary Heart Disease: Practical Management of the Risk Factors. Philadelphia, W.B. Saunders Co., 1983, pp. 130–138.
3. Barboriak, J.J., Anderson, A.J., and Hoffman, R.G.: Interrelationships between coronary artery occlusion, high density lipoprotein cholesterol and alcohol intake. J. Lab. Clin. Med. *94*:348, 1979.
4. Hartung, G.H., Reeves, R.S., Krock, L.P., et al.: Effect of alcohol and exercise on plasma HDL cholesterol subfractions and apolipoprotein A-I(APOA-I) in middle-aged men. Circulation *72*(Suppl. III):452, 1985.

415 A-T, B-T, C-F, D-F, E-T   *(Braunwald, pp. 1242, 1256; Fig. 37–39)*

Left ventricular aneurysm complicates AMI in approximately 12 to 15 per cent of patients who survive the acute insult. Formation of the aneurysm is presumed to occur when intraventricular tension leads to expansion of the noncontracting, infarcted myocardial tissue.[1] In general, an anterior MI complicated by left ventricular aneurysm occurs due to total occlusion of a poorly collateralized left anterior descending artery.[2,3] The presence of multivessel disease, extensive collaterals, or a nonoccluded left anterior descending artery makes the development of an aneurysm much less likely. Aneurysms occur approximately four times more commonly at the apex and in the anterior wall than in the inferoposterior wall, and in general range from 1 to 8 cm in diameter.

Even when compared with mortality in patients having comparable left ventricular ejection fractions, the presence of a left ventricular aneurysm leads to a mortality that is up to six times higher than that of patients without aneurysm.[4] Death in such patients is often sudden and presumed to be secondary to a high incidence of ventricular tachyarrhythmias that originate from the aneurysmal tissue itself. Diagnosis of aneurysm is best made by echocardiographic study, by radionuclide ventriculography, or at the time of cardiac catheterization by left ventriculography. Interestingly, the classic evidence of aneurysm on electrocardiogram, persistent ST-segment elevation in the area of the infarction, actually indicates a large infarct but does not necessarily imply an aneurysm.[5] In appropriately selected patients, especially those in whom relative preservation of contractile performance of the left ventricle may be achieved, surgical aneurysmectomy may achieve clinical improvement with a relatively low risk of death.

REFERENCES

1. Schuster, E.H., and Bulkley, B.H.: Expansion of transmural myocardial infarction: A patho-physiologic factor in cardiac rupture. Circulation *60*:1532, 1979.
2. Forman, M.D., Collins, H.W., Kipelman, H.A., et al.: Determinants of left ventricular aneurysm formation after anterior myocardial infarction: A clinical and angiographic study. J. Am. Coll. Cardiol. *8*:1256, 1986.
3. Hirai, T., Fujita, M., Nakajima, H., et al.: Importance of collateral circulation for prevention of left ventricular aneurysm formation in acute myocardial infarction. Circulation *79*:791, 1989.
4. Meizlish, J.L., Berger, H.J., Plankey, M., et al.: Functional left ventricular aneurysm formation after acute myocardial infarction: Incidence, natural history, and prognostic implications. N. Engl. J. Med. *31*:1001, 1984.
5. Lindsay, J., Jr., Dewey, R.C., Talesnick, B.S., and Nolan, N.G.: Relation of ST-segment elevation after healing of acute myocardial infarction to the presence of left ventricular aneurysm. Am. J. Cardiol. *54*:84, 1984.

416 A-T, B-T, C-T, D-F, E-F   *(Braunwald, pp. 1496–1498)*

Constrictive pericarditis usually results from progressive scarring and thickening of the pericardium with subsequent obliteration of the pericardial space due to an inflammatory process of the pericardium. The end-stage constricted pericardium is a fibrotic, thickened, adherent structure in which the visceral and parietal layers have become fused. This stiffened structure restricts diastolic filling and therefore leads to elevation and equalization of diastolic pressures in all four chambers of the heart. In general, cardiac filling occurs only early in diastole when the intracardiac volume is less than that defined by the stiffened pericardium. Because of the elevation of systemic venous pressure in this disorder, this early diastolic filling occurs more rapidly than in normal patients. Therefore, the characteristic dip-and-plateau waveform, in which rapid early diastolic filling is followed by an abrupt halt in filling leading to a plateau phase, is commonly seen in constriction. A prominent *y* descent results from the rapid early diastolic filling, and a clear *x* descent is usually present as well, leading to the characteristic "M" or "W" configuration of the venous waveform seen in this disorder. This may be compared with cardiac tamponade, in which the diastolic phase of venous return is blunted due to the presence of cardiac compression throughout the cardiac cycle. This results in a venous pressure tracing that shows a diminished or absent *y* descent and a predominant *x* descent.

417 A-T, B-T, C-F, D-T, E-F   *(Braunwald, pp. 1258–1263)*

Short-term and long-term survival following MI depends upon a variety of factors, but the single most important factor is the underlying state of the left ventricle.[1] One historical factor associated with poorer prognosis after infarction is diabetes mellitus, which leads to a three- to fourfold increase in risk.[2] Other negative factors include female sex, age greater than 70 years, hypertension, and prior angina or MI. Even when corrections are made for infarct size, a greater mortality is observed after anterior wall MI than after inferior MI.[3] Angina after MI usually is associated with a worse prognosis because it indicates the presence of residual myocardium at risk. In some instances, coronary artery spasm may cause postinfarction angina and the prognosis may then be relatively favorable. In at least one study, silent ischemia following MI on ambulatory monitoring has the same unfavorable prognosis as symptomatic ischemia.[4]

REFERENCES

1. DeBusk, R.F., for the Health and Public Policy Committee of the Clinical Efficacy Assessment Subcommittee: American College of Physicians: Evaluation of patients after recent acute myocardial infarction. Ann. Intern. Med. *110*:485, 1989.
2. Abbott, R.D., Donahue, R.P., Kannel, W.B., and Wilson, P.F.: The impact of diabetes on survival following myocardial infarction in men vs. women. The Framingham Study. JAMA *260*:3456, 1988.
3. Hands, M.E., Lloyd, B.L., Robinson, J.S., et al.: Prognostic significance of electrocardiographic site of infarction after correction for enzymatic size and infarction. Circulation *73*:885, 1986.
4. Tzivoni, D., Gavish, A., Zin, D., et al.: Prognostic significance of ischemic episodes in patients with previous myocardial infarction. Am. J. Cardiol. *62*:661, 1988.

418 A-F, B-T, C-T, D-T, E-T   *(Braunwald, pp. 1467–1469)*

It has been recognized that certain families appear to have an autosomal dominant transmission of recurrent myxomas. In addition, some patients with familial myxoma have a syndrome that involves a complex of abnormalities, including lentigines or pigmented nevi or both, primary nodular adrenal cortical disease with or without Cushing's syndrome, myxomatous mammary fibroadenomas, testicular tumors, and pituitary adenomas with gigantism or acromegaly. Patients who have two or more components of this complex usually present at a relatively young age. Either of two mnemonics are applied to their disease: NAME syndrome (*n*evi, *a*trial myxoma, *m*yxoid neurofibroma, and *e*phelides) or LAMB syndrome (*l*entigines, *a*trial, *m*yxoma, and *b*lue nevi). Approximately 7 per cent of all myxomas are found in persons with familial myxoma or the aforementioned complex of findings. These patients, in comparison to others, tend to be younger, have multiple myxomas of chambers other than the left atrium, and are more likely to have postoperative recurrence of myxoma.[1]

REFERENCE

1. McCarthy, P.M., Piehler, J.M., Schaff, H.V.: The significance of multiple, recurrent, and "complex" cardiac myxomas. Thorac. Cardiovasc. Surg. 91:389, 1986.

419 A-T, B-T, C-F, D-F   *(Braunwald, pp. 1254–1255)*

The development of angina in the postinfarction period is a complication that requires immediate evaluation. When postinfarction angina is accompanied by ST- and T-wave changes in the area where the infarction originally occurred, it may be due to occlusion of an initially patent vessel, reocclusion of a recanalized vessel, or coronary spasm in that location.[1] The presence of postinfarction angina means increased short-term and long-term mortality for the AMI patient.[2] In general, patients who develop spontaneous postinfarction angina early following the acute event should have cardiac catheterization and coronary arteriography to evaluate the need for and possibility of coronary angioplasty or, if necessary, coronary artery bypass graft surgery.[3]

It is difficult to distinguish postinfarction angina from extension of the underlying infarction. Infarct extension occurs in about 8 per cent of patients with AMI during the first 10 days.[4] Infarct extension is characterized by severe and prolonged chest discomfort, persistent ECG changes, and the reappearance of CK-MB in the patient's serum. Infarct extension leads to an increase in in-hospital mortality in the AMI setting. It appears to be more common in patients with diabetes, a previous MI, and an early-peaking CK-MB curve, and in obese females who have experienced a nontransmural infarction as their initial event.[5]

REFERENCES

1. Koiwaya, Y., Torii, S., Takeshita, A., et al.: Post-infarction angina caused by coronary arterial spasm. Circulation 65: 275, 1982.
2. Schuster, E.H., and Bulkley, B.H.: Early postinfarction angina. Ischemia at a distance and ischemia in the infarct zone. N. Engl. J. Med. 305:1101, 1981.
3. Epstein, S.E., Palmeri, S.T., and Patterson, R.E.: Evaluation of patients after acute myocardial infarction. Indications for cardiac catheterization and surgical intervention. N. Engl. J. Med. 307:1467, 1982.
4. Muller, J.E., Rude, R.E., Braunwald, E., et al.: Myocardial infarct extension: Occurrence, outcome, and risk factors in the Multicenter Investigation of Limitation of Infarct Size. Ann. Intern. Med. 108:1, 1988.
5. Marmor, A., Sobel, B.E., and Roberts, E.: Factors presaging early recurrent myocardial infarction ("extension"). Am. J. Cardiol. 48:603, 1981.

420 A-F, B-T, C-F, D-T, E-T   *(Braunwald, pp. 1504–1505)*

Because of the progressive nature of constrictive pericarditis, the majority of patients become symptomatic and come to medical attention due to weakness, peripheral edema, and/or ascites. The treatment for constrictive pericarditis is complete resection of the pericardium, including excision of the pericardium from the anterior and inferior surfaces of the RV as well as the diaphagmatic and anterolateral surfaces of the LV, extending upward to the great vessels and to or across the atrioventricular grooves. This procedure has been performed more successfully using an approach via median sternotomy rather than left thoracotomy and in patients who have had cardiopulmonary bypass to allow greater mobility of the heart. In most recent series, the average operative mortality has ranged between 7 and 19 per cent, with a clear correlation between the degree of the functional disability before the operation and the survival following repair.[1] Other factors that have an adverse influence upon overall outcome include diuretic use, renal insufficiency in the preoperative period, and a history of radiation pericarditis.[2]

It is generally agreed that patients should undergo pericardiectomy soon after the development of symptoms. Between 14 and 28 per cent of patients in the immediate postoperative period will develop a low-output syndrome. This occurs more commonly in patients with a marked degree of preoperative disability and high RV enddiastolic pressures, indicative of severe constriction.[3] Symptomatic improvement is seen in approximately 90 per cent of survivors of pericardiectomy, and 5-year survivals are in the 74 to 84 per cent range.

Patients with presumed tuberculosis pericarditis should receive a course of antituberculosis therapy before operation, which may be continued for 6 to 12 months after pericardiectomy if the diagnosis is confirmed. The time course for symptomatic improvement following pericardiectomy varies. Some patients may experience immediate decreases in symptomatology, while others may have a delayed or partial response that requires weeks or months for resolution of elevated jugular venous pressures and abnormal filling pressures.[4]

REFERENCES

1. Robertson, J.M., and Mulder, D.G.: Pericardiectomy: A changing scene. Am. J. Surg. *148*:86, 1984.
2. Siefort, F.C., Miller, C.D., Oesterle, S.N., et al.: Surgical treatment of constrictive pericarditis: Analysis of outcome and diagnostic error. Circulation *72*(Suppl. II):264, 1985.
3. McCaughlin, B.C., Schaff, H.V., Piehler, J.M., et al.: Early and late results of pericardiectomy for constrictive pericarditis. J. Thorac. Cardiovasc. Surg. *89*:340, 1985.
4. Viola, A.R.: The influence of pericardiectomy on the hemodynamics of chronic constrictive pericarditis. Circulation *48*:1038, 1973.

421 A-T, B-F, C-F, D-T, E-T *(Braunwald, pp. 1437–1439)*

Many viruses can cause an associated myocarditis. The myocarditis characteristically develops after a lag period of several weeks following initial systemic infection, which suggests that the myocarditis is due to an immunological response. Coxsackie viruses, in particular Coxsackie B, are the agents most frequently associated with viral myocarditis. Echovirus, which is similar to the Coxsackie virus, is also associated with myopericarditis, frequently during the course of an acute pleurodynia-like illness. Myocardial involvement during the course of mumps is rare, occurring in less than 10 per cent of adults affected with this virus, and even less frequently in children. Similarly, infectious mononucleosis is rarely associated with significant myocarditis. Neither variola nor vaccinia is associated with myocarditis. One-third of patients dying of influenza have associated myocarditis, indicating that cardiovascular involvement may be important in the mortality rate of this viral illness. Cardiac involvement occurs 1 to 2 weeks after the onset of the illness, manifested by signs and symptoms of congestive heart failure and pericarditis. Other viral illnesses in which myocarditis occurs include poliomyelitis and viral hepatitis, and illnesses involving the human immunodeficiency virus.

422 A-T, B-F, C-T, D-T, E-T *(Braunwald, p. 1589; Tables 46–9 and 46–10; Fig. 46–10)*

While perfusion lung scanning is generally a useful diagnostic test in screening for pulmonary embolism, a number of ambiguities associated with this procedure limit its usefulness. The designations "low," "moderate," "high," and "indeterminate" for perfusion lung scans are widely used, but these categories have not been standardized by a national body or organization. While prospective studies comparing ventilation-perfusion lung scans with pulmonary angiograms have been carried out, the results have usually been challenged due to potential selection biases in the patient populations studied. However, in the recent Prospective Investigation of Pulmonary Embolism Diagnosis (PIOPED) study, only 41 per cent of patients with positive pulmonary angiograms had a high-probability lung scan.[1] The PIOPED study, which recruited 931 patients, further underscores the importance of the clinical evaluation in predicting angiographic outcomes.[1,2] The presence of chest x-ray abnormalities in the regions of the perfusion defect makes the designation of "indeterminate" probability necessary and not infrequently limits the usefulness of the perfusion lung scan. Low-probability scans, in contrast, in which subsegmental and nonsegmental perfusion defects that may match ventilation defects are present, often are seen in conjunction with normal angiographic findings. In patients with low-probability scans pulmonary angiography generally is not warranted, unless there is a high level of clinical suspicion. In general, pulmonary angiography generally is reserved for patients with moderate probability or indeterminate lung scans or those in whom clinical suspicion remains high regardless of the perfusion lung scan findings.

REFERENCES

1. The PIOPED Investigators: Value of the ventilation/perfusion scan in acute pulmonary embolism: Results of the prospective investigation of pulmonary embolism diagnosis (PIOPED). JAMA *263*:2753, 1990.
2. Stein, P.D., Alavi, A., Gottschalk, A., et al.: Usefulness of noninvasive diagnostic tools for diagnosis of acute pulmonary embolism in patients with a normal chest radiograph. Am. J. Cardiol. *67*:1117, 1991.

423 A-F, B-T, C-F, D-F, E-T *(Braunwald, pp. 1315–1316)*

It is estimated that more than 300,000 angioplasties were done in 1993, a 10-fold increase over the number of PTCA procedures 1 decade earlier. Coronary angioplasty continues to undergo improvements and changes that result in improved outcome. Nevertheless, abrupt closure remains a major complication associated with PTCA in the catheterization laboratory. The current procedural success for PTCA is about 90 per cent with an acute closure rate of 2 to 10 per cent.[1,2] Closure is defined as a significant reduction in coronary flow that is recognizable before the patient leaves the laboratory, or soon thereafter. Clinical risk factors for closure include advanced age, female gender, unstable angina, diabetes, and chronic hemodialysis. Post-PTCA closure is usually caused by thrombosis or coronary dissection or both, not by vasospasm.

Treatment objectives for abrupt closure following PTCA include, first and foremost, restoration of adequate coronary blood flow, which may serve either as a bridge to bypass surgery or as the definitive therapy that was sought with the original PTCA procedure. Numerous strategies to treat abrupt closure have evolved recently, including specialized perfusion catheters, coronary stents and, in select cases, thrombolytic therapy.

REFERENCES

1. Landau, C., Lange, R.A., and Hillis, L.D.: Percutaneous transluminal coronary angioplasty. N. Engl. J. Med. *330*: 981, 1994.

2. De Feyer, P.J., de Jaegere, P.P., and Serruys, P.W.: Incidence, predictors and management of acute coronary occlusion after coronary angioplasty. Am. Heart J. *127*:643, 1994.

424 A-F, B-T, C-F, D-T, E-F *(Braunwald, pp. 1036–1037)*

The valve depicted in *A* is a stenotic aortic valve with three cusps. This is the most common form of aortic stenosis in the elderly and is an acquired type of aortic stenosis. If the valve illustrated were bicuspid (in which the cusps are situated anteriorly and posteriorly with commissures on either side), it would be a congenital defect. In acquired aortic stenosis, years of normal mechanical stress on the valve are thought to result in degenerative calcification. It is likely that the valve illustrated had suffered damage secondary to rheumatic fever because fusion of the commissures and development of calcific nodules on the cusps as shown are typical of rheumatic valvular disease. Because the apposition of the valve leaflets is otherwise good, it is unlikely that this individual had significant aortic regurgitation. Endocarditis would be unlikely to result in aortic stenosis of this type. Both diabetes mellitus and hypercholesterolemia increase the risk of aortic valve calcifications. Some patients with tricuspid aortic valves with commissural fusion are candidates for balloon valvuloplasty as shown in the accompanying photograph (*B*), which demonstrates reopening of the valve following balloon valvuloplasty (in this case, in vitro).

425 A-F, B-F, C-F, D-T, E-F *(Braunwald, pp. 1213–1215)*

Cell death that occurs following reperfusion of ischemic tissue that has not necessarily been irreversibly damaged by ischemia is a specific form of reperfusion injury.[1] Reperfusion may also accelerate necrosis of irreversibly injured myocytes, but it does not appear to add to the area of myocardium that is ultimately damaged.[2] Reperfusion following thrombolytic therapy is somewhat more likely to lead to hemorrhagic infarction than reperfusion by mechanical methods such as angioplasty.[3] Evidence to date suggests that this hemorrhagic event does not lead to extension of the evolving myocardial infarction. A variety of substances have been implicated in the pathophysiology of reperfusion injury, including the sudden exposure of ischemic tissue to calcium and oxygen, as well as toxicity from oxygen-derived free radicals. As of this writing, while some encouraging results from animal experiments have been reported, there is no *clinical* evidence to support the use of oxygen-derived free radical scavengers in the periinfarction setting.

One of the most common clinical sequelae of reperfusion is a change in cardiac rhythm. Sinus bradycardia may appear briefly in many patients, especially those with inferior infarction. Premature ventricular contractions are quite common at the time of reperfusion but are also noted frequently in patients with evolving MI and are thus *nonspecific* indicators of reperfusion. Increased incidences of ventricular tachycardia and accelerated idioventricular rhythm are observed after successful reperfusion and may serve as markers of successful thrombolytic therapy in some subjects[4]; however, they are far from specific.

REFERENCES

1. Weisfeldt, M.L.: Reperfusion and perfusion injury. Clin. Res. *35*:13, 1987.
2. Laffel, G.L., and Braunwald, E.: Thrombolytic therapy. A new strategy for treatment of acute myocardial infarction. N. Engl. J. Med. *311*:710, 1984.
3. Waller, B.F., Rothbaum, D.A., Pinkerton, C.A., et al.: Status of the myocardium and infarct-related coronary artery in 19 neocropsy patients with acute recanalization using pharmacologic (streptokinase, r-tissue type plasminogen activator), mechanical (percutaneous transluminal coronary angioplasty) or combined types of reperfusion therapy. J. Am. Coll. Cardiol. *9*:785, 1987.
4. Goldberg, S., Greenspan, A.J., Urban, P.L., et al.: Reperfusion arrhythmia: A marker of restoration of antegrade flow during intracoronary thrombolysis for acute myocardial infarction. Am. Heart J. *105*:26, 1983.

426 A-T, B-T, C-F, D-T, E-F *(Braunwald, pp. 1394–1395)*

Prior to any patient's embarking on an exercise program, a careful clinical examination is necessary; the severity and duration of specific underlying disorders may require special attention. In general, the presence of a poorly controlled systemic disease, an unstable condition, or any acute illness carries an unacceptable risk with exertional activities. Several specific cardiovascular contraindications to exercise exist. Among these are resting blood pressure >200/110 mm Hg, unpaced third-degree heart block, left ventricular outflow tract obstruction, cardiomyopathy, unstable ischemic syndromes including myocardial infarction, significant arrhythmias, active myocarditis within the last year, recent thromboembolic disorders, and aortic dissection.[1] It should be noted that while patients with underlying disorders of a more chronic nature may require special attention, such disorders rarely prohibit the patient from undertaking any physical exertion. Thus, patients with conditions such as diabetes, renal disease, anemia, obstructive lung disease, and orthopedic disabilities may perform rehabilitation programs with appropriate supervision.

Cardiac rehabilitation is especially useful in patients who have undergone recent coronary artery bypass grafting, although those who exhibit sternal instability after such a procedure should be prohibited from performing exercise involving the upper extremities or trunk.[2] The specific medical regimen that the patient brings to the rehabilitation program should also be known so that potential side effects of underlying medications may be taken into consideration. For example, individuals on anticoagulation must be observed carefully to avoid local trauma, and insulin-dependent diabetics must be made aware that their insulin requirements may decrease with the exercise program. Even though beta blockers alter the heart rate for given exercise intensities, the net effect of training is preserved in patients on such medications.[3]

REFERENCES

1. Council on Scientific Affairs: Physician-supervised exercise programs in rehabilitation patients with coronary heart disease. JAMA *245*:1463, 1981.
2. Metier, C.P., Pollock, M.L., and Graves, J.E.: Exercise prescription for the coronary artery bypass graft surgery patient. J. Cardiac Rehabil. *6*:85, 1986.
3. Beta blockers and exercise: A symposium. *In* Harrison, D.C. (ed.) Am. J. Cardiol. *55*:167D–171D, 1985.

427 A-T, B-T, C-F, D-F, E-F   *(Braunwald, pp. 1481–1485)*

Initial management of acute pericarditis should begin with an attempt to detect any underlying causes of the inflammatory process which might be amenable to specific therapy. Patients who have pain and fever during an acute phase of pericarditis should be placed on bed rest, since activity may lead to an increase or worsening of symptoms. In general such patients should be hospitalized, to exclude the possibility of an associated MI as well as to watch for the development of tamponade and to rule out any possibility that the pericarditis is due to an acute pyogenic process.

Treatment of the chest pain associated with pericarditis usually begins with a nonsteroidal anti-inflammatory agent such as aspirin or indomethacin. If patients fail to respond to such measures after 48 hours and pain remains severe, corticosteroid therapy may be employed using larger doses of prednisone, such as 60 to 80 mg daily in divided doses over 5 to 7 days. If symptoms subsequently abate during this time, the steroids may be tapered. Antibiotic therapy is reserved for patients who have documented purulent pericarditis. Oral anticoagulants should *not* be administered during the acute phase of pericarditis of any cause because of the increased possibility of resulting hemopericardium. Patients with acute pericarditis who require anticoagulant therapy for the presence of a prosthetic heart valve, for example, should be given intravenous heparin as their anticoagulant therapy in order to allow for prompt reversal with protamine should any difficulties arise. Such patients require close monitoring with both physical examination and echocardiography in order to detect the early development or accumulation of pericardial fluid.

428 A-T, B-T, C-F, D-F, E-T   *(Braunwald, pp. 1010–1011)*

The clinical and hemodynamic features of MS are dictated largely by levels of cardiac output and pulmonary vascular resistance. Several clinical features are commonly present. First, women tend to be affected more often than men. S_1 is usually loud, unless sufficient calcification and fibrosis have occurred to decrease the mobility of the valve. This is in contrast to mitral regurgitation in which the first heart sound is usually diminished. An S_3 is rarely heard in pure MS, since ventricular filling is slow and the LV wall has normal compliance. The presence of S_3 is an indication of coexisting cardiomyopathy or a regurgitant lesion. The left ventricle in MS usually has normal or slow filling due to the impaired flow of blood across the stenotic mitral valve. Thus, a presystolic lift or a presystolic wave is highly unlikely to be found on physical examination in MS. The LV is rarely hyperdynamic and is usually normal in size.

One hallmark of MS is the presence of presystolic accentuation of the diastolic murmur in patients in sinus rhythm because transvalvular blood flow is accelerated by atrial contraction. Such a murmur may also occur occasionally in patients with atrial fibrillation due to increased blood flow velocity across a mitral valve orifice that begins to narrow after the onset of LV contraction. Conditions other than MS that may mimic the crescendo presystolic murmur include aortic regurgitation, in which an Austin-Flint murmur may extend to S_1. In a hypertrophied restrictive ventricle the combination of S_3 and S_4 may be loud enough to simulate a presystolic murmur. In both tricuspid stenosis and left atrial myxoma a narrowed orifice may contribute to a crescendo presystolic murmur.

429 A-T, B-T, C-F, D-T, E-F   *(Braunwald, pp. 1493–1495; 1505)*

Preparation of patients for pericardiocentesis should include administration of intravascular fluids to allow for volume expansion and thus to delay the appearance of right ventricular diastolic collapse and subsequent hemodynamic deterioration. The major risk of percutaneous cardiocentesis is laceration of the heart or great vessels. The use of a subxyphoid approach under fluoroscopic guidance in the catheterization laboratory has greatly decreased the likelihood of such complications. In the large series describing the Stanford experience,[1] pericardial fluid was obtained in more than 80 per cent of patients studied. Of note, the probability of successfully obtaining such fluid was directly proportional to the size of the pericardial effusion present. Fluid was obtained in 93 per cent of patients with effusions present both anteriorly and posteriorly on echocardiogram but in only 58 per cent of those with an isolated small posterior effusion.

Cardiac tamponade associated with malignant effusions or with prior radiation therapy can often be managed using pericardiocentesis in combination with local or systemic chemotherapy and may therefore allow patients with end-stage disease to avoid the stress of major surgery. Certain situations make pericardiocentesis either more complicated or less likely to succeed. These include acute traumatic hemopericardium in which blood continues to enter the pericardial space rapidly, small pericardial effusions such as those that are solely posterior, the presence of clot and fibrin in the pericardial space, and the presence of a loculated effusion.

REFERENCE

1. Krikorian, J.G., and Hancock, E.W.: Pericardiocentesis. Am. J. Med. *65*:808, 1978.

430 A-T, B-F, C-F, D-T, E-T   (Braunwald, pp. 1483–1484; Table 43–3; Fig. 43–3)

Acute pericarditis is believed to cause an actual current of injury by a superficial myocardial or epicardial inflammatory process and leads to electrocardiographic changes that may be extremely useful in confirming the diagnosis. Four stages of abnormalities of the ST segments and T waves may be distinguished in classic acute pericarditis. The first stage of ECG changes is virtually diagnostic of acute pericarditis. This change includes ST-segment elevation, in which the segment is concave upward; this occurs in all leads except aV_r and V_1. In addition, the ST-segment axis usually varies between 30 and 60 degrees in acute pericarditis, in contrast to acute anterior MI, in which ST-segment axis varies from 100 to 120 degrees.[1] The T waves during this stage are usually upright. PR-segment depression occurs early in acute pericarditis in approximately 80 per cent of patients. The return of ST segments to baseline, accompanied by T-wave flattening, comprises stage II and usually is seen before the occurrence of T-wave inversion. This should be contrasted with the early evolution of T-wave changes in acute MI. The third electrocardiographic stage of acute pericarditis is characterized by inversion of the T waves, so that the T-wave vector is directed opposite to that of the ST segment. The fourth and final stage represents reversion of the T-wave changes to normal and may occur between weeks and months following the acute event.

While all four stages are detected in approximately half of patients with acute pericarditis, about 90 per cent of patients will demonstrate some electrocardiographic abnormalities that allow characterization of an acute chest pain episode as pericarditis, Stage I changes of pericarditis must be differentiated from normal early repolarization.[2] In this regard, an ST-segment/T-wave ratio >0.25 in lead V_6 has been noted to be more consistent with acute pericarditis while a ratio <0.25 is more suggestive of normal early repolarization.[3]

REFERENCES

1. Kouvaras, G., Soufras, G., Chronopoulos, G., et al.: The ST segment as a differential diagnostic feature between acute pericarditis and acute inferior myocardial infarction. Angiology *41*:207, 1990.

2. Wanner, W.R., Schaal, S.F., Bashore, T.M., et al.: Repolarization variant vs. acute pericarditis. A prospective electrocardiographic and echocardiographic evaluation. Chest *83*:180, 1983.

3. Ginzton, L.E., and Laks, M.M.: The differential diagnosis of acute pericarditis. Circulation *65*:1004, 1982.

431 A-T, B-T, C-F, D-T, E-F   (Braunwald, p. 1042; Fig. 32–32)

Although AS in adults has a long latent period some symptoms eventually develop, most commonly in the sixth decade of life. The most frequent symptoms consist of angina pectoris, syncope, and heart failure. When symptoms become manifested, prognosis for untreated AS is poor; survival curves show that the interval from the onset of symptoms to the time of death is approximately 5 years for patients with angina, 3 years in those with syncope, and 2 years in patients with heart failure.[1] Angina is present in approximately two-thirds of patients with critical AS and associated with coronary artery disease in approximately 50 per cent. In these patients angina may be due to associated coronary artery disease, but in general it is caused by a combination of increased oxygen needs of the hypertrophied myocardium and a reduction of oxygen delivery due to excessive compression of the coronary vessels during diastole.

Syncope is usually orthostatic and occurs most commonly following exertion. Most commonly it is due to reduced cerebral perfusion caused by systemic vasodilatation in the presence of a fixed cardiac output. Sudden death occurs with increased frequency in patients with critical AS and almost invariably in those who have been previously symptomatic. Asymptomatic patients frequently present during an episode of transient atrial fibrillation. Because of the decrease in diastolic compliance of the hypertrophied ventricle these patients are critically dependent upon the atrial contraction to deliver appropriate preload and to maintain cardiac output. Thus, when atrial fibrillation (AF) develops, patients may have impaired filling of the LV with a decrease in cardiac output and tolerate AF poorly. Also, an increased ventricular rate during AF further compromises diastolic filling of coronary arteries leading to impaired cardiac performance.

REFERENCE

1. Frank, S., Johnson, A., and Ross, J., Jr.: Natural history of valvular aortic stenosis. Br. Heart J. *35*:41, 1973.

432 A-T, B-T, C-F, D-F, E-F   (Braunwald, pp. 1329–1330)

Several randomized trials have been done to compare PTCA and CABG for treatment of patients with multivessel coronary disease. The Randomized Intervention Treatment of Angina (RITA) Study enrolled more than 1000 patients at cardiac centers in Great Britain between 1988 and 1991.[1]

Patients with poor MI or depressed left ventricular function were also included in the trial. This 5-year prospective study compared PTCA and CABG with the composite endpoint of death and nonfatal myocardial infarction. At the 2.5-year follow-up, no difference in the primary endpoint was found between the two treatment groups. Additionally, there was no difference in the primary endpoint among patients with one-, two-, or three-vessel disease regardless of treatment strategy. The RITA trial investigators thus concluded that both strategies resulted in similar exercise capacity and yielded a similar risk of death or nonfatal AMI during the early years of follow-up. However, the PTCA group in this study proved more likely to have angina, unstable angina, and repeated coronary angiograms.

The Emery University Angioplasty versus Surgery (EAST) Trial was a single-center trial of PTCA versus CABG.[2] The endpoint of the trial was a clinical composite adverse outcome that included death, Q-wave MI, or large ischemic thallium defect during the 3-year follow-up period. The mortality rate was 7.1 per cent among the PTCA group and 6.2 per cent among the CABG group, which was not statistically significant. Furthermore, as expected, in-hospital costs were markedly higher for the bypass surgery cohort ($26,130) compared with the PTCA cohort ($18,157), but the PTCA group underwent repeat interventions more often, and the overall costs for both groups at the 3-year point proved similar.

The Bypass Angioplasty Revascularization Investigation (BARI) trial is the largest of the randomized trials of PTCA and CABG. Though the 5-year survival favored CABG in 300 diabetic patients receiving therapy for diabetes, no significant difference in mortality was observed in the remaining 1500 patients for the two treatments.[3] Furthermore, in a recent metaanalysis of the randomized trials of CABG versus PTCA, a trend was demonstrated toward an overall adverse outcome after discharge in patients treated with PTCA.[4]

In conclusion, most studies comparing PTCA and CABG in multivessel disease have not demonstrated significant differences in mortality or in the rate of MI in treatment groups. Moreover, patients treated with PTCA have lower initial expenditures in these studies, but have more frequent revascularization and recurrence of angina in subsequent months which translates into similar overall expenditures for the two treatments.

REFERENCES

1. RITA Trial Participants: Coronary angioplasty versus coronary artery bypass surgery: The randomized intervention treatment of Angina (RITA) Trial. Lancet 241:573, 1993.
2. King, S.B., Lembo, N.J., and Weintraub, W.S.: A randomized trial comparing coronary angioplasty with coronary bypass surgery: Emory Angioplasty versus Surgery Trial (EAST). N. Engl. J. Med. 33:1044, 1994.
3. Sherman, D.L., and Ryan, T.J.: Coronary angioplasty versus bypass grafting. Cost-benefit considerations. Med. Clin. North Am. 79:1085, 1995.
4. Sim, I., Gupta, M., McDonald, K., et al.: A meta-analysis of randomized trials comparing coronary artery bypass grafting with percutaneous transluminal coronary angioplasty in multi-vessel coronary artery disease. Am. J. Cardiol. 76: 1025, 1995.

433 A-T, B-T, C-F, D-T, E-T (Braunwald, pp. 1414–1416)

Asymmetric septal hypertrophy most commonly refers to the presence of an abnormally thickened intraventricular septum compared with the left ventricular free wall, which is frequently familial and associated with disarray of ventricular septal myocardial fibers. However, echocardiographically, disproportionate septal hypertrophy may be documented in several other situations. In neonates and infants the predominance of the right ventricle relative to the left ventricle may result in the appearance of an enlarged ventricular septum.[1] This usually disappears by the age of 1 to 2 years. However, in individuals with other etiologies for right ventricular pressure overload, such as pulmonic stenosis or primary pulmonary hypertension, there may be persistent septal hypertrophy. Abnormal thickness of the septum relative to the free wall may also occur in coronary artery disease; for example, following infarction of the free wall there may be compensatory hypertrophy of the septum and inferior wall.[2] Other conditions that may present similar patterns of disproportionate septal hypertrophy include lentiginosis, Turner syndrome, hyper- and hypothyroidism, hyperparathyroidism, and Friedreich's ataxia.[1,3] Although beriberi may be associated with dilated cardiomyopathy, it is not associated with asymmetric septal hypertrophy.

REFERENCES

1. Larter, W.E., Allen, H.D., Sahn, D.J., and Goldberg, S.J.: The asymmetrically hypertrophied septum. Further differentiation of its causes. Circulation 53:19, 1976.
2. Maron, B.J., Savage, D.D., Clark, C.E., et al.: Prevalence and characteristics of disproportionate ventricular septal thickening of patients with coronary artery disease. Circulation 57:250, 1978.
3. Wilson, R., Gibson, T.C., Terrien, C.M., Jr., and Levy, A.M.: Hyperthyroidism and familial hypertrophic cardiomyopathy. Arch. Intern. Med. 143:378, 1983.

434 A-T, B-F, C-T, D-F (Braunwald, pp. 1539–1541)

Penetrating chest wounds, whether due to gunshots or stabbings, frequently involve damage to cardiac structures. All of these injuries are associated with significant bleeding into the pericardial space, as well as intramyocardial hemorrhage. Thus, posttraumatic pericarditis symptoms are common. Although these are not functionally limiting, they are nonetheless associated with a pericardial type of pain. Because the ventricles are larger than the atria, they are more commonly involved in penetrating wounds. However, survival is better with injuries to the ventricles than to the atria. Wounds involving thin-walled structures such as the atria and pulmonary artery rarely seal off spontaneously and therefore are associated with more bleeding and volume loss. Because of this acute complication, delay in performing a thoracotomy in patients with rapidly developing tamponade and excessive pericardial bleeding is ill-advised. A late complication of penetrating chest wounds is rupture of the interventricular septum, although frequently these defects are of minor hemodynamic significance. Laceration of the coronary artery is also a common occurrence with penetrating chest wounds, and because of its anterior location, the left coronary artery is most commonly involved. Following laceration of a coronary artery, myocardial infarction frequently develops even if rapid reanastomosis is performed.

435 A-F, B-F, C-T, D-T, E-F   (Braunwald, p. 1246)

In the past, VPBs, R-on-T phenomena, and repetitive VPB patterns are all thought to be warning arrhythmias. However, more recent data suggest that these findings occur in many patients who do not develop ventricular fibrillation, while ventricular fibrillation may develop in 40 to 83 per cent of patients without any warning arrhythmia.[1,2] This poor correlation between VPBs and ventricular fibrillation may in part explain the lack of a reduction in mortality in antiarrhythmic therapy trials of VPBs in the setting of AMI.[2] Recent data suggest that routine prophylactic lidocaine, which has been commonly used to treat warning arrhythmias in the presence of AMI can no longer be recommended.[2,3] Lidocaine is appropriate therapy for patients in whom sustained or symptomatic ventricular arrhythmias emerge. In patients for whom lidocaine is unsuccessful, or when lidocaine is contraindicated for other reasons, procainamide is an appropriate second choice. Interestingly, this drug appears to be effective at a lower dose in AMI patients than in patients with chronic heart disease, probably because of an increased sensitivity of myocardial tissue to the drug.[4]

The Cardiac Arrhythmia Suppression Trial (CAST) studied the drugs flecainide, encainide, and moricizine in AMI patients who were asymptomatic or mildly symptomatic and had documented frequent or repetitive VPBs. The trial was initiated because of the identified relationship between frequent and repetitive VPBs and sudden cardiac death in AMI after hospital discharge. This trial was terminated prematurely because of the marked increase in sudden cardiac death or arrest in the treatment group.[5]

REFERENCES

1. Lee, K.J., Wellens, H.J.J., Dorsnar, E., and Durrer, D.: Observations on patients with primary ventricular fibrillation complicating acute myocardial infarction. Circulation 52: 755, 1973.
2. Wyse, D.G., Kellen, J., and Rademaker, A.W.: Prophylactic versus selective lidocaine for early ventricular arrhythmias of myocardial infarction. J. Am. Coll. Cardiol. 12: 507, 1988.
3. Hine, L.K., Laird, N., Hewitt, P., and Chalmers, T.C.: Meta-analytic evidence against prophylactic use of lidocaine in acute myocardial infarction. Arch. Intern. Med. 149:2694, 1989.
4. Kessler, K.M., Kayden, D.S., Estes, S.M., et al.: Procainamide pharmacokinetics in patients with acute myocardial infarction or congestive heart failure. J. Am. Coll. Cardiol. 7:1131, 1986.
5. The Cardiac Arrhythmia Suppression Trial (CAST) Investigators: Preliminary report: Effect on encainide and flecainide on mortality in a randomized trial of arrhythmia suppression after myocardial infarction. N. Engl. J. Med. 321:405, 1989.

436 A-T, B-F, C-T, D-F, E-F   (Braunwald, p. 1302)

Nitrates are important agents for treatment of ischemic heart disease. They directly relax vascular smooth muscle by activating intracellular guanylate cyclase and causing an increase in cyclic guanosine monophosphate, which triggers smooth muscle relaxation. It is also possible that nitrates may activate the vasodilator prostaglandin system (PGI_2). Nitrates act directly on smooth muscle and therefore do not require an intact endothelium. The vasodilating effect of nitrates is present in both arteries and veins but appears to predominate in the venous circulation. The decrease in venous tone lessens the return of blood to the heart and reduces preload and ventricular dimensions, which in turn diminishes wall tension. As well as decreasing wall tension and myocardial oxygen demand, nitrates also increase oxygen supply by dilating coronary arteries. This dilatation is also present in vessels containing atherosclerotic plaques, presumably because the pathological atherosclerotic changes are eccentric and normal vascular smooth muscle, which can respond to nitrates, is present in a portion of the plaque. Quantitation of the direct vasodilatory effect of nitrates on coronary vessels have been performed by intracoronary administration and a direct effect of varying magnitude has been universally demonstrated.

437 A-F, B-F, C-T, D-F, E-T   (Braunwald, pp. 1097–1099; Table 33–15)

Patients at risk for endocarditis include those with congenital heart disease (both before and after operation), with mitral valve prolapse and significant mitral regurgitation, with rheumatic valvular heart disease and other acquired forms of valvular disease, with hypertrophic obstruction cardiomyopathy, with a history of infective endocarditis, with transvenous pacemakers, with ventriculoatrial shunts for hydrocephalus, and renal dialysis patients with shunts. Patients at particularly high risk are those with prosthetic valves, conduits, patches, and surgically created shunts. Patients who ordinarily do *not* require prophylaxis are those with isolated ostium secundum ASD, patients more than 6 months after repair of such a defect without a patch, patients more than 6 months after ligation of a patent ductus arteriosus, and patients following coronary artery bypass surgery.

The prophylactic antibiotic regimen is determined by the organisms likely to be encountered and also by the potential risk. Thus, patients with prosthetic valves, conduits, patches, and shunts are at much higher risk and should receive an intravenous antibiotic regimen whenever possible.[1]

REFERENCE

1. Dajani, A.S., Bisno, A.L., Chung, K.J., et al.: Prevention of bacterial endocarditis. JAMA 264:2919, 1990.

438 A-T, B-T, C-F, D-F, E-T *(Braunwald, pp. 1333–1335; Fig. 38–22)*

The findings at cardiac catheterization in patients with unstable angina vary, in part depending upon whether coronary disease has been identified previously. For example, patients with new-onset unstable angina and no prior history of angina or myocardial infarction have a higher incidence of single-vessel disease than those with a prior history of angina (43 per cent versus 27 per cent). Similarly, patients with new-onset unstable symptoms have a lower incidence of three-vessel disease (23 per cent versus 35 per cent).[1] The LAD coronary artery is the most commonly affected vessel in patients with stable or unstable angina. Autopsy studies confirm that patients with unstable angina have more severe and extensive coronary artery disease than patients with chronic stable angina. In addition, postmortem angiography and coronary arteriography both demonstrate specific lesion morphologies characteristic of unstable angina.[2] Thus, eccentric stenoses with scalloped or overhanging edges occur more commonly in unstable angina, while stenoses with concentric or symmetric narrowing and smooth borders are more common in patients with chronic stable angina.

Fissuring of an underlying atherosclerotic plaque is one mechanism by which acute coronary syndromes are precipitated.[3] Atherosclerotic plaques with an eccentrically situated lipid pool covered by a cap of fibrous tissue and endothelium seem most susceptible to fissuring events. Such episodes presumably predispose to the development of an occlusive thrombus, which are identified in many patients with unstable angina.[3] Intracoronary thrombi have been documented in up to three-quarters of patients who have persistent angina following their admission.[4]

REFERENCES

1. Roberts, K.B., Califf, R.M., Harrell, F.E., Jr., et al.: The prognosis for patients with new-onset angina who have undergone cardiac catheterization. Circulation 68:970, 1983.

2. Fuster, V., Stein, B., Ambrose, J.A., et al.: Atherosclerotic plaque rupture and thrombosis. Evolving concepts. Circulation 82(Suppl. II):47, 1990.
3. Davies, M.J., and Thomas, A.C.: Plaque fissuring—the cause of acute myocardial infarction, sudden ischemic death, and crescendo angina. Br. Heart J. 53:363, 1985.
4. Freeman, M.R., Williams, A.E., Chisholm, R.J., and Armstrong, P.W.: Intracoronary thrombus and complex morphology in unstable angina. Relation to timing of angiography and in-hospital cardiac events. Circulation 80:17, 1989.

439 A-F, B-T, C-T, D-F, E-F *(Braunwald, pp. 1420–1421)*

In patients with hypertrophic cardiomyopathy (HCM) the physical examination may be quite variable. However, the apical precordial impulse is usually abnormally prominent. Because of decreased diastolic compliance, a prominent presystolic apical impulse is frequently felt, which correlates with the presence of a prominent *a* wave in the jugular venous pulse. A characteristic but less frequently recognized abnormality is a triple apical impulse, the third impulse being a late systolic bulge associated with end-systolic contraction. A systolic murmur along the lower left sternal border is frequently present. The murmur of mitral regurgitation in association with systolic anterior motion of the mitral valve is also common. However, the murmur of aortic regurgitation is very rare without coexisting aortic valve disease or following an episode of infective endocarditis. An S_3 is frequently audible because HCM patients are usually young and because there is rapid ventricular filling.

It is important to emphasize the features of physical examination that permit differentiation of HCM from fixed aortic valve disease. The character of the carotid pulse is the most useful feature in this regard.[1] In aortic stenosis there is obstruction to left ventricular emptying from the beginning of systole, causing the carotid upstroke to be slowed and of low amplitude (pulsus parvus et tardus). With HCM, however, initial ejection of blood from the left ventricle is unimpeded and in fact is more robust than usual. Therefore, the arterial upstroke initially is brisk, followed by a more sustained plateau, giving rise to the classic "spike-and-dome" configuration.

REFERENCE

1. Maron, B.J., Wolfson, J.K., Ciro, E., and Spirito, P.: Relation of electrocardiographic abnormalities and patterns of left ventricular hypertrophy identified by two-dimensional echocardiography in patients with hypertropic cardiomyopathy. Am. J. Cardiol. 51:189, 1983.

440 A-T, B-T, C-F, D-T, E-F *(Braunwald, pp. 1213–1215)*

Among the various mechanisms potentially responsible for tissue damage following ischemia and reperfusion are oxygen-derived free radicals. Under normal conditions, oxygen free radicals are not normally found in the cell in significant concentrations. These molecules are characterized by an odd number of electrons, which makes them chemically reactive. There are three principal oxygen radicals: the superoxide anion ($\cdot O_2^-$), hydrogen peroxide (H_2O_2), and the hydroxyl radical ($\cdot OH$). During severe ischemia, several mechanisms appear to increase the production of oxygen radicals: dissociation of intramitochondrial electron transport, ischemia-induced calcium influx activating arachidonic acid metabolism, ischemia converting the normal myocardial enzyme xanthine dehydrogenase to xanthine oxidase (which in the presence of xanthine produces oxygen radicals), and activation of complement with accumulation of neutrophils, which release oxygen radicals.[1,2]

These radicals damage cell membranes by a variety of mechanisms, impair cell enzymes, and contribute to cell death. The superoxide anion can be dismutated to hydrogen peroxide by the superoxide dismutase enzymes. Hydrogen peroxide then may be converted via catalase and other perioxidases to O_2 and thereby deactivated. However, the superoxide anion can also, in the presence of iron, be converted to the hydroxyl radical, which is a potent oxidizing species. Thus, interventions directed at preventing oxygen-derived free radical injury have focused on administration of superoxide dismutase to convert these radicals to hydrogen peroxide followed by antioxidant treatment to convert the H_2O_2 to oxygen. Furthermore, administration of xanthine oxidase inhibitors to prevent this enzyme's action has been suggested. Finally, limiting iron availability and iron-containing enzyme availability to convert the superoxide anion to the hydroxyl radical has also been suggested. Currently, several clinical trials are under way to investigate the efficacy of these measures to limit oxygen free radicals in terms of myocardial protection during reperfusion.

REFERENCES

1. Hammond, B., and Hess, M.L.: The oxygen free radical system: Potential mediator of myocardial injury. J. Am. Coll. Cardiol. 6:215, 1985.
2. Rossen, R.D., Swain, J.L., Michael, L.H., et al.: Selective accumulation of the first component of complement and leukocytes in ischemic canine heart muscle. Circ. Res. 57:119, 1985.

441 A-F, B-T, C-F, D-T, E-T   (Braunwald, p. 1314; Fig. 38–6)

Several studies have addressed recently the use of PTCA or thrombolytic therapy in the setting of chronic stable angina. The Veterans Affairs ACME Trial was the first completed randomized study comparing PTCA with medical therapy in patients with stable angina.[1] In this trial, a total of 212 patients with single-vessel disease and exercise-induced ischemia were enrolled. During the 6-month follow-up period, no between-group differences were demonstrated in the frequency of cardiac death or MI, though patients treated with PTCA had a better exercise capacity and less angina during the study. In another recent randomized trial of PTCA, medical therapy, and CABG in patients with proximal LAD disease, there was no difference in the combined endpoint of cardiac death, MI, or refractory angina requiring revascularization between PTCA and medical therapy.[2] CABG, however, proved superior to PTCA and medical therapy in this study. The recent advent of coronary stenting, which has a lower rate of restenosis than PTCA, has not yet been compared to the other treatment options in a randomized trial.

The Duke University database, which includes more than 9000 patients referred for catheterization between 1984 and 1990, provides important survival data in patients with CAD.[3] The adjusted 5-year survival for patients with single-vessel disease in the Duke experience is similar for patients treated with either PTCA or medical therapy (95 per cent PTCA versus 94 per cent medical therapy); in patients with two-vessel diseases, 5-year survival was 91 per cent versus 86 per cent, respectively; and in patients with three-vessel disease, survival was 81 per cent versus 72 per cent. These observations suggest that PTCA may be superior to medical therapy in patients with multivessel disease.

The results of PTCA in patients with left ventricular dysfunction had been disappointing. Several studies of PTCA in such patients have reported a high initial success rate. However, long-term results have proven less favorable. In one study, the 2-year survival among patients treated with PTCA with an ejection fraction <0.40 and multivessel disease was only 75 per cent.[4] Data from the National Heart, Lung and Blood Institute registry show a 4-year survival in patients with ejection fractions <0.25 of only 45 per cent.[5] It is believed that the failure of multivessel PTCA to achieve complete revascularization accounts for such poor outcomes.[6] However, in patients with borderline left ventricular dysfunction and milder degrees of ischemia, PTCA may provide adequate revascularization whether or not it is anatomically complete.[7]

REFERENCES

1. Parisi, A.F., Folland, E.D., Hartigan, P., for the Veterans Affairs ACME Investigators: A comparison of angioplasty with medical therapy and the treatment of single vessel artery disease. N. Engl. J. Med. 326:10, 1992.
2. Heub, W.A., Bellotti, G., Almeida, S., et al.: The Medicine, Angioplasty or Surgery Study (MASS). A prospective randomized trial of medical therapy, balloon angioplasty or bypass surgery for single proximal left anterior descending artery stenosis. J. Am. Coll. Cardiol. 26:1600, 1995.
3. Mark, D.B., Nelson, C.L., Califf, R.M., et al.: Continuing evaluation of therapy for coronary artery disease: Initial results from the era of coronary angioplasty. Circulation 89:2015, 1994.
4. Ellis, S.G., Cowley, M.J., DiSciascio, G., et al.: Determinants of two-year outcome after coronary angioplasty in patients

with multivessel disease on the basis of comprehensive preprocedural evaluation: Implications for patient selection. Circulation 83:1905, 1991.
5. Holmes, D.R., Jr., Detre, K.M., Williams, D.O., et al.: Long-term outcome of patients with depressed left ventricular function undergoing percutaneous transluminal coronary angioplasty. The NHLBI PTCA Registry. Circulation 87:21, 1993.
6. Serota, H., Deligonul, U., Lee, W.-H., et al.: Predictors of cardiac survival after PTCA in patients with severe left ventricular dysfunction. Am. J. Cardiol. 26:931, 1995.
7. Gersh, B.J.: Coronary revascularization in the 1990s. A Cardiologist's perspective. Can. J. Cardiol. 10:661, 1994.

442 A-T, B-F, C-T, D-T, E-F (Braunwald, pp. 1319–1320)

The frequency of perioperative complications has increased in recent years because of the increasing percentage of high-risk patients who are currently undergoing operation.[1] MI occurs in 2 to 5 per cent of elective revascularization procedures.[2] While a perioperative MI leads to a higher mortality rate, most infarcts in this setting are small and may be managed successfully. Patients commonly show some impairment of cognitive function in the perioperative period. This phenomenon does *not* suggest that a stroke has occurred, and requires that the physician reassure the patient and family of its generally transient nature.[3] While the mechanisms are not well understood, hypertension occurs in up to one-third of patients following coronary artery surgery. It is important that this complication be adequately controlled to prevent increased myocardial oxygen demand. The presence of new fascicular conduction defects in the postoperative patient is a general sign of diffuse myocardial disease and heralds a worse prognosis. The cause of death in this setting is usually left ventricular failure or ventricular arrhythmia. Obesity predisposes to a number of postoperative complications, including sternotomy dehiscence, impaired leg wound healing, hypertension, and bronchoconstriction.[4] However, obesity does not appear to independently increase operative mortality.

REFERENCES

1. Christakis, G.T., Ivanov, J., Weisel, R.D., et al.: The changing pattern of coronary artery bypass surgery. Circulation 80(Suppl. I):151, 1989.
2. Daily, P.O.: Early and 5-year results for coronary artery bypass grafting. A benchmark for percutaneous transluminal coronary angioplasty. J. Thorac. Cardiovasc. Surg. 96:67, 1989.
3. Shaw, P.J., Bates, D., Cartlidge, N.E.F., et al.: Early intellectual dysfunction following coronary bypass surgery. Q.J. Med. 58:59, 1986.
4. Koshal, A., Hendry, P., Roman, S.V., and Keon, W.J.: Should obese patients not undergo coronary artery surgery? Can. J. Surg. 28:331, 1985.

443 A-T, B-T, C-T, D-F (Braunwald, pp. 1213–1215)

During reperfusion of ischemic myocardium, significant additional myocardial injury occurs due to a variety of mechanisms. Myocytes that appear to be ischemic upon reperfusion often suddenly develop ultrastructural changes of irreversible cell death, including explosive cell swelling and widespread architectural disruption, as if an acceleration of normal ischemic damage were occurring. It appears that reperfusion predominantly accelerates necrosis of irreversibly injured myocardium,[1] although during reperfusion there is significant cell swelling with resulting vascular compression. This may damage some reversibly injured cells.

Two mechanisms are thought to be responsible for reperfusion-induced injury. The reintroduction of oxygen to ischemic cells causes formation of oxygen-derived free radicals. These radicals disrupt cell membranes, impair enzyme function, and may result in cellular calcium overload. The increase in cell calcium then impairs mitochondrial function, disabling energy production and resulting in loss of cell integrity. Thus interventions directed at preventing formation of oxygen free radicals may be helpful in preventing reperfusion injury.

Because of the microvascular damage present in severely ischemic myocardium, hemorrhage is likely to occur upon reperfusion. Some areas of the myocardium are so severely ischemic that there is an absence of reflow, termed the "no-reflow phenomenon." These areas appear to result from ischemia-induced microvascular damage and myocardial contracture of such severity as to be nonreperfusable. However, the no-flow phenomenon does not appear to enhance myocyte death, because the zone of reflow is always contained within areas in which myocytes are already necrotic at the time of onset of reperfusion.[2]

REFERENCES

1. Jennings, R.B., Sommers, H.M., Smyth, G.A., et al.: Myocardial necrosis induced by temporary occlusion of a coronary artery in the dog. Arch. Pathol. 70:68, 1960.
2. Braunwald, E., and Kloner, R.A.: Myocardial reperfusion: A double-edged sword? J. Clin. Invest. 76:1713, 1985.

444 A-F, B-T, C-T, D-F, E-T (Braunwald, p. 1319)

A steady improvement in operative mortality for the CABG procedure has been documented in recent years, despite the fact that the operative population includes a larger percentage of patients with poor ventricular function, comorbid disease, or advanced age.[1] Even in patients with significant impairment of ventricular function, excellent operative results have been attained in the past decade.[2] It is clear that patients with small stature have an operative mortality that is significantly increased and often have less than complete relief of angina. This is probably secondary to their smaller cardiac and coronary artery size. While operative mortalities as low as 0.2 per cent have been reported, multiinstitutional results have demonstrated hospital death rates of 6.5 per cent for community hospitals and 2.1 to 3.7 per cent death rates in university hospitals.[3]

The use of IMA grafts has been associated with both reduced long-term mortality and reduced in-hospital mortality (see Braunwald, Fig. 38–13, p. 1318). Improvement in anesthetic techniques, as well as myocardial preservation, conduit selection and preservation, blood banking methods, hemodynamic monitoring, arrhythmia control, and intraaortic balloon assistance, have all contributed to the improved operative mortalities reported. Patients with poor left ventricular function, intractable ischemia, or cardiogenic shock are specific candidates for intraaortic balloon pumping, which may decrease operative mortality in these high-risk groups.

REFERENCES

1. Califf, R.M., Harrell, F.E., Lee, K.L., et al.: The evolution of medical and surgical therapy for coronary artery disease. A 15-year perspective. JAMA *261*:2077, 1989.
2. Bounous, E.P., Mark, D.B., Pollack, B.G., et al.: Surgical survival benefits for coronary disease patients with left ventricular dysfunction. Circulation *778*(Suppl. I):151, 1988.
3. Kirklin, J.W., Naftel, D.C., Blackstone, E.H., and Pohost, G.M.: Summary of a consensus concerning death and ischemic events after coronary artery bypass grafting. Circulation *79*(Suppl. I):81, 1989.
4. Bolooki, H.: Emergency cardiac procedures in patients in cardiogenic shock due to complications of coronary artery disease. Circulation *79*(Suppl. I):137, 1989.

445 A-T, B-T, C-T, D-F, E-T   *(Braunwald, pp. 1012; 1024–1025)*

Doppler echocardiography is the usual noninvasive procedure for quantitating and assessing the presence of both stenotic and regurgitant lesions of cardiac valves. Figure *A* is an example of a continuous-wave Doppler echocardiogram in combined mitral stenosis (MS) and mitral regurgitation (MR). In Figure *B*, pulsed wave Doppler measurement of normal mitral valve flow is displayed. Diastolic flow toward the transducer (above the baseline) is present; an early diastolic peak and an end-diastolic peak resulting in "M" configurations similar to the mitral valve pattern on M-mode echocardiography may be noted. Normally, no systolic flow signals are detected on Doppler examination of the mitral valve. The mitral valve peak diastolic velocity normally is <1.3 m/sec. MS results in high diastolic velocity (usually >1.5 m/sec). The difference in diastolic pressure between the LA and LV is increased and the rapidity of LA emptying is reduced in patients with mitral stenosis, as shown in *A*. This reduced rate of pressure equalization appears as a slower decline of the velocity signals during diastole.

The diagnosis of MR by pulsed wave Doppler examination consists of the detection of systolic turbulence when the probe samples the LA. In the example shown in Figure *A*, it can be seen that there is a high-velocity signal moving away from the transducer as indicated by the signal below the baseline with a velocity of 4.4 m/sec. Doppler echocardiography is quite sensitive for detecting MR that is due to rheumatic deformity, which causes thickening and calcification of the edges of the valve leaflets and a wide regurgitant jet directed to the left atrium parallel to the long axis of the heart. In contrast, the regurgitation signals of mitral valve prolapse, papillary muscle dysfunction, or prosthetic valve dysfunction are more difficult to detect, since these lesions cause small localized jets that "hug" the left atrial wall. Color-flow imaging may be more successful in detecting these forms of MR.

Assessment of MR by echocardiography is at best semiquantitative. The systolic jet of mild MR is detected only immediately above the mitral valve leaflet. As MR becomes more severe the turbulence becomes greater in the LA and can be detected further back in the LA. It should be noted that because the pressure gradient between the LV and LA in systole is much greater than between the LA and LV in diastole, signals produced by MR occur at a much higher flow velocity than those produced by MS.

446 A-T, B-T, C-T, D-F   *(Braunwald, pp. 1088–1089)*

Two-dimensional echocardiography has had considerable success in demonstrating the presence of vegetations during endocarditis. Factors important for the detection of valvular vegetations include the size of the lesion (3 mm or larger), its location, duration of the disease (vegetations are usually not seen before 2 weeks of the disease), the presence of abscess of the myocardium or valvular ring, and aneurysm of the sinus of Valsalva. Echocardiography is also useful in identifying rupture of the ventricular septum, flail leaflets, and fluttering of the mitral valve during diastole. Doppler echocardiography is of particular value in detecting early valvular regurgitation and assessing its severity. The ability of echocardiography to demonstrate vegetations is related primarily to the size of the lesions. Recent studies strongly suggest that transesophageal echocardiography (TEE) has an improved sensitivity for the diagnosis of smaller vegetations.[1,2] Fungal endocarditis is much more likely to yield echocardiographically visible vegetations than is bacterial endocarditis. In endocarditis caused by the less virulent organisms—especially *Streptococcus viridans*—vegetations documented by echocardiography are quite rare. Although it is typical for successful therapy to result in a decrease in the size of a vegetation, therapy may be associated with an increase or no change in the size of vegetations. In fact, in right-sided endocarditis it is not uncommon for vegetations to persist for years following curative therapy.[3]

REFERENCES

1. Mugge, A., Daniel, W.G., Frank, G., et al.: Echocardiography in infective endocarditis: Reassessment of prognostic im-

plications of vegetation size determined by the transthoracic and the transesophageal approach. J. Am. Coll. Cardiol. 14:631, 1989.

2. Steckelberg, J.M., Murphy, J.G., Ballard, D., et al.: Emboli in infective endocarditis: The prognostic value of echocardiography. Ann. Intern. Med. 114:635, 1991.

3. Neimann, J.L., Fischer, M., Kownator, S., and Faivre, G.: Echocardiographic follow-up of vegetations in infectious endocarditis. Arch. Mal. Coeur Vaiss 75:1329, 1982.

447 A-T, B-T, C-T, D-T   (Braunwald, pp. 934–935)

Clinical manifestations of Ebstein's anomaly of the tricuspid valve are variable because the spectrum of pathology varies widely and because of variations in the presence of associated malformations. The most common important associated cardiac defect is pulmonic stenosis or atresia. In addition, ostium primum atrial septal defect, ventricular septal defect, and physiologically corrected transposition of the great arteries all sometimes accompany Ebstein's anomaly.

The usual clinical manifestations of Ebstein's anomaly in infancy are cyanosis, a cardiac murmur, and congestive heart failure. However, beyond infancy the onset of symptoms tend to be exertional dyspnea and fatigue as well as cyanosis. Approximately one-fourth of patients suffer episodes of paroxysmal supraventricular tachycardia. Evidence of tricuspid regurgitation and wide splitting of the first and second heart sounds are characteristic features of the cardiac examination. Electrocardiographic abnormalities in Ebstein's anomaly may include right bundle branch block and the Wolff-Parkinson-White (WPW) syndrome. The latter case is usually type B WPW, with a left bundle branch block pattern and predominant S waves in the right precordial leads. The risk of paroxysmal supraventricular tachycardia appears to be increased in patients with the WPW pattern on the ECGs.[1] In addition, the ECG may show giant P waves, a prolonged P-R interval, and a prolonged terminal QRS depolarization with variable degrees of right bundle branch block.

Radiographic studies usually demonstrate right atrial enlargement in the presence of a small right ventricle. M-mode echocardiography demonstrates increased right ventricular dimensions, paradoxical ventricular septal motion, and an increase in tricuspid valve excursion. These findings may be seen in other forms of right ventricular overload. However, more specific findings for Epstein's anomaly include a delay in tricuspid valve closure relative to mitral closure and a decrease in the E-F slope of the tricuspid valve, an abnormal anterior position of the tricuspid valve during diastole, and tricuspid valve echoes detected when the transducer is placed laterally. Leftward and inferior displacement of the tricuspid valve and its abnormal position in relation to the mitral valve may be demonstrated by two-dimensional echocardiography (see Braunwald, Fig. 29–57, p. 935). Doppler examination may detect the presence of tricuspid regurgitation.

At cardiac catheterization an intracavitary ECG recorded proximal to the tricuspid valve shows a right ventricular type of complex, while the pressure recorded is that of the right atrium, demonstrating the presence of an "atrialized" portion of the right ventricular. It is common for significant arrhythmias to occur during catheterization, since the heart is unusually irritable in this condition. Selective right ventricular angiography may show the position of the displaced tricuspid valve, the size of the right ventricle, and the configuration of the outflow portion of the right ventricle, further confirming the diagnosis.

REFERENCE

1. Kastor, J.A., Goldreier, B.N., Josephson, M.E., et al.: Electrophyiologic characteristics of Ebstein's anomaly of the tricuspid valve. Circulation 52:987, 1975.

448 A-F, B-F, C-T, D-F, E-T   (Braunwald, p. 1315)

Despite the advancement and rapid improvement of PTCA, restenosis continues to be a major limiting factor for the long-term success of the procedure. Additionally, restenosis leads to adverse economic outcomes due to the need for repeat hospitalizations and repeat interventions. The most widely used definition for restenosis is a >50 per cent vessel diameter stenosis and/or >50 per cent late loss of the acute luminal gain.[1,2] The incidence of restenosis in most studies is 30 to 40 per cent depending on certain clinical anatomical variables, and usually occurs within 6 months of the procedure.

The pathogenesis of restenosis is not completely understood and appears to be multifunctional. Based on pathological examination of restenosed arteries, restenosis is believed to be due to neointimal thickening due in part to proliferation and migration of smooth muscle cells. The elastic properties of the vessel undergoing angioplasty also contribute to restenosis, since elastic recoil following PTCA reduces the immediate acute gain achieved. However, with the recent advent of stenting, the elastic recoil phenomenon has become less of a problem and maintenance of the immediate gain has proven more feasible.

Clinical variables that are associated with an increased incidence of restenosis include diabetes, male gender, smoking, and hemodialysis.[2] Anatomical variables that promote restenosis include total occlusion, left anterior descending coronary artery location, saphenous vein grafts, multivessel disease, and long lesions.[3] Procedural variables contributing to restenosis include greater residual stenosis left following PTCA, undersizing of PTCA, balloon for the reference artery, and severe intimal dissections.

REFERENCES

1. Kuntz, R.E., and Baim, D.: Defining coronary restenosis. Circulation *88*:1310, 1993.
2. Weintraub, W.S., Kosinski, A.S., Brown, C.L., and King, S.B.: Can restenosis after coronary angioplasty be predicted from clinical variables? J. Am. Coll. Cardiol. *21*:6, 1993.
3. LeFeuvre, C., Bonan, R., Lesperance, J., et al.: Predictor factors of restenosis after multivessel percutaneous transluminal coronary angioplasty. J. Am. Coll. Cardiol. *73*:840, 1994.

449 A-F, B-T, C-F, D-T   *(Braunwald, pp. 1168–1169)*

The clinical history presented is consistent with myocardial ischemia, most likely involving the right coronary artery and the inferior wall. The sudden decrease in chest discomfort associated with reductions in heart rate and blood pressure are consistent with coronary artery reperfusion. In this case it appeared that reperfusion caused activation of the Bezold-Jarisch reflex, which is a reflex that leads to bradycardia and hypotension.[1] The afferent limb of this reflex involves the vagus nerves and its efferent limb, coronary parasympathetic components. A similar phenomenon can be demonstrated experimentally by intracoronary injection of veratrum alkaloids as well as other metabolically active substances documenting the direct reflex arc from the coronary artery itself.

The term Anrep effect, also called "homeometric autoregulation," is applied to a positive inotropic effect following abrupt elevation of systolic aortic and left ventricular pressures. This effect occurs during the first minutes after aortic pressure is abruptly elevated, with the end-diastolic pressure then tending to fall as stroke volume and stroke work recover. Homeometric autoregulation is most marked in the anesthetized state. A variety of observations support the concept that the phenomenon is related, at least in part, to recovery from transient subendocardial ischemia. Thus, the Anrep effect would have been associated with an increase rather than a reduction in systolic pressure. A ruptured abdominal viscus would not be associated with a sudden decrease in chest pain.

REFERENCE

1. Jarisch, A., and Zotterman, Y.: Depressor reflexes from the heart. Acta Physiol. Scand. *16*:31, 1948.

450 A-T, B-F, C-T, D-F   *(Braunwald, pp. 1432–1433)*

Löeffler's endocarditis is a cardiac syndrome associated with eosinophilia, occurring in temperate climates. The typical patient with Löeffler's endocarditis is a male in his 40's who has had persistent eosinophilia with >1500 eosinophils/mm^3 for at least 6 months, with evidence of organ involvement.[1] Cardiac involvement is seen in approximately 75 per cent of patients with hypereosinophilia. The combination of hypereosinophilia and cardiac involvement is also part of the Churg-Strauss syndrome, which can be differentiated by the coexisting presence of asthma, nasal polyposis, and necrotizing vasculitis.

The pathology of Löeffler's endocarditis involves biventricular mural endocardial thickening with histological findings demonstrating an acute inflammatory eosinophilic myocarditis, thrombosis, fibrinoid change and inflammation of intramural coronary vessels, mural thrombosis, and fibrotic thickening. Clinically, patients have weight loss, fever, cough, skin rash, and congestive heart failure. Cardiomegaly is present early in the course, even in the absence of congestive heart failure, and the murmur of mitral regurgitation is common. Systemic embolism is frequent and may lead to neurological and renal dysfunction. Laboratory examination is remarkable for an elevated erythrocyte sedimentation rate and an increased eosinophil count. The echocardiogram frequently demonstrates localized thickening of the posterobasal LV wall with absent or remarkably limited motion of the posterior leaflet of the mitral valve. The hemodynamic consequences of the dense endocardial scarring are those of a restrictive cardiomyopathy with abnormal diastolic filling leading to a restrictive picture with "square root sign." A characteristic feature is the presence of largely preserved systolic function, with near-obliteration of the apex of the ventricles when studied angiographically. Medical treatment of Löeffler's endocarditis is moderately effective, with administration of both steroids and hydroxyurea improving survival substantially.

REFERENCE

1. Olsen, E.G., and Spry, C.J.: Relation between eosinophilia and endomyocardial disease. Prog. Cardiovasc. Dis. *27*: 241, 1985.

451 A-F, B-T, C-F, D-F, E-T   *(Braunwald, pp. 885–886)*

Cyanosis, which is defined as a bluish discoloration of skin and mucous membranes, is due to increased levels of reduced hemoglobin in excess of 3 gm/dl. Two forms of cyanosis are distinguished: peripheral and central cyanosis. Peripheral cyanosis is due to increased oxygen extraction from normally saturated arterial blood as a result of cutaneous vasoconstriction. Central cyanosis results from arterial blood desaturation and is most commonly seen in cyanotic heart disease in which systemic venous blood is shunted to the arterial circulation. Additionally, the amount of bluish discoloration in central cyanosis is dependent not only on the degree of arterial desaturation but also on the absolute amount of reduced hemoglobin and the oxyhemoglobin saturation of venous blood, which are in turn dependent on the extent of oxygen extraction from the tissues. Thus, cyanosis may appear or worsen with physical exertion due to decreased venous oxygen saturation and/or an increase in right-to-left shunting across a defect due primarily to a fall in the peripheral arterial resistance during exercise.

Differential cyanosis is characterized by the presence of normal oxygen saturation in the upper body and cyanosis in the lower part of the body, and is due usually to the presence of aortic coarctation and right-to-left shunting by means of a patent ductus arteriosus. Patients with cyanotic heart disease often assume the squatting position to relieve shortness of breath. Squatting decreases cyanosis and improves arterial oxygen saturation by increasing the systemic arterial resistance and thereby reducing the degree of right-to-left shunt and also by pooling of desaturated venous blood in the lower extremities.[1] Hypoxic spells can be seen in patients with cyanotic heart disease, especially in young children with tetralogy of Fallot. The spells are characterized by anxiety, hyperpnea, and a sudden increase in cyanosis and are caused by an abrupt decrease in pulmonary blood flow due to a sudden fall in systemic resistance or increase in right ventricular outflow obstruction. Treatment consists of oxygen administration, placing the child in the knee-chest position, and administration of drugs that increase the peripheral resistance and hence decrease the amount of right-to-left shunting.

REFERENCE

1. Guntheroth, W.G., Morgan, B.C., and Mullens, G.L.: Physiologic studies of paroxysmal hyperpnea in cyanotic congenital heart disease. Circulation 31:70, 1965.

452 A-F, B-T, C-F, D-T   (Braunwald, pp. 1060–1061)

This woman with rheumatic heart disease presents an interesting problem. It is clear that she has mitral stenosis (MS) based on the opening snap, loud S_1, and holodiastolic rumbling murmur, but it is unclear what coexisting valvular disease she may have. Many patients with severe MS have an early blowing diastolic murmur along the left sternal border and a normal pulse pressure. In 90 per cent of these patients the murmur is due to aortic regurgitation (AR), and it is usually of little clinical importance. However, approximately 10 per cent of patients with MS have severe rheumatic AR. This can usually be recognized by the peripheral signs of AR such as widening pulse pressure, water hammer pulses, and signs of LV enlargement on x-ray and ECG.

In patients with multivalvular disease, a proximal valvular lesion often masks a distal lesion. Thus, significant AR may be missed in patients with severe MS. The widened pulse pressure in particular may be absent in the presence of severe MS. Furthermore, the Austin-Flint murmur may be

mistaken for the diastolic rumbling murmur of MS. These two murmurs may be distinguished at the bedside by means of amyl nitrate inhalation, which diminishes the Austin-Flint murmur but augments the murmur of MS. Isometric handgrip and squatting augment both the diastolic murmur of AR and the Austin-Flint murmur but have little effect on the diastolic rumbling murmur of MS. In this patient the responses to amyl nitrite and handgrip are consistent with the presence of an Austin-Flint murmur.

The fact that the ECG in the patient described shows evidence of left ventricular hypertrophy and left-axis deviation in addition to left atrial enlargement is inconsistent with simple MS and suggests either AR or aortic stenosis (AS). The presence of the murmur of AR makes the latter the more likely diagnosis. There is no evidence for tricuspid stenosis or mitral regurgitation.

Further evaluation to confirm the diagnosis would probably include echocardiography and cardiac catheterization. Diastolic fluttering of the anterior leaflet of the mitral valve is an important clue to the presence of AR. Furthermore, a two-dimensional Doppler echocardiographic examination would be helpful because the Doppler is relatively sensitive (>90 per cent detection) for AR.

Patients such as this woman are most effectively treated by combined aortic and mitral valve replacement. This is usually associated with a higher risk and poorer survival than replacement of one of these two valves.[1] Kirklin reported a 5-year survival rate of 70 per cent for double-valve replacement compared to 80 per cent for single-valve replacement.[2] In general, patients with more dilated ventricles, especially those with a combination of AR and MR, fared worse than those patients with the other combinations.

REFERENCES

1. Baxley, W.A., and Soto, B.: Hemodynamic evaluation of patients with combined mitral and aortic prosthesis. Am. J. Cardiol. 45:42, 1980.
2. Kirklin, J.W., and Barratt-Boyes, B.G.: Combined aortic and mitral valve disease with or without tricuspid valve disease. In Cardiac Surgery, New York, John Wiley and Sons, 1986, pp. 431–446.

453 A-F, B-T, C-F, D-T   (Braunwald, p. 1011)

The opening snap (OS) of the mitral valve is thought to be caused by a sudden tensing of the valve leaflets after the valve cusps have completed their opening excursion. The OS is usually heard in valves that have not become completely calcified and therefore is accompanied by an accentuated S_1. The mitral OS follows A_2 by 0.04 to 0.12 sec and the A_2-OS interval varies inversely with the left atrial pressure.[1] A short A_2-OS interval (<0.08 sec) is a reliable indicator of tight MS and usually signifies significant left atrial pressure elevation. However, the reverse is not the case, since a long A_2-OS interval may be present in significant MS. This may occur when the time interval between the actual opening of the mitral valve and the OS is prolonged due to valvular calcification.

The A_2-OS interval can be altered by various maneuvers. Specifically, differentiation of tricuspid stenosis (TS) from MS can be aided by the fact that both the diastolic murmur and the OS of TS are accentuated during inspiration and reduced during expiration, while little change or the opposite occurs in MS. Furthermore, sudden standing with the resultant decrease in venous return causes a lowering of left atrial pressure and therefore widens the A_2-OS interval.[2] This maneuver is particularly useful in distinguishing the A_2-OS from a split S_2, which narrows on standing. However, the most reliable maneuver is exercise. This causes the A_2-OS interval to narrow, particularly in moderate or severe MS as there is a rapid elevation of the left atrial pressure resulting in the OS moving toward A_2.

REFERENCES

1. Ebringer, R., Pitt, A., and Anderson, S.T.: Hemodynamic factors influencing opening snap interval in mitral stenosis. Br. Heart J. *32*:350, 1970.
2. Surawicz, B.: Effect of respiration and upright position on the interval between the two components of the second heart sound and that between the second sound and mitral opening snap. Circulation *16*:422, 1957.

454 A-F, B-T, C-F, D-T   *(Braunwald, pp. 1492–1493)*

Cardiac catheterization is the test of choice to establish hemodynamic importance of pericardial effusion and tamponade. A number of characteristic cardiac catheterization findings confirm the diagnosis of cardiac tamponade. Simultaneous recordings of intrapericardial and RA pressure tracings in tamponade reveal that they are virtually identical and track together; except in instances of low-pressure cardiac tamponade, both are elevated as well. The RA pressure tracing displays a prominent systolic *x* descent and a small or absent systolic *y* descent in cases of cardiac tamponade. RV diastolic pressures are equal to RA and intrapericardial pressures and do not display the characteristic dip-and-plateau configuration that is seen in constrictive pericarditis (see Braunwald, p. 1496). The systolic pressures demonstrated on RV and pulmonary artery tracings are the summed result of the pressure developed by the RV and the intrapericardial pressure and are therefore often moderately elevated in the range of 35 to 50 mm Hg. The pulmonary capillary wedge pressure and the LV diastolic pressure are also often elevated and are equal to intrapericardial, RA, and RV diastolic pressures when simultaneous recordings are performed. In patients with severe underlying LV dysfunction, LV diastolic pressure may exceed that of the equalized intrapericardial and RA pressures.[1]

REFERENCE

1. Reddy, P.S., Curtiss, E.I., O'Toole, J.D., and Shaver, J.A.: Cardiac tamponade: Hemodynamic observations in man. Circulation *58*:265, 1978.

455 A-F, B-T, C-F, D-T   *(Braunwald, p. 1442)*

Chagas' disease is caused by the protozoan *Trypanosoma cruzi*. The major cardiovascular findings are extensive myocarditis with congestive heart failure. Typically, the disease becomes evident 20 to 30 years after the initial infection. Chagas' disease is prevalent in Central and South America, where approximately 10 to 20 million people are infected.

The disease is characterized by three phases: acute, latent, and chronic. During the acute phase, the disease is transmitted to humans by the bite of a reduviid bug, commonly called the kissing bug. Following inoculation, protozoa multiply and migrate widely through the body, and then enter a latent phase. Interestingly, about 30 per cent of infected individuals develop findings of chronic Chagas' disease, but many individuals with high parasite burdens do not develop the disease. Furthermore, it is not unusual to be unable to detect parasites in patients dying of Chagas' disease, so that an autoimmune mechanism for cardiac dysfunction may be involved.

Classic findings at autopsy include evidence of cardiac parasympathetic denervation. There is usually cardiac enlargement with dilatation and hypertrophy of cardiac chambers. The left ventricular apex is often thin and bulging, resembling an aneurysm. Thrombus formation is frequent and may occupy much of the apex.

Clinically, chronic progressive heart failure, predominantly right sided, is the rule in advanced cases. There is usually severe cardiomegaly, with the most common ECG abnormalities being *right bundle branch block* and left anterior hemiblock. T-wave abnormalities and atrioventricular block are also seen with some frequency. Ventricular arrhythmias are a prominent feature of chronic Chagas' disease.

Diagnosis is made using a complement-fixation test (Machado-Guerreiro test). At this time, no clinically effective treatment is available, although immunoprophylaxis with a vaccine is hoped for in the near future.

456 A-T, B-T, C-T, D-F   *(Braunwald, pp. 1412–1413, 1877)*

The consumption of alcohol may result in myocardial damage by three mechanisms: most commonly a direct effect of alcohol or its metabolites; a nutritional effect, occasionally with thiamine deficiency leading to beriberi heart disease; and rarely, toxic effects due to additives in the alcoholic beverage, such as cobalt.[1–3] It has become clear that even in the presence of normal nutritional status, alcohol can cause significant cardiomyopathy.[3] Alcohol results in acute as well as chronic depression of myocardial contractility and may produce acute demonstrable cardiac dysfunction even in normal individuals. It appears that prior cigarette consumption and coexisting hypertension augment the cardiomyopathic effects of alcohol.

The mechanism of cardiac depression produced by alcohol remains unclear. In several studies, alcohol and its metabolite acetaldehyde have been shown to interfere with a number of myocardial cellular functions including transport and binding of calcium, mitochrondrial respiration, lipid metabolism, protein synthesis, and myofibrillar ATPase.[1] Alcohol also is associated with systemic electrolyte imbalances (*hypokalemia*, hypophosphatemia, and hypomagnesemia), which may also play a role in alcohol-induced damage.

The gross and microscopic pathological findings of alcohol cardiomyopathy are nonspecific and are similar to those observed in idiopathic dilated cardiomyopathy.

REFERENCES

1. Regan, T.J.: Alcoholic cardiomyopathy. Prog. Cardiovasc. Dis. *27*:141, 1984.
2. Regan, T.J.: Alcoholic cardiomyopathy. *In* Zipes, D.P., and Rowlands, D.J. (eds.): Progress in Cardiology. Philadelphia, Lea & Febiger, 1989, p. 129.
3. McCall, D.: Alcohol and the cardiovascular system. Curr. Probl. Cardiol. *12*:351, 1987.

457 A-T, B-T, C-T, D-F *(Braunwald, pp. 1253–1254)*

The ECG demonstrates atrial fibrillation with a moderately rapid ventricular response, a common arrhythmia that occurs in between 10 and 15 per cent of patients with AMI. This should be contrasted with atrial flutter, which is a far less common atrial arrhythmia associated with AMI and which occurs in only 1 to 3 per cent of patients in this setting. While atrial fibrillation in patients with AMI is usually transient and occurs more commonly in patients with LV failure, it is seen more frequently following anterior infarction and appears to be caused by left atrial ischemia in most cases.[1] Atrial fibrillation is more common during the first 24 hours following infarction than later. It is associated with an increased mortality, in part because it occurs more frequently with extensive anterior wall infarctions. The rapid ventricular response and loss of atrial contribution to ventricular filling both may lead to a significant reduction in cardiac output.

In patients who are hemodynamically stable, the use of digitalis or verapamil to slow ventricular response has proved useful. However, electrical cardioversion is the treatment of choice in patients with clinical and/or hemodynamic evidence of decompensation. The management of atrial fibrillation in patients with AMI is often complicated by recurrence, especially when left atrial dilatation due to LV failure is the inciting event.

REFERENCE

1. Hod, H., Lew, A.S., Keltai, M., et al.: Early atrial fibrillation during evolving myocardial infarction: A consequence of impaired left atrial perfusion. Circulation *75*:146, 1987.

458 A-T, B-F, C-T, D-F, E-T *(Braunwald, pp. 904–906)*

In the majority of preterm infants under 1500 gm of birth weight, PDA persists for a prolonged period of time, and in approximately one-third of these infants a large shunt leads to significant cardiopulmonary deterioration.[1] Noninvasive evaluation may reveal evidence of significant right-to-left shunting before the appearance of physical findings suggesting ductal patency. Physical examination may reveal bounding peripheral pulses, an infraclavicular and interscapular systolic murmur (which occasionally is heard as a continuous murmur), a hyperactive precordium, hepatomegaly, and recurrent episodes of apnea and bradycardia with or without respirator dependency. On chest x-ray an increase in the cardiothoracic ratio is seen on sequential radiographs and may be accompanied by increased pulmonary arterial markings, perihilar edema, and ultimately generalized pulmonary edema. Echocardiography may demonstrate increases in LV end-distolic and LA dimensions. Cardiac catheterization is rarely necessary.

Management of the premature infant with a PDA depends upon the clinical presentation of the disorder. In an asymptomatic infant intervention is usually unnecessary, since the PDA will almost always undergo spontaneous closure and will not require surgical ligation and division. Infants with respiratory distress syndrome and signs of a significant ductal shunt usually are unresponsive to medical measures to control congestive heart failure and require closure of the PDA for survival. This usually may be accomplished pharmacologically, utilizing indomethacin to inhibit prostaglandin synthesis and achieve construction and closure of the ductus.[2] Approximately 10 per cent of infants are unresponsive to indomethacin and require surgical ligation.

REFERENCES

1. Friedman, W.F.: Patent ductus arteriosus in respiratory distress syndrome. Pediatr. Cardiol. *4*(Suppl. 2):3, 1983.
2. Gersony, W.M., Peckham, G.J., Ellison, R.C., et al.: Effects of indomethacin in premature infants with patent ductus arteriosus: Results of a national collaborative study. J. Pediatr. *102*:895, 1983.

459 A-T, B-T, C-F, D-T, E-T *(Braunwald, pp. 1316–1319)*

Coronary artery bypass surgery (CABG) has undergone many changes since it was first described by Garrett and DeBakey in 1964.[1] The number of CABG operations has increased from 180,000 in 1983 to 300,000 in 1993 and it is estimated that approximately 1 in every 1000 persons undergoes CABG on an annual basis, leading to annual expenditures for CABG of about $50 billion.[2]

Two principal types of bypass conduits are used routinely: saphenous vein grafts and internal mammary artery conduits. The saphenous vein is the preferred venous conduit and is used especially for distal branches of the right and circumflex coronary arteries. In emergency bypass operations, saphenous vein grafts are preferred because of the rapidity of vein graft harvest, and internal mammary conduits are not commonly used in this situation. About 8 to 12 per cent of saphenous vein grafts become occluded during the early perioperative period, usually due to thrombosis and by 1 year 15 to 30 per cent of vein grafts have become occluded. Causes of early vein occlusion vary from trauma to the vein during harvest, excessive surgical manipulation and/or overdistention of the saphenous vein.[3]

Internal mammary artery conduits are excellent bypass grafts and are used predominately for the left anterior descending artery. Internal mammary conduits are relatively immune to the development of intimal hyperplasia and atherosclerosis. Harvesting internal mammary arteries is time consuming due to the delicate nature of the artery and the amount of dissection needed for its retrieval. The diameter of the IMA graft is similar to the coronary artery and therefore changes in flow patterns across the anastomosis are minimal. Typically, saphenous vein grafts occlude at a rate of 2 to 4 per cent per year after the first year, yielding a patency rate of 40 to 60 per cent after 10 years. Beyond the first year, the histological appearance of occluded grafts is consistent with atherosclerosis. In contrast, IMA conduits have a patency rate of up to 90 per cent after 10 years.[4] Rarely, fibrointimal proliferation may occur in IMA grafts and cause late graft closure.[5] Patients receiving IMA conduits have a decreased risk of death, myocardial infarction, and repeat CABG.[4,5]

REFERENCES

1. Garrett, H.E., Dennis, E.W., and DeBakey, M.E.: Aortocoronary bypass with saphenous vein graft. Seven-year followup. JAMA 223:792, 1973.
2. Marwick, C.: Coronary bypass grafting economics, including rehabilitation. Curr. Opin. Cardiol. 9:635, 1994.
3. Bryan, A.J., and Angelini, G.D.: The biology of saphenous vein graft occlusion: Etiology and strategies for prevention. Curr. Opin. Cardiol. 9:641, 1994.
4. Lytle, B.W., and Cosgrove, D.M.: Coronary artery bypass surgery. Curr. Probl. Surg. 29:756, 1992.
5. Turina, M.: Coronary artery surgical technique. Curr. Opin. Cardiol. 8:919, 1993.

460 A-F, B-T, C-F, D-T, E-T   (Braunwald, pp. 1422–1423)

The most common physiological abnormality in hypertrophic obstructive cardiomyopathy (HCM) is not systolic but rather diastolic dysfunction. Thus, HCM is characterized by abnormal stiffness of the left ventricle during diastole, which results in impaired ventricular filling. This abnormality in diastolic relaxation results in elevation of the left ventricular end-diastolic pressure with associated elevations of left atrial, pulmonary venous, and pulmonary capillary pressures. Usually, the left ventricle is hypercontractile with a normal or supernormal ejection fraction. Although the generation of a pressure gradient due to subaortic obstruction would ordinarily imply that left ventricular ejection is slowed or impeded at some point during systole, actually there is rapid ventricular emptying and a normal or even high ejection fraction. Hemodynamic studies have shown that the majority of flow (at least 80 per cent) is unusually rapid in patients with HCM and is completed earlier in systole than normal, regardless of whether gradients are absent, provokable, or present. Thus, the symptoms in general are due to difficulty with diastolic filling rather than with systolic ejection. While there is a strong temporal and quantitative relationship between mitral valve systolic anterior motion and the subaortic gradient, symptoms do not necessarily correlate with the size of the gradient. Furthermore, there are significant variations on a daily basis in the extent of both the gradient and symptoms. Exertional and postexertional syncope and angina occur in some patients and are probably caused, at least in part, by systolic obstruction.

461 A-T, B-F, C-T, D-F   (Braunwald, pp. 1032–1033)

The auscultatory findings of the MVP syndrome are determined by the volume of the LV. The mitral valve begins to prolapse when the decrease in LV volume during systole reaches a critical point in which the mitral valve leaflets no longer coapt; at this instant the click occurs and the murmur commences. Thus, any maneuver that decreases LV volume will result in an earlier occurrence of prolapse during systole so that the click and onset of the murmur move closer to S_1. Conversely, any maneuver which increases LV volume will move the click and murmur toward S_2 and the murmur may actually disappear. Thus, during the straining phase of the Valsalva maneuver, upon sudden standing, and early during the inhalation of amyl nitrite, LV volume decreases and the click and murmur occur earlier in systole. Conversely, a sudden change in posture from standing to prone, leg raising, squatting, isometric exercise such as handgrip, and slowing of the heart rate with propranolol all increase LV volume and delay the click and murmur. When the onset of the murmur is delayed, both its duration and intensity are diminished because of a reduction in the severity of MR. However, with some maneuvers there is a discrepancy between the changes in the intensity and duration of the murmur. For example, following amyl nitrite the click occurs earlier and usually becomes softer, while the murmur becomes softer immediately but then after about 15 seconds becomes louder as a result of the reflex overshoot of blood pressure.

462 A-F, B-T, C-T, D-T, E-F   *(Braunwald, p. 929)*

Tetralogy of Fallot accounts for about 10 per cent of all types of congenital heart disease and is considered to be one of the most congenital cardiac defects associated with cyanosis after the first year of age.[1] There are four anomalies that constitute this malformation: (1) ventricular septal defect, (2) right ventricular outflow obstruction, (3) overriding of the aorta, and (4) right ventricular hypertrophy. The ventricular septal defect is usually located high in the septum below the right aortic valve cusp. Additionally, the aortic root may be displaced anteriorly and override the septal defect but, as in the normal heart, the aortic root is to the right of the origin of the pulmonary artery.

The clinical picture with tetralogy of Fallot depends on the degree of pulmonary right ventricular obstruction. The obstruction can be infundibular, which is the only obstruction in about 50 per cent of patients, and may coexist with valvular obstruction in another 25 per cent. When the obstruction is severe, pulmonary blood flow is markedly reduced and the degree of right-to-left shunting across the ventricular septal defect is increased, resulting in cyanosis and severe secondary polycythemia. Supravalvular and peripheral pulmonary artery stenosis can also be seen in association with tetralogy and may occur as single or multiple lesions.[2] Associated coronary anomalies are also not uncommon; the anterior descending artery may originate from the right coronary artery or a single right coronary artery may give off a left branch that passes anterior to the pulmonary trunk.[3]

REFERENCES

1. Pinsky, W.W., and Arciniegas, E.: Tetralogy of Fallot. Pediatr. Clin. North Am. *37*:179, 1990.
2. Feldt, R.H., Liao, P., and Puga, F.J.: Clinical profile and natural history of pulmonary atresia and ventricular septal defect. Prog. Pediatr. Cardiol. *I*:18, 1992.
3. Carvalho, J.S., Silva, C.M.C., Rigby, M.L., et al.: Angiographic diagnosis of anomalous coronary artery in tetralogy of Fallot. Br. Heart J. *70*:75, 1993.

463 A-F, B-F, C-F, D-5   *(Braunwald, pp. 194–195)*

In calculating aortic valve area in patients with combined AR and AS, it is important to use a measure for cardiac output that represents the *total* left ventricular output. Both the cardiac output measured by the Fick method, which is obtained by measurement of pulmonary artery saturation and pulmonary mixed venous oxygen saturation, and the output measured by the dye dilution method measure the *effective* cardiac output delivered to the body (i.e., the *forward* cardiac output). However, these measurements do *not* include the regurgitant flow that moves back and forth across the aortic valve. Thus, forward output alone will be smaller than total cardiac output and will give an inappropriately small measurement of the aortic valve area. Therefore, in order to accurately calculate valve area by the Gorlin formula, it is important to measure carefully the angiographic LV cardiac output (LV stroke volume × heart rate).

464 A-T, B-T, C-T, D-T, E-T   *(Braunwald, pp. 1542–1544)*

Traumatic injuries of the aorta, including complete aortic rupture, are most commonly associated with sudden high-speed deceleration injuries that result from motor vehicle accidents or other severe jolting injuries. Because they occur in the setting of other serious injuries and rarely have specific symptoms or signs, aortic injuries may be extremely difficult to diagnose without a high index of suspicion. Approximately two-thirds of patients with aortic rupture have clear-cut evidence of accompanying thoracic trauma, including chest or cardiac contusions, multiple rib fractures, hemorrhagic pleural effusions, and pulmonary contusions.[1] The specific physical examination for this injury, however, may be relatively unrevealing. A syndrome of "acute coarctation" with upper extremity hypertension, decreased blood pressure in the lower extremities, precordial systolic murmur, and a pulse lag between the radial and femoral arteries is nearly pathognomonic for the diagnosis but occurs uncommonly. In general, the diagnosis is best suspected from the chest x-ray, which is abnormal in >90 per cent of patients with traumatic aortic rupture. These abnormalities are due to the collection of blood and its continual leakage from the injury and are manifested in specific changes in mediastinal contour, and in the spatial relations of the intrathoracic structures.

The diagnosis of traumatic aortic rupture may be confirmed by the use of CT scanning with contrast injection; in patients about whom some doubt remains, thoracic aortography may be performed. While up to 90 per cent of patients with aortic rupture will die instantly, those patients who do reach the hospital alive with this injury have survival rates that approach 70 per cent in various series.[2] Survivors may have progressive hemorrhage at the site of the aortic tear and thus early, emergency surgical therapy is crucial to survival.

REFERENCES

1. Sturm, J.T., Billiar, T.R., Dorsey, J.S., et al.: Risk factors for survival following surgical treatment of traumatic aortic rupture. Ann. Thorac. Surg. *39*:418, 1985.
2. Atkins, C.W., Buckley, M.J., Daggett, W., et al.: Acute traumatic disruption of the thoracic aorta. A ten-year experience. Ann. Thorac. Surg. *31*:305, 1981.

465 A-T, B-T, C-T, D-F, E-T   *(Braunwald, pp. 904–906)*

The size of the patent ductus arteriosus (PDA) and the ratio of pulmonary to systemic vascular re-

sistance determine the pathophysiological consequences of this disorder. A large PDA leads initially to increased pulmonary blood flow with subsequent enlargement of the pulmonary arterial
circuit, left atrium, left ventricle, and descending
aorta, and eventually the development of congestive heart failure.[1] The development of pulmonary
arterial hypertension may herald the onset of bidirectional or reversed shunting through the ductus. If this occurs, differential cyanosis may develop with a relatively acyanotic right upper
extremity and cyanotic lower extremities because
of the persistence of the PDA, the onset of Eisenmenger's syndrome, and right-to-left shunting
through the ductus.

The physical findings in a patient with a large
left-to-right shunt through a PDA include vigorous
peripheral arterial pulses, a wide arterial pulse
pressure, and a hyperdynamic precordium. On auscultation, a high-pitched continuous murmur may
be heard, which is loudest at the left upper sternal
border or in the infraclavicular area. If the shunt is
large, the increased flow across the mitral valve
may create a diastolic flow rumble. When pulmonary vascular resistance arises, the left-to-right
shunt is diminished and the continuous murmur
may be replaced by a rough systolic murmur with
an accentuated pulmonary component of the second heart sound.

The ECG in this disorder shows either a normal
pattern or if the PDA is large, the development of
left ventricular hypertrophy with strain,[2] right ventricular hypertrophy may be present with pulmonary hypertension. Most commonly, sinus rhythm
is present. The chest x-ray usually reveals dilatation of the proximal pulmonary arteries and pulmonary plethora if the shunt is moderate to large
in size. The M-mode echocardiogram is nonspecific
in PDA and in general shows only left atrial, left
ventricular,   and   aortic   enlargement.   Two-
dimensional echocardiography, however, may allow diagnosis by direct visualization of the ductus.
Doppler analysis may further aid in quantifying the
magnitude of the left-to-right shunt as well as the
pulmonary artery pressure.

REFERENCES

1. Campbell, M.: Natural history of patent ductus arteriosus.
    Br. Heart J. 30:4, 1968.
2. Fisher, R.G., Moodie, D.S., Sterba, R., and Gill, C.C.: Patient
    ductus arteriosus in adults. Long-term follow-up: Non-
    surgical versus surgical treatment. J. Am. Coll. Cardiol. 8:
    280, 1986.

466 A-T, B-F, C-T, D-F, E-T   (Braunwald,
pp. 997–1003; Fig. 31–6)

Approximately 2 per cent of the pediatric population has elevations of systemic blood pressure.
Three points in particular with regard to hypertension in infants and children should be noted: (1)
The causes of hypertension in infants and children
differ markedly from those in adults. Infants and
children more commonly have secondary forms of
hypertension. Renal disease is by far the most common form of secondary hypertension. Examples of
sources of renal hypertension in infants and children include unilateral hydronephrosis, unilateral
pyelonephritis, unilateral tumors, unilateral multi-
cystic kidney, unilateral renal occlusion, renal artery stenosis, fibromuscular renal artery dysplasia,
and nephritis due to acute poststreptococcal disease, anaphylactoid purpura, or disseminated lupus
erythematosus. (2) The offspring of hypertensive patients are known to have an increased susceptibility
to blood pressure elevation. (3) Children with elevated blood pressure require the same surveillance
and treatment as those required in adults.

To measure blood pressure correctly, the inner
rubber bag should be wide enough to cover two-
thirds of the limb and three-fourths of the circum-
ference of the upper arm while leaving the antecubital pulse free. A cuff that is too small is likely
to produce spuriously *high* readings. Blood pressure increases with age; in 2-year-olds the 50th percentile is approximately 95/60 mm Hg while at age
10 the 50th percentile is 110/70.[1]

The workup for hypertension in infants and children should focus on identifying secondary causes
of hypertension.[2] Since renal disease is the most
common cause, typical tests should include urinalysis, complete blood count, serum electrolytes,
blood urea nitrogen, serum creatinine, echocardiogram, ECG, and chest x-ray. It has been shown that
echocardiograms   allow   careful   delineation   of
changes in myocardial function at an early age and
can be used to follow children with both mild hypertension and children of parents with significant
hypertension. This can then be used to decide
whether or not to initiate therapy at any particular
point. In children, even more so than in adults,
treatment of borderline hypertension (between 5
and 10 mm Hg beyond the 90th percentile value
for age) is an issue because of difficulties with compliance and potential long-term side effects of
chronic treatment. In general, drug therapy is initiated if diastolic blood pressure is >85 mm Hg in
children younger than 12 years, and >90 mm Hg
in children older than 12. If left ventricular hypertrophy is evident by echocardiogram, drug therapy
is advisable even with lower diastolic pressures. An
oral thiazide diuretic is usually the initial drug of
choice. Converting enzyme inhibitors such as captopril and enalapril and the calcium channel blockers are drug choices that may be better tolerated.

REFERENCES

1. Colan, S.D., Fujii, A., Borow, K.M., et al.: Noninvasive de-
    termination of systolic, diastolic and end-systolic blood
    pressure in neonates, infants, and young children: Com-
    parison with central aortic measurements. Am. J. Cardiol.
    52:867, 1983.
2. Rocchini, A.P.: Childhood hypertension: Etiology, diagnosis
    and treatment. Pediatr. Clin. North Am. 31:1259, 1984.

467 A-T, B-T, C-T, D-F, E-T *(Braunwald, pp. 1536–1538)*

The treatment of myocardial contusion is quite similar to that of acute myocardial infarction (AMI). Therefore, a period of bed rest of approximately 3 days is recommended, followed by progressive ambulation based on consideration of the patient's clinical symptoms. The chest pain is readily treated with a variety of analgesics, including the nonsteroidal antiinflammatory agents. Patients should *not* be anticoagulated because this may precipitate or exacerbate intramyocardial or intrapericardial hemorrhage. Such hemorrhage is a particular problem in these patients, since undiagnosed lacerations of the pericardium and/or the RV which clot spontaneously may rebleed in the presence of systematic anticoagulation and cause cardiac tamponade. Finally, because of the large variety of arrhythmias that occur in patients with myocardial contusion, they should be monitored. The prognosis for patients who survive the initial injury is excellent, primarily because they are usually relatively young, and unlike patients with AMI secondary to coronary atherosclerosis, their coronary arteries are usually normal. Cardiac catheterization is not necessary in uncomplicated cases.

468 A-T, B-F, C-T, D-F, E-F *(Braunwald, pp. 1564–1568)*

Initial therapy for acute aortic dissection includes immediate admission to an intensive care unit, where careful hemodynamic monitoring is carried out. The earliest therapeutic goals include elimination of pain as well as reduction of systolic arterial pressure. This correlates directly with the degree of stress on the vascular wall which is exerted by LV ejection. The most common pharmacological approach is the simultaneous use of the vasodilator sodium nitroprusside to lower arterial pressure and of a beta-adrenoreceptor blocking agent to reduce wall stress acutely. In patients in whom sodium nitroprusside is poorly tolerated or ineffective, trimethaphan, a ganglionic blocking agent, may be used instead. Lowering of arterial pressure and reduction of left ventricular ejection force allows for temporary stabilization in appropriate surgical candidates, and is the treatment of choice for those patients in whom surgery is not indicated. Following stabilization by such measures, definitive angiography to establish a diagnosis of the extent of the dissection should be performed. The appearance of a life-threatening complication such as aortic rupture, aortic regurgitation, cardiac tamponade, or compromise of a vital organ mandates immediate surgical therapy.

The general consensus regarding definitive subsequent therapy for aortic dissection has evolved over the last several decades. It may be summarized as follows: surgical results are in general superior to medical results in acute proximal dissection, while medical therapy is the preferred treatment in cases of uncomplicated acute distal dissection[1] (see Braunwald, Table 45–4, p. 1566). Patients with distal aortic dissection are in general older and have increased operative risk due to the coincident presence of severe ischemic heart disease or pulmonary disease. Medical therapy in this population has proved quite effective and differs sharply with the natural history of patients with proximal aortic dissection, in whom progression may lead to devastating complications and consequences in a short time.

REFERENCE

1. Cigarroa, J.E., Isselbacher, E.M., DeSanctis, R.W., and Eagle, K.A.: Diagnostic imaging of suspected aortic dissection. Old standards and new directions. N. Engl. J. Med. *328:* 35–43, 1993.

469 A-T, B-F, C-T, D-F *(Braunwald, pp. 1582–1583)*

The primary hypercoagulable states may be defined by specific laboratory abnormalities and are suggested clinically when thrombosis occurs at an early age, at unusual anatomical sites, in a recurrent fashion without apparent precipitating factors, or when a family history of thrombosis exists. Antithrombin III deficiency is probably the most common of the primary hypercoagulable states[1] and is marked clinically by the occurrence of recurrent pulmonary emboli and deep venous thrombosis (DVT). Antithrombin III is the major inhibitor of thrombin in the circulation. Protein C, which consumes factors Va and VIIIa and stimulates fibrinolysis (as well as protein S, a cofactor for activated protein C), may predispose to recurrent venous thromboembolic disease if the protein C level is decreased or absent in the circulation. The "lupus anticoagulant" is most commonly associated with a prolongation of the partial thromboplastin time, but paradoxically leads to an increased risk of venous thromboembolic disease. Either defective release of tissue plasminogen activator or an excess of tissue plasminogen activator inhibitor may also lead to a defective fibrinolytic state, which is associated with venous thrombosis. While oral contraceptive use is associated with coronary emboli and deep venous thrombosis, the association is clinical and without specific laboratory abnormalities and is therefore considered a *secondary* hypercoagulable state.[1]

REFERENCE

1. Schafer, A.I.: The hypercoagulable states. Ann. Intern. Med. *102:*814, 1985.

470 A-T, B-F, C-T, D-F *(Braunwald, pp. 1246–1247)*

The rhythm displayed is an example of accelerated idioventricular rhythm (AIVR), which is commonly defined as a ventricular escape rhythm with a rate between 60 and 100 beats/min. This rhythm is frequently referred to as "slow ventricular tachycardia" and may be seen in up to 20 per cent of patients with AMI, most commonly in the first 2 days after the acute infarction. In addition, AIVR is the most common arrhythmia noted following reperfusion of an occluded coronary artery by fibrinolytic therapy.[1] Approximately one-half of all episodes of AIVR are initiated by the occurrence of a premature beat; the other half of episodes are caused by sinus slowing or gradual speeding of a ventricular pacemaker with the emergency of an AIVR as an escape rhythm.[2] In general, episodes of AIVR are of short duration and may show variation in rate. Unlike more rapid forms of ventricular tachycardia, episodes of AIVR are in general thought not to affect prognosis in the setting of AMI.[1] It should be noted, however, that AIVR can occasionally accelerate to a more rapid ventricular tachycardia, which may require treatment. If an AIVR emerges which compromises hemodynamic function in any manner, treatment by accelerating the sinus rate with atropine or atrial pacing or by suppressing the ventricular pacemaker with lidocaine may be undertaken. However, no definitive evidence exists that AIVR by itself may lead to an increase in the incidence of either ventricular fibrillation or mortality.[3]

REFERENCES

1. Cercek, B., and Horvat, M.: Arrhythmias with brief, high-dose intravenous streptokinase infusion in acute myocardial infarction. Eur. Heat J. *6*:109, 1985.
2. Lichstein, E., Ribas-Mineolier, C., Gupta, P.K., and Chadda, K.D.: Incidence and description of accelerated idioventricular rhythm complicating acute myocardial infarction. Am. J. Med. *58*:192, 1975.
3. Bigger, J.T., Jr., Dresdale, R.J., Heissenbuttel, R.H., et al.: Ventricular arrhythmias in ischemic heart disease: Mechanism, prevalence, significance and management. Prog. Cardiovasc. Dis. *19*:255, 1977.

471 A-T, B-T, C-T, D-F *(Braunwald, pp. 1422–1423)*

Among the characteristic features of hypertrophic cardiomyopathy (HCM) is the variability of the left ventricular outflow gradient. Therefore, it is important when evaluating such a patient to perform a variety of dynamic maneuvers to bring out the murmur. Three basic mechanisms may be utilized to accentuate the systolic murmur, which reflects the severity of the obstruction: (1) increased contractility, (2) decreased preload, and (3) decreased afterload. Increases in contractility and decreases in preload or afterload all tend to augment the murmur. Perhaps the most helpful maneuver is sudden standing from a squatting position. Squatting results in an increase in venous return and an increase in aortic pressure, which increases the ventricular volume, diminishes the gradient, and decreases the intensity of the murmur. Sudden standing following this has the opposite effects and

results in accentuation of the gradient and murmur. Similarly, during the strain phase of the Valsalva maneuver the murmur increases, owing to decreased preload and afterload. Other interventions that increase contractility, such as premature atrial contraction with postextrasystolic potentiation, exercise, tachycardia, hypovolemia, and use of isoproterenol and digitalis, all increase the gradient and the murmur. Amyl nitrite, which markedly diminishes preload and afterload, will also increase the gradient and murmur.

A decrease in the gradient may result from any intervention that increases preload or decreases contractility. Thus, the Müller maneuver (i.e., a deep inspiration against a closed glottis), which is the opposite of the Valsalva maneuver, results in a lessening of the dynamic obstruction to LV outflow by increasing preload and afterload. Similarly, during the overshoot phase of the Valsalva maneuver, there is an increase in preload and afterload and a decrease in the murmur. Other interventions that tend to decrease the murmur include phenylephrine, beta-adrenoceptor blockade, and isometric handgrip.

472 A-T, B-T, C-T, D-F *(Braunwald, pp. 1256–1527)*

This 52-year-old man has the classic findings associated with a large anterior MI complicated by development of an LV aneurysm. The frequency of development of LV aneurysms after AMI depends on the incidence of transmural MI and congestive heart failure in the population studied. Over 80 per cent of LV aneurysms are located anterolaterally near the apex, with approximately 5 to 10 per cent located posteriorly. Most anterior aneurysms are true aneurysms, whereas nearly half of posterior aneurysms are false aneurysms, also known as pseudoaneurysms. These represent localized myocardial rupture in which the hemorrhage is limited by pericardial adhesions, with no myocardium present in the wall. About three-fourths of patients with aneurysms have multivessel coronary artery disease. Approximately 50 per cent of patients with moderate or large aneurysms will present with symptoms of heart failure, with or without associated angina. Thirty per cent have severe angina alone, and approximately 15 per cent have symptoms related to ventricular arrhythmias. Thrombi are found in about 50 per cent of patients with LV aneurysms, and embolic events occur with some frequency, usually within the first 4 to 6 months following infarction. Thus, it is prudent to administer anticoagulants, usually warfarin compounds, during this time period.

The most sensitive technique for diagnosis is biplane ventriculography. Although persistent ST-segment elevation on the ECG, a bulge on the cardiac silhouette, radionuclide ventriculography, and two-dimensional echocardiography all can suggest ventricular aneurysms, they rarely provide accurate assessment of the effect of the aneurysm on systolic function.

The treatment of choice in symptomatic patients is aneurysmectomy, which is indicated in patients with congestive heart failure, refractory ventricular tachycardia, recurrent thromboembolism, and refractory angina. It is helpful, if possible, to wait after the MI for the aneurysm to mature, to a point at which there is sufficient scar tissue to allow adequate surgical repair. The prognosis for patients with aneurysmectomy is significantly better than for those without, with an improvement of at least one New York Heart Association functional class in 70 to 80 per cent of the patients as well as improvement in the ejection fraction. However, preservation of contractile function in the nonaneurysmal left ventricle that remains is crucial and best correlates with outcome.[1]

REFERENCE

1. Brawley, R.K., Magovern, G.J., Jr., Gott, V.L., et al.: Left ventricular aneurysmectomy. Factors influencing postoperative results. J. Thorac. Cardiovasc. Sur. 85:712, 1983.

473 A-T, B-T, C-T, D-F   *(Braunwald, pp. 1412–1413)*

This 55-year-old man has congestive heart failure. There are several possible etiologies for his left ventricular dysfunction based on the clinical history. These include coronary artery disease exacerbated by his cigarette smoking and hypertension, primary hypertensive disease with evidence on chest x-ray and ECG for left ventricular hypertrophy, and alcohol-induced cardiomyopathy. Chronic excessive consumption of alcohol may itself cause hypertension. It has been observed clinically that the toxic effects of alcohol are more dramatic in hypertensive individuals and those with left ventricular hypertrophy. Alcoholic heart disease causes abnormalities of both systolic and diastolic function.[1] Two basic patterns have been observed: left ventricular dilatation with impaired systolic function and left ventricular hypertrophy with diminished compliance and normal or increased contractile performance. Left ventricular size is substantially increased in both. Frequently, these individuals have atrial fibrillation and ventricular arrhythmias as well as congestive heart failure. Angina pectoris does not usually occur unless there is concomitant coronary artery disease or aortic stenosis. Physical examination usually reveals elevated diastolic pressure, secondary to excessive peripheral vasoconstriction. There is frequently cardiomegaly, and S_3 and S_4 gallop sounds are common. An apical systolic murmur consistent with mitral regurgitation due to papillary muscle dysfunction is also found frequently, as in this individual.

The natural history of alcoholic cardiomyopathy depends on the drinking habits of the patient. Total abstinence in the early stages of the disease frequently leads to resolution of the manifestations of congestive heart failure and the return of the heart size to normal. Continued alcohol consumption leads to further myocardial damage and fibrosis with development of refractory heart failure. Thus, the key to treatment is complete abstinence. In this particular individual, who presented relatively early in the course of the illness, it is important that he curtail his drinking. It is also important to prescribe thiamine for the small possibility that thiamine deficiency may be contributing to the heart failure (see also Braunwald, pp. 461–462).

REFERENCE

1. Dancy, M., Leech, G., Bland, J.M., et al.: Preclinical left ventricular abnormalities in alcoholics are independent of nutritional status, cirrhosis, and cigarette smoking. Lancet 1: 1122, 1985.

474 A-T, B-T, C-T, D-F   *(Braunwald, pp. 1163–1166, 1169)*

Blood flow to the myocardium is determined by the perfusion pressure gradient and the vascular resistance of the appropriate myocardial bed. This is influenced by factors extrinsic to the bed (particularly compressive forces within the myocardium) and by metabolic, neural, and humoral factors intrinsic to the bed. Intramyocardial pressure is determined primarily by the ventricular pressure throughout the cardiac cycle. Because the ventricular pressure is so much higher in systole than it is in diastole, myocardial compressive forces acting on intramyocardial vessels are much greater during this phase of the cardiac cycle. Therefore, the endocardium, which is subjected to higher systolic pressures, has a smaller systolic flow than the subepicardium. However, total flow is greater in the subendocardium than the subepicardium because there is enhanced basal vasodilatation in the subendocardium. Interventions that reduce the perfusion gradient during diastole, when the majority of subendocardial flow occurs, lower the ratio of subendocardial to subepicardial flow and may cause the subendocardium to become ischemic. Thus, an increase in ventricular end-diastolic pressure such as occurs with stenotic lesions or a decrease in diastolic time as occurs with an increase in heart rate will decrease subendocardial flow disproportionately. Since the subendocardium has higher metabolic demands and hence lower basal vascular tone, the reserve for vasodilatation is less than in the subepicardium. Therefore, as perfusion is reduced, the deeper layers of the myocardium become ischemic sooner than the more superficial ones.[1]

The subendocardium is susceptible to ischemia due to the combination of limited reserve of vasodilatation, entrinsic compression from the higher wall stress to which it is subjected, and the increased metabolic demands.[2] This susceptibility accounts for the ST-segment depression on the ECG that is observed with episodes of transient ischemia.

REFERENCES

1. Klocke, F.J., Mates, R.E., Canty, J.M., Jr., and Ellis, A.K.: Coronary pressure-flow relationships. Controversial issues and probable implications. Cir. Res. *56*:311, 1985.
2. Klocke, F.J.: Measurements of coronary flow reserve: Defining pathophysiology versus making decisions about patient care. Circulation *76*:1183, 1987.

475 A-F, B-T, C-F, D-F, E-F *(Braunwald, pp. 1464–1466; Fig. 42–1)*

The apical four-chamber view shown demonstrates a large left atrial myxoma. A proposed echocardiographic classification system for left atrial myxomas would classify this lesion as a class IV tumor, because it is both large and apparently prolapsed.[1] Echocardiography is especially helpful in differentiating between left atrial thrombus and myxoma. Thrombus usually produces a layered appearance and is generally situated in the more posterior portions of the atrium. In contrast, left atrial myxoma is often mottled in appearance and only rarely occurs in the posterior atrium. In some atrial myxomas, including the one demonstrated here, echolucent areas are seen within the tumor mass, which correspond pathologically to areas of hemorrhage within the tumor. This too may help distinguish a myxoma from thrombus.

Cardiac myxoma may produce a large variety of noncardiac findings, which include all of those listed as well as cachexia, arthralgias, rash, clubbing, and even changes in behavior patterns.[2] A variety of laboratory findings in addition to an elevated ESR may be present, including an increased or decreased platelet count, polycythemia, leukocytosis, and anemia. The most common primary cardiac tumor of the left atrium is a benign myxoma, and in most instances these are solitary. Signs and symptoms similar to those of mitral valve disease may be present owing to interference of the mass with normal mitral valvular function (see Braunwald, Table 42–2, p. 1464). Physical examination may demonstrate pulmonary congestion and an increased first heart sound. It is believed that the loud S_1 occurs in patients with left atrial myxoma because of late onset of mitral valve closure as a consequence of tumor prolapse through the valvular orifice.[3] In many instances, an early diastolic sound that has been termed a tumor "plop" may be present, although this may be positional and may be confused with an opening snap or a third heart sound unless the diagnosis is suspected.

REFERENCES

1. Charuzi, Y., Bolger, A., Beeder, C., and Lew, A.S.: A new echocardiographic classification of left atrial myxoma. Am. J. Cardiol. *55*:614, 1985.
2. Fisher, J.: Cardiac myxoma. Cardiovasc. Rev. Rep. *9*:1195, 1983.

3. Gershick, A.H., Leech, G., Mills, P.G., and Leatham, A.: The loud first heart sound in left atrial myxoma. Br. Heart J. *52*:403, 1984.

476 A-T, B-T, C-F, D-F, E-T *(Braunwald, pp. 1044–1045; Fig. 32–35)*

By 1990, more than 1000 patients had undergone percutaneous aortic valvuloplasty.[1] The procedure is usually performed using a retrograde approach, although in patients with peripheral vascular disease a transseptal approach may be employed. Orifice improvement is usually less marked than that seen with mitral valvuloplasty but is often adequate to decrease or relieve symptoms of critical aortic stenosis.[2] A procedural mortality of 5 per cent is noted for aortic valvuloplasty, and systemic emboli, increased aortic regurgitation, and vascular injury at the access site (in 5 to 10 per cent of patients) are complications sometimes noted. Aortic valvuloplasty is perhaps best used in patients with symptomatic, critical aortic stenosis in whom surgical aortic valve replacement would be a high-risk procedure. In such patients it may sometimes be used as a "bridge" to valve replacement. More widespread use of the technique is unwarranted, principally because of the long-term complications, the most frequent of which is restenosis. Specifically, a 2-year mortality of 30 to 40 per cent is observed in aortic valvuloplasty patients and repeat valvuloplasty or valve replacement is required in 35 to 40 per cent of survivors.

REFERENCES

1. Block, P.C., and Palacios, I.F.: Aortic and mitral balloon valvuloplasty: The United States experience. *In* Topol, E.J. (ed.): Textbook of Interventional Cardiology. Philadelphia, W.B. Saunders Company, 1990.
2. Safian, R.D., Berman, A.D., Diver, D.J., et al.: Balloon aortic valvuloplasty in 170 consecutive patients. N. Engl. J. Med. *319*:125, 1988.

477 A-T, B-T, C-T, D-F *(Braunwald, pp. 1627–1628)*

Available data suggest that t-PA will have a role in the treatment of pulmonary embolism. Initial interest in this agent was stimulated by experimental findings by Collen and colleagues of decreased hemorrhage and more fibrin-specific thrombolysis in rabbit and canine models of venous thrombosis. Clinical studies of the short-term efficacy and safety of acutely administered recombinant tissue plasminogen activator in acute pulmonary embolism have been completed.[1] In this study, patients with angiographically documented pulmonary embolism had significant clot lysis within 2 to 6 hours following administration of t-PA through a peripheral vein. Plasma fibrinogen levels in patients decreased 42 per cent from baseline, and superficial oozing from venipuncture or arterial puncture sites was noted commonly. In addition, two major hemorrhagic complications occurred requiring surgical intervention (pericardial tamponade and hemorrhage from a pelvic tumor). The rate of major bleeding in this study was 5 per cent, noted in conjunction with an 83 per cent moderate or marked improvement in clinical symptoms and signs within 6 hours. While a precise rule for t-PA in the treatment of pulmonary embolism has not adequately been defined as of this writing, it is probable that the drug will play a significant role in the future.

REFERENCE

1. Goldhaber, S.Z., Markis, J.E., Kessler, C.M., et al.: Perspectives on treatment of acute pulmonary embolism with tissue plasminogen activator. Semin. Thromb. Hemost. *13*: 221, 1987.

478 A-T, B-T, C-T, D-F   *(Braunwald, p. 1431)*

Clinical manifestations of heart disease are present in less than 5 per cent of patients with documented pulmonary sarcoidosis, although at autopsy in 20 to 30 per cent of sarcoid cases granulomas were found in the myocardium. The typical pathological feature of sarcoidosis is the presence of noncaseating granulomas which infiltrate the myocardium and eventually become fibrotic scars. The granulomas may involve any region of the heart, although the left ventricular free wall and interventricular septum are the most common sites. The extensive granular scar tissue in the interventricular septum leads to abnormalities in the conduction system. Involvement of cardiac valves is unusual. The murmur of mitral regurgitation is common. However, it appears to be caused by left ventricular dilatation rather than by direct sarcoid involvement of either papillary muscles or the valve.[1]

Sudden death is the most common cause of death in sarcoid heart disease, probably resulting from paroxysmal arrhythmias and AV block. Since the risk of sudden death appears to be greatest in patients with extensive myocardial involvement, it is reasonable to administer glucocorticosteroids in these patients when their disease is active. The diagnosis of sarcoid heart disease may be suspected in appropriate patients with bilateral adenopathy on chest x-ray, in whom there is clinical, echocardiographic, or ECG evidence of myocardial disease. Percutaneous myocardial biopsy may be particularly useful in establishing the diagnosis.

Treatment of myocardial sarcoidosis is difficult, with the arrhythmias being quite refractory to standard therapy. Permanent pacing may be helpful, especially in patients with advanced heart block.

REFERENCE

1. Roberts, W.C., McAllister, H.A., and Ferras, V.J.: Sarcoidosis of the heart. A clinicopathologic study of 35 necropsy patients (Group I) and review of 78 previously described necropsy patients (Group II). Am. J. Cardiol. *63*:86, 1977.

479 A-T, B-F, C-T, D-T, E-T   *(Braunwald, pp. 1486–1492)*

The accumulation of fluid within the pericardial space leads to an increase in intrapericardial pressure. This may result in cardiac tamponade, which is characterized by an elevation of intracardiac pressures, progressive limitation of ventricular filling, and a reduction of stroke volume and cardiac output. Tamponade has been associated with most forms of pericarditis. Neoplastic disease, such as that demonstrated in the case illustrated, is the most common cause of tamponade identified (see Braunwald, Table 43–4, p. 1489).

The echocardiogram is an extremely useful study in patients with known or suspected cardiac tamponade. The presence and extent of pericardial effusion is best assessed by echocardiography. In most instances, including this case, the absence of a pericardial effusion by echocardiography would exclude the diagnosis of cardiac tamponade. However, in the postoperative cardiac surgical patient, loculated fluid or thrombus may cause cardiac compression and/or tamponade in the absence of obvious pericardial effusion. Several other echocardiographic findings are correlated with the hemodynamic presence of cardiac tamponade. Pulsus paradoxus is associated with both a sudden leftward septal motion and an exaggeration of the usual increase in right ventricular size during inspiration.[1] Diastolic right atrial and right ventricular compression or collapse are early signs during the development of cardiac tamponade[2] (see Braunwald, Fig. 43–9, p. 1491). Left atrial collapse may also be caused by a collection of pericardial fluid behind the left atrium, while right ventricular diastolic collapse may be absent when right ventricular hypertrophy is present. Therefore, while pericardial effusion, inspiratory increase in right ventricular dimensions, and right atrial and ventricular diastolic collapse all strongly suggest tamponade, they are not definitive, nor do they precisely predict the severity of cardiac tamponade.[3] Cardiac catheterization remains the choice to evaluate the hemodynamic importance of a pericardial effusion and suspected cardiac tamponade.

REFERENCES

1. Kronzon, I., Cohen, M.J., and Winer, H.E.: Contribution of echocardiography to the understanding of the pathophysiology of cardiac tamponade. J. Am. Coll. Cardiol. *1*:1180, 1983.
2. Singh, S., Wann, L.S., Schuchard, G.H., et al.: Right ventricular and right atrial collapse in patients with cardiac tamponade—a combined echocardiographic and hemodynamic study. Circulation *70*:966, 1984.
3. Martin, J.B., and Kerber, R.E.: Can cardiac tamponade be diagnosed by echocardiography? Circulation *60*:737, 1979.

480 A-T, B-T, C-T, D-F   *(Braunwald, pp. 1467–1471)*

Primary tumors of the heart are relatively rare, with benign tumors representing approximately 75 per cent of these tumors. The majority of benign cardiac tumors are myxomas, followed in frequency by lipomas, papillary fibroelastomas, rhabdomyomas, fibromas, and other rare tumors. Among the malignant tumors, the most common are sarcomas, and of these the angiosarcoma and rhabdomyosarcoma are the most common forms.

Although it is difficult to differentiate benign from malignant tumors, certain findings may be helpful clinically. The presence of distant metastases, local mediastinal invasion, evidence of rapid growth in tumor size, hemorrhagic pericardial effusion, precordial pain, location of the tumor on the right as opposed to the left side of the heart, and extension into the pulmonary veins are all suggestive of a malignant rather than a benign tumor.

Furthermore, infiltration of the myocardium is much more common in malignant than benign tumors. Benign tumors are more likely to occur on the left side of the interatrial septum and to grow slowly. Symptoms produced by benign and malignant tumors are difficult to differentiate, since both cause fever, arthralgias, and abnormalities of red and white blood cells. Cardiac symptoms caused by tumors are primarily determined by mechanical interference. Myxomas that are located on the left side are more likely to produce mitral valve symptoms, while malignant tumors more commonly found on the right side of the heart tend to produce signs of right-sided failure such as peripheral edema.

481 A-T, B-F, C-T, D-F   (Braunwald, pp. 1144–1146)

Chylomicrons are the largest of the lipoproteins and are composed mostly of triglycerides. They transport dietary triglyceride and cholesterol from the gut to the bloodstream. The chylomicrons are formed from cholesterol and partially digested triglycerides in the intestinal villi. In the cells of the intestinal wall cholesterol is esterified into cholesterol ester, mainly cholesterol oleate, through the enzymatic action of acyl cholesterol acyl transferase (ACAT). The resulting triglyceride particles complex with apolipoproteins and enter the systemic circulation via the lymphatic circulation. In the bloodstream, the chylomicrons bind to lipoprotein lipase, an enzyme on the endothelium that hydrolyzes the triglycerides, releasing free fatty acids. The non protein-enriched chylomicron remnants travel to the liver, where they are taken up by a receptor that recognizes apoprotein E. The presence of chylomicrons in fasting plasma is abnormal and is part of the criteria for the diagnosis of type I and type V hypolipoproteinemia. Chylomicronemia per se is not thought to result in premature coronary disease, although the accumulation of remnant particles as a consequence of chylomicron metabolism may be atherogenic.

482 A-T, B-T, C-T, D-T, E-T   (Braunwald, pp. 1505–1507)

Coxsackie virus group B and echovirus type 8 are the viruses most commonly associated with pericarditis in adults.[1] A variety of infections from other viruses may cause acute pericarditis and/or accompanying myocarditis; common entities in this group include mumps, influenza, infectious mononucleosis, poliomyelitis, varicella, and hepatitis B. It should be emphasized that there are no distinctive clinical features of viral pericarditis and that it is probable that many cases of community-acquired idiopathic pericarditis are due to unrecognized viral infection. Spring and fall are the peak seasons for the development of viral or idiopathic pericarditis, coincident with an increased incidence of enterovirus epidemics. Many patients with viral pericarditis report a prodromal syndrome of an upper respiratory tract infection, which they may describe as the "flu," just prior to the onset of chest pain. In older patients, the diagnosis of viral pericarditis is one of exclusion. Other causes that must be considered include pericarditis due to rheumatoid disorders, recent MI, tuberculosis, and neoplasm.

The illness is usually of short duration and self-limited, although it may follow a dramatic course. In between 15 and 40 per cent of patients a recurrence of pericarditis may follow the acute illness after several weeks, and in a small number of patients such recurrences may continue in the months and years that follow the initial insult.[2] While uncommon, several complications of acute viral or idiopathic pericarditis may occur, including an associated myocarditis, the development of pericardial effusion with or without cardiac tamponade, recurrence, and the late development of constrictive pericarditis.

REFERENCES

1. Celers, J., Celers, P., and Bertocchi, A.: Non-polio enterovirus in France from 1974 to 1985. Pathol. Biol. 36:1221, 1988.
2. Fowler, N.O., and Harbin, A.D.: Recurrent pericarditis: Follow-up of 31 patients. J. Am. Coll. Cardiol. 7:300, 1986.

483 A-T, B-T, C-T, D-F   (Braunwald, p. 1134)

Low-density lipoproteins (LDLs) are the major cholesterol-carrying components of the plasma. LDLs are mainly formed from VLDL breakdown, although they may also be synthesized directly. The major lipid components of LDL are triglyceride and esterified cholesterol. Apo B-100 is the predominant protein present in LDL and comprises approximately 25 per cent of the LDL mass. After LDLs are formed in the liver they are bound by the specific receptors in a variety of tissues, including the liver. In familial hypercholesterolemia there is a decreased number of LDL receptors; however, over 80 per cent of patients with elevated LDL do not have this single-gene disorder but rather have polygenic hypercholesterolemia. Therefore, elevations of LDL due to a primary receptor defect are relatively uncommon. Apo A-I is a major apolipoprotein of high-density lipoproteins (HDLs). It may be "antiatherogenic" because it facilitates the uptake of HDL particles in a receptor-mediated reverse transport pathway for cholesterol.

484 A-T, B-F, C-T, D-F *(Braunwald, pp. 1303–1304)*

Nitroglycerin administered sublingually is the drug of choice in the treatment of angina pectoris. The usual sublingual dosage of nitroglycerin is 0.3 to 0.6 mg, and most patients respond within 5 minutes to one or two 0.3-mg tablets. The development of tolerance is rarely a problem with intermittent sublingual usage. Even in patients who have been on chronic nitrates the rapidity of the increase in nitrate levels achieved through buccal absorption usually overwhelms the "tolerant state." However, among the causes for inadequate responses to orally administered nitrates are poor absorption due to dryness of the mouth and a delay in the dissolution of the tablet. This can be remedied by use of either a spray or tablets that contain a moisture gel that can be placed directly on the gum. Nitrates also undergo degradation when left in the open, especially when exposed to light, and it is likely that in this case, the light on the windowsill caused loss of potency of her pills.

In patients with stable angina, nitrate tolerance appears to develop during four-times-daily therapy with oral isosorbide dinitrate, so that the improvement in exercise tolerance disappears within a matter of a few days. This can be prevented by allowing prolonged drug-free intervals. Thus, one recommendation would be to have the patient take a pill at dinner and not take another until breakfast. This long drug-free interval allows recovery of the response to nitrates. Nitrate tolerance is particularly common with transdermal discs, because they continuously deliver a small dosage and because nitrate levels are maintained constantly.

485 A-F, B-T, C-F, D-T *(Braunwald, pp. 1498–1501; Table 43–7; Fig. 43–7)*

The clinical presentation of patients with chronic constrictive pericarditis is determined in part by the degree of elevation of systemic venous and right atrial pressures. In patients with a modest elevation in such pressures, symptoms due to systemic venous congestion may predominate, including edema, ascites, and discomfort due to passive hepatic congestion. When right and left heart filling pressures reach the 15 to 30 mm Hg level, symptoms of pulmonary venous congestion may appear, along with pleural effusions and elevation of the diaphragm due to ascites, all of which contribute to tachypnea and dyspnea. The most important

clinical finding in constriction is the elevation of jugular venous pressure, which may be obscured if the patient is examined in the supine position. While elevated jugular venous pressure is a clue to the presence of the disorder, other causes of increased venous pressure must be excluded. Inspiratory increases in venous pressure (*Kussmaul's sign*) may be seen in some patients; this sign does not occur in cardiac tamponade.

In pure or classic constrictive pericarditis, the presence of pulsus paradoxus is uncommon, although if pericardial fluid is present as well (effusive-constrictive pericarditis), this sign may be observed. Most patients with chronic constrictive pericarditis have an unobtrusive but diffuse precordial movement due to systolic retraction of the apical cardiac impulse. The most distinctive auscultatory finding in constrictive pericarditis is the presence of the *diastolic* pericardial knock, an early diastolic sound that may be heard at the left sternal border and corresponds in timing to the sudden cessation of ventricular filling due to the rigid, constricting pericardium. Pericardial knocks are in general earlier and of higher frequency than the typical S_3 gallop sounds, and may on occasion be confused with the opening snap of mitral stenosis. Most patients with constrictive pericarditis demonstrate hepatomegaly along with prominent hepatic pulsations and other evidence of hepatic dysfunction due to passive liver congestion. Younger patients with competent venous valves may have little or no lower extremity edema. In contrast, older patients with longstanding constrictive pericarditis may have large accumulations of fluid throughout the lower torso and abdominal cavity.

REFERENCE

1. Meyer, T.E., Sareli, P., Marcus, R.H., et al.: Mechanism underlying Kussmaul's sign in chronic constrictive pericarditis. Am. J. Cardiol. **64**:1069, 1989.

486 A-T, B-F, C-T, D-F *(Braunwald, pp. 1171–1174)*

The normal coronary vascular bed has the ability to reduce its resistance to approximately 20 per cent of basal levels during maximal exercise. The basic principles of fluid mechanics indicate that the pressure drop across a stenosis varies directly with the length of the stenosis and inversely with the fourth power of the radius. Thus changes in the radius are much more important than changes in the length of the stenosis. Furthermore, it can be shown that significant changes in flow do not occur until stenoses are greater than 80 per cent of the original diameter of the vessel. However, the resistance to flow triples as the severity of the stenosis increases from 80 to 90 per cent.[1] As a consequence, even a slight change in the severity of such a stenosis can cause a dramatic alteration in the coronary perfusion pressure distal to the obstruction.

In such a tight stenosis, when flow across the stenosis rises, passive collapse[2] may occur. This is due to substantial energy losses from turbulence (proportional to the square of the flow) which result in an exponential rise in the pressure gradient across the stenosis. Thus at any flow rate, the gradient rises with the degree of stenosis. Therefore, as the transstenotic pressure gradient increases, the distal perfusion pressure will fall significantly, leading to a fall in intraluminal pressure and collapse of the vessel, thereby further augmenting the severity of stenosis.

REFERENCES

1. Klocke, F.J.: Measurements of coronary blood flow and degree of stenosis: Current clinical implications and continuing uncertainties. J. Am. Coll. Cardiol. 1:31, 1983.
2. Epstein, S.E., Cannon, R.O., III, and Talbot, T.L.: Hemodynamic principles in the control of coronary blood flow. Am. J. Cardiol. 56:4E, 1985.

487 A-T, B-T, C-T, D-T (Braunwald, pp. 1583–1584; Table 46–3)

The NIH consensus development statement regarding the prevention of venous thrombosis and pulmonary embolism[1] notes that clinically significant pulmonary embolism occurs in approximately 1.6 per cent of the general surgical population. This body therefore recommended prophylaxis in all general surgical patients who meet any of the following criteria: (1) age 40 and over, (2) surgical procedures longer than 1 hour's duration, (3) obesity, (4) known cancer, or (5) prior pulmonary embolism or DVT. The presence of any of these should dictate the use of 5000 units of heparin subcutaneously every 8 to 12 hours beginning before surgery commences and continuing at least until the patient is ambulatory.

Patients at higher risk should receive a combination of heparin and dihydroergotamine (H-DHE), which has been shown in a variety of clinical trials to be more effective than either drug alone in the prophylaxis of venous thromboembolism.[2] In 1985, the FDA approved one fixed dose of heparin (5000 units) in combination with 0.5 mg of DHE to be administered subcutaneously 2 hours prior to surgery and then every 12 hours for 5 to 7 days. Because of the selective vasoconstrictive effect on veins and venules from the dihydroergotamine preparation, the drug is believed to help counteract venous stasis by accelerating venous return from the legs. However, it should not be used in patients undergoing vascular surgery or in those who have suspected bowel or coronary ischemia.

REFERENCES

1. NIH Consensus Development Statement: Prevention of venous thrombosis and pulmonary embolism. JAMA 256: 744, 1986.
2. Gent, M., and Roberts, R.S.: A meta-analysis of the studies of dihydroergotamine plus heparin in the prophylaxis of deep vein thrombosis. Chest 89:3965, 1986.

488 A-F, B-T, C-F, D-T (Braunwald, pp. 1340–1343)

The treatment of Prinzmetal's variant angina is similar to that of chronic stable angina in some respects, but several drugs useful in patients with stable angina may provoke paradoxical clinical deterioration in those with Prinzmetal's angina. Patients with both forms of angina are successfully treated with nitrates, which are direct vascular smooth muscle dilators. However, the response in patients with variant angina to beta blockers is variable. In some patients with fixed stenoses beta blockers, by reducing myocardial oxygen demands, will lessen symptoms. In others, however, blockade of beta$_2$ receptors, which are involved in coronary dilation, allows unopposed alpha-adrenoceptor receptor activity leading to coronary vasoconstriction, which may prolong episodes of vasospasm.[1]

In contrast to the beta blockers, the calcium channel antagonists are universally effective in preventing coronary artery spasm associated with variant angina.[2] The three currently available calcium channel antagonists, nifedipine, diltiazem, and verapamil, are all equally effective, although some idiosyncratic responses have been documented. Prazosin, a selective alpha$_1$-adrenoreceptor blocker, has also been found to be of some value. Aspirin, which improves symptoms and decreases infarction in unstable angina, may actually increase the frequency of ischemic episodes in patients with Prinzmetal's angina, because it inhibits synthesis of the naturally occurring vasodilator prostaglandin I$_2$.[3]

REFERENCES

1. Robertson, R.M., Wood, A.J.J., Vaughn, W.K., and Robertson, D.: Exacerbation of vasotonic angina pectoris by propranolol. Circulation 65:281, 1982.
2. Schroeder, J.S., Lamb, I.H., Bristow, M.R., et al.: Prevention of cardiovascular events in variant angina by long-term diltiazem therapy. J. Am. Coll. Cardiol. 1:1507, 1983.
3. Miwar, K., Kambara, H., and Kawai, C.: Effect of aspirin in large doses on attacks of variant angina. Am. Heart J. 105: 351, 1983.

489 A-T, B-T, C-T, D-F (Braunwald, pp. 1035–1037)

In the adult with acquired AS, stenosis of a tricuspid aortic valve is usually on a congenital, rheumatic, or degenerative basis. Rheumatic stenosis results from adhesions along the commissures of the cusps leading to retraction and stiffening of the free borders of the cusps with calcific nodules present on both surfaces. Since there is commissural fusion with associated retraction, the rheumatic valve is often regurgitant as well as stenotic. In degenerative or senile calcific AS, the immobility of the aortic valve is due to deposition of calcium at the valve bases rather than at the tips. This currently appears to be the most common cause of AS in adults in the United States; it is probably due to trauma secondary to normal mechanical stress on the valve. Common associated findings in patients with this form of AS include calcification of the mitral annulus and the coronary arteries, but co-existing AR is uncommon. Both diabetes mellitus and hypercholesterolemia appear to be risk factors for the development of calcific AS.[1] Other causes of AS in adults include rheumatoid involvement of the valve and, very rarely, ochronosis.[2]

REFERENCES

1. Deutscher, S., Rockette, H.E., and Krishanswami, V.: Diabetes and hypercholesterolemia among patients with calcific aortic stenosis. J. Chronic Dis. 37:407, 1984.
2. Ptacin, M., Sebastian, J., and Bamrah, V.S.: Ochronotic cardiovascular disease. Clin. Cardiol. 8:441, 1985.

490 A-T, B-T, C-T, D-T (Braunwald, pp. 1007–1009)

In normal adults the mitral valve orifice is 4 to 6 cm^2. When the orifice is reduced to approximately 2 cm^2, which is consistent with mild MS, blood flow from the LA to the LV occurs only with the development of an abnormal pressure gradient. When the mitral valve opening is reduced further, to approximately 1 cm^2, critical MS is considered to exist. In this setting, a pressure gradient of approximately 20 mm Hg is recorded, and therefore in the presence of normal LV diastolic pressure, a mean left atrial pressure of approximately 25 to 30 mm Hg is required to maintain normal cardiac output at rest. The severity of mitral valve obstruction is determined by both the transvalvular gradient and the flow rate. The transvalvular flow rate depends directly on the cardiac output and inversely on the heart rate. An increase in heart rate shortens the time for diastole proportionately more than systole and diminishes the time for flow across the mitral valve. Therefore, at any given level of cardiac output (flow rate), tachycardia augments the transmitral valvular pressure gradient.

Hydrodynamic considerations indicate that for any given orifice size the transvalvular gradient is a function of the *square* of the transvalvular flow rate[1] (i.e., a doubling of the flow rate will quadruple the pressure gradient). Thus, a patient with moderate mitral stenosis (e.g., a valve area 2 cm^2) at rest would be able to generate a flow of 300 ml/sec of diastole with a diastolic pressure gradient of less than 20 mm Hg. However, with exercise and a doubling of the heart rate, the time for diastole will be at least halved. The flow rate would now have to be approximately 600 ml, which would require a much greater diastolic pressure gradient resulting in symptoms of dyspnea and congestive heart failure.

Atrial contraction augments the presystolic transmitral valvular gradient by approximately 30 per cent in patients with MS. A loss of atrial contraction by the development of atrial fibrillation decreases cardiac output by approximately 20

per cent. Furthermore, the rapid ventricular rate common in atrial fibrillation raises the transvalvular pressure gradient. Thus, the importance of sinus rhythm in patients with MS is determined by both effects on transvalvular flow rate and the ability to raise the presystolic transmitral valve gradient.

REFERENCE

1. Gorlin, R., and Gorlin, S.G.: Hydraulic formula for calculation of the area of stenotic mitral valve, other cardiac valves and central circulatory shunts. Am. Heart J. 41:1, 1951.

491 A-T, B-T, C-T, D-F (Braunwald, pp. 1144–1146)

Type IV hyperlipoproteinemia is characterized by increased VLDL, normal or increased cholesterol level, and increased triglycerides. The metabolic defect appears to be an oversynthesis of triglyceride and VLDL by the liver. The genetic disorders that are associated with this disorder include familial hypertriglyceridemia and familial combined hyperlipidemia. Secondary causes of type IV pattern are common and include excess dietary calories or alcohol, renal failure, diabetes mellitus, hepatocellular disease (glycogen-lipid storage disease), and dysproteinemias. Diabetes is frequently associated with elevated triglycerides; this appears to be due to the elevated insulin levels. Reduced lipoprotein lipase activity occurs in myxedema and renal failure and may account for the elevated triglyceride levels in these conditions. Although neurofibromatosis is associated with an increased incidence of cardiovascular disease, it is not associated with hyperlipoproteinemia.

492-B, 493-B, 494-A, 495-C (Braunwald, pp. 1150–1151; 1707–1708)

Prescribed medications are among the common contributing factors to abnormal serum lipids. Commonly used medications in patients with cardiovascular disease which elevate cholesterol, LDL, triglyceride, and VLDL include thiazide diuretics and beta blockers. Beta blockers have also been shown to lower the HDL fraction of total cholesterol.[1] Although thiazide diuretics have multiple effects, their dominant effects are to increase LDL, VLDL, and triglycerides. Oral contraceptives tend to increase levels of serum cholesterol, but the overall effect on lipids likely is a function of the relative amounts of estrogen and progesterone in different preparations.[2] Estrogens tend to raise HDL cholesterol and VLDL levels, while progesterone analogs decrease elevated levels of triglycerides and also decrease HDL. Many other drugs including alpha-adrenoreceptor blockers such as prazosin, calcium channel antagonists, angiotensin-converting enzyme inhibitors, and centrally acting antihypertensive drugs such as clonidine and guanabenz have no significant effect on plasma lipoproteins.

REFERENCES

1. Leren, P., Foss, P.O., Helgeland, A., et al.: Effect of propranolol and prazosin on blood lipids. The Oslo Study. Lancet *2*:4, 1980.
2. Ernster, V.L., Bush, T.L., and Huggins, G.R.: Benefits and risks of menopausal estrogens and progestin hormone use. Prev. Med. *17*:201, 1988.

496-A, 497-C, 498-B, 499-D   (Braunwald, pp. 907–911)

Persistent truncus arteriosus is a rare, serious congenital anomaly in which a single vessel forms the outlet of both ventricles, giving rise to the systemic, pulmonary, and coronary arteries. Persistent truncus arteriosus is always accompanied by a VSD and usually by a right-sided aortic arch. The VSD results from an absence or underdevelopment of the distal portion of the pulmonary infundibulum. This malformation should be distinguished from "pseudotruncus arteriosus," which is the severe form of tetralogy of Fallot with pulmonary atresia, in which the single aorta arises from the heart in the presence of a remnant of pulmonary artery. Differentiation between truncus arteriosus and tetralogy of Fallot by ultrasound may be difficult. The diagnosis may be suspected at cardiac catheterization if the catheter fails to enter the central pulmonary arteries from the RV. Selective angiocardiography and retrograde aortography are necessary to establish the diagnosis and reveal the common trunk arising from the heart, as well as the origin of the pulmonary arteries from this trunk.

Anomalous origin of the coronary artery from the pulmonary artery is a rare malformation which is usually characterized by the *left* coronary artery having its source from the posterior sinus of the pulmonary artery. The most common clinical presentation of this anomaly is the occurrence of MI and subsequent congestive heart failure in an infant. The syndrome usually becomes manifested between 2 and 4 months of age with angina-like symptoms that may be misinterpreted as colic. The diagnosis of anomalous origin of the coronary artery gains support from electrocardiographic demonstration of Q waves in association with ischemic ST-segment alterations and T-wave inversions in lateral chest leads. The diagnosis may be established using retrograde aortography to demonstrate drainage of the left coronary artery into the pulmonary artery. Ventricular arrhythmias may complicate this disorder. Management of infants with anomalous pulmonary origin of the coronary artery depends in part on the degree of left-to-right shunting that is present. The surgical outcome and ultimate prognosis depend on how much myocardial damage the patient has suffered preoperatively.

Coronary arteriovenous fistula also is an unusual anomaly composed of a communication between the coronary system and a cardiac chamber, usually the RV, RA, or coronary sinus. In approximately 55 per cent of cases, the right coronary artery is involved. A majority of these communications lead to a small degree of left-to-right shunting, and patients are most often asymptomatic. Diagnosis thus occurs most commonly because of a loud, superficial continuous cardiac murmur. The ECG and chest x-ray are usually normal in this disorder. Significantly enlarged coronary arteries may be visualized by two-dimensional echocardiography, and occasionally the diagnosis can be made by a combination of this technique and Doppler flow analysis. The usual treatment of this disorder involves closure of the fistula even in asymptomatic patients in order to prevent subsequent symptoms or complications such as infective endocarditis.

Congenital aneurysm of an aortic sinus of Valsalva occurs most frequently in the right coronary sinus and in males, although it is an uncommon anomaly. When such an aneurysm ruptures, the resulting aorticocardiac fistula usually involves a communication with the RV, although when the noncoronary cusp is affected the fistula may drain into the RA. The presence of this disorder may be suspected in a patient with the sudden onset of chest pain, symptoms of decreased cardiac reserve, hyperdynamic pulses, and a loud, continuous, superficial murmur accentuated in diastole. The physical findings may occasionally be difficult to distinguish from those produced by a coronary arteriovenous fistula. ECG may show biventricular hypertrophy and chest x-ray may show generalized cardiac enlargement. Echocardiographic studies may be able to localize the aneurysm, as well as the perturbation in flow produced by the fistula. Diagnosis may be established definitively by retrograde aortography, and cardiac catheterization may reveal a left-to-right shunt at the ventricular level. Preoperative medical management involves treatment of congestive heart failure, arrhythmias, and endocarditis.

Aortic arch obstruction describes a variety of lesions that lead to interruption of a portion of the aortic arch, including localized juxtaductal coarctation, hypoplasia of the aortic isthmus, and frank aortic arch interruption. In contrast to the four lesions mentioned, aortic arch obstruction may exist without accompanying left-to-right shunting.

500-B, 501-C, 502-A, 503-D   (Braunwald, pp. 1106–1111)

Each of the cell types listed is involved in the process of atherogenesis, albeit in different ways. *Endothelial cells*, which represent a large and extensive lining of the entire vascular tree, form a highly selective, permeable barrier to the bloodstream and maintain a nonthrombogenic surface. They also actively manufacture and secrete several important vasoactive substances. Endothelial cells have a surface coat of heparan sulfate which helps maintain nonthrombogenicity and are capable of forming prostaglandin derivatives, in particular prostacyclin. The latter is a vasodilator which inhibits platelet aggregation.[1] In addition, endothelial cells secrete tissue plasminogen activator, which may lead ultimately to lysis of fibrin clots and regulation of the local hemostatic milieu, and endothelium-derived relaxing factor (EDRF), which causes vasodilation and also inhibits platelet aggregation. EDRF has recently been identified as nitric oxide or a closely related compound and may therefore be considered an endogenous nitrate. Thus, endothelial cells regulate or provide protection against the development of inappropriate thrombus formation through a variety of mechanisms.

The *smooth muscle cell* is originally derived from the media of the blood vessel and proliferates extensively in the arterial intima to form atherosclerotic plaques. The principal physiological role of this cell in the media of the artery is presumably to maintain arterial wall tone by a capacity to alter contractile state in response to a variety of substances. Thus, prostacyclin may induce relaxation and vasodilation, while numerous vasoactive agents such as epinephrine and angiotensin may cause smooth muscle contraction. Like the macrophage, the smooth muscle cell may become filled with cholesteryl ester and form a "foam cell." In advanced atherosclerotic lesions extensive proliferation of smooth muscle cells in the intima contributes significantly to the development of the mature atherosclerotic lesion.

Macrophages, derived from circulating blood monocytes, are capable of secreting a large number of biologically active substances as they participate in the inflammatory and immune responses. These cells synthesize and secrete a variety of growth factors that are probably critical in the proliferation of connective tissues and may be involved in development of atherosclerotic lesions. Macrophages become foam cells by extensive accumulation of cholesteryl ester and as such form the principal cells in the fatty streak, the initial lesion of the developing atherosclerotic plaque.

Platelets participate in an important and complex manner with both the endothelium and developing atherosclerotic plaque. Although platelets are capable of little or no protein synthesis, they contain numerous protein substances in their alpha granules which are released upon platelet activation. These include a variety of factors that participate in the coagulation cascade as well as several extremely potent growth factors or mitogens. Growth factors may play an important role in stimulating both vasoconstriction and subsequent proliferation in the injured vessel wall. In addition, the factors released that participate in the coagulation cascade play a role with platelets in the development of thrombi and as such are important clinically in the thrombotic sequelae of atherosclerotic disease.

Each of the cells mentioned plays an important part in the "response-to-injury" hypothesis favored by Ross and colleagues.[2] In this theory, some form of injury occurs to the endothelial cells lining the arterial wall. The subsequent interactions between the underlying portions of the blood vessel, the blood elements, and the various cells mentioned lead to a vascular response to injury and, if unchecked, may ultimately lead to a frank atherosclerotic lesion (*see Braunwald, Fig. 34–12, p. 1115*).

REFERENCES

1. Moncada, S., Herman, A.G., Higgs, E.A., and Vane, J.R.: Differential formation of prostacyclin (PGX or PGI$_g$) by layers of the arterial wall. An explanation for the antithrombotic properties of vascular endothelium. Thromb. Res. *11*:323, 1977.
2. Ross, R.: The pathogenesis of atherosclerosis—An update. N. Engl. J. Med. *314*:496, 1986.

504-C, 505-A, 506-A, 507-D, 508-B   *(Braunwald, pp. 1437–1444)*

Cardiac dysfunction in *diphtheria* usually occurs in unimmunized children, especially in the western United States, and appears to be a result of abnormal myocardial lipid metabolism due to the diphtheria toxin.[1] Pathologically, extensive fat vacuolization and glycogen depletion are noted in myocytes. Cardiac involvement occurs in approximately 10 per cent of patients with diphtheria and is the most common cause of death from the disease. Heart disease is most easily detected by noting electrocardiographic changes, which may range from ST-segment and T-wave changes to arrhythmias and conduction disturbances, including complete heart block. The appearance of right or left bundle branch block or complete AV block is associated with mortality rates of greater than 50 per cent. In general, treatment for this disorder is not satisfactory. Patients receive diphtheria antitoxin and intravenous penicillin, as well as symptomatic treatment for arrhythmias and congestive failure due to myocardial dysfunction. However, no specific therapy is available. The prognosis is good if the child recovers from the acute episode of diphtheritic cardiomyopathy.

Infection by trypanosomal organisms, especially *Trypanosoma cruzi*, results in Chagas' disease, which occurs most commonly in the southern United States and is endemic in Latin America. Trypanosomal myocarditis is an unusual disease in that its most important clinical manifestation is a chronic myocarditis that may not occur until 10 to 30 years after the acute infectious process. There is no satisfactory treatment for the illness. Another trypanosome, *Trypanosoma rhodesiense*, which causes African sleeping sickness, may produce myocardial hemorrhage and a slow degenerative disease resulting in myocardial failure. Cardiac involvement with this parasite is usually mild and is overshadowed by the concomitant encephalitis.

In newborns, Coxsackie B and rubella viruses are the most common causative agents of *infective my-*

ocarditis. Coxsackie B leads to an illness of sudden onset characterized by systemic signs of infection and occasionally cardiac failure. The diagnosis of this viral myocarditis is first suggested by ECG findings that may include atrial or ventricular arrhythmias as well as by marked cardiomegaly and pulmonary vascular congestion on the chest x-ray. When the virus can be isolated from pharyngeal secretions or other body fluids, the diagnosis is strongly suggested. Although general supportive measures are of little benefit in this disorder, the vast majority of children recover from acute episodes of myocarditis with few or no sequelae. After infancy, other agents that may cause such a viral myocarditis include Coxsackie A, influenza, adenovirus, and echovirus. In addition, many of the common viral infectious diseases of childhood, such as mumps and measles, may be associated with a mild myocarditis. Rarely, a child may develop sequelae, such as a permanent conduction defect or a mild cardiac enlargement from viral myocarditis. In some cases, a more severe chronic cardiomyopathy may result. There do not appear to be any predictive criteria to identify which children will ultimately suffer more severe complications.[2]

REFERENCES

1. Challoner, D.R., and Prols, H.G.: Free fatty acid oxidation and carnitine levels in diphtheritic guinea pig myocardium. J. Clin. Invest. *51*:2071, 1972.
2. Taliercio, C.P., Seward, J.B., Driscoll, D.J., et al.: Idiopathic dilated cardiomyopathy in the young: Clinical profile and natural history. J. Am. Coll. Cardiol. *6*:1126, 1985.

509-D, 510-B, 511-E, 512-A   *(Braunwald, pp. 1039–1042)*

The diagnosis of *aortic stenosis* (AS) by clinical examination rests on several physical findings. Among these are the location and radiation of the murmur and thrill, presence of an aortic ejection sound, characteristics of the aortic component of the second sound, coexisting presence of a regurgitant diastolic murmur, and characteristics of the arterial pulse in both the carotid and peripheral vessels. In the most common form of AS (the acquired nonrheumatic form), the murmur is commonly heard over the second right intercostal space radiating to the neck. An aortic ejection sound is uncommon, and the aortic component of the second heart sound is diminished or absent. A regurgitant diastolic murmur is occasionally heard especially in patients with coexisting hypertension; the carotid pulses are delayed in upstroke and are of diminished volume.

Examination findings in patients with acquired AS due to rheumatic fever are quite similar. One exception is the increased incidence of coexisting aortic regurgitation (AR) due to commissural fusion and retraction of the aortic valve leaflets.

Hypertrophic cardiomyopathy (HCM) is characterized by its prevalence throughout all age groups in contrast to calcific AS, which is observed more frequently in the elderly. In HCM the systolic murmur is frequently audible along the sternal border and radiates well to the apex. Features characteristic of HCM are a normal aortic component of the second heart sound, absence of a murmur of AR, and frequent coexistence of mitral regurgitation (MR). It should also be noted that in HCM the arterial pulse is usually brisk and sometimes bisferiens (classically a spike-and-dome configuration is noted).

In *congenital subaortic stenosis* the presence of a fibrous ring below the aortic valve gives rise to a discrete murmur, which is similar to that in valvular AS. Ejection sounds are rare, the aortic component of the second sound is variably present, AR is common, and again, the upstrokes are delayed with diminished amplitude.

In *congenital supravalvular* AS the murmur and thrill are most prominent in the first right intercostal space. In this lesion the right carotid and brachial pulses may have normal rates of rise while the left carotid and brachials exhibit slow rates of rise. The peripheral pulses are abnormally strong, and the blood pressure may be higher in the right arm than the left arm. This is thought to be due to the streaming of the aortic outflow jet toward the innominate artery with increased flow to the right side. In this lesion aortic ejection sounds are also rare. The aortic component of the second heart sound is usually normal. AR is uncommon.

In *congenital AS* a common finding is the presence of an aortic ejection sound, which is due to the sudden upward displacement (doming) of the pliant aortic leaflet whose upward motion ceases suddenly, giving rise to a click.

Frequently in aortic outflow tract disease, murmurs are heard at the apex which resemble those produced by MR. In the most common situation a patient with degenerative (senile) calcific AS has a harsh systolic ejection quality murmur in the right second intercostal space which changes in character as the stethoscope is inched toward the apex. This is termed the *Gallavardin phenomenon* and is caused by the selective radiation of high-frequency components of the AS murmur to the apex. This finding is most common in elderly patients because in degenerative calcific AS commissural fusion does not occur and the nonfused cusps may vibrate and produce high-frequency sounds.

REFERENCE

1. Perloff, J.K.: Clinical recognition of aortic stenosis. The physical signs and differential diagnosis of the various forms of obstruction to left ventricular outflow. Prog. Cardiovasc. Dis. *10*:323, 1968.

513-B, 514-A, 515-C, 516-E   *(Braunwald, pp. 1084–1086)*

Janeway lesions are small macular lesions which are distinguished from Osler nodes by the fact that they are painless and nontender and are most often present in the thenar and hypothenar eminences of the hand and soles of patients with subacute infective endocarditis. They appear much less often on the tips of the fingers or plantar surfaces of the toes. Lesions on the hands and feet blanch with pressure and with elevation of the extremities. In cases of acute valvular infections the lesions tend to be purple and hemorrhagic.

Osler nodes are small raised, nodular, tender lesions present most often in the pulp spaces of the terminal phalanges of the fingers. They may also be present on the backs of the toes, the soles, and the thenar and hypothenar eminences. The most characteristic feature of these lesions is their tenderness. Lesions may be fleeting in some cases, disappearing within a few hours after they have developed; however, they usually persist for 4 to 5 days. Although almost completely restricted to the subacute form of endocarditis, Osler nodes are occasionally present in acute valvular infection. Prevalence of both Osler nodes and Janeway lesions has decreased in recent years, most likely because of early institution of antibiotic therapy and a decrease in both endothelial destruction and frequency of embolic events.

The ocular signs in infective endocarditis include both retinal petechiae and *Roth spots*. These are located in the nerve layer of the retina and look like hemorrhagic exudates. They consist of aggregations of cytoid bodies; histologically they have been shown to be composed of perivascular accumulation of lymphocytes with or without surrounding hemorrhage.

Similarly, embolic events to the myocardium cause a localized inflammatory reaction consisting of collections of lymphocytes and mononuclear cells termed *Bracht-Wächter lesions*. These lesions may eventually replace enough of the muscle to contribute to the congestive heart failure seen in chronic endocarditis.

Subungual or splinter hemorrhages are uncommon in patients with infective endocarditis. The characteristic features of the splinter hemorrhage are its linear form and the fact that its distal end does not reach the anterior nail bed; the latter distinguishes this lesion from a true splinter. In some cases, the toes may also be involved but because of the strong association with trauma, splinter hemorrhages are relatively nondiagnostic.

517-C, 518-E, 519-A, 520-D   *(Braunwald, pp. 1140–1142)*

There are many drugs that have been utilized for treatment of lipid disorders. Part of the explanation for this diversity is the relative lack of effectiveness of any single drug and the fact that several different pathways are responsible for the lipid abnormalities. Although there have been many approaches to treating hyperlipidemia, a national committee has recently provided specific guidelines for elevated

cholesterol levels.[1] For example, diet therapy is always recommended initially, but it is usually associated with only a 10 per cent reduction in cholesterol. Patients who have LDL cholesterol levels above 160 mg/dl should be treated with drugs in addition to diet. Patients with total cholesterol above 300 mg/dl often require therapy with more than a single drug.

Nicotinic acid is a B vitamin that is effective in all types of hyperlipoproteinemia except type I. It decreases LDL by about 25 per cent by blocking hepatic VLDL synthesis. This is associated with numerous side effects, including cutaneous flushing and gastrointestinal symptoms. Gastrointestinal side effects include gastritis, making it contraindicated in patients with peptic ulcer disease. It also causes abnormalities of liver function, impairment of glucose tolerance, and hyperuricemia, which is usually a significant problem only in patients with preexisting gout or diabetes.

Neomycin sulfate is an aminoglycoside antibiotic that has been shown to decrease LDL by unknown means. It is not well absorbed in the gastrointestinal tract and has both potential nephrotoxic and hepatotoxic effects, so it is not frequently utilized.

Cholestyramine and *colestipol* are quaternary ammonium salts that act as ion exchange resins and bind bile salts in the intestine. This binding results in interruption of the enterohepatic circulation and causes an increased loss of cholesterol in the stool. Cholestyramine and colestipol are particularly effective in type II hyperlipoproteinemia. They are difficult to administer due to frequent side effects, predominantly involving gastrointestinal distress. They may bind concomitantly administered medications such as digitalis, phenobarbital, thiazides, warfarin, and tetracycline, and therefore may be associated with a decrease in the prothrombin time in patients taking warfarin.

Probucol is another drug that lowers LDL but also has the side effect of lowering HDL. Its mechanism of action is unknown at this time, but it is thought to increase clearance of LDL via the scavenger or macrophage pathways. It is most frequently used in conjunction with other agents such as the bile acid sequestrants.

Gemfibrozil is a fibric acid derivative that is effective in lowering VLDL, LDL, and triglycerides. Although the exact mechanism of action is unknown, it does appear to increase lipoprotein lipase activity. The most common side effects are nausea and gastrointestinal discomfort, although impaired glucose intolerance has also been noted. All fibric acid derivatives may potentiate the effects of coumarin anticoagulants so that patients on warfarin may have an increased prothrombin time and must be carefully monitored.

REFERENCE

1. Report of the National Cholesterol Education Program expert panel on detection, evaluation and treatment of high

blood cholesterol in adults. Arch. Intern. Med. *148*:36, 1988.

521-C, 522-A, 523-B   *(Braunwald, pp. 1304–1308)*

The physician should be aware that many drugs can affect the uptake and metabolism of beta blockers. Cimetidine reduces the hepatic metabolism of beta blockers, resulting in prolongation of the serum half-life and increased plasma levels. This is particularly true for the lipophilic beta blockers such as propranolol and metoprolol, in contrast to the hydrophilic blockers such as atenolol and nadolol, which are not as extensively metabolized. The barbiturates induce hepatic microsomal enzymes, and therefore enhance metabolism of beta blockers and reduce their plasmic levels. Although lidocaine has no effect on beta blockers, propranolol reduces the hepatic clearance of lidocaine and may result in increased lidocaine levels.

Aluminum hydroxide gel, a common form of antacid, can delay or reduce gastrointestinal absorption of beta blockers, causing diminished plasma levels. This is particularly important with respect to hydrophilic beta blockers such as atenolol and nadolol, which normally are not as readily absorbed from the gastrointestinal tract and whose action is more affected by concomitant administration of these antacids. Calcium carbonate antacids do *not* alter absorption.

There are a number of interactions of the beta blockers with commonly administered drugs. The hypotension, bradycardia, and negative inotropy associated with verapamil may be additive with beta blockers, and concomitant usage requires careful patient monitoring. Aminophylline, which increases cyclic AMP by inhibiting phosphodiesterase, is antagonized by concurrent use of beta blockers. This effect may contribute to the bronchoconstriction observed in patients with asthma. Propranolol may also induce hypoglycemia and exacerbate the effects of antidiabetic agents, particularly long-acting drugs. Finally, the withdrawal syndrome observed in patients on clonidine, resulting in increased epinephrine release, may be exacerbated by beta blockade due to resulting unopposed alpha-adrenoceptor tone.

524-E, 525-C, 526-C, 527-D   *(Braunwald, pp. 1061–1066; Table 32–11; Figs. 32–49 through 32–52)*

The development of artificial cardiac valves has dramatically improved the surgical outcome for all patients with valvular heart disease. The valves can be classified into mechanical prostheses and bioprosthetic tissue valves as well as into the various subtypes of discs, balls, and cages that are utilized to approximate normal valve function.

Mechanical prosthetic valves are classified into two groups: caged ball and tilting disc valves. The Starr-Edwards caged ball valve was one of the earliest valves and has a long record of predictable performance. However, its major disadvantage is a bulky cage design, which makes it unsuitable for patients with a small LV cavity or a small aortic annulus. Furthermore, the flow characteristics and action of the ball in the cage result in low-level hemolysis and elevation of lactate dehydrogenase. Tilting disc valves have become more widely employed, primarily because they are less bulky and may have a lower profile than the caged ball valve. The Lillehei-Kaster valve is a pivoting disc valve that has a relatively high incidence of thrombosis, precluding its use for smaller aortic orifices or in the mitral position. The St. Jude valve has two semicircular discs that pivot between open and closed positions without need for supporting struts. It has a lower transvalvular gradient than other caged ball or tilting disc types and appears to have particularly favorable hemodynamic characteristics in the smaller sizes, making it especially useful in children and in the mitral position in adults, in whom it appears to be the least thrombogenic of all mechanical prostheses.

All of the mechanical prosthetic valves are extremely durable, lasting up to 20 years, but they are associated with a high incidence of thromboembolism, greatest in the first postoperative year. Without anticoagulation the incidence of thromboembolism is three- to sixfold higher than in properly anticoagulated patients.[1] Despite treatment with anticoagulants, the incidence of thromboembolic complications with the best mechanical prosthesis is still 1 to 2 nonfatal events per 100 patient years. The incidence is significantly higher for prostheses in the mitral than in the aortic position. Thrombosis of mechanical prostheses in the tricuspid position is extremely high, most likely due to the lower transvalvular pressure gradients, and for this reason bioprostheses are preferred at this site. Furthermore, administration of warfarin carries its own mortality and morbidity, estimated at 0.2 and 2.2 per 100 patient years, respectively.

Because of the high risk of thromboembolism inherent in the mechanical prosthetic valves, tissue valves have been developed. Among the tissue valves that are currently available, the Hancock valve is a porcine heterograft valve, as is the Carpentier-Edwards. There also is an Ionescu-Shiley pericardial xenograft consisting of bovine pericardium. This valve appears to have a relatively high primary failure rate due to calcification and tearing at the attachments to the struts and is therefore not widely used. Recently, human homograft valves have been utilized with increasing success.

The porcine heterografts require anticoagulation during the first 3 months while the sewing ring becomes endothelialized. Thereafter, anticoagulants are not required for porcine valves in the aortic position and the thromboembolic rate is approximately 1 to 2 per 100 patient years without these drugs.[2] Patients with these valves in the mitral valve position who are in sinus rhythm generally do not require anticoagulant treatment. However, in patients in atrial fibrillation these valves are associated with an increased incidence of thromboembolism most likely due to LA thrombi. Anticoagulation is, in general, advocated.

In terms of selecting artificial valves, the relative risks and benefits of durability, endocarditis, hemodynamics, high versus low profile, and thromboembolism must be evaluated. In general, tissue valves are preferred over mechanical prostheses in patients in whom anticoagulation is difficult or in whom it is especially hazardous because they are prone to hemorrhage or are noncompliant. The common recommendation is to employ mechanical prosthetic valves in patients under the age of 65 to 70 who have no contraindications to anticoagulants. Bioprostheses are recommended for patients with coexisting disease that is likely to make them prone to hemorrhage, those who are noncompliant, those unable to take anticoagulants for other reasons, women who may become pregnant, and those in advanced age.

REFERENCES

1. Harker, L.A.: Antithrombotic therapy following mitral valve replacement. *In* Duran, C., et al. (eds.): Recent Progress in Mitral Valve Disease. London, Butterworth's, 1984, pp. 340–348.
2. Zussa, C., Ottino, G., diSumma, M., et al.: Porcine cardiac bioprostheses: Evaluation of long-term results in 990 patients. Ann. Thorac. Surg. 39:243, 1985.

528-C, 529-B, 530-A, 531-A   *(Braunwald, pp. 1503–1504; Table 43–8; Fig. 43–21)*

Clinical distinction between patients with constrictive pericarditis and those with restrictive physiology due to such diseases as amyloidosis, hemochromatosis, and the hypereosinophilic syndrome may be difficult. Both restrictive cardiomyopathy and constrictive pericarditis may show the electrocardiographic changes of atrial fibrillation, left atrial abnormality, diffuse low voltage, and T-wave flattening. The presence of atrioventricular block and conduction disturbances may favor the diagnosis of restrictive cardiomyopathy. While findings at cardiac catheterization may be of some help in differentiating these two conditions, some patients will defy all analyses and a final diagnosis of one entity or the other will not be possible. In both conditions, RV and LV diastolic pressures are elevated, stroke volume and cardiac output are decreased, and LV end-diastolic volume is normal or decreased, with impaired diastolic filling. A frame-by-frame analysis of LV filling in one study has been used as a method to differentiate between constrictive pericarditis and restrictive cardiomyopathy,[1] demonstrating that early diastolic filling tends to be excessively rapid (80 per cent in the first half of diastole) in constrictive pericarditis in

contrast with that seen in restrictive cardiomyopathy.

A diagnosis of restrictive cardiomyopathy is more likely when marked RV systolic hypertension is present (pressure >60 mm Hg) and is also suggested when LV and RV diastolic pressures at rest or during exercise differ by more than 5 mm Hg.[2] It should be noted, however, that some patients with restrictive cardiomyopathy may have hemodynamics at rest and during exercise which are indistinguishable from constrictive pericarditis, including sustained and complete equilibration of RV and LV pressures as well as the presence of a dip-and-plateau pattern in the ventricular waveform.[3] Angiography in these conditions reveals a straightening of the right heart border in both cases, as well as thickening of the heart border due to either pericardial or myocardial thickening. Echocardiographic examination in some patients with restrictive cardiomyopathy may reveal abnormal ventricular myocardial thickening with a peculiar "sparkling" appearance if amyloidosis is present. However, in general, echocardiography is not capable of distinguishing between these two entities in a definitive manner. Endomyocardial biopsy may prove useful in the diagnosis of amyloidosis or hemochromatosis[4] but does not provide an adequate method for distinguishing between constriction and restriction on a consistent basis.

REFERENCES

1. Tyberg, T.I., Goodyer, A.V.N., Hurst, V.W., et al.: Left ventricular filling in differentiating restrictive amyloid cardiomyopathy and constrictive pericarditis. Am. J. Cardiol. 47:791, 1981.
2. Meaney, E., Shebatai, R., and Bhargava, V.: Cardiac amyloidosis, constrictive pericarditis and restrictive cardiomyopathy. Am. J. Cardiol. 38:547, 1976.
3. Lorell, B.H., and Grossman, W.: Profiles in constrictive pericarditis, restrictive cardiomyopathy, and cardiac tamponade. *In* Grossman, W., and Baum, D.S. (eds.): Cardiac Catheterization, Angiography, and Intervention. 4th ed. Philadelphia, Lea & Febiger, 1991, pp. 633–653.
4. Eagle, K.A., and Southern, J.F.: A 62-year-old woman with rightsided congestive heart failure. N. Engl. J. Med. 319: 932, 1988.

532-E, 533-D, 534-B, 535-C, 536-A   *(Braunwald, pp. 1780–1783)*

The spondyloarthropathies, including ankylosing spondylitis, Reiter's syndrome, and psoriatic arthritis, have a predilection for arthritis of the sacroiliac and lumbosacral joints. These diseases are associated with the histocompatibility antigen HLA-B27 and are predominantly found in men. *Ankylosing spondylitis* is the most common of these syndromes to involve the heart, and classically causes dilatation of the aortic valve ring with fibrous thickening and inflammation. The aorta in ankylosing spondylitis is histologically similar to syphilitic aortitis, including adventitial scarring, intimal proliferation, and narrowing of the vasa vasora. Aortic regurgitation results from thickening of the valvular cusps and dilatation of the aortic root.[1] Conduction system disorders, due to fibrous infiltration in the atrioventricular node and the bundle, may be seen in ankylosing spondylitis as well.

Reiter's syndrome is a form of nonpurulent, reactive arthritis, often following enteric or urogenital infections. Reiter's syndrome is often associated with uveitis/conjunctivitis and nongonococcal urethritis. The cardiac complications of Reiter's syndrome are similar to those of ankylosing spondylitis.

The etiology of the cardiac dysfunction in patients with *progressive systemic sclerosis/scleroderma* is unclear. It may be difficult to discern whether the cardiac complications are due to primary myocardial disease or problems related to systemic or pulmonary hypertension. Nonetheless, there are classical changes associated with this syndrome. The myocardium often becomes fibrotic and necrotic with the development of contraction band necrosis.[2] Pericardial effusions and adhesions may lead to symptomatic pericarditis. Conduction defects, along with valvular abnormalities, including thickening of the mitral and aortic valves, may also occur. Systemic vasculitis syndromes may directly affect the cardiovascular system, depending on the size and type of vessel that is inflamed.

Giant cell arteritis/large vessel arteritis predominantly causes inflammation of the aorta, its major branches, and coronary arteries. Weakening of the vessels may lead to dilatation, aneurysm formation, and valvular insufficiency. The vascular pathology often reveals granuloma formation. Treatment of giant cell arteritis initially involves large doses of steroids. If no improvement is seen in 6 to 8 weeks, cytotoxic therapy may be instituted.

Behçet's syndrome is a multisystem disorder highlighted by recurrent oral and genital ulcers and uveitis. The ulcers are often painful and necrotic, and eye involvement occasionally progresses to blindness. The etiology of the disease is unclear, but appears to involve endothelial dysfunction, and vasculitis is present in most individuals.[3] Venous and arterial thrombosis may occur, along with aneurysm formation of the large vessels. Diffuse aortitis in Behçet's syndrome can lead to valvular insufficiency and aortic root dilation.[4] Laboratory abnormalities may include an elevated erythrocyte sedimentation rate or C-reactive protein and antibodies to human oral mucosa proteins.

REFERENCES

1. O'Neil, T.W., King, G., Graham, J.M., et al.: Echocardiographic abnormalities in ankylosing spondylitis. Ann. Rheum. Dis. *51*(6): 705, 1992.
2. Anuari, A., Graninger, W., Schneider, B., et al.: Cardiac involvement in systemic sclerosis. Am. Heart J. *35*:1356, 1992.
3. Mendelsohn, M.E., and Loscalzo, J.: The endotheliopathies: Endothelial dysfunction in clinical disorders. *In* Thrombosis and Hemorrhage. Boston, Little, Brown & Company, 1993.
4. Tai, Y.T., Fong, P.C., Ng, W.F., et al.: Diffuse aortitis complicating Behçet's disease leading to severe aortic regurgitation. Cardiology *79*:156, 1991.

537-B, 538-A, 539-E, 540-D, 541-C *(Braunwald, pp. 1464–1471)*

Benign cardiac myxomas are the most common type of primary adult cardiac tumor. Most myxomas occur sporadically and three-quarters occur in females. About 7 per cent of myxomas occur in an autosomal dominant pattern and may be part of a syndrome that involves a complex of abnormalities, including blue nevi, lentigines, or a variety of endocrine tumors. Most myxomas occur in the left atrium and over 90 per cent are solitary.[1] Signs and symptoms suggestive of cardiac myxoma include dyspnea, syncope, mitral valve dysfunction, and embolic phenomena. Constitutional symptoms associated with myxoma, including fever and weight loss, may be due to the synthesis and secretion of interleukin-6.[2]

Approximately 25 per cent of all cardiac tumors are malignant, and the vast majority of these are part of the sarcoma family. While cardiac sarcomas may be seen at any age, they are more common between the third and fifth decades, show no sex preference, and are found most frequently in the right atrium. These tumors are usually aggressive, with distant metastases and obstruction of cardiac flow as frequent complications. Because the right atrium is more commonly affected, presentations of the disease may include right-sided heart failure or superior vena cava obstruction. Surgery and chemotherapy remain the mainstays of treatment; however, the long-term prognosis remains poor.

Rhabdomyomas are the most common pediatric cardiac tumors, occurring primarily in patients less than 1 year old. They occur equally in the right and left ventricle, and approximately a third involve the atrium. Rhabdomyomas are strongly associated with tuberous sclerosis, a familial condition including seizures, mental retardation, adenoma sebaceum, and multiple hamartomas.[3] Some believe that rhabdomyomas are actually myocardial hamartomas rather than true neoplasms.

Lipomatous tumors are subendocardial or subpericardial growths occurring in the ventricles, atria, and interatrial septum. The lesions are usually well encapsulated and contain fibrous connective and muscular tissue, as well as fatty tissue. Lipomas occur equally in males and females and range in diameter from 1 to 15 cm. Most produce symptoms by obstruction or compression. AV or intraventricular conduction disturbances may be noted. Lipomatous hypertrophy of the interatrial septum may be seen in obese, elderly females and most often appears as an echocardiographically detected protrusion into the right atrium. Various atrial arrhythmias may accompany this entity, but the exact relationship is unclear.

Papillary fibroelastomas are the most common tumors of cardiac valves. These tumors may involve adjacent endocardial tissue and may occur on any valve or papillary muscle or chordae tendineae. Most often, the atrial surface of atrioventricular valves and the ventricular surface of semi-lunar valves are affected. In adults, the mitral and aortic valves are more commonly affected by these benign tumors. Papillary fibroelastomas are likely the result of endocardial trauma or organized thrombus, and most cause symptoms by embolization or obstruction.

REFERENCES

1. Carney, J.A.: Differences between nonfamilial and familial cardiac myxoma. Am. J. Surg. Pathol. *9*:53, 1985.
2. Seguin, J.R., Beigbeder, J.Y., Hvass, U., et al.: Interleukin-6 production by cardiac myxomas may explain constitutional symptoms. J. Thorac. Cardiovasc. Surg. *103*:599, 1992.
3. Bass, J.L., Breningstall, G.N., and Swaiman, K.F.: Echocardiographic incidence of cardiac rhabdomyoma in tuberous sclerosis. Am. J. Cardiol. *55*:137, 1985.

542-A, 543-A, 544-D, 545-B, 546-B   *(Braunwald, pp. 918–921)*

Discrete subaortic stenosis accounts for between 8 and 10 per cent of all cases of congenital aortic stenosis (AS) and is seen more commonly in males than in females. The disorder is characterized by a membranous diaphragm that encircles the left ventricular outflow tract beneath the base of the aortic valve. While the diastolic murmur of aortic regurgitation is heard more commonly in this disorder and an ejection sound is rarely appreciated, distinction of subvalvular from valvular AS is difficult by clinical means alone. Dilatation of the ascending aorta is common in this condition, but calcification of the valve itself is not observed. Echocardiography has proved extremely useful in the diagnosis of this disorder and in identifying the coexistence of hypertrophic subaortic stenosis or in differentiating between these two disorders. The definitive diagnosis, however, is provided by recording pressure tracings as a catheter is withdrawn across the outflow tract or by direct visualization of the site of obstruction with LV angiography. The mild aortic regurgitation that is commonly appreciated in patients with discrete subaortic stenosis appears to be a result of thickening of the valve and decreased mobility of valve cusps due to trauma created by a high-velocity stream of blood flowing through the subaortic diaphragm. Discrete subaortic stenosis of any degree merits consideration for elective repair. Operative repair is frequently curative.[1]

Supravalvular AS is a congenital narrowing of the ascending aorta, which originates at the superior margin of the sinuses of Valsalva above the level of the coronary arteries. Three anatomical types of supravalvular AS are recognized, the most common of which is the hourglass type in which thickening and disorganization of the aortic media leads to a constriction or annular ridge at the superior margin of the sinuses of Valsalva. Less commonly a membrane is noted, with a small central opening stretched across the lumen of the aorta. A

third form occurs in which uniform hypoplasia of the ascending aorta is also noted. What makes the clinical picture of supravalvular obstruction unique is its association with idiopathic infantile hypercalcemia, a disease that may be related to abnormal vitamin D metabolism.[2] "Williams syndrome" is a term applied to the constellation of clinical findings that includes the cardiac abnormalities of supravalvular aortic stenosis and a multisystem disorder. The disorder includes a peculiar elfin facies (see Braunwald, Fig. 29–36, p. 920), mental retardation, auditory hyperacusis, narrowing of peripheral, systemic, and pulmonary arteries, inguinal hernia, strabismus, and abnormalities of dental development. Some patients may show an association of valvular pulmonary stenosis or peripheral pulmonary artery stenosis, and rarely mitral valve abnormalities may occur. However, tricuspid stenosis is not a part of this syndrome or of the disease discrete subaortic stenosis. While the physical findings in supravalvular AS resemble those in valvular AS for the most part, the presence of an especially prominent transmission of a thrill or murmur into the jugular notch, a late systolic or continuous murmur due to peripheral pulmonary artery stenoses, or a significant difference between the arterial pressures recorded in the upper extremities may suggest the diagnosis of supravalvular AS. This last finding occurs due to selective streaming of blood into the innominate artery from the constricting lesion.[3]

Echocardiography is extremely valuable in localizing the site of obstruction of supravalvular AS, and retrograde aortic catheterization may be used to quantitate precisely the degree of hemodynamic abnormality present. Operative repair of this disorder is most successful when little or no hypoplasia of the ascending aorta and arch is present and when the obstruction is discrete and significant. In these instances, the aortic lumen may be widened by the insertion of a fabric patch. In patients with a markedly hypoplastic ascending aorta, however, operative repair usually succeeds only in displacing the pressure gradient distally and is therefore not advised.

REFERENCES

1. Newfeld, E.A., Muster, A.J., Paul, M.H., et al.: Discrete subvalvular aortic stenosis in childhood, Am. J. Cardiol. *38*: 53, 1976.
2. Taylor, A.B., Stern, R.H., and Bell, N.H.: Abnormal regulation of circulating 25-hydroxy vitamin D in the Williams syndrome. N. Engl. J. Med. *306*:972, 1982.
3. Goldstein, R.E., and Epstein, S.E.: Mechanism of elevated innominate artery pressures in supravalvular aortic stenosis. Circulation *42*:23, 1970.

547-C, 548-B, 549-D, 550-A   *(Braunwald, pp. 1804–1805)*

Numerous cardiac medications can cause hematological complications. As with the administration of any drug, the practitioner must be keenly aware of possible side effects of such medications to the patient. Most often, discontinuation of the offending drug results in resolution of symptoms.

Heparin is a widely used medication for cardiovascular patients. Heparin-induced thrombocytopenia (HIT) is a potentially serious problem, with a reported incidence of up to 30 per cent.[1] Two types of HIT have been described. Type I HIT is mild (platelet counts ranging from 100,000 to 150,000/mm³), occurs during the first few days of heparin treatment, and may resolve even with the continuation of the medication. In contrast, type II HIT produces a more severe thrombocytopenia (often 60,000/mm³), begins after 4 to 14 days of heparin therapy, and will resolve only with the discontinuation of the medicine. The pathogenesis of the thrombocytopenia in type II HIT is related to IgG binding to platelets which leads to platelet aggregation and microthrombotic complications. Platelet counts often return to baseline after 5 to 7 days, but will decline again if rechallenged with heparin.

A positive direct Coombs' test is seen in up to 10 per cent of patients who receive the antihypertensive agent alpha-methyldopa. In these patients, the IgG antibody is directed against the Rh complex of red cells. Hemolysis may be severe, but improves within several weeks after cessation of the medication. The direct Coombs' test may remain positive for up to a year despite withdrawal of the drug.

Methemoglobinemia may result from exposure to a wide variety of agents, including nitroglycerin, sulfonamides, and lidocaine, all chemicals that can oxidize ferrous (Fe^{2+}) hemoglobin to the ferric (Fe^{3+}) state. Patients with methemoglobinemia have an oxygen dissociation curve which is shifted to the left, have normal PO_2 levels, and appear cyanotic because of the decreased oxygen-carrying capacity of the ferric hemoglobin. Patients with methemoglobinemia may complain of nonspecific symptoms such as dizziness, fatigue, and headache or may present with respiratory distress, seizures, and arrhythmias. Blood with high levels of methemoglobin is chocolate brown colored. The syndrome is usually corrected by discontinuation of the offending agent; however, exchange transfusions or methylene blue therapy may be necessary.

Procainamide, along with drugs such as hydralazine, isoniazid, and chlorpromazine, may cause a syndrome resembling systemic lupus erythematosus (SLE). The syndrome consists of polyarthralgias, pleuritis, a photosensitive rash, and other systemic symptoms of SLE. Nephritis and CNS disease are rare with drug-induced lupus. Patients with drug-induced lupus are ANA positive with antibodies to histones, but rarely have hypocomplementemia or antibodies to DNA. Discontinuation of the offending drug will likely result in improvement of symptoms within a few days to weeks. A short course of glucocorticoids may be helpful if symptoms are severe. ANA levels may remain elevated for years.

REFERENCES

1. Schmitt, P.B., and Adelman, B.: Heparin-associated thrombocytopenia: A critical review and pooled analysis. Am. J. Med. Sci. *305*:208, 1993.
2. Chong, B.H.: Heparin-induced thrombocytopenia. Br. J. Haematol. *89*:431, 1995.

551-C, 552-B, 553-D, 554-A, 555-D   (Braunwald, pp. 1592–1598)

The treatment of pulmonary embolism continues to evolve. Heparin has long been considered the "traditional" therapy, but thrombolytic agents have had a varying and increasing role over the years. Heparin is a porcine- or bovine-derived glycosaminoglycan that acts by binding to antithrombin III and inhibits the procoagulant factors including thrombin, Xa, IXa, XIa, and XIIa. Heparin prevents additional thrombus formation and promotes endogenous fibrinolysis; however, it does not directly dissolve thrombus. Activated partial thromboplastin times (aPTT) should be measured and maintained at least 1.5 to 2 times control values for the treatment of a blood clot with heparin. A plasma heparin level may be useful when the PTT is elevated at baseline (e.g., lupus anticoagulant), or when monitoring patients with DVT/PE who require large quantities of heparin.[1] For initiation of heparin therapy and maintenance dosing, consider following the "Raschke" weight-based nomogram (Braunwald, Table 46–13, p. 1593).

Protamine may be used to reverse the anticoagulant effects of heparin. The dose of protamine is based on the amount of heparin given to the patient (~1 mg/100 units of heparin). Protamine should be given with caution to patients who are taking NPH insulin. The major complication of heparin therapy is hemorrhage. Thrombocytopenia, osteopenia, osteoporosis, and elevated liver enzymes may all be seen with heparin usage. In addition, heparin may cause aldosterone depression a few days after the initiation of the drug. This effect can result in hyperkalemia, especially in patients with renal failure or diabetes.

30 years ago, trials were conducted to compare the efficacy of urokinase to that of heparin in dissolving pulmonary clots.[3] These studies showed that thrombolytic therapy with heparin and urokinase reduced mortality and recurrent PE when compared to heparin alone. In recent studies, it has been shown that patients with normal right ventricular function who present with small to moderate pulmonary emboli do well if given anticoagulation alone.[3] For those who present with right ventricular dysfunction, there is now an increasing literature on the efficacy of using thrombolytic agents.[4] Streptokinase (given as an initial loading dose and followed by a drip for 24 hours), urokinase (given as a loading dose and followed by a continuous infusion for 12 to 14 hours) and rt-PA (given as a 2-hour infusion) are all FDA-approved regimens for the treatment of pulmonary embolism.

These agents work primarily by dissolving the thrombus, and unlike myocardial infarction regimens for thrombolytic therapy, patients with PE may be treated effectively up to 2 weeks after the onset of signs or symptoms.

Dextran, not heparin or the thrombolytic agents, is a polysaccharide anticoagulant that inhibits leukocyte plugging, platelet adhesion, and erythrocyte aggregation. In some cases, dextran may be used clinically as an anticoagulant, especially if there is a contraindication to the use of more traditional agents. In general, neither heparin nor thrombolytic agents need to be administered with an antiplatelet agent.

REFERENCES

1. Levine, M.N., Hirsh, J., Gent, M., et al.: A randomized trial comparing activated thromboplastin time with heparin assay in patients with acute venous thromboembolism requiring large daily doses of heparin. Arch. Intern. Med. 154:49, 1994.
2. Urokinase pulmonary embolism trial: A national cooperative study. Circulation 47 and 48 (Suppl. II): 1, 1973.
3. Wolfe, M.W., Lee, R.T., Feldstein, M.L., et al.: Prognostic significance of right ventricular hypokinesis and perfusion lung scan defects in pulmonary embolism. Am. Heart J. 127:1371, 1994.
4. Goldhaber, S.Z.: Contemporary pulmonary embolism thrombolysis. Chest 107:45S, 1995.

556-D, 557-C, 558-B, 559-B, 560-A *(Braunwald, pp. 992–993)*

Type II glycogen storage disease (Pompe's disease) is an autosomal recessive disorder that results from a deficiency of a lysosomal enzyme that hydrolyzes glycogen into glucose. This results in deposition of excessive amounts of glycogen in a generalized fashion, but especially in the heart, the skeletal muscles, and the liver. The clinical consequences include cardiomegaly—often of a marked degree—and the subsequent development of congestive heart failure. The disease usually is detected in the early neonatal period and is marked by a failure to thrive, progressive hypotonia, lethargy, and a weak cry.[1] The ECG may demonstrate extremely tall and broad QRS complexes, with a P-R interval that is commonly less than 0.09 sec. This shortening of the P-R interval may be caused by facilitated atrioventricular conduction as a consequence of the glycogen deposition. The differential diagnosis includes other causes of cardiac failure in the early months of life, including endocardial fibroelastosis, anomalous pulmonary origin of the left coronary artery, the variety of fixed and dynamic forms of LV outflow tract obstruction, coarctation of the aorta, and myocarditis. The presence of skeletal muscular *hypotonia* and short P-R interval helps to suggest the diagnosis of glycogen storage disease type II. The disease is uniformly fatal, and patients usually die within the first year of life.

The mucocutaneous lymph node syndrome (Kawasaki disease) was first described in Japan in 1967 and has subsequently been reported both in Asia and throughout Europe and North America. The disease usually occurs in children between the ages of 2 and 10 years and is commonly associated with a fever lasting 5 days or longer that is unresponsive to antibiotics, as well as bilateral congestion of the ocular conjunctivae and fissuring of the lips, injected oropharangeal mucosa, and strawberry tongue. These manifestations may then be followed by a rash and edema of the hands and feet, accompanied by palmar and plantar erythema. The disease progresses to a phase of cutaneous desquamation within approximately 2 weeks. Other noncardiovascular complications of the illness may include arthritis, pulmonary infiltrates, and hydrops of the gallbladder. In addition, cervical adenopathy, diarrhea, and a variety of laboratory abnormalities may become apparent.

The etiology of Kawasaki disease continues to be obscure, although some evidence for a viral cause has been accumulated. Cardiovascular involvement in the disorder may include myocarditis and pericarditis resulting in congestive heart failure and/or arrhythmias. Coronary angiitis, which may include the development of coronary artery aneurysms, is also noted. These cardiac complications are primarily responsible for the associated acute mortality of 1 to 3 per cent in the disease. Approximately half of the children who develop coronary artery aneurysms during the acute phase of Kawasaki disease have normal-appearing vessels by angiography 1 to 2 years following the illness.[2] No treatment has proven effective in the prevention of coronary artery aneurysms, although a variety of agents have been utilized. Apparently, corticosteroid therapy during the acute phase of the illness is detrimental, while high-dose salicylate treatment is advised in all patients. Recently, investigators have had success using gamma globulin during the acute phase, with substantial reduction in the formation of coronary arterial aneurysms.[3] In general, coronary angiography is recommended in patients with symptoms of cardiovascular involvement and/or signs of such involvement by physical examination or laboratory evaluation.

REFERENCES

1. Hwang, G., Meng, C.C., Lin, C.Y., and Hsu, H.C.: Clinical analysis of five infants with glycogen storage disease of the heart—Pompe's disease. Jpn. Heart J. 27:25, 1986.
2. Kato, H., Ichinose, E., Matsunaga, S., et al.: Fate of coronary aneurysms in Kawasaki disease: Serial coronary angiography and long-term follow-up study. Am. J. Cardiol. 49: 1758, 1982.
3. Newburger, J.W., Takahasi, M., Burns, J.C., et al.: The treatment of Kawasaki syndrome with intravenous gamma globulin. N. Engl. J. Med. 315:341, 1986.

561-A, 562-C, 563-A, 564-D, 565-B *(Braunwald, pp. 1112–1114; Figs. 34–10 and 34–11)*

The fatty streak is the earliest lesion of atherosclerosis and can usually be found in the aorta of young children. On gross inspection, a fatty streak has a yellow discoloration due to the large amount of lipid deposited in the foam cells that comprise the lesion. These foam cells are principally lipid-laden macrophages, together with a small number of lipid-filled smooth muscle cells that accumulate beneath the macrophage layer as the lesions enlarge.[1] The lipid that is present is in the form of cholesteryl ester or cholesterol. Analyses of the distribution of fatty streaks in coronary arteries of children and young adults reveal that they occupy the same anatomical sites as the more advanced lesions (fibrous plaques) of atherosclerosis. Over time, fatty streaks enlarge to occupy an increasing surface area of the coronary arteries, and these sites often precede the formation of advanced lesions. Data such as these lend support to the notion that the fatty streak is in many instances—if not in most—the precursor to the advanced occlusive form of atherosclerosis. Using monoclonal antibodies directed against cell-specific markers, the fatty streak has been demonstrated to consist principally of lipid-laden macrophages, regardless of its site of origin (see Braunwald, Fig. 34–10, p. 1112).

The more advanced lesion of atherosclerosis is usually termed the "fibrous plaque." Fibrous plaques appear grossly white, and often protrude into the lumen of the artery.[2] Therefore, they are more likely to become involved in thrombosis, hemorrhage, and/or calcification. Fibrous plaques consist of a variety of cells, especially large numbers of intimal smooth muscle cells, along with macrophages. Lipid deposition in both of these cell types occurs in the fibrous plaque. In addition, fibrous plaques seem to be covered consistently by a fibrous tissue cap. The fibrous plaque lesion appears to be composed of several layers. The fibrous cap of each lesion involves a smooth muscle cell and connective tissue matrix, which is exceedingly dense. Beneath this may be found a mixture of smooth muscle cells, macrophages, and lymphocytes. Large amounts of connective tissue are also found in this cellular sublayer. Still deeper in the fibrous plaque, there is frequently a zone of necrotic tissue, which may contain areas of cholesterol and calcification, as well as enlarged foam cells. Interestingly, the material that constitutes a fibrous plaque varies, depending upon the individual risk factors present in a given patient. For example, it is common that fibrous plaques observed in the femoral arteries of heavy cigarette smokers are extremely fibrous, with relatively little lipid, while those from individuals with hypercholesterolemia often have large areas of lipid deposition within the plaque.[2]

The general pattern of distribution of advanced atherosclerotic lesions in humans shows a predilection for the abdominal aorta, with lesions most prominent near the ostia of major branches. The renal arteries appear to be spared from atherosclerosis except at their ostia. Coronary arteries generally demonstrate a more intense involvement with atherosclerosis, and lesions are often located within their first 6 cm. Understanding the cell types and patterns that constitute both the developing and mature lesions of atherosclerosis is important to formulating hypotheses of both atherogenesis and of the conversion of a plaque from the quiescent to the clinically active state.

REFERENCES

1. Masuda, J., and Ross, R.: Atherogenesis during low-level hypercholesterolemia in the nonhuman primate: I. Fatty streak formation. Arteriosclerosis 10:164, 1990.
2. Masuda, J., and Ross, R.: Atherogenesis during low-level hypercholesterolemia in the nonhuman primate: II. Fatty streak conversion to fibrous plaque. Arteriosclerosis 10:178, 1990.

566-A, 567-C, 568-B, 569-A, 570-B   *(Braunwald, pp. 924–926; 1054–1056; 1059–1060)*

Tricuspid stenosis (TS) is most commonly rheumatic in origin and almost never occurs as an isolated lesion but rather usually accompanies mitral valve disease, with involvement of the aortic valve frequently noted as well. The pathophysiology of the lesion is quite similar to that of mitral stenosis (MS). The lesion results in a characteristic low-cardiac-output state which presents as fatigue and right-sided heart failure, including uncomfortable hepatomegaly, abdominal swelling due to ascites, and anasarca. While MS is usually present with TS, the characteristic symptoms associated with that lesion are usually absent. Thus the absence of symptoms of pulmonary congestion in a patient with tight MS should suggest the possibility of TS. The physical findings are subtle and are notable for signs of right-sided heart failure in the presence of clear lung fields. Auscultation usually reveals signs of MS, and these often overshadow the more subtle findings of TS. The diastolic murmur of TS is commonly heard best along the lower left sternal border in the fourth intercostal space and is usually softer, higher pitched, and shorter in duration than the murmur of MS. The management of severe TS is surgical and requires mitral valvulotomy or valve replacement in patients in whom tricuspid orifice areas are less than approximately 2.0 cm². In general, tissue valves are used preferentially in the tricuspid position because of the risk of thrombosis with mechanical prostheses.

The most common form of pulmonic stenosis (PS) is congenital. A much rarer form of PS results from carcinoid plaques, present in the outflow tract of the right ventricle in patients with malignant carcinoid. These can cause constriction of the pulmonic valve ring, retraction and fusion of the cusps, and PS with or without accompanying pulmonic regurgitation. Carcinoid heart disease also involves the tricuspid valve and most commonly leads to tricuspid regurgitation. However, some degree of TS is sometimes noted with carcinoid involvement of the tricuspid valve.[1]

Most adults with mild to moderate PS are asymptomatic, and it is only in the more severe forms of the disease that symptoms of dyspnea and fatigue secondary to an inadequate cardiac output response to exercise are noted. Patients with severe grades of PS may develop tricuspid regurgitation and frank RV failure. The severity of PS is grouped according to the peak systolic pressure gradient between the RV and the pulmonary artery. Gradients of 50 to 79 mm Hg are considered moderate, while those greater than 80 mm Hg are severe. In most patients, valvular PS is a relatively stable or at most slowly progressive disease. The physical examination in patients with PS is notable for a systolic thrill present along the left upper sternal border of the chest, a prominent systolic ejection murmur heard most clearly in the location of the thrill, and often an associated ejection click. In contrast to the inspiratory increase in most right-sided cardiac sounds, the intensity of the pulmonic click in PS *decreases* with inspiration.[2] Increasing degrees of severity of PS lead to increases in both the length and the intensity of the murmur, with peaking of the murmur occurring later in systole in the more severe forms of the lesion. A normal pulmonic component of the second heart sound and a murmur that is less than grade 4 out of 6 in intensity suggests a gradient that is less than 80 mm Hg and hence at most moderate PS. Echocardiography can usually define the lesion, and Doppler echocardiography allows accurate estimation of the gradient across the pulmonary valve in many cases. In adults the use of percutaneous balloon valvuloplasty for typical valvular PS is both safe and effective and is now considered by many cardiologists to be the treatment of choice for this lesion.[3] Interestingly, studies have shown no significant restenosis in follow-up catheterizations of patients initially treated with balloon valvuloplasty.

REFERENCES

1. Ross, E.M., and Roberts, W.C.: The carcinoid syndrome. Comparison of 21 necropsy subjects with carcinoid heart disease. Am. J. Med. *79*:339, 1985.
2. Feldman, T., and Borow, K.M.: Adults with pulmonic stenosis: Management. Cardiovasc. Med. *9*:711, 1984.
3. Block, P.C., and Palacios, I.F.: Aortic and mitral balloon valvuloplasty: The United States experience. *In* Topol, E.J. (ed.): Textbook of Interventional Cardiology. Philadelphia. W.B. Saunders Company, 1990.

571-B, 572-B, 573-A, 574-B   *(Braunwald, pp. 1613–1614)*

Cor pulmonale is most commonly caused by chronic obstructive pulmonary disease (COPD). This term includes the diseases of chronic bronchitis, emphysema, and bronchial asthma. However, atopic asthma does *not* produce chronic cor pulmonale. In most patients with COPD, chronic bronchitis and emphysema coexist, but cor pulmonale is restricted to those with functionally significant airway disease (i.e., bronchitis, with or without emphysema).[1]

A common classification scheme places chronic bronchitis at one extreme and emphysema at the other in the continuum of COPD. Classically, patients with chronic bronchitis are termed "blue bloaters" and have chronic cough and sputum production, recurring respiratory infections, secondary erythrocytosis, and repeated bouts of right heart failure. Physiologically, these patients have hypoxemia and hypercapnea at rest, normal diffusion capacity, elevated residual volumes, and functional residual capacity, with relatively normal values for total lung capacity and pulmonary compliance. On chest x-ray, these patients usually have moderately hyperinflated lungs, increased bronchovascular markings, and rather commonly, cardiomegaly.

In contrast, patients with predominant emphysema, classically described as "pink puffers," present with dyspnea, while cough and sputum production are considerably less prominent. Erythrocytosis is uncommon, and right heart failure tends to occur only as a terminal event. Because these patients hyperventilate, the alveolar-arterial gradient for oxygen is abnormally elevated, but arterial oxygen tension is usually normal or slightly depressed and hypercapnea is rare. Standard spirometric indices are usually similar to those observed in chronic bronchitis, but the pink puffer has an abnormally low diffusing capacity and greatly increased lung volumes and pulmonary compliance. Because of this, the cardiac silhouette frequently appears smaller than normal. Because the primary pathological defect in this illness is destruction of the alveolar septa, these patients initially have normal or near-normal pulmonary artery pressures at rest, and it is only with severe loss of lung parenchyma that secondary changes occur in the vasculature leading to resting pulmonary artery hypertension and cor pulmonale. In contrast, patients with chronic bronchitis become hypoxic early in the course of their illness and therefore have elevated pulmonary pressures at rest.

REFERENCE

1. Murphy, M.L., Dinh, H., and Nicholson, D.: Chronic cor pulmonale. Dis. Mon. *35*:653, 1989.

575-A, 576-C, 577-D, 578-A, 579-B   *(Braunwald, pp. 964; 1041–1042; 1698)*

A illustrates a parasternal short-axis two-dimensional echocardiographic image at the level of the aortic valve in which a bicuspid (but otherwise normal) aortic valve is present. *B* illustrates a parasternal two-dimensional echocardiographic image of valvular aortic stenosis with thickening of the aortic valve leaflets and a decrease in aortic valve leaflet separation, or "doming."

A bicuspid aortic valve is probably the most common congenital cardiac anomaly. Most frequently, the bicuspid valve is functionally normal early in life but may become thickened, fibrotic, calcified, and stenotic during adulthood[1] (Figs. 32–26 and 32–27, p. 1036). By the age of 45, approximately half of all bicuspid valves show some degree of stenosis. The bicuspid valve is also a common cause of congenital valvular aortic stenosis (AS), a lesion that may be associated with coarctation of the aorta and, less frequently, atrial septal defect or isolated pulmonic stenosis. Thus in young or middle-aged adults, the presence of isolated valvular AS is usually congenital in origin rather than due to rheumatic disease. Interestingly, aortic valve prolapse may be noted in association with a bicuspid aortic valve,[2] and may occasionally lead to aortic regurgitation that requires valve replacement. Two-dimensional echocardiography is quite useful in making the diagnosis of bicuspid aortic valve, although the diagnosis can occasionally be confusing due to the presence on echocardiography of a fused commissure resembling a third leaflet.[3] All patients with known bicuspid aortic valve require antibiotic prophylaxis against infective endocarditis.

The changes causing AS that occur in a bicuspid valve resemble those occurring in senile degenerative calcific stenosis of a tricuspid aortic valve, which is illustrated in B. Senile calcific AS has a pathophysiology similar to stenosis occurring upon a bicuspid valve but presents several decades later. The natural history of this form of AS includes a long latent period during which a gradual increase in LV outflow tract obstruction occurs, leading to a similarly gradual increase in the pressure load on the LV while the patient remains asymptomatic.

In untreated patients, the appearance of any of the cardinal symptoms of AS heralds a poor prognosis. Thus, survival curves show that the interval from the onset of symptoms to the time of death is approximately 5 years in patients with angina, 3 years in patients with syncope, and 2 years in patients with congestive heart failure (see Braunwald, Fig. 32–32, p. 1042).[4] Approximately two-thirds of patients with critical AS have angina, which usually is similar clinically to angina that is observed in patients with coronary artery disease. It occurs because of the increased oxygen needs of the hypertrophied myocardium and/or reduction of oxygen delivery due to excessive compression of coronary vessels.[5]

Medical management of AS includes careful counseling of patients regarding the hazards of endocarditis and the need for endocarditis prophylaxis prior to both dental and invasive procedures, as well as discussions regarding the potential symptoms that may arise in the asymptomatic patient. It is crucial that patients understand that the earliest appearance of symptoms should be reported to their physician. In addition, noninvasive assessment of the severity of obstruction by Doppler echocardiography should be performed at regular intervals. In most adults with AS, aortic valve replacement should be recommended when symptoms appear and documented hemodynamic evidence of critical obstruction is present.

Ankylosing spondylitis leads to a dilatation of the aortic valve ring with fibrous thickening and scarring, as well as focal inflammatory lesions involving the aortic valve cusps. Dilatation of the sinuses of Valsalva and focal degenerative changes in the ascending aorta may also be involved. Aortic regurgitation may result from shortening and thickening of the valve cusps and their displacement by aortic root dilatation (see Braunwald, Fig. 56–6, p. 1780).

REFERENCES

1. Passik, C.S., Ackermann, D.M., Pluth, J.R., and Edwards, W.D. Temporal changes in the causes of aortic stenosis. A surgical pathologic study of 646 cases. Mayo. Clin. Proc. *62*:119, 1987.
2. Shapiro, L., Thwaites, B., Westgate, C., and Donaldson, R.: Prevalence and clinical significance of aortic valve prolapse. Br. Heart J. *54*:179, 1985.
3. Brandenburg, R.O., Tajik, A.J., Edwards, W.D., et al.: Accuracy of two-dimensional echocardiographic diagnosis of congenitally bicuspid aortic valve—echocardiographic-anatomic correlation in 115 patients. Am. J. Cardiol. *51*: 1469, 1983.
4. Ross, J., Jr., and Braunwald, E.: The influence of corrective operations on the natural history of aortic stenosis. Circulation *37*:(Suppl. V):61, 1968.
5. Lombard, J.T., and Selzer, A.: Valvular aortic stenosis: A clinical and hemodynamic profile of patients. Ann. Intern. Med. *106*:292, 1987.

580-C, 581-C, 582-D, 583-A   *(Braunwald, pp. 1243–1244)*

Rupture of the interventricular septum in the presence of AMI usually occurs secondary to anterior infarction and in patients with multivessel coronary artery disease.[1] Patients with an anterior infarction that leads to rupture tend to have a septal defect that is apical in location, whereas inferior infarctions are associated with perforation of the basal septum. Partial or total rupture of a papillary muscle in the setting of AMI usually is due to damage to the posteromedial papillary muscle resulting from inferior wall infarction. Such a papillary muscle rupture occurs with relatively small infarctions in approximately half of the cases, in contrast to rupture of the ventricular septum, which almost always occurs with larger infarct.[2]

Clinically, patients with both lesions develop a new murmur, which is usually holosystolic. The murmur associated with rupture of the interventricular septum is often more obvious, but clinical distinction between the two entities in question may be difficult. In both lesions, the murmur may decrease or disappear as arterial blood pressure falls with the progressive hemodynamic compromise that invariably ensues. The use of echocardiography to identify partial or complete rupture of a papillary muscle and ventricular septal defect is often helpful.[3] However, the definitive diagnosis and distinction between acute ventricular septal rupture and mitral regurgitation is accomplished by insertion of a pulmonary artery balloon catheter, which allows the detection of a "step-up" in oxygen saturation in blood samples from the right ventricle and pulmonary artery in patients who have developed an acute ventricular septal rupture.[4] Patients with both lesions may develop tall v waves in the pulmonary papillary wedge tracing; therefore, this finding is not useful in distinguishing between the two lesions. Hemodynamic monitoring of right and left ventricular filling pressures, as well as measurement of cardiac output and systemic vascular resistance, are helpful guides during vasodilator therapy. The latter may allow stabilization of a patient's condition prior to diagnostic catheterization and subsequent surgical repair.

REFERENCES

1. Radford, M.J., Johnson, R.A., Daggett, W.M., et al.: Ventricular septal rupture: A review of clinical and physiologic features and an analysis of survival. Circulation *64*:545, 1981.
2. Nishimura, R.A., Schaff, H.V., Shub, C., et al.: Papillary muscle rupture complicating acute myocardial infarction: Analysis of 17 patients. Am. J. Cardiol. *51*:373, 1983.
3. Come, P.C., Riley, M.F., Weintraub, R., et al.: Echocardiographic detection of complete and partial papillary muscle rupture during acute myocardial infarction. Am. J. Cardiol. *56*:787, 1985.
4. Meister, S.G., and Helfant, R.H.: Rapid bedside differentiation of ruptured interventricular septum from acute mitral insufficiency. N. Engl. J. Med. *287*:1024, 1972.

584-C, 585-B, 586-A, 587-B *(Braunwald, pp. 1503–1504; Table 43–8 and Fig. 43–21)*

The clinical and hemodynamic features of restrictive heart disease such as that which may be caused by cardiac amyloidosis are very similar to those of chronic constrictive pericarditis.[1] Endomyocardial biopsy, CT scanning, and magnetic resonance imaging may be useful in differentiating the two diseases. The typical hemodynamic feature present in both conditions is the deep and rapid early decline in ventricular pressure at the onset of diastole, with a rapid rise to a plateau in early diastole, termed the "square root" sign. In the atrial tracings, the dip and plateau is manifested as a prominent "y descent" followed by a rapid rise in pressure. The x descent may also be prominent, and the combination results in a characteristic M or W waveform in the atrial pressure tracing. Both systemic and pulmonary venous pressures are usually elevated. Patients with restrictive heart disease may have left ventricular filling pressures that exceed right ventricular filling pressures by more than 5 mm Hg, and this difference can be accentuated by exercise. This may be because in restrictive disease, as opposed to constrictive disease, the "encasement" of the heart is relative. Furthermore, the pulmonary artery systolic pressure may be

greater than 60 mm Hg in patients with restrictive cardiomyopathy but is usually lower in constrictive pericarditis. Finally, the plateau of the right ventricular diastolic pressure is usually at least one-third of the peak right ventricular systolic pressure in patients with constrictive pericarditis, while it is more commonly less than one-third in patients with restrictive cardiomyopathy.

REFERENCE

1. Lorell, B.H., and Grossman, W.: Profiles in constrictive pericarditis, restrictive cardiomyopathy, and cardiac tamponade. *In* Grossman, W., and Baim, D.S. (eds): Cardiac Catheterization, Angiography, and Intervention. 4th ed. Philadelphia, Lea & Febiger, 1991, pp. 633–653.

588-C, 589-A, 590-B, 591-B, 592-C *(Braunwald, pp. 1572–1574)*

Takayasu's arteritis, which is also referred to as "aortic arch syndrome," "pulseless disease," "reversed coarctation," "young female arteritis," and "occlusive thromboaortopathy," is a disease of unknown etiology characterized by marked fibrous and degenerative scarring of the elastic fibers of the vascular media. The disease may be subclassified depending upon sites of involvement and commonly involves the aorta and carotid arteries. The disease is much more common in women than it is in men, and in most patients the disease has its onset during the teenage years.[1] Patients not uncommonly present initially with a systemic illness characterized by fever, malaise, weight loss, night sweats, arthralgias, pleuritic pain, anorexia, and fatigue. Regardless of whether or not a patient goes through this initial phase, after a latent period, symptoms and signs referable to the obliterative and inflammatory changes in affected blood vessels begin to appear. These often include diminished or absent pulses, narrowing of affected arteries, hypertension, and in approximately one-fourth to one-third of patients, heart failure, which is usually seen in very young patients as a consequence of systemic hypertension.

A minority of patients have involvement primarily of the abdominal aorta and may therefore have abdominal angina, lower extremity claudication, and hypertension due to renal arterial involvement. More commonly, patients manifest symptoms and signs due to upper extremity arterial involvement. Common laboratory abnormalities include elevated sedimentation rate, low-grade leukocytosis, and mild normocytic anemia. A typical pattern is often seen on arteriography and may include a "rat-tail" appearance of the thoracic aorta (see Braunwald, Figs. 45–24 and 45–25, pp. 1573–1574).

Therapy of this disorder includes treatment with steroids of patients with documented systemic symptoms and/or clinical progression of the disease. In patients who remain unresponsive, cyclophosphamide may be added. In addition, platelet-inhibitory agents such as aspirin and dipyridamole are often used to treat the symptoms of transient ischemia as well as to prevent progression of the disease, although clinical trials of efficacy of these agents have not yet been performed. Survival in general depends on the degree and number of complications that develop during the course of the illness. The use of corticosteroid therapy, cytotoxic agents, and appropriate surgery has led to excellent 5-year survival rates.

Giant cell arteritis is a disease of unknown etiology characterized by granulomatous inflammation of the media of small- to medium-caliber arteries with a special predilection for vessels of the head and neck. The disease is also known as "granulomatous arteritis" and "temporal arteritis" and is seen primarily in elderly people. Clinically, the classic triad of severe headache, fever, and marked malaise characterize the illness. The headaches are often extremely severe and are typically localized over the involved temporal arteries. Claudication of the jaw muscles during chewing is present in up to two-thirds of patients and is considered to be very suggestive of the illness.[2] Involvement of the ophthalmic artery leads to visual symptoms in between 25 and 50 per cent of patients and may result in irreversible blindness. The syndrome of polymyalgia rheumatica, consisting of diffuse muscular aching and stiffness, occurs in close to 40 per cent of patients with giant cell arteritis.[3] In a minority of cases, involvement of the aorta or its major branches may lead to symptoms and signs similar to those of Takayasu's arteritis, although interestingly, renal artery involvement is almost never seen in this disorder.

Patients with giant cell arteritis appear ill and almost always have fever. Affected vessels feel abnormal to palpation and are tender, allowing experienced examiners to make the diagnosis of temporal arteritis at the bedside by identifying an indurated, beaded, tender, temporal artery. Laboratory tests often reveal a very high sedimentation rate, normochromic normocytic anemia, and elevated acute phase reactants. Biopsy of an involved temporal artery allows confirmation of the diagnosis.

Management of granulomatous arteritis includes early intervention with high-dose steroid therapy (60 to 80 mg of prednisone per day). Steroids may be titrated against the sedimentation rate and clinical symptoms and gradually tapered to a maintenance dose, which is typically continued for 1 to 2 years. Early administration of steroid therapy is crucial to the prevention of involvement of the ophthalmic arteries and possible blindness.

REFERENCES

1. Shelhamer, J.H., Volkman, D.J., Parillo, J.E., et al.: Takayasu's arteritis and its therapy. Ann. Intern. Med. 103:121, 1985.
2. Huston, K.A., and Hunder, G.G.: Giant cell (cranial) arteritis: A clinical review. Am. Heart J. 100:99, 1980.
3. Chuang, T., Hunder, G.G., Ilstrup, D.M., and Kurland, L.T.: Polymyalgia rheumatica. Ann. Intern. Med. 97:672, 1982.

593-C, 594-A, 595-A, 596-B   *(Braunwald, pp. 1022–1024, 1041)*

The systolic murmur is the most prominent auscultatory finding in mitral regurgitation (MR), but it must be differentiated from the systolic murmur heard in aortic stenosis (AS), tricuspid regurgitation, and ventricular septal defect. In most cases the systolic murmur of MR commences immediately after a soft S_1 and extends to S_2. The murmur may persist beyond S_2, obscuring A_2 in some instances because of a persistent pressure difference between the left ventricle and the left atrium. The holosystolic murmur in chronic MR is usually constant in intensity, blowing, high-pitched, and loudest at the apex. The murmur of AS, on the other hand, has a crescendo-decrescendo pattern, is usually much less musical than the murmur of MR, and is followed by a single S_2. However, these murmurs can frequently be confused with each other; several dynamic maneuvers are helpful in their differentiation.

The dynamic maneuvers can be conceptualized as altering either preload (the left ventricular end-diastolic pressure or volume) or afterload (left ventricular systolic pressure). In general, the intensity of regurgitant murmurs is reduced while that of stenotic murmurs is increased by a fall in afterload. Regurgitant murmurs are minimally affected by alterations in preload while stenotic murmurs are significantly affected by changes in preload. Thus, handgrip, which increases the peripheral resistance, tends to have little effect on the murmur of AS but will increase the murmur of MR. Amyl nitrite, which causes an immediate and marked drop in blood pressure, will make an MR murmur softer while an AS murmur will become louder due to the increased velocity of LV ejection following the reflex increase in cardiac output. During slow atrial fibrillation, with significant beat-to-beat variation in left ventricular stroke volume, there will be marked beat-to-beat changes in the intensity of the murmur of AS but little change in the murmur of MR; similar findings occur with ventricular premature beats. The murmurs of AS and MR are both usually diminished during the strain phase of the Valsalva maneuver due to a decrease in the preload with resulting decrease in total cardiac output and blood flow.[1]

REFERENCE

1. Dalen, J.E., and Alpert, J.S.: Valvular Heart Disease. 2nd ed. Boston, Little, Brown & Company, 1987.

597-C, 598-C, 599-C, 600-C, 601-C   *(Braunwald, pp. 935–940; 944–946)*

In complete transposition of the great arteries, the aorta arises from the right ventricle while the pulmonary artery arises from the left ventricle. Because the origin of the aorta is to the right and anterior to the main pulmonary artery, this disorder is often termed dextro or D-transposition. Complete transposition is a common and potentially lethal form of congenital heart disease. The resulting anatomical disarrangement results in two separate and parallel circulations that usually communicate through an atrial septal defect. In addition, two-thirds of the patients have a patent ductus arteriosus and about one-third have an associated ventricular septal defect. Infants with complete transposition are particularly susceptible to the early development of pulmonary vascular obstructive disease.[1] They usually present at birth with dyspnea and cyanosis as well as progressive hypoxemia and congestive heart failure. Cardiac murmurs are of little diagnostic significance and are actually absent in up to one-half of infants with complete transposition.

Electrocardiographic findings include right axis deviation, right atrial enlargement, and right ventricular hypertrophy. Echocardiography may be extremely useful in making the diagnosis of complete transposition. Cardiac catheterization with angiography allows confirmation of the anatomical arrangement of the great arteries and establishes the presence of associated lesions. Palliative balloon atrial septostomy at the time of catheterization in the newborn serves to enlarge the interatrial communication and improves oxygenation. While medical management of this disorder is often of limited value and is primarily symptomatic, the development of corrective surgical operation for infants born with transposition has greatly improved their prognosis.[2] Operative repair using the Mustard technique or the Senning procedure allows atrial rerouting of blood flow with clinical improvement that is usually quite dramatic. While the procedures are usually well tolerated, there appears to be a high incidence of early and later postoperative dysrhythmias in these repairs.

Total anomalous pulmonary venous connection is the result of persistent communication of all of the pulmonary veins either to the right atrium directly or to the systemic veins and their tributaries. Because all pulmonary venous blood therefore returns to the right atrium, an interatrial communication is an integral part of this malformation in viable infants. The anatomical varieties of total anomalous pulmonary venous connection are subdivided based on the level of abnormal drainage[3] (see Braunwald, Fig. 29–66 and Table 29–10, p. 944). The physiological consequences and subsequent clinical manifestations of this disorder depend upon the size of the interatrial communication that is present as well as upon the height of the pulmonary vascular resistance. Most patients with total anomalous pulmonary venous connection develop symptoms during the first year of life and 80 per cent die before age 1 if left untreated.

Infants with this disorder have early onset of severe dyspnea, pulmonary edema, right heart failure, and cyanosis. Cardiac murmurs are usually not a prominent finding. Multiple heart sounds are often heard, including a prominent S_1 followed by an ejection sound and a fixed and widely split S_2, as well as an S_3 and S_4. The ECG usually shows right-axis deviation and right atrial and ventricular hypertrophy. In some instances, echocardiographic identification of anomalous pulmonary venous connection to the systemic veins, coronary sinus, or right atrium may be made. Analysis of oxygen saturations at cardiac catheterization as well as selective pulmonary arteriography will establish the diagnosis. Balloon atrial septostomy may provide dramatic palliation for infants with this disorder.[4] Unless pulmonary vascular disease has developed prior to correction, the results of operation for total anomalous pulmonary venous connection in patients beyond infancy are generally favorable.[5] Surgical correction usually involves anastomosis between the pulmonary venous channels and left atrium as well as closure of the atrial septal defect.

REFERENCES

1. Rabinovitch, M., Keane, J.F., and Norwood, W.I.: Vascular structure and lung biopsy tissue correlated with pulmonary hemodynamic findings after repair of congenital heart defects. Circulation 69:655, 1984.
2. Castaneda, A.R., Norwood, W.I., Jonas, R.A., et al.: Transposition of the great arteries and intact ventricular septum: Anatomical repair in the neonate. Ann. Thorac. Surg. 38:438, 1984.
3. Lucas, R.V., Jr., Lock, J.E., Tandon, R., and Edwards, J.E.: Gross and histologic anatomy of total anomalous pulmonary venous connections. Am. J. Cardiol. 62:292, 1988.
4. Ward, K.E., Mullins, C.E., Huhta, J.C., et al.: Restrictive interatrial communication in total anomalous pulmonary venous connection. Am. J. Cardiol. 57:1131, 1986.
5. Lamb, R.K., Qureshi, S.A., Wilkinson, J.L., et al.: Total anomalous pulmonary venous drainage. 17-year surgical experience. J. Thorac. Cardiovasc. Surg. 96:368, 1988.

602-D, 603-B, 604-B, 605-D (Braunwald, p. 1099; Tables 33–16 and 33–17)

There is considerable dispute concerning the selection of appropriate prophylactic antibiotics to prevent infective endocarditis in patients with cardiac disease. However, a few rules have been agreed upon. First, the procedures for which chemoprophylaxis is necessary include those that may cause substantial bacteremia, such as dental and oral surgical procedures, open-heart surgery, tonsillectomy, gastrointestinal and genitourinary operations, instrumentation or biopsies, nasal intubation, rigid bronchoscopy, and incision and drainage of abscesses. Patients at particularly high risk for endocarditis (such as those with surgically created shunts, prosthetic valves, conduits, and patches) should also receive prophylaxis for percutaneous liver biopsy, gastrointestinal endoscopy, barium enema, complicated vaginal delivery, bladder catheterization, and diagnostic cardiac catheterization.

Second, the specific prophylactic program should be directed at the organisms most likely to be involved in transient bacteremia. Thus, the bacterium present in blood following dental manipulation and operations of the upper respiratory tract is predominantly *Streptococcus viridans*, although some staphylococci may also circulate. Transient bacteremia associated with procedures involving the urinary, gastrointestinal, and genital tracts usually includes gram-negative bacteria and occasionally staphylococci.

Based on these general recommendations, guidelines for prophylaxis have been established and recently updated by the American Heart Association.[1] Patient No. 1 is not at risk and would not need prophylaxis (see Table 33–15, p. 1098). Patient No. 2, who is to undergo dental extraction, is at high risk for endocarditis because of having an aortic valve prosthesis. This patient should therefore probably receive intravenous prophylaxis (see Table 33–16, p. 1098). Patient No. 3, undergoing general anesthesia with known hypertrophic cardiomyopathy, would be most appropriately covered with an intravenous antibiotic regimen such as that listed in B in the question. Patient No. 4, who will undergo genitourinary surgery, does not require chemoprophylaxis for the implanted pacemaker.

Patients at high risk who are allergic to penicillin may be treated with vancomycin for procedures associated with significant bacteremia. For patients allergic to penicillin who are undergoing simple procedures such as dental work, erythromycin orally is appropriate chemoprophylaxis.[1]

REFERENCE

1. Dajani, A.S., Bisno, A. L., Chung, K.J., et al.: Prevention of bacterial endocarditis. JAMA *264*:2919, 1990.

606-C, 607-A, 608-D, 609-B   *(Braunwald, pp. 1800–1804)*

The cardiovascular system is the target of a variety of chemotherapeutic complications. The most notable class of chemotherapeutic agents causing cardiotoxicity is the anthracyclines (doxorubicin, daunorubicin, and idarubicin). These drugs may cause acute cardiac complications, manifested by atrial and ventricular arrhythmias and chronic congestive heart failure and cardiomyopathy. Heart failure due to anthracycline therapy is dose related and may be adversely affected by concurrent risk factors, including age, previous heart disease, hypertension, irradiation, and other cardiotoxic drugs.

Patients receiving 5-fluorouracil may experience acute chest pain syndromes and myocardial infarction due to vasoocclusive events.[1] The mechanism of these adverse side effects is unclear. Ifosfamide and cyclophosphamide are alkylating agents used in many cancer treatment protocols. These agents

have been related to congestive heart failure, which often develops within 2 weeks of therapy. Histological characteristics of the cardiomyopathy include myocardial edema and necrosis. Cardiomyopathy is most often due to an acute drug reaction, not to cumulative dosage. Pericarditis and supraventricular and ventricular arrhythmias have also been noted with the alkylating agents. Busulfan, another alkylating agent, is associated with pulmonary infiltrates and fibrosis, along with endocardial fibrosis. Interleukins, chemotherapeutic agents which are potent modulators of the immune system, are associated with capillary leak syndrome, hypotension, noncardiogenic pulmonary edema, and nephrotoxicity.[2]

REFERENCES

1. de Forni, M., and Armand, J.P.: Cardiotoxicity of chemotherapy. Curr. Opin. Oncol. *6*:340, 1994.
2. Osanto, S., Cluitman, F.H.M., Franks, C.R., et al.: Myocardial injury after interleukin-2 therapy. Lancet *2*:48, 1988.

610-B, 611-A, 612-B, 613-B, 614-D   *(Braunwald, pp. 898–901; 904–906)*

A complete atrioventricular canal defect consists of a constellation of findings including an ostium primum atrial septal defect, a ventricular septal defect in the posterior basal portion of the ventricular septum, and a common atrial-ventricular orifice. This latter structure usually has six leaflets. In approximately 35 per cent of cases, accompanying cardiovascular lesions are present, including tetralogy of Fallot, transposition of the great arteries, total anomalous pulmonary venous connection, pulmonic stenosis, double-outlet RV, and persistent left superior vena cava. The malformation is commonly associated with Down syndrome. Patients usually present during the first year of life with a history of poor weight gain and frequent respiratory infections. Heart failure in infancy is extremely common and often requires aggressive medical therapy. Two-dimensional echocardiography is usually diagnostic (see Braunwald, Fig. 29–14, p. 900). However, hemodynamic study is frequently indicated in patients with common AV canal because the level of pulmonary vascular resistance has important prognostic implications. Infants with the complete form of the AV canal defect are at high risk for obstructive pulmonary vascular disease. The diagnosis may also be established during LV angiography, at which time the relationship between the anterior components of the left atrioventricular valve and the aorta leads to a "gooseneck" deformity. In most medical centers, primary repair of the abnormality is the preferred therapeutic approach, especially in patients with growth failure, severe pulmonary hypertension, or intractable heart failure.[1]

In the fetal circulation, most of the output of the RV bypasses the unexpanded lungs and travels from the pulmonary trunk through the ductus arteriosus to the descending aorta just distal to the left subclavian artery. Patency of the ductus arteriosus after birth occurs most commonly in females, and in the offspring of pregnancies in which the mother had rubella infection in the first trimester. While the lesion may coexist with coarctation of the aorta, ventricular septal defect, pulmonic stenosis, or aortic stenosis, it is most commonly seen in an isolated form. A characteristic continuous "machinery" murmur and thrill are noted on physical examination at the upper left sternal border. However, the presence of a diastolic, high-pitched decrescendo murmur, characteristic of aortic regurgitation, is not heard in either this disorder or in complete atrioventricular canal defect.

The clinical diagnosis of persistent patent ductus arteriosus may be subtle, and full-term infants not uncommonly survive for a number of years, either undiagnosed or with minimal symptoms. The leading causes of death in children with this anomaly as they progress are infective endocarditis and heart failure. The lesion may be visualized directly by two-dimensional echocardiography. If accompanying lesions are suspected, or pulmonary vascular disease needs evaluation, cardiac catheterization may be indicated. Operative ligation of the ductus is a low-risk procedure and may be made safer by aggressive medical therapy of any accompanying heart failure prior to the operation.

REFERENCE

1. Clapp, S.K., Perry, B.L., Farooki, Z.O., et al.: Surgical and medical results of complete atrioventricular canal: A ten-year review. Am. J. Cardiol. 59:454, 1987.

615-B, 616-A, 617-D, 618-D   (Braunwald, pp. 1304–1308)

The beta blockers constitute a cornerstone of therapy for chronic stable angina.[1] Their widespread use is partially explained by the wide variety of agents available and the ability to select for particular characteristics important to individual patient management. The beta blockers can be characterized on the basis of several of their actions. There are two types of beta receptors, designated $beta_1$ and $beta_2$, which are present in different proportions in different tissues. $Beta_1$ receptors predominate in the heart and their stimulation leads to an increase in heart rate and AV conduction and contractility. $Beta_2$ stimulation results in bronchial dilation, vasodilation, and glycogenolysis. The beta blockers currently available have been classified according to their relative cardioselectivity: the nonselective beta blocking drugs (propranolol, timolol, pindolol, and nadolol) block both $beta_1$ and $beta_2$ receptors, whereas relatively cardioselective beta blockers (atenolol, metoprolol, and acebutolol) produce selective blockade of $beta_1$ receptors. There are no commercially available $beta_2$ selective blockers.

These drugs can also be characterized by their membrane-stabilizing ability—a quinidine-like effect—measured by the reduction in the rate of rise of the cardiac action potential (of uncertain clinical significance).

The presence of intrinsic sympathomimetic activity may also distinguish types of beta blockers and is characteristic of pindolol and acebutolol, which are partial agonists and produce blockade by shielding beta receptors from more potent beta agonists. Thus, these agents produce low-grade beta stimulation when sympathetic activity is low (for instance, at rest), while during stress and exercise, the agonists behave more like conventional beta blockers.

The major determinant of absorption and metabolism of the beta blockers is their lipid solubility or hydrophobicity. The lipid-soluble beta blockers (propranolol, metoprolol, and pindolol) are readily absorbed from the gastrointestinal tract, are metabolized predominantly by the liver, have a relatively short half-life, and are more likely to cause central nervous system side effects. The water-soluble beta blockers (atenolol, metoprolol, and nadolol) are not as readily absorbed from the gastrointestinal tract, are not as extensively metabolized in the liver, have relatively long plasma half-lives, and therefore accumulate in renal failure. Finally, a beta blocker, labetolol, is now available that also possesses alpha adrenergic receptor blocking activity; this may make it particularly useful as an antihypertensive agent.

REFERENCE

1. Rogers, W.J.: Use of beta blockers in the treatment of ischemic heart disease: A comparison of the available agents. Cardiovasc. Rev. Rep. 5:311, 1984.

Parts IV and V
Broader Perspectives on Heart Disease and Relation Between Heart Disease and Disease of Other Organ Systems

CHAPTERS 48 THROUGH 63

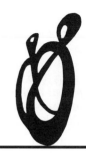

DIRECTIONS: Each question below contains five suggested responses. Select the ONE BEST response to each question.

619. True statements about inherited disorders of rhythm and conduction include all of the following EXCEPT:

    A. Familial conduction disturbances of the sinus mode have been recognized
    B. Familial conduction disturbances of the bundle branches have been recognized
    C. Rheumatic diseases are associated with congenital heart block
    D. Ward-Romano syndrome is inherited as an autosomal recessive disorder
    E. Jervell and Lange-Nielsen syndrome is characterized by syncope, congenital deafness, and sudden death

620. The most common glomerulopathy associated with infectious endocarditis is:

    A. interstitial nephritis
    B. minimal change disease
    C. membranous glomerulonephritis
    D. focal/segmental proliferative glomerulonephritis
    E. crescentic glomerulonephritis

621. A 40-year-old man presents to the office with shortness of breath on exertion, edema, and hand arthritis. On examination, his vital signs are normal. His sclera are icteric and his skin has a gray hue. Lungs have rales at the bases; carotids have a normal upstroke. The cardiac

impulse is displaced laterally and there is an audible S_3. His abdomen is distended with evidence of ascites and hepatosplenomegaly. There is peripheral edema. Laboratory studies reveal a blood sugar of 225 mg/dl and a transferrin saturation of 70 per cent. Which of the following statements about this condition is true:

    A. It may be inherited as an autosomal dominant disease
    B. Cardiac involvement is the presenting manifestation in about 15 per cent of patients
    C. Early cardiac death is common, due primarily to accelerated atherosclerosis
    D. Ventricular hypertrophy and conduction delays are typical electrocardiographic findings
    E. Echocardiography often shows a thickened ventricle with a "granular sparkling" appearance

622. Peptide growth factors likely play a role in the development of cardiac hypertrophy and heart failure. Each of the following are true concerning cardiac growth factors EXCEPT:

    A. Insulin-like growth factor-1 (IGF-1) has been shown to play a role in the hypertrophic response of the myocardium
    B. Angiotensin II can lead to increased myocardial contractility and growth

C. Receptor antagonists to endothelin 1 have been shown to limit the development of myocardial hypertrophy

D. Transforming growth factor-beta (TGF-β) works by increasing messenger RNA during cardiac hypertrophy

E. Angiotensin I receptor antagonists have been linked to the regression of cardiac hypertrophy

623. A 30-year-old woman with no history of hypertension, hyperlipidemia, diabetes mellitus, or other risk factors for atherosclerosis presents with symptoms consistent with angina pectoris. Examination revealed angioid streaks in the left eye and raised yellow papules in the axillary region. The rest of the physical examination is within normal limits. True statements regarding this condition include all of the following EXCEPT:

A. Arterial and venous thrombosis are prevalent

B. There is an increased risk of bleeding

C. Restrictive cardiomyopathy may develop

D. Myocardial infarction is a common cause of death

E. Mitral valve prolapse is associated with this condition

624. True statements about the diagnosis of pulmonary emboli include all of the following EXCEPT:

A. Arterial blood gas measurement may be misleading in the diagnosis of acute pulmonary emboli

B. The electrocardiographic findings consistent with pulmonary emboli include right heart strain and tachycardia

C. Pulmonary infarction due to pulmonary emboli may be visualized on the chest x-ray

D. A narrow splitting of the second heart sound (S_2) is often heard in cases of large pulmonary emboli

E. Fibrin degradation products have been found to be elevated in some patients with pulmonary embolism

625. Each of the following statements about the evaluation of coronary artery disease in women is true EXCEPT:

A. The initial presentation of coronary artery disease in women is more often angina, whereas men more commonly present with myocardial infarction

B. Women are typically 10 years older than men at the time of initial presentation of coronary artery disease

C. Women have repolarization abnormalities (ST/T wave changes) on the resting electrocardiogram more commonly than men

D. Men are more likely to experience renal and vascular complications associated with coronary angiography

E. Exercise stress testing in women has a higher false-positive rate compared with men

626. True statements about homocystinuria include all of the following EXCEPT:

A. Heterozygosity for homocystinuria is associated with an increased incidence of atherosclerosis

B. Mental retardation may be present

C. Foods rich in pyridoxine should be encouraged

D. Cystathionine beta-synthase deficiency is present in homocystinuria

E. Platelet dysfunction is a likely cause for the vascular complications

627. True statements regarding the immediate postoperative period for patients after coronary artery bypass graft (CABG) surgery include all of the following EXCEPT:

A. Serum potassium levels fluctuate, especially in diabetics

B. Serum glucose levels are frequently elevated, in part due to increased catecholamine and cortisol secretion

C. Alveolar dysfunction is common, often due to left-to-right intrapulmonary shunting of blood

D. Hypocalcemia and hypomagnesemia are frequently seen

E. Mild metabolic acidosis or alkalosis are common and usually do not require correction

628. True statements regarding estrogen and estrogen replacement therapy (ERT) in women include all of the following EXCEPT:

A. In postmenopausal women, ERT results in higher HDL and lower LDL levels

B. Functional estrogen receptors have been identified in vascular smooth muscle

C. Unopposed estrogen usage has been associated with a twofold increase in endometrial cancer in women with an intact uterus

D. Smoking and advanced age are risk factors for thromboembolism in women taking oral contraceptives

E. Tamoxifen, an estrogen agonist/antagonist, has been shown to have positive effects on lipoproteins and coronary artery disease in women

629. True statements about peripartum cardiomyopathy (PPCM) include all of the following EXCEPT:

A. Symptoms of PPCM most commonly occur in the immediate postpartum period
B. Clinical and hemodynamic findings in PPCM are indistinguishable from those of other forms of dilated cardiomyopathy
C. The incidence of PPCM is greatest in primiparous white women of European extraction
D. Approximately 50 per cent of PPCM patients show complete or near-complete recovery within the first 6 months after delivery
E. Subsequent pregnancies in women with PPCM carry an increased risk for relapse

630. True statements about supravalvular aortic stenosis (AS) include all of the following EXCEPT:

A. Supravalvular AS is a component of Williams syndrome
B. Supravalvular AS may be asymptomatic
C. Supravalvular AS is not seen as an isolated, sporadic anomaly
D. Supravalvular AS may be associated with peripheral pulmonic stenoses
E. Hypercalcemia may be associated with supravalvular AS

631. A 75-year-old male presents to the emergency department complaining of dizziness and chest pain. Vital signs include a heart rate of 90 beats/min and a blood pressure of 140/86 mm Hg in both arms. No abnormalities are detected in the cardiac and pulmonary examination. Splenomegaly is noted on abdominal examination. The electrocardiogram reveals mild ST elevations in the lateral leads. Laboratory data are notable for a white blood cell count of 22,000, hemoglobin of 21 gm/dl, and platelet count of 690,000. What should be the initial management of this patient?

A. thrombolytic agents
B. phlebotomy with colloid volume replacement
C. iron therapy
D. immediate cardiac catheterization
E. bone marrow biopsy

632. Common findings in the obese cardiac patient include all of the following EXCEPT:

A. decreased cardiac output
B. elevated preload
C. decreased sensitivity to insulin
D. eccentric ventricular hypertrophy
E. increased ectopy

633. The presence of underlying heart disease in the mother may influence both maternal and fetal outcome. Each of the following maternal cardiovascular disorders are usually well tolerated during pregnancy EXCEPT:

A. atrial septal defect (ASD)
B. ventricular septal defect (VSD)
C. Marfan syndrome
D. coarctation of the aorta
E. patent ductus arteriosus (PDA)

634. A 30-year-old male presents to the emergency room in heart failure after falling from his bicycle. He has no history of rheumatic fever, heart murmur, or family history of heart disease. Physical examination is notable for a young man in moderate distress with a heart rate of 110 beats/min and a blood pressure of 100/50 mm Hg. There is evidence of moderate jugular venous distention. The carotid examination is normal. Cardiac findings include a continuous murmur throughout the lower sternum with a palpable thrill. S_1 and S_2 are audible. Lungs have bibasilar rales and there is no peripheral edema. Echocardiogram reveals a fistulous tract between the aorta and the right ventricle. The following statements about this entity are true EXCEPT:

A. It is often associated with a congenital anomaly of the aortic valve
B. It is more common in females
C. It may present suddenly, often following chest trauma
D. It is often accompanied by a ventricular septal defect
E. Patients with Marfan syndrome have a higher incidence

635. True statements about trisomy 21 (Down syndrome) and cardiovascular disease include all of the following EXCEPT:

A. The risk of Down syndrome increases exponentially with maternal age
B. Congenital heart defects are seen in 40 to 50 per cent of cases of Down syndrome
C. Endocardial cushion defects are the most characteristic cardiac anomalies of Down syndrome

D. Patients with this syndrome have a tendency to develop pulmonary hypertension in the setting of increased right-sided flow

E. Postoperative survival in Down syndrome patients is worse than survival for unaffected patients with similar defects

---

636. True statements about the inheritance of familial hypertrophic cardiomyopathy (FHC) include all of the following EXCEPT:

A. About half of patients with FHC have first-degree relatives who are affected

B. It is a disease primarily of the myocyte mitochondria

C. Mutations that alter the charge of the beta-myosin heavy chain carry a worse prognosis

D. Pedigree screening for FHC should include an echocardiogram

E. Mutations of cardiac troponin T have been described in familial FHC

---

637. Each of the following lesions may be considered amenable to a *reparative* cardiac operation EXCEPT:

A. patent ductus arteriosus
B. ventricular septal defect
C. aortopulmonary window
D. tetralogy of Fallot
E. ventricular aneurysm

---

638. True statements concerning the management of acute myocardial infarction in the elderly include all of the following EXCEPT:

A. Angiotensin-converting enzyme inhibitors have been shown to reduce fatal and non-fatal events following infarction in the elderly

B. It has been shown that elderly patients with a myocardial infarction benefit from receiving thrombolytic agents

C. Elderly patients are less likely than younger patients to benefit from beta blockade for secondary prevention

D. Central nervous system toxicity from lidocaine is more common in older populations

E. Heparin-induced bleeding is a more common problem in older female populations

---

639. Preoperative factors associated with a significantly increased risk for development of cardiac complications after major noncardiac surgery in patients over 40 years of age include all of the following EXCEPT:

A. presence of an S_3
B. stable class II angina

C. myocardial infarction within 3 months
D. severe mitral stenosis
E. more than 5 PVCs/min on the preoperative ECG

---

640. Hemolytic anemia in patients with valvular heart disease is associated with all of the following EXCEPT:

A. spherocytes
B. low haptoglobin levels
C. hemosiderinuria
D. iron deposits in the kidney
E. helmet cells

---

641. True statements regarding hypertension in the elderly include all of the following EXCEPT:

A. Clinical studies have established the effectiveness of therapy for mild diastolic hypertension in the elderly

B. Clinical studies have not yet established the effectiveness of therapy for isolated systolic hypertension in the elderly

C. Elderly patients less often respond to beta blocker therapy for hypertension

D. The presence of left ventricular hypertrophy (LVF) in elderly hypertensive patients is an independent risk factor for coronary disease

E. Hypertensive hypertrophic cardiomyopathy of the elderly occurs primarily in females

---

642. True statements about the role of platelets in hemostasis include all of the following EXCEPT:

A. Platelet adhesion is the initial event in "primary hemostasis"

B. Platelets initially adhere to collagen fibrils on the endothelial lining of the vessel

C. Activation of platelets leads to release of granular constituents

D. Specific platement membrane receptors participate in the processes of platelet adhesion and aggregation

E. Arachidonic acid derivatives formed in platelets may recruit additional circulating platelets for the developing platelet aggregate

---

643. Anorexia nervosa may be associated with all of the following conditions EXCEPT:

A. bradycardia
B. mitral valve prolapse
C. hypocholesterolemia
D. hypertension
E. arrhythmias

644. True statements with regard to metastatic disease involving the heart include all of the following EXCEPT:

A. Metastases rarely involve the valves or endocardium
B. The most common primary tumor producing cardiac metastases is bronchogenic carcinoma
C. A chylous pericardial effusion is characteristic of metastatic breast carcinoma
D. More than 50 per cent of patients with malignant melanoma have cardiac metastases that are usually clinically silent
E. A solitary cardiac mass is more likely to be benign than metastatic

645. True statements about cardiovascular defects associated with teratogen exposure include all of the following EXCEPT:

A. The most common teratogen exposed to human embryos and fetuses is ethanol
B. Lithium ingestion during pregnancy has been associated with Ebstein's anomaly
C. Subvalvular aortic stenosis is classically seen in fetuses exposed to vitamin D
D. Warfarin in early pregnancy can cause abnormalities of cartilage formation and exhtracellular matrix metabolism
E. Ventricular septal defects may be seen in the fetal hydantoin syndrome

646. Radiotherapy for malignant disease may affect the heart in all of the following ways EXCEPT:

A. pericarditis
B. coronary artery disease
C. valvular stenosis
D. conduction abnormalities
E. asymmetrical septal hypertrophy

DIRECTIONS: Each question below contains suggested answers. For EACH of the alternatives listed you are to respond either True (T) or False (F). In a given item, ALL, SOME, OR NONE OF THE ALTERNATIVES MAY BE CORRECT.

647. In addition to the "major manifestations" of acute rheumatic fever, including carditis, polyarthritis, chorea, erythema marginatum, and subcutaneous nodules, other supporting evidence for this condition includes:

A. prolonged QT-interval
B. fever
C. elevated C-reactive protein
D. normochromic, normocytic anemia
E. rising streptococcal antibody titers

648. The following statements concern hypertension in pregnancy:

A. Hypertension complicates about 10 per cent of pregnancies
B. Elevated blood pressure during pregnancy or in the post-partum period without a history of hypertension/preeclampsia is associated with hypertension later in life
C. Arteriolar vasodilators (hydralazine) and alpha$_2$-adrenergic receptor agonists (methyldopa) are frequently used in the treatment of pregnant hypertensive patients
D. Preeclampsia usually occurs at the end of the second trimester in multiparous women
E. Severe hypertension near term or during delivery should be treated with magnesium sulfate alone

649. True statements with respect to *heterozygous* familial hypercholesterolemia include:

A. It is a relatively common disorder with a gene frequency of 1 in 500 persons in the population
B. It is inherited as a recessive trait
C. Tendon xanthomas and arcus corneae are common but nonspecific findings
D. Cutaneous planar xanthomas are a specific finding that occur in one-third of patients
E. The fundamental defect is the presence of only half the normal number of LDL receptors in the individual's cells

650. True statements about inherited forms of atrial septal defect (ASD) include which of the following?

A. Two mendelian forms of isolated ASD have been recognized
B. Secundum ASD is common in both the familial forms of ASD and the Holt-Oram syndrome
C. One form of familial ASD is associated with ventricular tachycardia
D. ASD of the sinus venosus type is most common in the Ellis–Van Creveld syndrome
E. Short stature is one finding in Holt-Oram syndrome

651. Correct pairings of anesthetic agents and their side effects include:

A. Halothane—decreased blood pressure
B. Thiopental—depressed myocardial contractility
C. Succinylcholine—bradycardia
D. Ketamine—depressed myocardial contractility
E. Morphine—venodilation

652. True statements about perioperative myocardial infarction (MI) in the coronary artery bypass graft (CABG) patient include which of the following?

A. Perioperative MI occurs in between 5 and 15 per cent of patients undergoing CABG surgery
B. In patients dying of a perioperative MI, autopsy studies usually reveal thrombotic occlusion of the bypass graft
C. CPK levels are often elevated in the post-cardiac surgery patient
D. The echocardiogram is the most reliable tool for diagnosing a perioperative MI
E. Prolonged pump time (>75 minutes) is not correlated with an increased likelihood of perioperative MI

653. A 60-year-old male was admitted to the hospital with an acute anterior myocardial infarction. Nitroglycerin, morphine sulfate, metoprolol, aspirin, and streptokinase were given in the early hours of treatment and his chest pain was relieved. His hospital course was complicated by rising serum creatinine and urea nitrogen. In addition, he developed a purple, net-like discoloration on his lower extremities. Which of the following is (are) true regarding this patient:

A. A kidney biopsy should be performed to obtain a diagnosis
B. The urinalysis is likely to reveal proteinuria without cells or casts
C. Elevated serum complement levels are typical
D. Transient eosinophilia may be present
E. End-stage renal failure may develop

654. True statements with regard to cardiac involvement in systemic lupus erythematosus (SLE) include:

A. Pericarditis is the most common cardiac finding
B. Libman-Sacks lesions are caused by active myocarditis
C. Libman-Sacks lesions rarely produce serious valvular regurgitation during the acute phase of the disease

D. In pregnant women with active SLE, fetal tachycardia and atrial fibrillation are caused by transplacental transfer of abnormal antibodies

655. Which of the following statements regarding hereditary hemorrhagic telangiectasia (HHT; Osler-Rendu-Weber disease) and cardiovascular disease is true?

A. HHT is exceedingly rare
B. Telangiectases are often present on the tongue and lips in this disorder
C. Recurrent sinusitis occurs in this disorder
D. Pulmonary arteriovenous malformations are often present in patients with HHT
E. The gene for HHT has been mapped to the short arm of chromosome 3

656. Characteristics of familial hypertriglyceridemia include:

A. inheritance as an autosomal dominant trait
B. development of eruptive xanthomas and pancreatitis following alcohol ingestion
C. normal cholesterol levels
D. a 5- to 10-fold increased incidence of atherosclerosis

657. True statements about inherited forms of dilated cardiomyopathy include the following:

A. The frequency of hereditary forms of dilated cardiomyopathy is higher than that of hypertrophic cardiomyopathy
B. A positive family history for dilated cardiomyopathy is seen in less than 3 per cent of cases
C. Most inherited examples of dilated cardiomyopathy fit an autosomal recessive pattern
D. In some families with inherited dilated cardiomyopathy, associated skeletal myopathy is noted
E. While peripartum-dilated cardiomyopathy is usually sporadic, it has also been recognized in an inherited form

658. Compensatory adaptations to chronic anemia which occur in the cardiovascular system include:

A. increased left ventricular end-diastolic volume
B. decreased left ventricular afterload
C. increased levels of catecholamine and non-catecholamine inotropic factors in plasma
D. increased affinity of red cell hemoglobin for oxygen with a shift in the hemoglobin oxygen dissociation curve to the left

659. True statements with respect to alterations in cardiovascular function with aging include:

   A. There is a steady 1 to 2 per cent increase in the number of myocardial cells each year
   B. There is moderate hypertrophy of left ventricular myocardium
   C. In healthy elderly individuals there is a significant fall in stroke volume and ejection fraction due to a decrease in peak contractile force
   D. During exercise, heart rate increases less in older individuals, probably because of decreased catecholamine responsiveness

660. The effects of amiodarone on thyroid function include:

   A. inhibition of peripheral conversion of T_4 to T_3
   B. decrease in thyroid-stimulating hormone levels
   C. inhibition of thyroid organification with a decrease in thyroid clearance of iodide
   D. development of hyperthyroidism in 25 per cent of patients on therapy for longer than 12 weeks

661. Risk factors for the development of mediastinitis and sternal osteomyelitis after median sternotomy include:

   A. prolonged cardiopulmonary bypass time
   B. use of both internal mammary arteries as bypass vessels
   C. diabetes
   D. decreased postoperative cardiac output

DIRECTIONS: Each group of questions below consists of lettered headings followed by a set of numbered items. For each numbered item select the ONE lettered heading with which it is MOST closely associated. Each lettered heading may be used ONCE, MORE THAN ONCE, OR NOT AT ALL.

   A. Kartagener syndrome
   B. Holt-Oram syndrome
   C. LEOPARD syndrome
   D. Noonan syndrome

662. Webbed neck, pulmonic stenosis, left anterior hemiblock

663. Deafness, pulmonic stenosis, complete heart block

664. Lentigines, pulmonic stenosis, P-R prolongation

665. Sinusitis, dextrocardia, bronchiectasis

666. Abnormal scaphoid bone, ventricular septal defect, right bundle branch block

   A. Hyperparathyroidism
   B. Hypothyroidism
   C. Hyperaldosteronism
   D. Cushing's syndrome
   E. Hyperthyroidism

667. U-waves on the electrocardiogram

668. Cardiac myxoma

669. Means-Lerman scratch

670. Shortened Q-T interval

671. Pericardial effusion

   A. Streptokinase
   B. Anisoylated plasminogen-streptokinase activator complex (APSAC)
   C. Urokinase
   D. Tissue-type plasminogen activator

672. Both single and double chain forms demonstrate proteolytic activity

673. Synthesized in renal tubular epithelial cells as well as endothelial cells

674. Prolonged plasma half life

675. Single polypeptide of 414 amino acids

DIRECTIONS: Each group of questions below consists of four lettered headings followed by a set of numbered items. For each numbered item select

A if the item is associated with (A) *only*
B if the item is associated with (B) *only*
C if the item is associated with *both* (A) and (B) and
D if the item is associated with *neither* (A) nor (B)

Each lettered heading may be used ONCE, MORE THAN ONCE, OR NOT AT ALL.

A. Unfractionated heparin
B. Low molecular weight heparin
C. Both
D. Neither

676. Hyperkalemia

677. Bioavailability after subcutaneous injection >90 per cent

678. Inactivates clot-bound thrombin

679. Thrombocytopenia

680. Increases vascular permeability

See illustrations below for Questions 681–684.

A. Familial hypercholesterolemia
B. Type III hyperlipoproteinemia (familial dysbetaliproteinemia)
C. Both
D. Neither

681. *See A below*

682. *See B below*

683. *See C below*

684. *See D below*

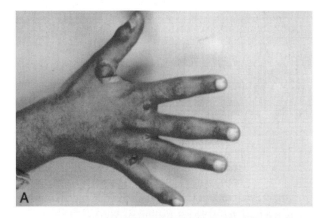

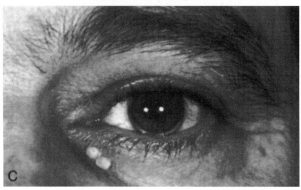

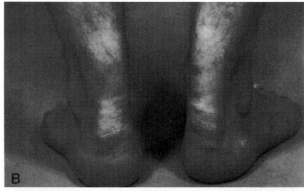

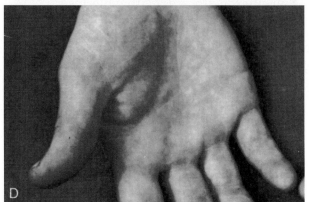

681–684, From Gotto, A.: Cholesterol Education Program: Clinician's Manual 1991, pp. 34–36. By permission of the American Heart Association, Inc.

A. Rheumatoid arthritis
B. Systemic lupus erythematosus
C. Both
D. Neither

685. Constrictive pericarditis

686. Associated with HLA-B27 antigen

687. Complete heart block

688. Cerebrovascular events

Match each photograph *below* with the condition it represents.

689. Fabry's disease

690. Subacute infective endocarditis

691. Amyloidosis

692. Scleroderma

A. Turner syndrome
B. Noonan syndrome
C. Both
D. Neither

693. Coarctation of the aorta

694. Normal karyotype

695. Pulmonic stenosis

696. Short stature, webbing of the neck, skeletal anomalies, and renal anomalies

---

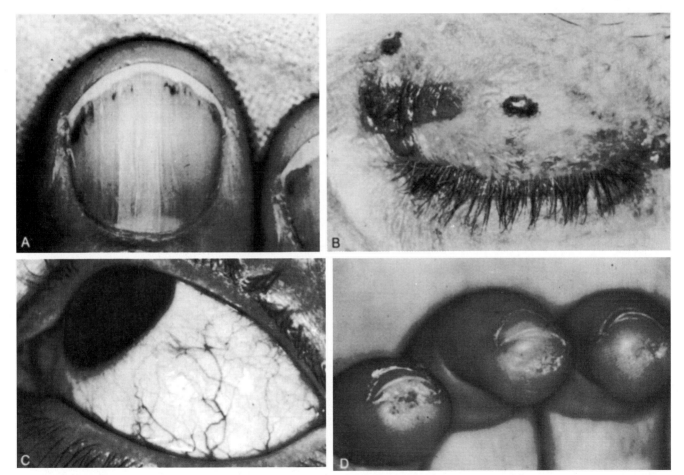

A, From Swartz, M.N., and Weinberg, A.N.: Infections due to gram-positive bacteria. *In* Fitzpatrick, T.B., et al. (eds.): Dermatology in General Medicine, New York, McGraw-Hill, 1970, p. 1436.

B, From Calkins, E.: Amyloidosis of the skin. *In* Fitzpatrick, T.B., et al. (eds.): Dermatology in General Medicine, New York, McGraw-Hill, 1979, p. 1065.

C, From Frost, P., and Spaeth, G.L.: Alpha galactosidase A deficiency, Fabry's disease. *In* Fitzpatrick, T.B., et al. (eds.): Dermatology in General Medicine, New York, McGraw-Hill, 1979, p. 1129.

D, From Eisen, A.Z., Uitto, J.J., and Bauer, E.A.: Scleroderma. *In* Fitzpatrick, T.B., et al. (eds.): Dermatology in General Medicine, New York, McGraw-Hill, 1979, p. 1307.

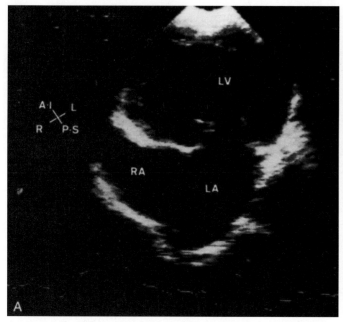

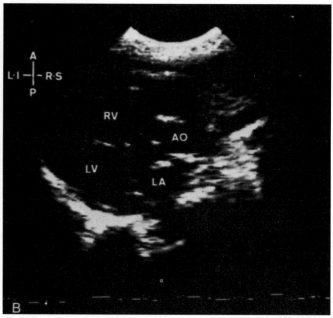

From Fulton, D.R., Geggel, R.L., and Pandian, N.G.: Two dimensional and Doppler echocardiographic evaluation. *In* Miller, D.D., et al. (eds.): Clinical Cardiac Imaging. New York, McGraw-Hill, 1988, p. 562.

From Fulton, D.R., Geggel, R.L., and Pandian, N.G.: Two dimensional and Doppler echocardiographic evaluation. *In* Miller, D.D., et al. (eds.): Clinical Cardiac Imaging. New York, McGraw-Hill, 1988, p. 561.

See illustrations above

    A. *See above*
    B. *See above*
    C. Both
    D. Neither

697. A ventricular septal defect may accompany this anomaly

698. D-Transposition of the great arteries may accompany this anomaly

699. The coronary arteries in this condition may have surgically important variations

700. Cyanosis and an ECG finding of left ventricular hypertrophy may be found in this condition

701. The Fontan procedure may be useful in this condition

    A. Sickle cell anemia
    B. Thalassemia
    C. Both
    D. Neither

702. Pericarditis

703. Pulmonary infarction

704. Second-degree heart block

705. Transfusional hemosiderosis

706. Chordae tendineae calcification

Parts IV and V

Broader Perspectives on Heart Disease and Relation Between Heart Disease and Disease of Other Organ Systems

CHAPTERS 48 THROUGH 63

ANSWERS

619-D *(Braunwald, p. 1667)*

Inherited forms for virtually every recognized conduction abnormality have been described, including those of the sinus node, atrioventricular node, and bundle branches. Complete heart block is known to be associated with rheumatic diseases and was first recognized when the children of mothers with lupus erythematosus were found to have complete heart block.[1] Risk appears to be highest in children of women with autoantibodies to a specific ribonucleoprotein in anti-Ro(ss-a),[2] implying that maternal genotype may determine genetic susceptibility to inflammation of the fetal heart. Interestingly, a genetic susceptibility to inflammation of the AV node is suggested by the high association of HLA-B27 in adults requiring permanent pacemakers.[3] Ward-Romano syndrome is characterized by a prolonged Q-T interval, sudden death, and an autosomal *dominant* inheritance pattern. Jervell and Lange-Nielsen syndrome is inherited as an autosomal *recessive* condition and is characterized by syncope and sudden death, but is associated with congenital deafness. Heterozygotes for this syndrome have normal hearing and cardiac rhythm; slight prolongation of the Q-T$_c$ interval may be detected.[4] Long Q-T$_c$ intervals are noted in approximately 1 in 100 deaf children, underscoring the need for routine ECG screening of any hearing-impaired child.

REFERENCES

1. Chameides, L., Truex, R.C., Vetter, V., et al.: Association of maternal systemic lupus erythematosus with congenital complete heart block. N. Engl. J. Med. *297*:1204, 1977.
2. Scott, J.S., Maddison, P.J., Taylor, P.V., et al.: Connective-tissue disease antibodies to ribonucleoprotein, and congenital heart block. N. Engl. J. Med. *309*:209, 1983.
3. Bergfeldt, L., Vallin, H., and Edhag, O.: Complete heart block in HLA B27 associated disease. Electrophysiological and clinical characteristics. Br. Heart J. *51*:184, 1984.
4. Fraser, G.R., Froggatt, P., and Murphy, T.: Genetical aspects of the cardioauditory syndrome of Jervell and Lange-Nielsen congenital deafness and electrocardiographic abnormalities. Ann. Hum. Genet. *28*:133, 1964.

620-D *(Braunwald, p. 1921)*

Renal failure accounts for a significant morbidity and mortality in patients with infective endocarditis. More than 60 per cent of patients with infective endocarditis have evidence of renal involvement, ranging from mild hematuria and proteinuria to overt nephrotic syndrome and renal failure. Deposition of circulating immune complexes in the glomeruli accounts for much of the kidney damage. The most common form of glomerulonephritis associated with endocarditis is focal/segmental proliferative nephritis. This widespread process includes areas of fibrosis, necrosis, and inflammation. In addition, areas of proliferation of renal endothelial, epithelial, and mesangial cells are prevalent. Deposits of IgG, IgM and C3 occur in mesangial and subendothelial cells. Infective endocarditis must be identified quickly and treated aggressively in an effort to limit the renal complications of this disease. Antibiotic therapy has decreased the incidence of proliferative glomerulonephritis associated with endocarditis from up to

80 per cent to less than 15 per cent.[1] Renal infarction, emboli, hemorrhage, cortical necrosis, and therapy-induced lesions (interstitial nephritis, toxic nephropathy, acute tubular necrosis) have also been implicated in the pathogenesis of renal failure associated with endocarditis.

REFERENCE

1. Neugarten, J., and Baldwin, D.S.: Glomerulonephritis in bacterial endocarditis. Am. J. Med. 77:297, 1984.

621-B   (Braunwald, pp. 1674–1675; 1790–1792)

Hemochromatosis is a disease that leads to abnormal deposition of iron in tissues. Genetic hemochromatosis is an autosomal recessive disorder linked to the A locus of the HLA complex on chromosome 6; acquired hemochromatosis is the result of excess iron load associated with another disease process (e.g., thalassemia) or increased ingestion of iron. Normal body content of iron is maintained by the proper absorption of iron in the intestines. In hemochromatosis, mucosal absorption is inappropriately high, which leads to elevated plasma iron levels and increased transferrin saturation. The extra iron load is deposited in virtually all organs, including the heart, pancreas, and liver. The classic presentation therefore is that of "bronze diabetes" due to excess iron deposition in the dermis and pancreas.

Other presenting findings include hypogonadism (impaired hypothalamic-pituitary function), hand arthropathy (often the small joints of the hands), and cirrhosis with an increased risk of hepatocellular carcinoma. Fifteen per cent of patients with hemochromatosis initially present with cardiac symptoms, most commonly congestive heart failure due to a dilated cardiomyopathy and reduced systolic function.[1] Electrocardiographic findings may include supraventricular arrhythmias, varying degrees of atrioventricular block, and low QRS voltage. Diagnosis is based on a detailed history, blood studies for iron, total iron-binding capacity (TIBC), transferrin saturation (iron/TIBC ratio), ferritin, and imaging studies of the liver (including a liver biopsy).[2] Treatment options include phlebotomy, chelating agents and supportive care.

REFERENCES

1. Porter, J., Cary, N., and Schofield, P.: Haemochromatosis presenting as congestive heart failure. Br. Heart J. 73:73, 1985.
2. Edwards, C., and Kushner, J.: Screening for hemochromatosis. N. Engl. J. Med. 328:1616, 1993.

622-E   (Braunwald, pp. 1641–1643)

Recently, some of the molecular mechanisms relevant to cardiac myocyte function, regulation, and growth have been discovered. Several growth factors have been implicated in the regulation of cardiomyocyte growth and development, thereby allowing increased understanding of the pathogenesis of cardiac dysfunction and the development of new therapeutic approaches to heart failure. Some of the cardiac growth factors that are thought to be involved in producing cardiac hypertrophy include angiotensin II, endothelin I, insulin-like growth factor-1 (IGF-1), and transforming growth factor-beta (TGF-β).

The renin-angiotensin system is one of the main regulators of intravascular volume and blood pressure. Angiotensinogen is activated by angiotensin I by the enzyme renin; angiotensin I is then converted to angiotensin II by the angiotensin-converting enzyme. Angiotensin II's effects of the heart occur through at least two distinct receptors that can affect both contractility and hypertrophy.[1] Endothelin I receptors also have been demonstrated on ventricular myocytes and are thought to participate in cardiac cell growth and hypertrophy. IGF-1 is a structurally similar compound to proinsulin and has recently been shown to be a growth factor for cardiac myocytes.[2] In addition to other functions, TGF-β and cytokines including cardiotrophin-1 have been shown to play a role in cardiac myocyte hypertrophy.

REFERENCES

1. Lindpaintner, K., and Ganten, D.: The cardiac renin-angiotensin system. Circ. Res. 68:905, 1991.
2. Sacca, L., Cittadini, A., and Fazio, S.: Growth hormone and the heart. Endocr. Rev. 15:555, 1994.

623-A   (Braunwald, p. 1673)

Pseudoxanthoma elasticum is a connective tissue disorder primarily affecting the eyes, skin, gastrointestinal system and the heart. The pattern of transmission of this disease is thought to be sporadic or by autosomal recessive inheritance.[1] Microscopic examination of affected tissue shows abnormal calcification of elastic fibers. The most obvious physical features are yellow macular/papular lesions primarily in areas of skin folds. Biopsy of these lesions is helpful in establishing a diagnosis. Funduscopic examination may reveal angioid streaking in one or both eyes. Angioid streaking may also be seen in patients with sickle cell disease, Paget's disease, hyperphosphatemia, Ehlers-Danlos syndrome, lead poisoning, and intracranial disorders. Gastrointestinal hemorrhage is common in pseudoxanthoma elasticum and is difficult to manage due to persistent bleeding of mucosal arterioles. Cardiovascular complications of this condition may be life threatening, including premature coronary artery disease.[2] Myocardial ischemia develops due to accelerated atherosclerosis causing progressive luminal narrowing and even complete vessel occlusion. Bypass surgery is often difficult to perform due to diffuse atherosclerosis, and arterial conduits used in surgery also become prematurely diseased (including internal mammary and radial arteries). Mitral valve prolapse and restrictive cardiomyopathy have been associated with pseudoxanthoma elasticum.

REFERENCES

1. Neldner, K.H.: Pseudoxanthoma elasticum. Clin. Dermatol. *6*:1, 1988.
2. Lebwohl, M., Halperin, J., Phelps, R.: Occult pseudoxanthoma elasticum in patients with premature cardiovascular disease. N. Engl. J. Med. *329*:1237, 1993.

624-D *(Braunwald, pp. 1585–1592)*

The differential diagnosis of pulmonary embolism (PE) ranges from diseases including acute myocardial infarction, asthma, and anxiety. Therefore, the diagnosis of PE is often a very difficult diagnosis to make, even to the most astute clinician. The most common symptoms of patients presenting with PE are dyspnea and pleuritic chest pain. Cardiovascular physical findings may include tachycardia and tachypnea, a right ventricular heave, an S_3 gallop, and increased pulmonic component of the second heart sound. While arterial blood gas studies may be useful in managing a patient's respiratory status, they do not tend to be of great value in the diagnosis of pulmonary embolism. It is important to recognize that normal values of the alveolar–arterial oxygen gradient do not exclude the diagnosis of PE.[1] The finding of a pleural effusion is a nonspecific sign, and analysis of the pleural find may be variable.

The classic manifestation of acute cor pulmonale secondary to PE seen on the electrocardiogram include S_1-Q_3-T_3, right bundle branch block, P pulmonale, and right-axis deviation. In a series of 49 patients presenting with acute PE, three-fourths had evidence of right ventricular strain on admission electrocardiograms.[2] Blood testing for elevated plasma D-dimers may be helpful in establishing a diagnosis of PE. This monoclonal antibody test is more than 90 per cent sensitive for detecting patients with PE proven by lung scan or by angiogram.[3,4] The chest x-ray may provide some clues to the diagnosis of PE, but more often than not is normal. Markedly diminished vascular markings, an engorged major hilar artery, the sudden appearance of a "plump" vessel, and the presence of a homogeneous wedge-shaped density in the peripheral region of the lung with the rounded, convex apex pointing toward the hilum ("Hampton's hump") may indicate the presence of pulmonary embolism and/or pulmonary infarction.

REFERENCES

1. Stein, P.D., Goldhaber, S.Z., and Henry, J.W.: Alveolar-arterial oxygen gradient in the assessment of acute pulmonary embolism. Chest *107*:139, 1995.
2. Sreeram, N., Cheriex, E.C., Smeets, J.L., et al.: Value of the 12-lead electrocardiogram at hospital admission in the diagnosis of acute pulmonary embolism. Am. J. Cardiol. *73*:298, 1994.
3. Bounameaux, H., de Moerloose, P., Perrier, A., and Reber, G.: Plasma measurement of D-dimer as diagnostic aid in suspected venous thromboembolism. An overview. Thromb. Haemost. *71*:1, 1994.
4. Goldhaber, S.Z., Simons, G.R., Elliott, C.G., et al.: Quantitative plasma D-dimer levels among patients undergoing pulmonary angiography for suspected pulmonary embolism. JAMA *270*:2819, 1993.

625-D *(Braunwald, pp. 1704–1706)*

Coronary artery disease is the leading cause of death in the United States for both men and women. The presentation, evaluation, and treatment of the disease, however, may differ between women and men.[1] Women are roughly 10 years older than men upon presentation and are more likely to complain of angina as their initial manifestation of coronary artery disease. Men, however, present more often with active myocardial infarction. Women are also more likely to have atypical chest pain complaints, often associated with coronary spasm, and more commonly have noncoronary causes for chest discomfort. Mortality rates from coronary artery disease are equal for women and men after myocardial infarction. The principles of diagnostic testing for coronary artery disease in women do not differ from those of men. However, interpretation and utility of the data vary. The resting electrocardiogram in women with suspected heart disease more often reveals repolarization changes (ST-T wave changes). There is a higher rate of false-positive exercise stress testing in women. When myocardial perfusion imaging is used (thallium scanning), some of the false-positive reports are thought to be secondary to breast attenuation. Exercise echocardiography is an alternative approach to the evaluation of chest pain in women. Women, more often than men, have vascular and renal complications following diagnostic coronary angiography.

REFERENCE

1. Douglas, P.S., and Ginsburg, G.S.: The evaluation of chest pain in women. N. Engl. J. Med. *334*:1311, 1996.

626-E *(Braunwald, p. 1673)*

Homocystinuria is caused by a deficiency of the enzyme cystathionine β-synthase. Patients with homocystinuria are similar phenotypically to those with Marfan syndrome. Patients may have tall stature, skeletal deformities, and mental retardation. Psychological disturbances and ectopia lentis may also be seen. These patients have a predilection for venous and arterial thromboses, and myocardial infarction, stroke, and pulmonary embolism are the most common causes of death in this disease. Heterozygotes for homocystinuria, who have no phenotypic features of the disease, have an increased risk of atherosclerosis.[1] The pathogenesis of the cardiovascular complications of this disease is complex and focuses on the actions of homocysteine on endothelial and smooth muscle cells.[2] Previous theories concerning abnormalities in platelet dysfunction have been discounted and studies show that platelet survival is normal in untreated patients.[3] Studies also suggest that elevated plasma homocysteine is a risk factor for the development of coronary artery disease independent of other risk factors.[4] Patients with the full homocystinuric phenotype may be treated with pyridoxine; patients unresponsive to pyridoxine should be given a low-protein diet in an effort to reduce methionine intake. Folate and vitamins B_6 and B_{12} should also be given to optimize the metabolism of sulfurated amino acids.[5]

REFERENCES

1. Selhub, J., Jacques, P.F., Bostom, A.G., et al.: Association between plasma homocysteine concentrations and extracranial carotid artery; stenosis. N. Engl. J. Med. 32:286, 1995.
2. Hajjar, K.A.: Homocysteine-induced modulation of tissue plasminogen activator binding to its endothelial cell membrane receptor. J. Clin. Invest. 91:2873, 1993.
3. Hill-Zobel, R.L., Pyeritz, R.E., Scheffel, U., et al.: Kinetics and biodistribution of 111-In-labeled platelets in homocystinuria. N. Engl. J. Med. 307:781, 1982.
4. Genest, J.J., Jr., McNamara, J.R., Upson, B., et al.: Prevalence of familial hyperhomocyst(s)inemia in men with premature coronary artery disease. Arterioscler. Thromb. 11: 1129, 1991.
5. Stampfer, M.J., and Manilow, M.R.: Can lowering homocysteine levels reduce cardiovascular risk? N. Engl. J. Med. 332:328, 1995.

627-C (Braunwald, pp. 1721–1722)

The first 48 hours after cardiovascular surgery involve electrolyte imbalances and fluid shifts. Serum potassium levels fluctuate significantly, especially in diabetics. Serum calcium, phosphorus, and magnesium levels are often decreased and demand close monitoring and replacement to limit cardiac arrhythmia potential.[1] Many patients demonstrate mild to moderate glucose intolerance in the immediate postoperative period owing to both the glucose contained in intravenous solutions and the surgically induced increase in catecholamines and cortisol production. Most nondiabetic patients do not require insulin therapy. In the period following rewarming, metabolic acidosis or alkalosis may be evident, but usually does not require further therapy in the absence of renal failure.[2] Most patients experience alveolar dysfunction during the immediate postoperative period due to right-to-left intrapulmonary shunting (atelectasis, pulmonary edema, pulmonary vasoconstriction). Respiratory muscle function and central respiratory drive are decreased postoperatively due to drug effects and mechanical dysfunction after thoracic surgery.

REFERENCES

1. Karen, A., and Tzivoni, D.: Magnesium therapy in ventricular arrhythmias. PACE 13:937, 1990.
2. Kirklin, J.W., and Barratt-Boyes, B.: Postoperative care. In Kirklin, J., and Barratt-Boyes, B. (eds.): Cardiac Surgery. New York, Churchill Livingstone, 1993, p. 195.

628-C (Braunwald, pp. 1707–1709)

It is widely known that menopause (estrogen deprivation) is associated with an increased car-

diovascular risk. Postmenopausal estrogen therapy in women has many favorable effects on the risk factors for cardiac disease. Exogenous estrogen in women has been shown to increase HDL and reduce total cholesterol, LDL, and VLDL.[1] Oral estrogen therapy appears to be more effective than transdermal delivery for this lipid effect due to first-pass hepatic metabolism. Estrogen also appears to play a direct role in regulation of vascular smooth muscle function.

Functional estrogen receptors have been demonstrated in vascular smooth muscle and are capable of altering gene transcription and potentially smooth muscle proliferation.[2] In addition, estrogen is a proven therapy for women with osteoporosis and may have a protective effect against stroke. Tamoxifen, the estrogen agonist/antagonist used by many women with breast cancer has beneficial effects on lipid profiles and postmenopausal coronary disease.

Unopposed estrogen therapy has been linked to endometrial hyperplasia and up to an eightfold increased risk for uterine carcinoma in women with an intact uterus. Therefore, for women with an intact uterus, progestins are often prescribed in an effort to offset the estrogen effect on the endometrium. However, progestins may ameliorate the favorable effect of estrogen on the lipid profile. Long-term estrogen use has also been linked to the development of breast cancer, especially in cases with known personal or family histories of breast cancer. Thus, careful monitoring is mandatory for any patient on estrogen therapy and, as with any therapy, the risks and rewards must be discussed with the patient prior to initiation of treatment.

REFERENCES

1. Lobo, R.A.: Hormones, hormone replacement therapy, and heart disease. In Douglas, P.S. (ed.): Cardiovascular Health and Disease in Women. Philadelphia. W.B. Saunders Company, 1993, p. 153.
2. Karas, R.H., Patterson, B.L., and Mendelsohn, M.E.: Human vascular smooth muscle cells contain functional estrogen receptor. Circulation 89:1943, 1994.

629-C (Braunwald, pp. 1851–1852; Fig. 59–6)

Peripartum cardiomyopathy (PPCM) is a form of dilated cardiomyopathy that occurs for the first time in the antepartum or postpartum period and is clinically indistinguishable from other forms of dilated cardiomyopathy. Symptoms usually occur during the first month after delivery or in the month immediately before delivery (see Braunwald, Fig. 59–6, p. 1851). Occasionally the disease may occur earlier in the last trimester or later in the postpartum period.[1] The incidence of PPCM appears to be greater in *multiparous black women* who are over 30 years of age and in women carrying twin pregnancies.[1,2] The etiology of PPCM is unknown, although recent data from endomyocardial biopsy studies of such patients suggest a greater incidence of myocarditis in this disorder than in other forms of dilated cardiomyopathy.[3] A bimodal population of outcomes is noted in PPCM: approximately 50 per cent of patients show complete or near-complete recovery during the first 6 months after delivery, while the remaining patients demonstrate either continual clinical deterioration or persistent left ventricular dysfunction and chronic heart failure.[1,2,4] Subsequent pregnancies in patients with PPCM with persistent cardiac dysfunction should be discouraged because of the high likelihood of relapse.[5] Patients who have recovered from an episode of PPCM also have a higher risk for relapse during subsequent pregnancies and must be carefully counseled before subsequent pregnancies are initiated.

REFERENCES

1. Homans, D.C.: Peripartum cardiomyopathy. N. Engl. J. Med. *312*:1432, 1985.
2. Ribner, H.S., and Silberman, R.L.: Peripartal cardiomyopathy. *In* Elkayam, U., and Gleicher, N. (eds.): Cardiac Problems in Pregnancy: Diagnosis and Management of Maternal and Fetal Disease. 2nd ed. New York, Alan R. Liss, Inc., 1990, p. 115.
3. Midei, M.C., DeMent, S.H., Feldman, A.M., et al.: Peripartum myocarditis and cardiomyopathy. Circulation *81*:922, 1990.
4. Carvalho, A., Brandao, A., Martinez, E.E., et al.: Prognosis in peripartum cardiomyopathy. Am. J. Cardiol. *64*:540, 1989.
5. St. John Sutton, M., Cole, P., Saltzman, D., et al.: Risks of cardiac dysfunction in peripartum cardiomyopathy (PPCM) with subsequent pregnancy. Circulation *80*(Suppl. 11):320, 1989.

630-C *(Braunwald, pp. 1661–1662)*

Congenital supravalvular AS has been documented in at least four settings. The lesion has been seen as (1) a sporadic anomaly; (2) in association with peripheral pulmonic stenoses (and inherited as an autosomal dominant trait); (3) as a component of Williams syndrome; and (4) in isolated form inherited with an autosomal dominant inheritance. The lesion may be asymptomatic and is then often recognized because of the presence of a systolic ejection murmur loudest in the suprasternal notch. The Williams syndrome is usually sporadic but may also occur as a variable autosomal dominant condition. This disorder includes infantile hypercalcemia, "elfin" facies, short stature, mental deficiency, multiple peripheral pulmonic stenoses, and supravalvular AS.[1] Mitral valve prolapse, hypertension, and bicuspid aortic valve have all been described in this syndrome as well. Isolated supravalvular AS has now been recognized as a distinct autosomal dominant entity as well.[2] In addition to the association of hypercalcemia with supravalvular AS in Williams syndrome, undetected hypercalcemia during vulnerable periods of gestation has been suggested as one cause of the sporadic form of supravalvular AS.

REFERENCES

1. Preus, M.: The Williams syndrome. Objective definition and diagnosis. Clin. Genet. *23*:422, 1984.
2. Ensing, G.J., Schmidt, M.A., Hagler, D.J., et al.: Spectrum of findings in a family with nonsyndromic autosomal dominant supravalvular aortic stenosis. A Doppler echocardiographic study. J. Am. Coll. Cardiol. *13*:413, 1989.

631-B *(Braunwald, pp. 1792–1794)*

Polycythemia vera is a myeloproliferative disorder characterized by increased production of all myeloid elements.[1] Increased levels of red blood cells, white blood cells, and platelets occur due to disregulation of clonal growth. Polycythemia vera begins in middle adult life and is more common in males. Patients with this disorder often present with symptoms associated with increased blood volume and viscosity and subsequent decreased transportation of oxygen to target organs. In addition to thrombosis from high viscosity, hemorrhage may occur due to both local ischemia and to the presence of dysfunctional platelets. Patients may complain of headache, dizziness, visual disturbances, syncope, dyspnea, and chest pain. Patients may also note fevers, sweats, and pruritis (which, curiously, may worsen with hot water showers). Splenomegaly is found in later stage disease and is associated with extramedullary hematopoiesis. Along with elevations in hemoglobin, white blood cell count, and platelet count, increases in red cell mass, leukocyte alkaline phosphatase, lactate dehydrogenase, and serum B_{12} levels also are common in this disease. Bone marrow evaluation shows erythroid hyperplasia or panhyperplasia.

Long-term therapy for polycythemia vera is controversial. However, the initial management of the symptomatic patient should focus on decreasing the blood volume by phlebotomy and replacement with colloid. Lowering the hematocrit to less than 45 per cent has been shown to improve blood flow.[2] Bone marrow suppression with agents such as hydroxyurea, melphalan, busulfan, and chlorambucil may be helpful. Secondary polycythemia is defined as an elevated hematocrit with increased erythropoietin secretion in response to another stimulus (i.e., cyanotic heart disease, pulmonary disease). The treatment of patients with secondary polycythemia includes phlebotomy and identification of correction of the stimulus.

REFERENCES

1. Fruchtam, S.M., and Berk, P.D.: Polycythemia vera and agnogenic myeloid metaplasia. *In* Handin, R.I., Lux, S.E., and Stossel, T.P. (eds.): Blood: Principles and Practice of Hematology. Philadelphia, J.B. Lippincott, 1995.
2. Thomas, D.J., Marshall, J., Russell, R.W., et al.: Effect of hematocrit on cerebral blood flow in man. Lancet *2*:941, 1977.

632-A *(Braunwald, pp. 1905–1907)*

In addition to its metabolic consequences, which include glucose intolerance, hypertriglyceridemia and hyperaminoacidemia, obesity has marked effects on the cardiovascular system. It is estimated that over 34 million American adults are obese with a body mass index (weight in kilograms/height in meters squared) of over 27. Obesity is accompanied by an increase in preload and cardiac output and a slight elevation in hematocrit. The increased cardiac output is due to an elevated stroke volume and left ventricular end-diastolic volume. Heart rate is not directly related to weight gain.

Pathological examination of heart tissue in obese individuals reveals left ventricular dilation and hypertrophy, often in an eccentric pattern. The heart is heavy due to increased muscle mass, not fatty infiltration into the tissue. Ventricular ectopy is a frequent finding in obese patients, likely secondary to autonomic dysfunction. Hypertension is very common in obese patients and may lead to both concentric and eccentric hypertrophy. Patients may also develop an increased resistance to insulin and glucose intolerance, and there is also a direct correlation between obesity and elevated cholesterol levels.[1]

Central obesity is considered to be an independent risk for the development of coronary artery disease. Many of the ill effects of obesity, however, may be reversed with weight loss. Weight loss of as little as 8 kg has been shown to decrease left ventricular mass and chamber enlargement.[2] In addition, exercise capacity, blood pressure and preload improve with weight loss. Rapid weight loss has been associated with cardiac arrhythmias, associated with electrolyte abnormalities, cardiac atrophy, or myocardial protein imbalance.

REFERENCES

1. Foster, W.R., and Burton, B.T. (eds.): Health implications of obesity: NIH consensus development conference. Ann. Intern. Med. *103*:979, 1985.
2. MacMahon, S.W., Wilcken, D.E., and MacDonald, G.J.: The effect of weight reduction on left ventricular mass: A randomized controlled trial in young, overweight hypertensive patients. N. Engl. J. Med. *314*:334, 1986.

633-C *(Braunwald, pp. 1846–1848, 1850–1851)*

Congenital heart disorders in the mother may influence both maternal and fetal outcome. Careful management often allows an excellent obstetric result in this population. This fact must be tempered with an increased incidence of both fetal wastage and prematurity in cyanotic mothers and an increased risk for congenital heart disease in the offspring of mothers with such disorders.[1] ASD is a common form of maternal congenital heart disease (CHD) and frequently presents during pregnancy, when a murmur may first be heard. The condition is usually well tolerated during pregnancy, even among patients with large left-to-right shunts. Similarly, patients with isolated VSD usually tolerate pregnancy well. Occasionally, congenital heart failure or arrhythmias may be precipitated in patients

with uncorrected lesions,[2] and a marked reduction in blood pressure during delivery may lead to shunt reversal in patients with pulmonary hypertension. Because of the early diagnosis and surgical correction of PDA, this lesion is now relatively rare among pregnant women. In general, maternal outcome in patients with PDA is favorable. As with PDA, coarctation of the aorta is a relatively rare finding in the pregnant mother because surgical correction is usually performed before the childbearing age.[3] In uncomplicated coarctation, pregnancy is usually safe for the mother, although fetal development may be impaired to some degree and maternal complications such as hypertension, congestive heart failure, angina, and aortic dissection have all been reported.[4] Because of such complications and because infants of mothers with uncorrected coarctation seem to have a higher incidence of congenital heart disease than those who have undergone repair,[1] correction of aortic coarctation is advised before pregnancy whenever possible.

Marfan syndrome is one congenital disorder that is poorly tolerated during pregnancy. The incidence of aortic dissection and maternal death appears to be increased in pregnant patients with the Marfan syndrome and is in part correlated with the extent of underlying cardiac involvement.[5] Present recommendations include advising against conception in women with significant cardiac involvement from Marfan syndrome, including asymptomatic dilatation of the aorta. If the condition in such patients is discovered after pregnancy begins, early abortion is advised. However, in patients without cardiac complications and with a normal aortic diameter, strict management may allow successful pregnancy and delivery.

REFERENCES

1. Whittemore, R., Hobbins, J.C., and Engle, M.A.: Pregnancy and its outcome in women with and without surgical treatment of congenital heart disease. Am. J. Cardiol. *50*: 641, 1982.
2. Lee, W., Shah, P.K., Amin, D.K., et al.: Hemodynamic monitoring of cardiac patients during pregnancy. *In* Elkayam, U., and Gleicher, N. (eds.): Cardiac Problems in Pregnancy: Diagnosis and Management of Maternal and Fetal Disease. 2nd ed. New York, Alan R. Liss, Inc., 1990, p. 47.
3. McFaul, P.B., Dorman, J.C., Lamki, H., et al.: Pregnancy complicated by maternal heart disease. A review of 519 women. Br. J. Obstet. Gynecol. *95*:861, 1988.
4. Wachtel, H.L., and Czarnecki, S.W.: Coarctation of the aorta and pregnancy. Am. Heart J. *72*:251, 1966.
5. Pyeritz, R.E.: Maternal and fetal complications of pregnancy in the Marfan syndrome. Am. J. Med. *71*:784, 1981.

634-B *(Braunwald, pp. 1669–1672)*

Sinus of Valsalva aneurysm is a rare congenital anomaly due to a failure of fusion between the aortic media and the heart at the level of the annulus fibrosis of the aortic valve. This entity has also been associated with ankylosing spondylitis, syphilis, endocarditis, and Marfan syndrome and is more common in Orientals and men. The defect gradually gives way to the high aortic pressures and forms an aneurysm, and over time, may rupture into a cardiac chamber. Rupture occurs most often in the second and third decades of life. Ruptured sinuses of Valsalva may occur spontaneously or may be secondary to trauma or endocarditis. Nonruptured aneurysms are usually asymptomatic and silent on examination. Rupture produces symptoms in about 40 per cent of patients: slow rupture is often silent and produces a small fistula and shunt with a predisposition for endocarditis, while sudden rupture often causes sharp chest pain with rapid decompensation and heart failure. Aneurysmal enlargement and rupture may cause coronary occlusion, conduction abnormalities, and valvular insufficiency.

Physical examination of a ruptured sinus of Valsalva reveals a continuous murmur and thrill on the lower/mid sternum (similar to a patient ductus arteriosus, coronary arterovenous fistula, ventricular septal defect). Electrocardiogram may show evidence of right heart strain and the chest x-ray often shows cardiac enlargement or elevated pulmonary pressures. Most commonly, aneurysms form in the right coronary sinus and rupture into the right ventricular infundibulum. These fistulas are associated with ventricular septal defects in 50 per cent of cases.[1] Right coronary sinus aneurysms may also rupture into the right atrium and left ventricle. Aneurysms originating in the noncoronary sinus rupture most often into the right ventricle and right atrium. Left coronary sinus rupture is less common and may form a fistulous tract into the left heart. Aortic insufficiency is detected in about half of the cases and vegetations on various valves are found in about one-sixth of cases. Other complications of rupture include pulmonic stenosis, tricuspid regurgitation, mitral regurgitation, and arrhythmias.

Before the advent of noninvasive cardiac imaging, the diagnosis of sinus of Valsalva aneurysms/ rupture was made by cardiac catheterization. Two-dimensional echocardiography, along with color flow imaging and Doppler, has now become the chosen method for diagnosis. M-mode echocardiography may also be helpful in the detection of aneurysms. Transesophageal echocardiography allows for excellent location and hemodynamic assessment of sinus of Valsalva aneurysms, and intracardiac ultrasound imaging has also been shown to be helpful in defining the anatomy and physiology of intracardiac fistulas.[2] Surgical repair involves opening the involved chamber and the aortic root to allow for closure of the fistula and inspection of the aorta. Life expectancy of patients undergoing surgical repair approaches that of the health population. There is a low risk of recurrence, but late aortic insufficiency is a risk, especially in right sinus of Valsalva to right ventricular fistula with associated VSD.[3] Transcatheter closure of ruptured aneurysms of the sinus of Valsalva has been reported recently.[4]

REFERENCES

1. Dev, V., Goswami, K., et al.: Echocardiographic diagnosis of aneurysm of the sinus of Valsalva. Am. Heart J. *126*:930–936, 1993.
2. McKenney, P., Shemin, R., and Wiegers, S.: Role of transesophageal echocardiography in sinus of Valsalva aneurysm. Am. Heart J. *123*:228–229, 1992.
3. van Son, J., Danielson, G., et al.: Long-term outcome of surgical repair of ruptured sinus of Valsalva aneurysm. Circulation *90*:II-20–II-28, 1994.
4. Cullen, S., Somerville, J., and Redington, A.: Transcatheter closure of a ruptured aneurysm of the sinus of Valsalva. Br. Heart J. *71*:479–480, 1994.

635-E (Braunwald, pp. 1656–1657)

Trisomy 21 occurs in approximately 1 in every 600 births, and increases exponentially in relation to maternal age. Women over the age of 45 have a 4 per cent chance of delivering a child with this syndrome. Morbidity and mortality in Down syndrome patients are most commonly caused by congenital heart defects, hematological malignancies, and duodenal atresia. Congenital heart disease is detected in between 40 and 50 per cent of Down's patients and most characteristically is seen as an endocardial cushion defect. An increased predisposition to pulmonary hypertension in the setting of increased right-sided flow exists in Down syndrome patients with septal defects.[1]

Approximately one-third of the congenital heart defects in Down syndrome patients are quite complex, and these patients tend to be the most ill of those with Down syndrome. Mitral valve prolapse and aortic and/or pulmonary valve cusp fenestrations are also seen with increased frequency in trisomy 21. As surgical follow-up data have become available, it has become clear that early and late postoperative survival statistics in patients with Down syndrome are no different from those in unaffected patients with similar cardiac defects.[2]

REFERENCES

1. Clapp, S., Perry, B.L., Farooki, Z.Q., et al.: Down's syndrome, complete atrioventricular canal and pulmonary vascular obstructive disease. J. Thorac. Cardiovasc. Surg. *100*:115, 1990.
2. Schneider, D.S., Zahka, K.G., Clark, E.B., et al.: Patterns of cardiac care in infants with Down syndrome. Am. J. Dis. Child. *143*:363, 1989.

636-B (Braunwald, pp. 1664–1665)

Familial hypertrophic cardiomyopathy (FHC) is a cardiac condition that is increasingly better understood at the molecular level. FHC is a disease of the sarcomere, affecting the thick and thin filaments, which results in myocardial hypertrophy, myofibril disarray and fibrosis and mediointimal proliferation of small coronary arteries. Approximately half of the patients with idiopathic FHC have first-degree relatives who are affected, and transmission is felt to be autosomal dominant. There are a wide variety of presentations of FHC, especially due to age dependency of the trait.[1] Numerous mutations have been identified for this disease. About 50 per cent of all FHC mutations occur on the cardiac β-myosin heavy chain, and these patients carry a worse prognosis in terms of age of detection, electrocardiographic abnormalities, and sudden death.[2,3] Mutations in α-tropomyosin, cardiac troponin T, and the gene coding for cardiac myosin binding protein-C have also been linked to FHC.[4,5] Pedigree screening is essential and includes a thorough history and physical examination along with an echocardiogram and electrocardiogram. Molecular screening for mutations may assist in the diagnosis.

REFERENCES

1. Epstein, N.D., Lin, H.J., and Fananapazir, L.: Genetic evidence of dissociation (generational skips) of electrical from morphologic forms of hypertrophic cardiomyopathy. Am. J. Cardiol. 66:627, 1990.
2. Watkins, H., Seidman, J.G., and Seidman, C.E.: Familial hypertrophic cardiomyopathy: A genetic model of cardiac hypertrophy. Hum. Mol. Genet. 4:1721, 1995.
3. Watkins, H., Rosenzweig, A., Hwang, D.S., et al.: Characteristics and prognostic implications of myosin missense mutations in familial hypertrophic cardiomyopathy. N. Engl. J. Med. 326:1108, 1992.
4. Watkins, H., MacRae, C., Thierfelder, L., et al.: A disease locus for familial hypertrophic cardiomyopathy maps to chromosome 6q3. Nat. Genet. 3:333, 1993.
5. Bonnie, G., Carrier, L., Bercovici, J., et al.: Cardiac myosin binding protein-C gene splice acceptor site mutation is associated with familial hypertrophic cardiomyopathy. Nat. Genet. 11:438, 1995.

637-E   (Braunwald, pp. 964–971, 1347–1348)

In current cardiac surgery, most procedures have a low hospital mortality. Reparative operations in general are ones that are most likely to yield excellent or prolonged palliation or cure and are least likely to require repeat operation. Included among these are closure of patent ductus arteriosus, closure of aortopulmonary windows, closure of atrial septal and ventricular septal defects, simple repair (opening) of mitral stenosis, and simple repair of tetralogy of Fallot. (A more complicated reconstruction of tetralogy of Fallot, such as use of a transannular patch, is not considered a simple repair).

Excisional procedures are less common in cardiac surgery than in most other fields of surgery; they include removal of trial myxomas as well as excision of left ventricular aneurysms. In many cases, such excisional procedures are accompanied by a reconstructive process. However, surgical treatment of ventricular aneurysm cannot be considered a simple reparative operation.

In some institutions simple cardiac repairs, including pulmonary, aortic, and mitral valvotomy, as well as closure of patent ductus arteriosus, are now successfully carried out via percutaneous approaches in the cardiac catheterization laboratory.

638-C   (Braunwald, p. 1697)

Elderly patients have myocardial infarctions that may differ from those in younger populations. There is an increase in congestive heart failure, ventricular rupture and mortality with acute myocardial infarction in the elderly. The size of the infarction is often no greater with increased age, but there is a higher degree of left ventricular dysfunction following the event. However, despite atypical and delayed presentations of myocardial ischemia, along with an increased risk of bleeding, there is a survival benefit with the use of thrombolytic agents in older age groups.[1] Like with younger populations, contraindications to thrombolytic agents in the elderly include hypertension, history of stroke, and gastrointestinal bleeding.

The Global Utilization of Streptokinase and Tissue Plasminogen Activator for Occluded Coronary Arteries I (GUSTO I) trial revealed a significantly increased risk of intracranial bleeding in patients over 75 years old who received tissue plasminogen activator therapy. Recent studies indicate a survival benefit and lower risk of cerebrovascular accidents in older patients who undergo primary angioplasty rather than receive thrombolytic therapy.[2] Toxicity of other drugs may also be more pronounced in older populations. Central nervous system side effects from lidocaine are more common in the elderly,[3] and heparin-induced bleeding is more common in older women.[4] Remodeling changes after infarction may differ in the elderly patient due to changes in the inflammatory response, decreased ability of the area to undergo hypertrophy, and increased collagen content of the heart tissue. However, elderly patients benefit as much as younger patients from beta blocker therapy for secondary prevention.[5] In addition, in patients over 65 years old who had myocardial infarctions and an ejection fraction of less than 40 per cent, angiotensin-converting enzyme inhibitors reduce fatal and nonfatal events just as they do for patients under age 65.[6]

REFERENCES

1. Gore, J., Becker, R., Tiefenbrunn, A., et al.: The National Registry of Myocardial Infarction (NRMI) Investigators: Current trends in the treatment of elderly patients with acute myocardial infarction. J. Am. Coll. Cardiol. 21:481A, 1993.
2. Grines, C.L., Griffin, J.J., Brodie, B.R., et al.: The secondary primary angioplasty for myocardial infarction study (PAMI-II): Preliminary Report. Circulation 90(Suppl. I): 433, 1994.
3. Lie, K.L., Wellens, H.J., van Capelle, F.J., et al.: Lidocaine in the prevention of primary ventricular fibrillation. N. Engl. J. Med. 291:1324, 1974.
4. Jick, H., Sloan, D., and Borda, I.T.: Efficacy and toxicity of heparin in relation to age and sex. N. Engl. J. Med. 297: 284, 1988.
5. Gundersen, T., Abrahamsen, A.M., Kjekshus, J., et al.: Timolol-related reduction in mortality and reinfarction in patients ages 65–75 years surviving acute myocardial infarction. Circulation 66:1179, 1982.
6. Pfeffer, M.A., Braunwald, E., Moye, L.A., et al.: Effect of captopril on mortality and morbidity in patients with left ven-

tricular dysfunction after myocardial infarction. N. Engl. J. Med. *327*:669, 1992.

639-B *(Braunwald, pp. 1764–1766)*

Because many patients over the age of 40 who are scheduled for elective surgery are likely to have coronary artery disease and other cardiac illnesses, it is useful to estimate their preoperative risk for a cardiac event. Certain cardiovascular problems, such as recent myocardial infarction (<3 months), inadequately treated congestive heart failure, and severe mitral or aortic stenosis, are absolute contraindications to *elective* surgery. Relative contraindications to surgery include a history of MI (within 3 to 6 months of the surgery), angina pectoris, mild heart failure, cyanotic congenital heart disease, and coagulation abnormalities. Several criteria have been suggested for estimation of cardiac risk.[1,2] Included are age greater than 70 years, recent myocardial infarction, signs of congestive heart failure, S_3 gallop, jugular venous distention, abnormal ECG (including rhythm other than sinus or more than 5 PVCs/min), and abnormal arterial blood gases with Pco_2 greater than 50 mm Hg, BUN greater than 50 mg/dl, and creatine greater than 3 mg/dl. Notably, statistically nonsignificant factors include smoking, glucose intolerance, hyperlipidemia, hypertension, peripheral atherosclerotic vascular disease, stable class I or II angina, and a remote MI.[1]

It should be noted that these criteria are useful only for risk stratification. The history and examination of the patient, including prior responses to surgery, development of unstable angina, and abnormalities on chest x-ray consistent with heart failure, should initially alert the clinician to cardiac risk. Furthermore, it is clear that any correctable abnormality, including anemia, hypovolemia, polycythemia, hypoxemia, electrolyte abnormalities, hypertension, and arrhythmias, should be treated preoperatively when identified.

REFERENCES

1. Goldman, L., Caldera, D.L., Nussbaum, S.R., et al.: Multifactorial index of cardiac risk in noncardiac surgical procedures. N. Engl. J. Med. *297*:845, 1977.
2. Zeldin, R.A.: Assessing cardiac risk in patients who undergo noncardiac surgical procedures. Can. J. Surg. *27*:402, 1984.

640-A *(Braunwald, p. 1790)*

Microangiopathic hemolytic anemia may be seen in patients with native cardiac valvular disease or with valvular prostheses. The incidence of hemolysis is greater with mechanical valves than with porcine valves, greater with small valves than with large valves, greater with valves in the aortic position than with valves in lower flow areas such as the mitral valve, and greater when there is a paravalvular leak. The peripheral blood smear from patients with valvular hemolysis may reveal frag-mented red blood cells, burr cells, and schistocytes. Spherocytes are commonly found in patients with *extra*vascular hemolysis, including immune-mediated hemolysis. In addition to the findings on the blood smear, plasma and urine hemoglobin levels are elevated, haptoglobin is low, and the reticulocyte count and serum lactic dehydrogenase levels are high. When evidence exists for intravascular hemolysis, one must always consider causes other than the presence of a valvular prosthesis, including disseminated intravascular coagulation and thrombotic thrombocytopenic purpura.

641-B *(Braunwald, p. 1699)*

Data from three major trials indicate clearly that effective therapy for even mild diastolic hypertension leads to a reduction in mortality and cardiovascular events.[1-3] Similar results have also recently been published on the effectiveness of therapy for isolated systolic hypertension in older populations. In the SHEP study of systolic hypertension in the elderly,[4] treatment of isolated systolic hypertension was shown to reduce the incidence of both stroke and major cardiovascular events. The SHEP trial thus validates the treatment of isolated hypertension in the elderly, an approach recommended since 1984 by the Joint National Committee on Detection, Evaluation, and Treatment of High Blood Pressure.[5] Beta blocker therapy may be less effective in older patients, and calcium channel antagonists and/or angiotensin-converting enzyme inhibitors therefore may be especially appropriate for use in this population. Recent data from the Framingham Study have proved the importance of LVH as an independent risk factor for coronary disease in older, hypertensive subjects.[6] Hypertrophic cardiomyopathy in the setting of hypertension in elderly patients represents an interesting syndrome.[7] The vast majority of patients with this disease are female, and the presenting symptom is usually dyspnea or chest pain. Diagnosis is made by echocardiography; therapy is based on the use of beta blocker or calcium channel blocker therapy, with avoidance of vasodilators, which may exacerbate symptoms.

REFERENCES

1. Hypertension Detection and Follow-up Program Cooperative Group: Five-year findings on the Hypertension Detection and Follow-up Program: Mortality by race, sex and age. JAMA *242*:2572, 1979.
2. European Working Party on High Blood Pressure in the Elderly: Mortality and morbidity results from the European Working Party on High Blood Pressure in the Elderly Trial. Lancet *1*:1349, 1985.
3. Management Committee of the Australian Therapeutic Trial in Mild Hypertension: Treatment of mild hypertension in the elderly. Med. J. Aust. *2*:398, 1981.
4. Prevention of Stroke by Antihypertensive Drug Treatment in Older Persons with Isolated Systolic Hypertension. Final results of the Systolic Hypertension in the Elderly Program (SHEP). JAMA *265*:3255, 1991.

5. Joint National Committee on Detection, Evaluation, and Treatment of High Blood Pressure: The 1984 report of the Joint National Committee on Detection, Evaluation, and Treatment of High Blood Pressure. Arch. Intern. Med. *144*: 1045, 1984.
6. Levy, D., Garrison, R.J., Savage, D.D., et al.: Left ventricular mass and incidence of coronary heart disease in an elderly cohort. Ann. Intern. Med. *110*:101, 1989.
7. Topol, E.J., Traill, T.A., and Fortuin, N.J.: Hypertensive hypertrophic cardiomyopathy of the elderly. N. Engl. J. Med. *312*:277, 1985.

642-B   *(Braunwald, pp. 1810–1811)*

In their unactivated state, platelets circulate as smooth-surfaced discs that do not interact with the endothelial cells lining blood vessels. The events of primary hemostasis may be initiated by exposure of *subendothelium* by vascular injury. Platelet adhesion is the initial event in primary hemostasis and is a complex process that involves the interaction of specific platelet membrane receptors, subendothelial collagen, and adhesive glycoproteins (including von Willebrand's factor), and fibronectin. The process of platelet activation and secretion is complex and culminates in both phosphorylation of intraplatelet regulatory proteins and the formation of specific eicosanoids derived from arachidonic acid. These eicosanoids are capable of extending the processes of platelet activation and vasoconstriction during hemostasis. Degranulation of platelet occurs following activation. It leads to the release of further constituents and mediators such as ADP, which are capable of recruiting circulating platelets to the developing platelet aggregate.

These events, known as "primary hemostasis," serve as an initial defense against hemorrhage following vascular injury. They are especially important in capillaries and arterioles, in which shear forces are higher and the formation of a platelet plug is therefore critical for effective hemostasis. The "secondary hemostatic" system includes the plasma coagulation system, which leads to the generation of fibrin strands capable of interdigitating with the platelet plug and further strengthening the local hemostatic response.

643-C   *(Braunwald, p. 1907)*

Anorexia nervosa is an eating disorder seen primarily in young, white, previously healthy women from middle to upper-income homes. In this disorder, the patients struggle to limit food intake because of an overwhelming fear of being fat. The prevalence of anorexia nervosa is between 0.5 and 1.5 per 100,000 persons, and is felt to be on the rise. Cardiac complications of this condition are frequent. Electrolyte abnormalities, including hypomagnesemia, hypocalcemia, and hypokalemia may result in arrhythmias and even sudden death.[1] Cardiac output and left ventricular mass may be diminished, and these patients are often hypertensive.[2] Bradycardia, prolonged Q-T interval, ectopic

rhythms, and nonspecific electrocardiographic changes may also be noted. Mitral valve abnormalities may be detected. Laboratory abnormalities may include electrolyte disturbances, prerenal azotemia, and hypercholesterolemia. Hormonal imbalance may also be detected. Heart failure may occur during the refeeding stage due to profound hypophosphatemia.

REFERENCES

1. Isner, J.M., Roberts, W.C., Heymsfield, S.B., and Yager, J.: Anorexia nervosa and sudden death. Ann. Intern. Med. *102*:49, 1985.
2. de Simone, G., Scalfi, L., Galderisi, M., et al.: Cardiac abnormalities in young women with anorexia nervosa. Br. Heart J. *71*:287, 1994.

644-C   *(Braunwald, pp. 1795–1797)*

Metastatic tumors to the pericardium or heart are much more common than are primary tumors of the heart. Cardiac metastases are present at autopsy in approximately 6 per cent of patients with malignant disease, while primary cardiac tumors occur in less than 1.0 per cent of autopsies. Usually the metastases involve the pericardium and the myocardium, with the valves and endocardium rarely affected. Solitary metastases to the heart are rare, and a solitary cardiac tumor is usually a benign tumor. Many cardiac metastases are clinically silent. For instance, in malignant melanoma, approximately 60 per cent of patients have cardiac metastases, yet cardiac symptoms are rare. The most common clinical manifestations of metastatic disease are secondary to the effects of pericardial effusion, such as tamponade, tachyarrhythmias, AV block, and congestive heart failure. The most common primary tumor producing cardiac metastases in carcinoma of the bronchus, with carcinoma of the breast, malignant melanoma, lymphoma, and leukemias following in order of frequency.[1]

Signs and symptoms of pericarditis, pericardial effusion, and tamponade are typical in patients with carcinoma of the lung and breast as well as in Hodgkin's disease, non-Hodgkin's lymphoma, and leukemia involving the heart. The finding of a chylous pericardial effusion is usually characteristic of lymphomatous involvement.

Pericardial symptoms are best treated by effective therapy of the primary tumor with chemotherapy or radiation therapy. When these prove ineffective, recurrent pericardiocentesis or surgical construction of a pericardial window may provide symptomatic relief. In rare cases, analysis of pericardial fluid may help produce the diagnosis in otherwise unsuspected situations. Pericardial fibrosis secondary to radiation therapy may mimic chronic constrictive pericarditis or chronic effusive pericardial disease, especially in patients with carcinoma of the lung, Hodgkin's disease, or non-Hodgkin's lymphoma, who commonly undergo radiation to the thorax. It has become clear that radiation-induced pericarditis may occur 8 years or more following therapy. Therefore, in patients with recurrent symptoms of pericardial disease who have also received radiation, differentiation from recurrent disease is somewhat difficult.

REFERENCE

1. Schoen, F.J., Berger, B.M., and Guerina, N.G.: Cardiac effects of noncardiac neoplasms. Cardiol. Clin. 2:657, 1984.

645-C   (Braunwald, pp. 1663–1664)

Teratogens are exogenous substances that adversely affect the development of an embryo or fetus. Teratogens can include drugs, microorganisms, chemicals, and exposures (such as radiation). The cardiovascular system in the developing fetus may be adversely affected by teratogens. The most common teratogenic exposure for the human embryo and fetus is ethanol. Alcohol's deleterious effects are directly proportional to the quantity consumed, and the time of exposure to the fetus is critical, with first-trimester ingestion being the most harmful. Cardiovascular features of the *fetal alcohol syndrome* include ventricular septal defects, atrial septal defects, tetralogy of Fallot, and aortic coarctation.[1]

Lithium ingestion during pregnancy has been linked to both Ebstein's anomaly and tricuspid atresia. Hypervitaminosis D (associated with idiopathic infantile hypercalcemia) is associated with *supra*valvular aortic stenosis. In addition, this entity is associated with mental retardation, elfin facies, auditory hyperacusis, and peripheral pulmonary stenosis.

Warfarin is a common drug and therefore is often prescribed to women of childbearing age. The teratogenic effects of warfarin differ based on the time of exposure to the fetus. If warfarin exposure occurs during the sixth through the ninth week of gestation, the compound acts to inhibit enzymes involved in extracellular matrix metabolism and cartilage formation. In contrast, exposure during the second and third trimesters of pregnancy has been linked to spontaneous abortion, stillbirth, and central nervous system defects. About 10 per cent of fetuses exposed in later pregnancy have congenital heart disease, including patent ductus arteriosus and pulmonic stenosis. Cardiovascular manifestations of the fetal hydantoin syndrome include septal defects, pulmonic stenosis, and a single umbilical artery.

REFERENCE

1. Jones, K.L.: Fetal alcohol syndrome. Pediatr. Rev. 8:122, 1986.

646-E   (Braunwald, p. 1799)

Radiotherapy is presently offered, alone or in combination with chemotherapy, as a form of treatment for patients with a wide variety of malignancies. The heart, like many organs, may be adversely affected by radiation.[1] Much of the data regarding radiation effects on the heart originated from studies of children who were treated with radiotherapy for Hodgkin's and non-Hodgkin's lymphoma. Radiotherapy may cause myocardial damage by directly damaging cells and thereby decreasing cardiac tissue mass and by causing endothelial damage, which can result in ischemia and fibrosis. Pericarditis, which may be accompanied by an effusion and even tamponade, may occur anytime after radiotherapy treatment, from 3 months to 18 years.[2] Radiation therapy has been associated with accelerated coronary artery disease due to scarring and fibrosis within the coronary vessel. In addition, myocardial fibrosis with cardiomyopathy, conduction abnormalities, and valvular regurgitation and stenosis have been linked to radiation treatments. However, radiotherapy is not associated specifically with asymmetrical septal hypertrophy.

REFERENCES

1. Arsenian, M.A.: Cardiovascular sequelae of therapeutic thoracic radiation. Prog. Cardiovasc. Dis. 33:299, 1991.
2. Hancock, S.L., Donaldson, S.S., and Hoppe, R.T.: Cardiac disease following treatment of Hodgkin's disease in children and adolescents. J. Clin. Oncol. 11:1208, 1993.

647 A-F, B-T, C-T, D-T, E-T   (Braunwald, pp. 1770–1772)

The diagnosis of acute rheumatic fever is based on the five major manifestations listed: carditis, arthritis, chorea, subcutaneous nodules, and erythema marginatum. In addition, several other symptoms, laboratory findings, and data are commonly seen in this condition and are considered "minor manifestations." Nonspecific arthralgias, especially of large joints, and fever may occur. Elevated acute-phase reactants can occur due to tissue inflammation. In the acute phase of the disease, the erythrocyte sedimentation rate and C-reactive protein may be elevated. Electrocardiographic findings with acute rheumatic fever may include a prolonged P-R interval, tachycardia, atrioventricular block, and changes consistent with myocarditis. Patients often develop a leukocytosis and a normochromic, normocytic anemia. Antistreptococcal antibodies may be helpful; however, only about 11 per cent of patients have positive throat cultures for group A streptococci at the time of diagnosis of acute rheumatic fever.[1] A positive throat culture does not distinguish between a recent infection or chronic oropharyngeal colonization. Therefore, rising antistreptococcal antibody levels may provide a more reliable method of confirming infection.

REFERENCE

1. Dajani, A.S.: Current status of nonsuppurative complications of group A streptococci. Pediatr. Infect. Dis. J. 10: S25, 1991.

648 A-T, B-T, C-T, D-F, E-F   *(Braunwald, pp. 1852–1853)*

Hypertension is found in 8 to 10 per cent of all pregnancies and is defined as a diastolic blood pressure of greater than 90 mm Hg (on more than one occasion).[1] Hypertension during pregnancy is classified as chronic hypertension, preeclampsia/eclampsia, or transient hypertension. Each entity places the mother and fetus at increased risk for morbidity and mortality. Chronic hypertension is defined as an elevated blood pressure (>140/90 mm Hg) before pregnancy, before the 20th week of gestation, or hypertension that persists after pregnancy (after the 42nd day). Chronic hypertension may be associated with slowed fetal growth, abruption, or renal failure. Preeclampsia/eclampsia may be a life-threatening complication of pregnancy.

In addition to hypertension, preeclampsia may be associated with edema, proteinuria, low platelet count, hemolysis, elevated hepatic enzymes, abdominal pain, and headache. Eclampsia occurs when the preeclamptic patient develops a convulsion. Preeclampsia most often occurs after the 20th week of the first pregnancy and close to term in patients who are multiparous. Transient hypertension is defined as elevated blood pressure during pregnancy or in the peripartum period without a history of elevated blood pressure or signs/symptoms of preeclampsia. These patients, however, carry an increased risk of developing hypertension in the future.[1]

The treatment of hypertension during pregnancy is paramount in preventing complications for the mother and fetus.[2] Alpha-adrenergic receptor agonists (e.g., methyldopa) are the most widely used antihypertensive agents during pregnancy, and are often used in combination with arteriolar vasodilators (e.g., hydralazine). Beta-adrenergic receptor antagonists are considered safe in the later stages of pregnancy. Angiotensin-converting enzyme (ACE) inhibitors have been shown to be teratogenic and should not be used in pregnant patients.[3] The treatment of severe hypertension in pregnancy often includes intravenous hydralazine, diazoxide, labetalol. Intravenous magnesium sulfate is given acutely for preeclampsia/eclampsia. Delivery of the fetus is often the best method of treating pregnancy-associated hypertension.

REFERENCES

1. Lindheimer, M.D.: Hypertension in pregnancy. Hypertension *22*:127, 1993.
2. Sibai, B.M.: Treatment of hypertension in pregnant women. N. Engl. J. Med. *335*:257, 1996.
3. Rosa, F.W., Bosco, L.A., Graham, C.F., et al.: Neonatal anuria with maternal angiotensin-converting enzyme inhibition. Obstet. Gynecol. *74*:371, 1989.

649 A-T, B-F, C-T, D-F, E-T   *(Braunwald, pp. 1142–1143)*

Familial hypercholesterolemia is one of the few examples of an autosomal dominant disorder in which homozygotes survive infancy. Heterozygotes number about 1 in 500 persons in the population, making this disease one of the most common caused by a single mutant gene. The inherited defect in familial hypercholesterolemia involves the gene coding for the cell surface low-density lipoprotein (LDL) receptor. Heterozygotes inherit one mutant gene and one normal gene and therefore produce only half the normal number of receptors. Homozygotes inherit two copies of the mutant gene and so have virtually no LDL receptors. Physicians rarely see homozygotes, who occur at a frequency of 1 in 1 million.

Familial hypercholesterolemia heterozygotes commonly present with tendon xanthomas, which are nodules that may involve the Achilles tendon and various extensor tendons of the forearm and leg. They consist of deposits of cholesterol derived from deposition of LDL particles. Cutaneous planar xanthomas occur only in homozygotes and usually present within the first 6 years of life. These xanthomas are yellow to bright orange and occur over areas of trauma. Both the heterozygous and homozygous forms of familial hypercholesterolemia are associated with an increased incidence of coronary artery disease due to the elevated levels of LDL, the latter far more severe than the former. The disease may be detected by assaying the density of functional LDL receptors on circulating lymphocytes.[1]

REFERENCE

1. Cuthbert, J.A., East, C.A., Bilheimer, D.W., and Lipsky, P.E.: Detection of familial hypercholesterolemia by assaying functional low-density lipoprotein receptors on lymphocytes. N. Engl. J. Med. *314*:879, 1986.

650 A-T, B-T, C-F, D-F, E-F   *(Braunwald, pp. 1660–1662; Table 49–6; Fig. 49–6)*

Atrial septal defect (ASD) most often is a sporadic occurrence, but may be inherited as an isolated cardiac lesion or may be one of a constellation of findings present in an inherited syndrome. Two forms of isolated familial ASD have been recognized, both associated with a secundum type of defect. In one form, atrioventricular (AV) conduction delay is also noted.[1] The presence of an ASD and an A-V conduction delay in a patient should therefore prompt a detailed family history and evaluation of immediate relatives. If patients with ASD due to aneuploidy or one of the autosomal dominant familial forms of the disease are excluded, the recurrence risk of ASD is approximately 3 per cent. This is in marked contrast to the 50 per cent likelihood of ASD seen in the autosomal dominant disorder Holt-Oram syndrome. This condition is marked by upper limb dysplasia and accompanying ASD, which is usually of the secundum type. Ventricular septal defect and conduction abnormalities are also occasionally associated with this syndrome.[2] The diagnosis of the Holt-Oram syndrome may be subtle and requires careful inspection of the upper extremities with specific attention to the thumbs and thenar eminences. Skeletal changes may be recognized only by radiographic examination.

The Ellis-Van Creveld syndrome is a rare autosomal recessive disorder found in Amish people as a result of both a founder effect and consanguinity. The syndrome includes congenital heart disease in the majority of homozygotes and consists of an *ostium primum* ASD.[3] Defects thought to be due to abnormal embryonic blood flow, such as coarctation of the aorta, left heart hypoplasia, or patent ductus, are also seen in approximately one-fifth of patients with this syndrome. To date, there is no familial form of ASD that has been reported in association with ventricular tachycardia.

REFERENCES

1. Pease, W.E., Nordenberg, A., and Ladda, R.L.: Genetic counseling in familial atrial septal defect with prolonged atrioventricular conduction. Circulation *53*:759, 1976.
2. Zhang, K-Z., Sun, Q-B., and Cheng, T.O.: Holt-Oram syndrome in China. A collective review of 18 cases. Am. Heart J. *111*:572, 1986.
3. McKusick, V.I., Egeland, J.A., Eldridge, R., et al.: Dwarfism in the Amish. I. The Ellis—van Creveld syndrome. Bull. Johns Hopkins Hosp. *115*:306, 1964.

651 A-T, B-T, C-T, D-F, E-T   *(Braunwald, p. 1757)*

Changes in cardiovascular function during general anesthesia are due to many factors, including direct effects of the anesthetic agents on the heart and indirect effects mediated primarily by the nervous system. In addition, depending on the anesthetic's effects on respiration, there may be resulting changes in oxygen and carbon dioxide content, which exert indirect effects on myocardial contractility and cardiac irritability. In general, the dominant effects of all the anesthetic agents are to decrease cardiac contractility and lower blood pressure. Specifically, inhalation agents, which enter the bloodstream by way of the alveoli, are known to cause moderate decreases in cardiac function. Nitrous oxide causes about a 15 per cent decrease in cardiac output but does not cause significant hypotension because there is reflex vasoconstriction. Halothane also causes a reduction in myocardial contractility but is not associated with substantial reflex vasoconstriction so that it is commonly associated with falls in arterial pressure.

Of the narcotic analgesics, morphine is well tolerated, although it can cause venodilatation, thus decreasing preload and cardiac output. It does not have major effects on myocardial contractility per se. The short-acting barbiturates, including thiopental, cause a fall in blood pressure because of the combination of depressive actions on myocardial contractility and sympathetic tone. Ketamine, another intravenous anesthetic, is useful because it does *not* cause cardiovascular depression.

Frequently, in addition to inhalation and intravenous anesthetics, a muscle relaxant is added.

Succinylcholine can cause bradycardia, while tubocurarine and metocurine result in falls in mean arterial pressure, mild elevations in heart rate, and little if any change in cardiac output.

By skillful adjustment of the relative proportions of inhalation anesthetics, narcotic analgesics, and muscle relaxants, the anesthesiologist can modify the effects of anesthesia on the cardiovascular system. It should be noted that the level of anesthesia determines the sympathetic responses that are possible. In patients with cardiovascular disease, the depth of anesthesia is very important to the long-term outcome of surgery. Thus, increases in blood pressure during lightening of anesthesia can lead to dangerous effects on cardiac function, and it is important to monitor blood pressure carefully as anesthetic agents are withdrawn.

652 A-T, B-F, C-T, D-F, E-F   *(Braunwald, pp. 1723–1725; Tables 52–8 and 52–9)*

Ischemia in the perioperative cardiac surgical patient is a frequent finding.[1] However, only 5 to 15 per cent of patients undergoing CABG surgery actually suffer a perioperative MI.[2] Perioperative MI may be due to a variety of factors, ranging from the presence of diffuse underlying atherosclerotic disease to technical problems, such as inadequate myocardial preservation intraoperatively or difficulties with graft anastomoses. Diagnosis of AMI following cardiac surgery is more difficult because of the usual elevation in CPK levels and the frequent finding of nonspecific ST-T wave abnormalities on the electrocardiogram (ECG).

The ECG, however, remains the most reliable tool for diagnosing a perioperative MI. The single most important criterion on the ECG is the presence of new and persistent Q waves on serial ECGs once the early postoperative rewarming period is completed.[2] Bedside echocardiograms may also be helpful, especially when a regional wall motion abnormality not present on a preoperative study is detected. An elevated CPK-MB (>30 IU/liter) provides further support for the diagnosis of perioperative MI (see Table 52–9, p. 1724). Prolonged pump times (>75 minutes) and increased total ischemic time (>50 minutes) both are correlated with the development of perioperative MI in patients undergoing CABG surgery. In some studies, an increased number of bypass grafts is correlated with increased risk of MI, although this is not a universal finding.[4] In general, patients with perioperative MI have an increased hospital mortality (~10 per cent) compared with patients who remain free of such insults (~1 per cent).[5]

REFERENCES

1. Gray, R.J., Harris, W.S., Shah, P.K., et al.: Coronary sinus blood flow and sampling for detection of unrecognized myocardial ischemia and injury. Circulation *56*(Suppl. II): 58, 1977.

2. London, M.J., Hollenberg, M., Wong, M.G., et al.: Intraoperative myocardial ischemia. Localization by continuous 12-lead electrocardiography. Anesthesiology 69:232, 1988.
3. Albert, D.E., Cliff, R.M., LeCoq, D.A., et al.: Comparative rates of resolution of QRS changes after operative and nonoperative acute myocardial infarcts. Am. J. Cardiol. 51:378, 1983.
4. Chaitman, B.R., Alderman, E.L., Sheffield, L.T., et al.: Use of survival analysis to determine the clinical significance of new Q waves after coronary bypass surgery. Circulation 67:302, 1983.
5. Bateman, T.M., Matloff, J.M., and Gray, R.J.: Myocardial infarction during coronary artery bypass surgery—benign event or prognostic omen? Int. J. Cardiol. 6:259, 1984.

653 A-F, B-T, C-F, D-T, E-T   (Braunwald, p. 1922)

The patient described in this question probably suffered from atheroemboli to his kidneys, likely precipitated by the administration of thrombolytic agents. Because of their proximity to the aorta, the kidneys commonly are targets for atheroemboli. Atheroemboli usually are produced by mechanical manipulation of the aorta via catheters or surgery. It is believed that anticoagulants, which occasionally precipitate an episode of atheroemboli, expose atheromatous plaques by disrupting the overlaying fibrin-platelet formation.[1] Atheroemboli often cause acute renal failure with a stepwise decline in function. Patients may progress to end-stage renal disease, while others may recover full kidney function. The emboli may lodge in terminal arteries of the kidney causing localized glomerular ischemia, or may compromise large renal arteries and result in the loss of entire kidney function.

The urinalysis is often unremarkable, with only mild proteinuria and a bland sediment. Rarely, lipid droplets in the urine can be seen with cholesterol emboli. Peripheral eosinophilia and low serum complement levels may also be seen. Livido reticularis, the purple discoloration described in this patient, occurs in 50 per cent of patients and is due to areas of impaired perfusion, most often in the lower extremities. Other cutaneous manifestations of atheroembolic disease include gangrene, purple toes, and purpura. Back pain and systemic hypertension also may be present. Often, the diagnosis of renal embolization can be made on clinical grounds alone. However, if there is cutaneous involvement, biopsies of the skin and muscle may be helpful and are considered safe. Kidney biopsies may provide useful information, but carry a significant complication rate. Perfusion scanning and renal arteriography may show defects from large emboli.

The management of atheroemboli centers around supportive care, which may include hemodialysis. Large emboli may be amenable to surgical or catheter removal.

REFERENCE

1. Queen, M., Biem, H.J., Moe, G.W., and Sugar, L.: Development of cholesterol embolization syndrome after intravenous streptokinase for acute myocardial infarction. Am. J. Cardiol. 65:1042, 1990.

654 A-T, B-F, C-T, D-F   (Braunwald, pp. 1778–1779)

Systemic lupus erythematosus (SLE) is an autoimmune disease causing a diffuse microvasculitis, so that the heart is almost always involved at autopsy. Cardiac manifestations are frequently overshadowed by associated renal and dermatological findings. Pericarditis is found in approximately 70 per cent of cases at autopsy and is the most common cardiac lesion of SLE. During acute disease flares, pericardial inflammation may extend into the sinoatrial and AV nodes, causing acute heart block, while massive inflammation may lead to large effusions and tamponade.

Myocarditis is proportional to the severity of the systemic disease process but is usually subclinical. The myocarditic lesions consist of fibrinoid necrosis of interstitial tissues and blood vessels. There is rarely gross myocardial dysfunction except in the setting of hypertension and edema secondary to renal disease.

Endocarditis is a common cardiac manifestation of SLE. The most characteristic finding is the Libman-Sacks lesion, which is a wart-like collection of degenerating valve tissue which extrudes beyond the endothelium. These lesions are found most commonly in the angles of the AV valves and on the underside of the base of the mitral valve. They may lead to marked scarring or deformity, and can be distinguished from the fibrinoid necrosis that is common in myocarditis. Clinically important valvular disease in SLE is not uncommon, however, especially in a subset of patients with valvular thickening and deformity of a nonspecific nature.[2]

Infants born to women with active SLE may demonstrate congenital complete heart block. Several observations indicate that transplacental transfer of abnormal antibodies may be of pathogenic importance in these cases.[3] Thus, during examination of pregnant women with SLE, fetal bradycardia should be recognized as a possible complication of maternal SLE rather than fetal distress from other causes. Arrhythmias such as atrial flutter and fibrillation are rare, both in mothers with SLE and in their fetuses.

REFERENCES

1. Doharty, N.E., and Siegal, R.J.: Cardiovascular manifestations of systematic lupus erythematosus. Am. Heart J. 110:1257, 1985.
2. Galve, E., et al.: Prevalence, morphologic types, and evolution of cardiac valvular disease in systemic lupus erythematosus. N. Engl. J. Med. 319:817, 1988.
3. Litsey, S.E., Noonan, J.A., Connor, W.N., et al.: Maternal connective tissue disease and congenital heart block. N. Engl. J. Med. 309:209, 1983.

655 A-F, B-T, C-F, D-T, E-F   (Braunwald, p. 1676; Fig. 2–3, p. 17)

Hereditary hemorrhagic telangiectasia, or Osler-Rendu-Weber disease, is more common than has been appreciated previously, in part because of marked variability in the clinical presentation. The disease may be present in mild forms and may therefore go undiagnosed for long periods of time.[1] Widespread telangiectases and arteriovenous malformations are characteristic of HHT. Mucocutaneous telangiectases on the tongue, lips, and fingertips are common. Small and moderate-sized malformations may occur in the nose and lead to recurrent epistaxis. Similarly, such vascular malformations may cause recurrent gastrointestinal bleeding and occult anemia or, if located in the lung, hypoxemia, hemoptysis, polycythemia, and even paradoxical embolization through the right-to-left shunt.

Screening for pulmonary vascular malformations with auscultation and chest x-ray may be helpful, and the presence of a decreased arterial P_{O_2} suggests the need for angiography and attempted therapeutic balloon occlusion if a malformation is found.[2] Danazol therapy may be helpful in treating the epistaxis that occurs in this disorder.[3] The biochemical defect and the gene(s) involved in HHT have not been identified. However, the genetic abnormality in Von Hippel–Lindau syndrome, an autosomal dominant condition that also involves malformations and abnormal vascular growth, has been mapped to the short arm of chromosome 3.

REFERENCES

1. Peery, W.H.: Clinical spectrum of hereditary hemorrhagic telangiectasia (Osler-Weber-Rendu disease). Am. J. Med. 82:989, 1987.
2. Terry, P.B., White, J.L., Jr., Barth, K.H., et al.: Pulmonary arteriovenous malformations. Physiologic observations and results of therapeutic balloon embolization. N. Engl. J. Med. 308:1197, 1983.
3. Haq, A.U., Glass, J., Netchvolodoff, C.V., et al.: Hereditary hemorrhagic telangiectasia and danazol. Ann. Intern. Med. 109:171, 1988.

656 A-T, B-T, C-T, D-F (Braunwald, p. 1146)

Familial hypertriglyceridemia is a relatively common autosomal dominant disorder, in which the concentration of very-low-density lipoprotein (VLDL) is elevated in the plasma. These patients do not usually exhibit hypertriglyceridemia until puberty or early adulthood, at which time plasma triglyceride levels are moderately elevated in the range of 200 to 500 mg/dl. Associated conditions include obesity, hyperglycemia, hyperinsulinemia, hypertension, and hyperuricemia. Xanthomas are not a characteristic feature of this disorder. These individuals exhibit only a slightly increased incidence of atherosclerosis, and it is unclear whether or not this is caused by the hypertriglyceridemia, by associated decreases in HDL cholesterol, or by associated illnesses. Patients with hypertriglyceridemia can develop severe exacerbations, with increases in plasma triglyceride levels as high as 1000 mg/dl, when they are exposed to a variety of precipitating factors. These include excessive al-

cohol ingestion, poorly controlled diabetes, ingestion of birth control pills containing estrogen, and development of hypothyroidism.[1] These high levels of triglycerides may lead to pancreatitis and eruptive xanthomas.

The disorder appears to be genetically heterogeneous in that patients from different families may have different mutations. No consistent abnormality of lipoprotein structure or receptor function have been described at this time. The cardinal diagnostic feature is the presence of a moderate elevation in plasma triglyceride levels, with a normal cholesterol level. Lipoprotein electrophoresis shows an increase in the pre-beta fraction (type IV lipoprotein pattern). These individuals can be treated by controlling the exacerbating conditions, such as obesity, and restricting intake of fats and alcohol.

REFERENCE

1. Chart, A., and Brunzell, J.D.: Severe hypertriglyceridemia: Role of familial and acquired disorders. Metabolism 32: 209, 1983.

657 A-F, B-F, C-F, D-T, E-T (Braunwald, pp. 1665–1666)

Idiopathic dilated cardiomyopathy is common and more prevalent than the hypertrophic form of the disease. Familial forms of the myopathy have been described, although the frequency of inherited forms of this disorder is small. Estimates of a positive family history for dilated cardiomyopathy range between 7 and 30 per cent in most analysis, although a shared environmental cause is one alternative explanation for familial clustering of dilated cardiomyopathy.[1] Most familial examples of dilated cardiomyopathy fit an autosomal dominant pattern of inheritance.[2] In some families, a mild proximal skeletal myopathy of type I muscle fibers is seen to coexist with cardiac abnormalities.[3] In addition, peripartum cardiomyopathy has been recognized as an inherited disease in at least one large family,[4] although its occurrence is usually sporadic.

REFERENCES

1. Valantine, H.A., Hunt, S.A., Fowler, M.B., et al.: Frequency of familial nature of dilated cardiomyopathy and usefulness of cardiac transplantation in this subset. Am. J. Cardiol. 63:959, 1989.
2. Michels, V.V., Driscoll, D.J., and Miller, F.A., Jr.: Familial aggregation of idiopathic dilated cardiomyopathy. Am. J. Cardiol. 55:1232, 1985.
3. Caforio, A.L.P., Rossi, B., and Risaliti, R.: Type 1 fiber abnormalities in skeletal muscle of patients with hypertrophic and dilated cardiomyopathy. Evidence of mechanical myogenic myopathy. J. Am. Coll. Cardiol. 14:1464, 1989.
4. Voss, E.G., Reddy, C.V.R., Detrano, R., et al.: Familial dilated cardiomyopathy. Am. J. Cardiol. 45:456, 1984.

658 A-T, B-T, C-T, D-F (Braunwald, pp. 1786–1787)

Anemia is one of the most common causes of increased cardiac output and sometimes results in heart failure due to a high-output state. Several compensatory adaptations occur which result in maintenance of normal cardiac function in association with cardiac anemia. These include an increase in left ventricular end-diastolic volume due to an increase in preload, a reduction in systemic vascular resistance due to the decrease in blood viscosity resulting in a lowered afterload, and an increase in the levels of catecholamine and non-catecholamine inotropic factors in the plasma.[1-2]

In animal studies it has been demonstrated that myocardial oxygen deficiency exceeds the supply at any given hematocrit[3] (see Fig. 57–1, p. 1787). There are also changes in the affinity of red blood cells for oxygen with a shift in the hemoglobin oxygen dissociation curve *to the right*, so that more oxygen is released from hemoglobin as the P_{O_2} declines. This is thought to be due to an increase in the production of 2,3-diphosphoglycerate (2,3-DPG). At normal arterial P_{O_2}, arterial oxygen saturation remains high, despite the reduction in oxygen affinity. However, at lower P_{O_2} in the venous system, the elevated 2,3-DPG displaces the hemoglobin dissociation curve to the right, causing greater release from oxygen from the cells at any level of P_{O_2}. In terms of actual numbers, the position of the hemoglobin oxygen dissociation curve can be expressed by the value of P_{50} (i.e., the partial pressure of oxygen at which hemoglobin is 50 per cent saturated). A shift of the dissociation curve to the right as occurs with anemia increased the P_{50} value. As a consequence, an anemic individual with a 50 per cent reduction in red cell mass may suffer only a 27 per cent reduction in oxygen delivery.[4]

REFERENCES

1. Florenzano, F., Diaz, G., Regonesi, C., and Escobar, E.: Left ventricular function in chronic anemia: Evidence of non-catecholamine positive inotropic factor in the serum. Am. J. Cardiol. *54*:638, 1984.
2. Rossi, M.A., Carello, S.V., and Oliveria, J.S.M.: The effect of iron deficiency anemia in the rat on catecholamine levels and heart morphology. Cardiovasc. Res. *15*:313, 1981.
3. Baer, R.W., Vlahakes, G.J., Uhlig, P.N., and Hoffman, I.E.: Maximum myocardial oxygen transport during anemia and polycythemia in dogs. Am. J. Physiol. *252*:H1086, 1987.
4. Oski, E.G., Marshall, B.D., Cohen, P.J., et al.: Exercise with anemia. The role of the left or right shifted oxygen-hemoglobin equilibrium curve. Ann. Intern. Med. *74*:44, 1971.

659 A-F, B-T, C-F, D-T   *(Braunwald, pp. 1689–1693)*

Aging affects all organs of the body, including the heart. However, study of the normal aging process is difficult because of the high prevalence of cardiovascular disease in the American population. Recent studies in which coronary artery disease and other common cardiovascular diseases have been carefully excluded have revealed several interesting findings. First, there is moderate hypertrophy of left ventricular myocardium, probably in response to increased arterial stiffness and loss of cardiac myocytes with age. Although myocardial cells are unable to proliferate or increase in number, they can increase in size; this appears to be an adaptive response. Careful studies have shown that despite alterations in the contractile proteins leading to reductions in the velocity of contraction and lengthening of contraction and relaxation times, peak contractile force production is maintained at normal levels.

However, there are changes in beta adrenoceptor–mediated inotropic and chronotropic cardiovascular responses with aging due to a generalized desensitization. Thus, maximal heart rate during exercise and other cardiovascular responses to exercises are blunted. Maximal heart rate at peak exercise thus can be estimated by the formula: 200 minus patient age in years. In summary, there appears to be no change in cardiac output, stroke volume, or ejection fraction at rest with aging.[1] Preservation of these functions is due to adaptive responses in contraction time and calcium transients. These adaptations compensate for the increased LV stiffness secondary to hypertrophy and loss of elasticity of pericardium and other supporting structures.

REFERENCE

1. Gerstenblith, G., et al.: Echocardiographic assessment of a normal adult aging population. Circulation *56*:273, 1977.

660 A-T, B-F, C-T, D-F   *(Braunwald, p. 1894)*

Amiodarone, a potent antiarrhythmic agent, has two primary effects on thyroid function. First, it inhibits the peripheral conversion of T_4 to T_3, causing reduction in serum T_3 and a transient rise in TSH. Within a few days to weeks, however, a compensatory increase in serum T_4 levels occurs and TSH returns to normal. Clinically, these patients are euthyroid, even when the T_4 levels are elevated.[1] Amiodarone's second effect occurs because it contains a large amount of iodine (35 per cent by weight) so that when it is metabolized, there is a significant increase in the available inorganic iodide. This results in acute inhibition of thyroid organification and a decrease in clearance of iodide. In the United States, where there is a high level of iodide uptake, patients may develop hypothyroidism. In one study of 45 patients,[1] nearly 50 per cent of the patients had an increase in T_4, with 25 per cent having an elevated TSH level. Of these, 7 per cent also had a low level of T_4. In this series no subject developed hyperthyroidism, but 9 per cent developed clinical hypothyroidism.

REFERENCE

1. Borowski, G.D., Garofano, C.D., Rose, L.L., et al.: Effect of long-term amiodarone therapy on thyroid hormone levels and thyroid function. Am. J. Med. *78*:443, 1985.

661 A-T, B-T, C-T, D-T *(Braunwald, pp. 1732–1733)*

Poststernotomy mediastinitis and osteomyelitis are among the most serious complications of cardiac surgery. Roughly 2 per cent of patients undergoing median sternotomy develop this problem.[1] Patients most often present about 2 weeks after surgery with persistent fever (>101°F), leukocytosis, bacteremia, discharge, and erythema at the wound site. Risk factors for the development of mediastinal infection include prolonged cardiopulmonary bypass time, excessive bleeding necessitating reexploration for hemostatic control, decreased cardiac output following surgery, and the use of both internal mammary arteries.

Diabetes, immunosuppression, and other chronic states are additional risk factors. About half of the infections are caused by *Staphylococcus* species, while gram-negative organisms account for about 40 per cent of cases. The diagnosis of a sternal wound infection often requires surgical exploration and removal of material for Gram stain and culture. Imaging techniques including MRI and CT scanning also may be helpful. Intravenous antibiotics, along with possible débridement and irrigation, may be required for prolonged periods. Early diagnosis and initiation of treatment greatly enhance the prognosis. Mediastinal infections do not seem to change patency rates of the bypass grafts.

REFERENCE

1. Spencer, F.C., and Grossi, E.A.: Mediastinitis after cardiac operations. Ann. Thorac. Surg. *49*:506, 1990.

662-D, 663-C, 664-C, 665-A, 666-B *(Braunwald, pp. 1659–1663)*

Noonan syndrome is a genetic disorder with an inheritance that is consistent with an autosomal dominant pattern.[1] The entity is relatively common, and is characterized phenotypically by short stature, a unique facial appearance, mild mental retardation, webbing of the neck, cryptorchidism, and renal anomalies. Approximately half of all patients with Noonan syndrome have congenital heart disease, the most common lesion of which is valvular pulmonic stenosis, present in about 60 per cent of patients with cardiac involvement. Because of the relatively high frequency of Noonan syndrome, cardiologists encountering patients with congenital pulmonic stenosis should have a high index of suspicion regarding the possibility of underlying Noonan syndrome. The ECG in pulmonic stenosis associated with Noonan syndrome is often different from the pattern seen in usual pulmonary valve stenosis, and commonly displays left anterior hemiblock with a deep S wave in precordial leads. Approximately 20 per cent of patients with Noonan syndrome have an atrial septal defect or hypertrophic cardiomyopathy, primarily involving the left ventricle.

The *LEOPARD syndrome*[2] is a rare, single-gene complex of congenital malformations for which the acronym LEOPARD was formed. The mnemonic includes *L*, lentigines; *E*, electrocardiographic conduction defects; *O*, ocular hypertelorism; *P*, pulmonic valve stenosis; *A*, abnormalities of the genitals; *R*, retardation of growth; and *D*, deafness. The most common structural cardiac feature in this disorder is pulmonic stenosis, which may exist as an isolated anomaly or in combination with aortic stenosis. In addition, endocardial fibroelastosis and hypertrophic cardiomyopathy have been reported in the syndrome. The electrocardiographic conduction defects which are most commonly noted in the LEOPARD syndrome include P-R interval prolongation, QRS widening, left anterior hemiblock, and complete heart block. The most striking feature of the syndrome is the presence of diagnostic small, dark-brown spots, known as lentigines, which are concentrated over the neck and upper extremities. LEOPARD syndrome is transmitted in an autosomal dominant fashion, with cardiovascular abnormalities in at least 95 per cent of affected subjects. Approximately 80 per cent of patients have lentigines, while deafness and abnormalities of the genitals occur in about 20 per cent of patients.

Kartagener syndrome is an autosomal recessive disorder with a primary genetic defect that has been elucidated by electron microscopic investigation of cilia from affected individuals' bronchial mucosa or sperm. Dynein arms, which are protein structures that normally form cross bridges between adjacent microtubules in cilia and sperm tails, are abnormal in this disorder.[3] Several different mutations capable of producing the syndrome are recognized, and in each case, the mutant gene disrupts the synthesis either of the dynein protein itself or of a protein that binds dynein to the microtubules. Clinically, the syndrome consists of the triad of sinusitis, bronchiectasis, and situs inversus with dextrocardia. Cases of Kartagener syndrome usually come to attention in infancy due to recurrent upper respiratory infections or pneumonia, and development of classic sinusitis and chronic bronchiectasis occurs as childhood progresses. The majority of individuals with Kartagener syndrome have dextrocardia as the only cardiac manifestation, which leads to an abnormal 12-lead ECG when the leads are routinely placed, but has no other clinical consequences. On rare occasions associated cardiac anomalies may be present, including transposition of the great vessels or trilocular or bilocular heart.

Holt-Oram syndrome is a rare autosomal dominant disorder with varying degrees of clinical involvement and some constellation of clinical abnormalities in all affected individuals. The classic clinical manifestation of the syndrome is the simultaneous occurrence of congenital heart disease and an upper limb deformity. The most common cardiovascular abnormality is an atrial septal defect of the secundum type, with ventricular septal defect being next most common. While other types of congenital heart disease have been noted in this disorder, 70 per cent of affected individuals have either an atrial septal defect or a ventricular septal defect. Electrocardiographic abnormalities are frequently present as well and may include first-degree AV block, right bundle branch block, or bradycardia. Deformities of the thumb are the best-known features of the Holt-Oram syndrome with "digitalization of the thumbs" or hypoplasia or triphalangeal changes in the thumbs. However, these deformities are not pathognomonic for Holt-Oram syndrome.[4] The most specific upper extremity abnormalities in this disorder, an abnormal scaphoid bone and/or accessory carpal bones, may be detected on wrist radiography.

REFERENCES

1. Mendez, H.M.M., and Opitz, J.M.: Noonan syndrome: A review. Am. J. Med. Genet. *21*:493, 1985.
2. Seuanez, H., Mane-Garzon, F., and Kolski, R.: Cardiocutaneous syndrome (the "LEOPARD" syndrome). Review of the literature and a new family. Clin. Genet. *9*:266, 1976.
3. Afzelius, B.A.: A human syndrome caused by immotile cilia. Science *193*:317, 1976.
4. Lin, A.E., and Perloff, J.K.: Upper limb malformations associated with congenital heart disease. Am. J. Cardiol. *55*: 1576, 1985.

667-C, 668-D, 669-E, 670-A, 671-B *(Braunwald, pp. 1890–1900)*

Metabolic and electrolyte abnormalities have a distinct role in the pathogenesis of cardiovascular morbidity and mortality. Excess thyroid hormone levels may have a profound effect on the heart, resulting in tachycardia, palpitations, and hypertension (often with a widened pulse pressure).[1] Examination of the precordium reveals a hyperdynamic impulse with an accentuated first heart sound and pulmonic component of the second heart sound. Systolic murmurs are common and a Means-Lerman scratch, due to the rubbing of normal pleura and pericardial surfaces in the presence of a hyperdynamic heart, may be heard during expiration.

The cardiovascular manifestations of hypothyroidism may lead to a dilated heart with a decreased ejection fraction. Bradycardia, cardiac dilatation, hypotension, edema, and evidence of heart failure and shock are associated with severe hypothyroid states.[2] Myxedema may promote capillary leakage of protein into the interstitial space. This fluid accumulation can result in a pericardial effusion, with rare progression to cardiac tamponade. Distant heart sounds and low voltage on the surface electrocardiogram may be helpful, but an echocardiogram is the best way to make the diagnosis.

Cushing's syndrome, due to the excess production of glucocorticoids and androgens, has profound effects on the cardiovascular system. Accelerated atherosclerosis in these patients has been linked to the higher incidence of hypertension, hyperlipidemia, and hypercholesterolemia. Cardiac myxomas also have been associated with Cushing's syndrome.[3] There also appears to be an association between nodular adrenal hyperplasia, cutaneous pigmented lesions, and cardiac lesions. It is unclear whether these abnormalities are the result of a dysplastic, neoplastic or hyperplastic process.

Hyperaldosteronism is associated with excess aldosterone production from an adrenal or extra-adrenal source. Hypertension, hypokalemia, and metabolic alkalosis are common findings. Many of the cardiac findings associated with hyperaldosteronism are nonspecific and are secondary to the metabolic and electrolyte abnormalities. For example, U-waves and ventricular arrhythmias have been noted on the electrocardiogram secondary to hypokalemia.

Parathyroid hormone has a direct positive inotropic and chronotropic effect on the heart, likely due to increased calcium entry into cardiac cells.[4] Hypercalcemia associated with hyperparathyroidism may result in excess calcium deposition in the heart, hypertension, and shortening of the Q-T interval.

REFERENCES

1. Woeber, K.A.: Thyrotoxicosis and the Heart. N. Engl. J. Med. *327*:94, 1992.
2. Mackerrow, S.D., Osborn, L.A., Levey, H., et al.: Myxedema-associated cardiogenic shock treated with intravenous thyroxine. Ann. Intern. Med. *117*:1014, 1992.
3. Carney, J.A., Gordon, H., Carpenter, P.C., et al.: The complex of myxomas, spotty pigmentations, and endocrine overactivity. Medicine *64*:270, 1985.
4. Gafter, U., Battler, A., Eldar, M., et al.: Effect of hyperparathyroidism on cardiac function in patients with end-stage renal disease. Nephron *41*:30, 1985.

672-D, 673-C, 674-B, 675-A *(Braunwald, pp. 1821–1822)*

Tissue-type plasminogen activator (t-PA) is the major physiological activator of plasminogen and is synthesized predominantly in endothelial cells. The protein is synthesized in a single-chain form, which is subsequently converted to a two-chain form by proteolytic cleavage of a single plasmin-sensitive site. Both the single-chain and the two-chain forms have endogenous proteolytic activity. The alpha chain of t-PA is derived from the aminoterminal portion of single-chain t-PA and contains a pair of finger-like structures referred to as "kringle" domains. The lysine binding sites located on these kringle domains confer binding specifically for fibrin. Thus, t-PA is a relatively fibrin-specific activator which converts plasminogen to plasmin two or three times more efficiently in the presence of fibrin. The protease domain of t-PA contains a proteolytic site that converts plasminogen to plasmin. This portion is homologous with other serine proteases, such as urokinase and trypsin.[1]

Urokinase is a two-chain serine protease with a molecular weight of 33,000, and is synthesized in both renal tubular epithelial cells and in endothelial cells. While urokinase converts plasminogen to plasmin by hydrolyzing the same bond as that acted on by t-PA, the proteolytic activity of urokinase is not enhanced by the presence of fibrin. Therefore, urokinase may activate circulating plasminogen as effectively as plasminogen absorbed onto fibrin thrombi.

Streptokinase is a single polypeptide chain of 414 amino acids with a molecular weight of 50,000 that is produced by a strain of hemolytic streptococci. Streptokinase does not cause thrombolysis by intrinsic enzymatic activity. Instead, streptokinase activates the fibrinolytic system by combining with plasminogen to form a plasminogen activator complex which is then capable of converting plasminogen to plasmin. Plasmin then degrades fibrin and other procoagulant proteins and assists in dissolving the thrombus. Many individuals have circulating antibodies to streptokinase as a result of previous streptococcal infections. Therefore, a large dose of streptokinase is administered to neutralize these antibodies. Antistreptococcal antibodies may remain high up to 6 months after administration.[2]

Anisoylated plasminogen-streptokinase activator complex (APSAC) is the combination of acetylated human plasma-derived lys-plasminogen and purified streptokinase. An anisoyl group blocks the active site on APSAC. Deacylation occurs in vivo and allows for the conversion of plasminogen to plasmin. The plasma clearance for APSAC is roughly 70 minutes and does not require a prolonged infusion.

REFERENCES

1. Loscalzo, J., and Braunwald, E.: Tissue plasminogen activator. N. Engl. J. Med. *319*:925, 1988.
2. Battershill, P.E., Benfield, P., and Goa, K.L.: Streptokinase. A review of its pharmacology and therapeutic efficacy in acute myocardial infarction in older patients. Drugs Aging *4*:36, 1994.

676-A, 677-B, 678-D, 679-C, 680-A   *(Braunwald, pp. 1817–1818)*

Unfractionated heparin is a naturally occurring compound that works in vivo by combining with antithrombin III (an inhibitor of thrombin and factors X, IX, and XI). The conformational change which occurs in antithrombin allows for an accelerated interaction with the activated clotting factors' limiting thrombin generation and fibrin formation. Commercial heparin is extracted from porcine intestinal mucosa and bovine lung and does not inactivate clot-bound thrombin or factor VII. Heparin is not absorbed by the gastrointestinal tract and is therefore administered in intravenous or subcutaneous forms. The bioavailability of subcutaneous injections of heparin is only 30 per cent.

An activated partial thromboplastin time (APPT) test is used to determine the inhibitory effect of heparin on thrombin, factor X, and factor IX. For acute thrombosis or embolism, intravenous heparin is administered with a goal APPT of 1.5 to 2 times the control value. Subcutaneous heparin is often used for patients who require a lower level of anticoagulation. Heparin therapy's major complication is bleeding. There is up to a 30 per cent incidence of heparin-induced thrombocytopenia which may be associated with thromboembolic events and often resolves with discontinuation of the drug.[1] In addition, heparin may cause osteoporosis, elevated liver enzymes, increased vascular permeability, alopecia, and hypoaldosteronism (with hyperkalemia).

Low molecular weight (LMW) heparin (MW 4000 to 5000) also produces an anticoagulant effect by binding to antithrombin III. LMW heparin inhibits factor Xa and thrombin, and like unfractionated heparin, is inactivated by heparinase and does not inactivate clot-bound thrombin. LMW heparin binds less with platelet factor 4, plasma proteins, and endothelial cells, and therefore, has over a 90 per cent bioavailability when administered by subcutaneous injection. LMW heparin has reduced plasma clearance, a prolonged half-life, and a predictable anticoagulant response.

Patients may receive LMW heparin once daily and do not need daily laboratory monitoring. Periodic blood tests, including a platelet count and complete blood count, are recommended during the treatment course. LMW heparin has a weak effect on platelets, does not increase vascular permeability, and has only a limited interaction with von Willebrand factor. Therefore, patients using LMW heparin are unlikely to suffer bleeding complications.[2] Thrombocytopenia with thrombosis can occur with LMW heparin, but is less common compared with unfractionated heparin. LMW heparin has also been associated with increases in liver enzymes. Numerous studies are ongoing comparing the efficacy of LMW heparin with unfractionated heparin.[3]

REFERENCES

1. Schmitt, P.B., and Adelman, B.: Heparin-associated thrombocytopenia: A critical review and pooled analysis. Am. J. Med. Sci. *305*:208, 1993.
2. Hirsh, J., and Levine, M.N.: Low molecular weight heparin. Blood *79*:1, 1992.
3. Levine, M., Gent, M., Hirsh, J., et al.: A comparison of low-molecular weight heparin administered primarily at home with unfractionated heparin administered in the hospital for proximal deep-vein thrombosis. N. Engl. J. Med. *334*: 677, 1996.

681-A, 682-A, 683-C, 684-B   *(Braunwald, pp. 1142–1143)*

Familial hypercholesterolemia is an autosomal dominant trait caused by a single-gene mutation that leads to hypercholesterolemia and atherosclerosis and its complications. Heterozygotes for the condition number about 1 in 500 persons, while the homozygote form of the disease is rare, occurring in approximately 1 in 1 million subjects.[1] The single-gene mutation in this disorder leads to a defect in the production of the cell surface LDL receptor. Heterozygotes thus produce approximately one-half the normal number of receptors for this lipoprotein particle, while homozygotes with familial hypercholesterolemia produce few if any LDL receptors. These biochemical defects lead to dramatic clinical presentations; heterozygotes with this condition develop MI, typically in their fourth or fifth decade, while homozygotes usually develop MI before the age of 20. Characteristic dermatological lesions are noted in this disorder. Heterozygotes may develop nodular swellings involving the various tendons around the knee, elbow, dorsum of the hand, and ankle, which are known as *tendon xanthomas*, as shown in the figure for Question 682. Microscopically, these consist of large deposits of cholesterol, which apparently is derived from the deposition of LDL particles, both extracellularly and within scavenger macrophage cells. Tendon xanthomas are diagnostic, while deposition of cholesterol in the tissues of the eyelid and within the cornea, known respectively as *xanthelasma* (see figure for Question 684) and *arcus corneae*, may occur in adults with normal plasma lipid levels, as well as in other lipid disorders.

Patients with homozygous familial hypercholesterolemia disease have dramatic elevations in the plasma LDL level from birth, with levels typically six- to eightfold higher than normal. In addition, they demonstrate a specific and unique cutaneous xanthoma known as a *planar xanthoma*, which is often present at birth, and always develops within the first 6 years of life. Planar xanthomas are yellow and occur at points of trauma over the knees, elbows, and buttocks. In addition, they may be found in the interdigital webs of the hands, especially between the thumb and index finger. Tendon xanthomas, xanthelasma, and arcus corneae also occur in homozygotes. As already noted, coronary artery atherosclerosis in homozygote familial hypercholesterolemia is rapidly progressive and frequently fatal. Most homozygotes die before the age of 30.[2] The severe atherosclerosis that develops in this disorder occurs throughout the thoracic and abdominal aorta, and in the major pulmonary arteries in addition to the coronary arteries. Deposition of atheromatous material characteristically also involves the aortic valve and may lead to significant aortic stenosis, with subsequent congestive heart failure. It should therefore be noted that subjects with the homozygous form may present with clinical manifestations suggestive of rheumatic fever or connective tissue disease: painful joints, a persistently elevated sedimentation rate, and cardiac murmurs.

Diagnosis of the heterozygous form of familial hypercholesterolemia is suggested by the finding of an isolated elevation of plasma cholesterol with a normal fasting concentration of plasma triglycerides. While this pattern is the phenotypical type IIA hyperlipoproteinemia, several features distinguish the heterozygous form of familial hypercholesterolemia from other hyperlipidemias that create a similar plasma lipid pattern (such as polygenic hypercholesterolemia and multiple lipoprotein–type hyperlipidemia). These characteristics include a higher average level of plasma cholesterol (in the 350 to 400 mg/dl range), tendon xanthomas, and a characteristic family history. Diagnosis of the homozygous form is more easily established. The early appearance of cutaneous xanthomas, massive elevations of cholesterol (>600 mg/dl) with a normal triglyceride level, and early symptomatology referable to atherosclerosis all make the diagnosis readily apparent.

The approach to treatment of familial hypercholesterolemia includes specific dietary therapy, bile acid–binding resins, and the use of HMG-CoA reductase inhibitors. Treatment of homozygotes is much more difficult and may require dramatic measures, including plasma exchanges at monthly intervals in addition to the specific drug therapy just mentioned. In selected instances, portacaval anastamosis has been effective. Liver transplantation, which provides the recipient with a normal hepatic complement of LDL receptor, has also been successfully employed.[3]

Type III hyperlipoproteinemia, or familial dysbetalipoproteinemia, is a single-gene disorder that requires both the presence of a mutation in the gene for apolipoprotein E and contributory environmental or genetic factors.[4] In this disorder, the plasma concentrations of both cholesterol and triglycerides are elevated due to the accumulation of remnant-like particles that come from the partial metabolism of both VLDL and chylomicrons. This condition is characterized clinically by severe atherosclerosis involving the coronary arteries, the internal carotids, and the abdominal aorta and its branches. Interestingly, hyperlipidemia or the other clinical features of the disease are usually not seen until after the age of 20 years. Two specific dermatological lesions are characteristic of type III hyperlipoproteinemia. *Xanthoma striata palmaris* appears as orange or yellow discolorations of the palmar and digital creases, as illustrated in the figure for Question 684. In addition, bulbous cutaneous xanthomas in a variety of sizes known as tuberous or tuberoeruptive xanthomas are characteristically located over the elbows and knees in this disorder (not shown). Xanthelasmas of the eyelids may also occur in this disease, but, as noted, are not unique to familial dysbetalipoproteinemia. While about 1 per cent of Caucasian individuals are homozygotes for the allele of apoprotein E, which confers the biochemical abnormality of this disorder, only 1 in 100 of these homozygous individuals (1/10,000 of the general population) has clear-cut familial dysbetalipoproteinemia. The mechanism by which the remaining homozygotes for this disorder are able to compensate for the defective protein and thus avoid the clinical sequelae mentioned remains obscure. Diagnosis of this disorder is suggested by moderate elevations in both cholesterol and triglyceride levels to approximately 300 to 350 mg/dl. In addition, 80 per cent of patients exhibit palmar or tuberous xanthomas. The diagnosis is strongly supported by a "broad beta" band on lipoprotein electrophoresis, which results from the presence of the unique remnant particles just described. Definitive confirmation of the diagnosis rests upon specific analysis of the patient's VLDL fraction, which contains an abnormal remnant particle with a relatively high ratio of cholesterol to triglyceride, and specific extraction and analysis of the proteins present in this VLDL particle to confirm that apoprotein E-II is present.

REFERENCES

1. Brown, M.S., and Goldstein, J.L.: A receptor-mediated pathway for cholesterol homeostasis. Science 232:34, 1986.
2. Sprecher, D.L., Schaefer, E.J., and Kent, K.M., et al.: Cardiovascular features of homozygous familial hypercholesterolemia: Analysis of 16 patients. Am. J. Cardiol. 54:20, 1984.
3. Bilheimer, D.W., Goldstein, J.L., Grundy, S.C., et al.: Liver transplantation provides low density lipoprotein receptors and lowers plasma cholesterol in a child with homozygous familial hypercholesterolemia. N. Engl. J. Med. 29:385, 1984.
4. Mahley, R.W., and Angelin, B.: Type III hyperlipoproteinemia: Recent insights into the genetic defect of familial dysbetalipoproteinemia. Adv. Intern. Med. 29:385, 1984.

685-C, 686-D, 687-C, 688-B *(Braunwald, pp. 1776–1779)*

Rheumatoid arthritis (RA) and systemic lupus erythematosus (SLE) are chronic multisystem diseases with multiple cardiac manifestations. RA afflicts approximately 1 per cent of the population, with women being affected especially in their fourth and fifth decades of life, and three times more often than men. It is believed that there is both a genetic (HLA-DR4) and environmental link to the development of RA. In addition to the chronic polyarthritis, many extraarticular manifestations, including cardiac abnormalities, have been associated with RA.[1]

Pericarditis is the most common cardiac finding in patients with RA and is often associated with a pericardial and pleural effusion. Pericardial fluid in RA, like pleural fluid, has a low glucose, low complement level, and a leukocyte count between 100 and 30,000/ml. Although the pericardial effusion associated with RA is most often small, cases of tamponade associated with RA pericarditis have been reported.[2] In addition, constrictive pericarditis may occur. Valvular findings in RA include the presence of rheumatoid granulomata in the valve leaflets and valve rings. The mitral and aortic valves are more commonly affected, and rarely, patients may require valve replacement surgery. Myocardial ischemia and infarction have been linked to coronary vasculitis associated with RA. Aortitis and myocarditis may be evident in this disease. Cardiac conduction defects in RA are thought to be due to the formation of rheumatoid nodules in the conduction pathways of the heart. First-degree heart block is the most common conduction defect, but one may also see complete heart block. Treatment of RA focuses on pain relief and decreasing the inflammatory process. Nonsteroidal antiinflammatory agents, glucocorticoids, agents including gold, D-penicillamine, the antimalarial drugs and sulfa derivatives, and immunosuppressive compounds are often useful in the treatment of RA.

SLE is also more prevalent in women, usually of childbearing age. The disease is more common in the African American and Asian populations. The pathogenesis of the SLE syndrome involves the production of antibodies and immune complexes. There appears to be a genetic predisposition to the disease, and it has been linked to HLA-DR2 and DR3. Like RA, SLE is a widespread disease involving virtually every organ system, including the heart.[3]

Pericarditis is a common cardiac manifestation, often associated with pericardial effusions. Tamponade and constrictive pericarditis occur in rare instances. Immune complex disease with SLE has been linked to the development of active myocyte inflammation causing myocarditis and possibly heart failure. Libman-Sacks endocarditis involves the formation of noninfected verrucous vegetations on the cardiac valves. Mitral and aortic valve regurgitation are the most common findings on physical examination. There appears to be a higher incidence of coronary artery disease in patients with SLE, likely due to corticosteroid usage, coronary vasculitis, coronary artery spasm, and the hypercoagulable state associated with the antiphospholipid antibody syndrome. Numerous conduction abnormalities in SLE, including complete heart block, may occur due to active myocardial inflammation and fibrosis. Nonsteroidal antiinflammatory agents, glucocorticoids, antimalarial agents, and cytotoxic agents have been used in the treatment of SLE.

REFERENCES

1. Malone, S., Valentin, G., Giunta, A., et al.: Cardiac involvement in rheumatoid arthritis. Cardiology 83:234, 1993.
2. Escalonte, A., Kaufman, R.L., Quismorio, F.P., and Beardmore, T.D.: Cardiac compression in rheumatoid pericarditis. Semin. Arthritis Rheum. 20:148, 1990.
3. Doherty, N.E., and Siegel, R.J.: Cardiovascular manifestations of systemic lupus erythematosus. Am. Heart J. 110:1257, 1985.

689-C, 690-A, 691-B, 692-D *(Braunwald, pp. 1084–1085, 1427–1430, 1781)*

Dermatological manifestations of systemic disorders that have major cardiac involvement are relatively common and may provide specific clues to the underlying diagnosis. A classic example of such a disorder is *subacute infective endocarditis*, which has several lesions involving the skin, its appendages, and the eye that have for years been considered classic peripheral stigmata of the disorder. These include petechiae, Osler nodes, Janeway lesions, Roth spots, and subungual or "splinter" hemorrhages; the last are illustrated in Figure *A*. Subungual hemorrhages are uncommon but helpful in the diagnosis of infective endocarditis at the bedside. The differential diagnosis of this dermatological finding includes advanced age, trauma, and trichinosis. Osler nodes are small, raised, nodular, and painful red to purple lesions that are present in the pulp spaces of the terminal phalanges of the fingers. They, along with all the peripheral stigmata of infective endocarditis, are seen much less commonly since the advent of antibiotic therapy for this disorder. Janeway lesions are small, irregular, flat, and nontender macules occurring most often on the thenar and hypothenar eminences of the hands and soles of patients with subacute infective endocarditis. Roth spots, located in the retina, have the appearance of a "cotton wool" exudate and consist of aggregations of cytoid bodies.

Amyloidosis is a systemic illness that is due to deposition of unique fibrils of amyloid protein in a variety of organs; it has major cardiac sequelae, including restrictive cardiomyopathy, abnormalities of cardiac impulse formation and conduction, systolic dysfunction, and orthostatic hypotension. In general, patients will exhibit at least one and often several of these cardiac manifestations. There are a host of dermatological findings in amyloid disease. Perhaps the most common of these are lesions consisting of small papules that are especially seen on the face, scalp, neck folds, or intertriginous folds. In addition, small, smooth and yellowish papules may be seen in the areas around the eyes and mistaken for xanthomata. While they are characteristically rounded, they frequently exhibit a hemorrhagic component, as in Figure *B*, which is an important point in the differential diagnosis. In some patients, nodules of a larger size may appear.

Fabry's disease is a sex-linked disorder of glycosphingolipid metabolism that is due to a deficiency of the enzyme ceramide trihexosidase. The disorder is characterized by the accumulation of glycolipids within the myocardium, skin, and kidneys. Systemic hypertension, mitral valve prolapse, renovascular hypotension, and congestive heart failure are all common clinical manifestations of the disease. Fabry's disease may also be associated with a restrictive cardiomyopathy that may be difficult to distinguish from cardiac amyloidosis. Ocular signs in the disorder are common. Approximately 90 per cent of patients have corneal opacities, while two-thirds of patients have conjunctival vessel tortuosity as illustrated in Figure *C*. Hypertensive cardiovascular disease, renal failure, and

cerebrovascular disease are the major causes of death in this disorder.

Progressive systemic sclerosis, or scleroderma, presents as a progressive tightening and thickening of the skin, with Raynaud's phenomenon occurring at some time in almost all patients. Cardiac involvement is extremely common in this disorder and is a frequent cause of death, second only to involvement of the kidneys as a factor shortening survival. Scleroderma heart disease is primarily a myocardial process, leading to vascular insufficiency and fibrosis in the small vessels of the heart, which produces cardiomyopathy with both congestive heart failure and conduction system abnormalities. The CREST variant of this syndrome includes patients with calcinosis, Raynaud's phenomenon, esophageal dysmotility, sclerodactyly, and telangiectasia. Recurrent painful ulcerations of the fingertips, which may become infected, are a common problem in this disorder, and are illustrated in Figure *D*. These are believed to result from the vascular disorder that produces Raynaud's phenomenon in these patients. They must be cared for in a careful and meticulous manner to avoid serious infection and even digital loss.

693-A, 694-B, 695-B, 696-C *(Braunwald, pp. 1657, 1663)*

The *Turner* and *Noonan* syndromes share several superficial features, including shortness of stature, webbing of the neck, skeletal anomalies, renal abnormalities, and congenital heart disease. Because of these clinical similarities, Noonan syndrome is frequently referred to as "male Turner syndrome" or Turner phenotype with normal chromosomes. However, there are several striking genetic and clinical differences that can readily distinguish these two disorders. The Turner syndrome occurs exclusively in females due to the fact that in about 60 per cent of patients all cells are deficient in one of the two chromosomes (45,X). The remaining 40 per cent of patients are mosaics with the chromosomal pattern 45,X/46,XX. Most fetuses with the 45,X form of Turner syndrome die in utero and are aborted spontaneously. Of those that survive, cardiovascular abnormalities occur in 35 to 50 per cent.[1] Coarctation of the aorta is the most common abnormality that is encountered, accounting for 50 to 70 per cent of all cardiac anomalies. The coarctation is usually of the postductal type. Other abnormalities include bicuspid aortic valve, hypertrophic obstructive cardiomyopathy, atrial septal defect, mitral valve prolapse, and dextrocardia. Stenosis of the pulmonic valve is rarely if ever seen in Turner syndrome in contrast to Noonan syndrome. Patients with Turner syndrome also frequently develop hypertension, which is independent of the coarctation.

Noonan syndrome appears similar to Turner syndrome, although there is a unique facial appearance, with hypertelorism, strabismus, small chin, and low-set ears in patients with Noonan syndrome. In contrast to Turner syndrome, in Noonan syndrome both males and females are affected and the karyotype in both sexes is normal. Noonan syndrome is inherited as an autosomal dominant trait. Approximately 50 per cent of patients have congenital heart disease, with the most common lesion being valvular pulmonary stenosis, occurring in about 60 per cent of patients. Characteristically, the annulus of the pulmonary valve is normal, but the valves are thickened and immobile. Other findings include atrial septal defect and hypertrophic cardiomyopathy. Although diagnosis is difficult, the presence of ocular abnormalities (ptosis, hypertelorism, and epicanthus) in association with pulmonary artery stenosis should suggest Noonan syndrome.[2]

REFERENCES

1. Lacro, R.V., Lyons Jones, K., and Benirschke, K.: Coarctation of the aorta in Turner syndrome: A pathologic study of fetuses with nuchal cystic hygromas, hydrops fetalis and female genitalia. Pediatrics 81:445, 1988.
2. Mendez, H.M.M., and Opitz, J.M.: Noonan syndrome: A review. Am. J. Med. Genet. 21:493, 1985.

697-C, 698-A, 699-B, 700-A, 701-A   (Braunwald, pp. 929–934)

The two-dimensional echocardiogram illustrated in Figure A displays an apical, four-chamber view of tricuspid atresia, demonstrating a dense band in the tricuspid annulus and a large left ventricle. This anomaly is marked by the absence of the tricuspid orifice and the presence of an intraatrial communication and hypoplasia of the right ventricle, with a communication between the systemic and pulmonary circulations that is usually a ventricular septal defect. In approximately 60 to 70 per cent of patients with this disease the great arteries have normal relationships, and the remainder have D-transposition of these vessels. In addition, pulmonic stenosis or atresia may be present and other cardiac abnormalities may coexist, especially in patients with transposition. Clinically, the marked diminution in pulmonary blood flow usually leads to severe cyanosis (see Braunwald, Fig. 29–53, p. 932). In those infants in whom transposition coexists with a ventricular septal defect and an unobstructed pulmonary outflow tract, torrential pulmonary flood flow will occur, leading to heart failure rather than cyanosis as the predominant problem. The majority of infants with tricuspid atresia have pulmonary hypoperfusion and the clinical picture of cyanosis with electrocardiographic findings of LV hypertrophy, left-axis deviation, and RA enlargement.[1]

Echocardiographic examination in this disorder is usually diagnostic. At cardiac catheterization the RV cannot be entered from the RA. When the great arteries are normally related, pulmonary blood flow is found to be maintained via a ventricular septal defect or a patent ductus arteriosus. However, in complete transposition, the pulmonary artery blood flow is derived directly from the LV. Functional correction of tricuspid atresia has been accomplished by the Fontan procedure, which consists of construction of a prosthetic conduit between the RA and pulmonary artery and closure of the intraatrial communication (see Braunwald, Fig. 29–55, p. 934).[2]

The two-dimensional echocardiogram in Figure B is a parasternal long-axis view of tetralogy of Fallot, which demonstrates both overriding of the aorta and the presence of a ventricular septal defect. The two other components of this malformation are obstruction to RV outflow and RV hypertrophy. The clinical presentation in tetralogy of Fallot is determined principally by the degree of obstruction to pulmonary blood flow which exists in each patient. In general, infants with tetralogy of Fallot become symptomatic and cyanotic before the age of 1 year. There is a direct correlation between the time of onset of symptoms and the severity of pulmonary outflow tract obstruction that exists. Intense cyanotic spells related to sudden increases in venoarterial shunting and simultaneous decreases in pulmonary blood flow occur between 2 and 9 months of age and may be life-threatening. Physical examination of infants with tetralogy of Fallot usually reveals varying degrees of underdevelopment and cyanosis, commonly with clubbing of the terminal digits within the first year of life. An RV impulse and systolic thrill may often be appreciated along the left sternal border. A systolic flow murmur across the pulmonic valve is often present, and the intensity and duration of this murmur vary inversely with the severity of the pulmonic outflow tract obstruction. The ECG usually shows RV hypertrophy, which is occasionally accompanied by RA hypertrophy as well. A normal-size but boot-shaped heart ("coeur en sabot") with prominence of the RV and a concavity in the region of the underdeveloped RV outflow tract may be seen on roentgenographic examination. Echocardiographic examination is often diagnostic of this disorder. Cardiac catheterization with angiography is necessary to confirm the diagnosis, to quantitate the magnitude of shunting, to evaluate the architecture of the right-sided cardiac chambers, and to document the coronary artery anatomy prior to surgical repair. Coronary artery anatomy may have surgically important variations in this disorder, including origin of the anterior descending artery from the right coronary artery, or a single right or left coronary artery giving rise to the coronary vessels.[3]

The management of tetralogy of Fallot consists of total correction of the anomaly, with early definitive repair being advocated in most centers once infants are medically prepared for intracardiac surgery. Pulmonary arterial size is the single most important determinant in evaluating a patient for primary repair of the anomaly. In patients in whom marked hypoplasia of the pulmonary arteries is present, a systemic–pulmonary artery anastomosis may be used in a palliative manner to allow the infant to survive until childhood or adolescence, at which time total correction may be carried out at a lower risk.

REFERENCES

1. Bharati, S., and Lev, M.: Conduction system in tricuspid atresia with and without regular D-transposition. Circulation 56:423, 1977.
2. Fontan, F., Deville, C., Quaegebeur, J., et al.: Repair of tricuspid atresia in 100 patients. J. Thorac. Cardiovasc. Surg. 85:647, 1983.
3. Fellows, K.E., Freed, M.D., Keane, J.F., et al.: Results of routine preoperative coronary angiography and tetralogy of Fallot. Circulation 51:561, 1977.

702-B, 703-A, 704-B, 705-C, 706-D *(Braunwald, pp. 1787–1790)*

Chronic hemolytic anemias, such as sickle cell anemia and thalassemia, have a variety of accompanying cardiovascular problems, including cardiomegaly, congenital heart failure, and sudden death. In addition, the specific diseases in question may have characteristic cardiopulmonary complications. In *sickle cell disease*, frank cardiac decompensation usually occurs in patients who have co-existing complications of the disease such as renal failure, pulmonary thrombosis and infarction, and systemic infections, or underlying cardiovascular abnormalities that are dependent on the sickle cell process. Pulmonary infarction is a common complication of sickle cell anemia, and is thought to be due to thrombosis in situ rather than to embolization. Acute myocardial infarction may rarely complicate sickle cell disease, and this may involve the papillary muscle because of its susceptibility to hypoxia, since it is at the terminal portion of the coronary circulation. Cardiomegaly occurs in almost all patients with sickle cell anemia, despite the absence of other common causes of cardiomegaly. Multiple blood transfusions given as treatment for the underlying anemia may lead to myocardial iron deposition or hemosiderosis, which can contribute to the impairment of cardiac function that is noted in sickle cell disease. However, this complication occurs much more frequently in homozygous thalassemia (see below). In sickle cell disease there are no specific electrocardiographic abnormalities, but approximately 80 per cent of patients have an abnormal ECG. Arrhythmias, on the other hand, occur only rarely with sickle cell anemia, although they may be more prevalent during acute, painful crisis.[1]

The *thalassemias* are a group of inherited disorders that result from an imbalance in the production of hemoglobin chains and therefore a decreased production of hemoglobin A, leading to a hypochromic, microcytic anemia. Cardiac complications are the major cause of death in patients with thalassemia. Iron overload due to frequent transfusions is a common problem in thalassemia and often causes cardiomegaly. In addition, the iron deposition may lead to electrocardiographic abnormalities including arrhythmias and higher grades of heart block due to deposition of iron in the AV node and conduction system. Approximately half of all patients with thalassemia have episodes of pericarditis which may be recurrent and present in a classic manner. Roentgenographic evidence of cardiac enlargement in children regresses when hemoglobin is maintained above 10 mg/dl in this disorder, and supportive therapy with an adequate transfusion program, splenectomy, and early treatment of infections has prolonged the lives of patients with thalassemia.[2] Calcification of chordae tendineae is not seen in either sickle cell anemia or thalassemia.

REFERENCES

1. Maisel, A., Friedman, H., Flint, L., et al.: Continuous electrocardiographic monitoring in patients with sickle cell anemia during pain crisis. Clin. Cardiol. 6:339, 1983.
2. Yee, H., Mra, R., and Nyunt, K.M.: Cardiac abnormalities in the thalassemia syndromes. Southeast Asian J. Trop. Med. Public Health 15:414, 1984.